Hair Loss Disorders in Domestic Animals

Edited by

Lars Mecklenburg

Monika Linek

Desmond J. Tobin

With contributions by

Rosario Cerundolo

Linda Frank

Wilfried Meyer

Manon Paradis

Monika Welle

WILEY-BLACKWELL

A John Wiley & Sons, Ltd., Publication

Edition first published 2009

Blackwell Publishing was acquired by John Wiley & Sons in February 2007. Blackwell's publishing program has been merged with Wiley's global Scientific, Technical, and Medical business to form Wiley-Blackwell.

Editorial Office
2121 State Avenue, Ames, Iowa 50014-8300, USA

For details of our global editorial offices, for customer services, and for information about how to apply for permission to reuse the copyright material in this book, please see our website at www.wiley.com/wiley-blackwell.

Library of Congress Cataloguing-in-Publication Data

Hair loss disorders in domestic animals / edited by Lars Mecklenburg,
Monika Linek, Desmond J. Tobin ; with contributions by Rosario
Cerundolo . . . [et al.].
p. cm.
Includes bibliographical references and index.
ISBN-13: 978-0-8138-1082-9 (alk. paper)
ISBN-10: 0-8138-1082-5 (alk. paper)
1. Scabies. 2. Domestic animals—Diseases. I. Mecklenburg, Lars.
II. Linek, Monika. III. Tobin, Desmond John, 1965–
RL764.S28H35 2009
636.089′6546—dc22
2008049842

A catalog record for this book is available from the U.S. Library of Congress.

Set in 10/12pt Minion by Aptara® Inc., New Delhi, India
Printed in Singapore

Disclaimer

1 2009

Contents

Foreword

It is with greatest pleasure and enthusiasm that I am writing these introductory lines to what has turned out to be a much-needed, authoritative, and most informative new monograph on hair growth disorders in domestic animals—one of the major topics of clinical dermatology, not only in human but also in veterinary medicine.

The editors have done an admirable job in charting a difficult territory marred by the unavailability of sufficient analytical research, by confusion about key underlying biological principles, by often rather vague pathogenesis concepts, and by contradictory, misleading, or ill-advised terminology. Together with an excellent, international team of expert contributors, the editors are offering solid guidance and a fresh perspective on how to approach alopecias in domestic animals from the vantage point of modern skin and hair biology in a very systematic manner, and thus convincingly fill a void in the available veterinary literature.

As a clinical dermatologist with a special interest in basic hair biology and human hair pathology, I am fully aware of the importance and instructiveness of alopecia in domestic animals for dissecting the principles that control hair follicle cycling, and for studying how cycling disorders can lead to hair loss. I also realize the major, as yet insufficiently exploited potential of domestic animals as excellent models for the study of human hair disease. Therefore, the editors are to be congratulated for calling our attention to the multiple, but often neglected parallels between human and animal hair loss, and for the highly methodical, well-structured approach they are taking in presenting the topic at hand.

Mirroring the often merely historical and commonly descriptive rather than pathobiologically founded classification of human alopecias, the even less studied animal alopecias are notoriously difficult to classify. The editors and chapter authors have done a marvellous job in providing pragmatic guidance and a reasonable working classification that generally avoids to fall into the trap of drawing unadvisedly close parallels to suspected "analogous" human forms of alopecia, whose pathogenesis may well be distinct from what is conceived as a counterpart in domestic animals.

Thus, one does not have to be a prophet to predict that this unique new monograph—a most welcome enrichment of the veterinary dermatology literature—will soon also be consulted by many investigators across a wide range of the life sciences, who are interested in the principles that drive hair loss disorders in mammalian species or who are looking for instructive animal models of specific alopecias, beyond what mice and rats have long offered in this respect.

May this exquisite new book enjoy the exceptionally long "anagen" phase it deserves!

Ralf Paus, MD
Professor of Dermatology
Head, Experimental Dermatology
University of Lübeck, Germany
&
Professor of Cutaneous Medicine
School of Translational Medicine
University of Manchester, UK
May 2008

Preface

With the loss of its relevance as a thermal regulator in mammalian survival, the psychosocial significance of hair for humans has continuously increased. Therefore, it is not surprising that domestic animals with alopecia are increasingly presented by their owners to veterinarians for treatment. As with physicians, the veterinary clinician is confronted with a difficult task, since the pathogenesis of alopecia can be very complex and therapeutic possibilities very limited. The aim of this book is to help with the understanding and diagnosis of alopecia and to demonstrate what therapeutic options are available to both the veterinarian and client. As the diagnosis of alopecia frequently relies on a histopathological evaluation of the hair-bearing skin, this book is aimed not solely at practicing veterinarians, but also veterinary pathologists who work with skin biopsies from alopecic patients.

Above all, the diagnosis and treatment of alopecia should be grounded on a thorough understanding of hair follicle anatomy and physiology, and particularly on how this may differ between species. To this end, our book begins with a detailed introduction into the basics of hair follicle biology. Moreover, it provides an insight into the variety of spontaneous alopecic diseases in domestic animals. This will hopefully stimulate new thinking on the etiology and pathogenesis of alopecia, and aid researchers in their search and development of new therapeutics for alopecia.

As Hopwood claimed in 1957, "the urge to classify is a fundamental human instinct; like a predisposition to sin, it accompanies us into the world at birth and stays with us to the end" (Hopwood AT. *Proceedings of the Linnean Society of London* 1957;171:230). As is true for other diseases, the classification of alopecias continues to become more and more complex as new disease entities are described. Our system of classification significantly extends that of previous literature on veterinary alopecia, and reflects this increasing complexity. We consider that histopathologic and clinical features of disease are the most relevant parameters for classification and aim to be as descriptive and precise as possible in our system. This classification however remains in a state of flux, and will no doubt be further improved over the next decades. As was so well expressed by H.E.M. Kay (*The Lancet* 1974;11:586) when addressing lymphoma classification: "This system makes no claim to be comprehensive or even comprehensible, so there may well be scope for other classifications of classifications and ultimately, one hopes a classification of classifications of classifications. At that point we shall need a conference in the Caribbean."

Finally, we would like to thank all those who have enabled us to compile this book. Among many others, these are: Zeineb Alhaidari, Ellen Baumeister, Luc Beco, Kerstin Bergvall, Jan Declercq, Claude Favrot, Raffaella Finocchiaro, Marion Gähle, Szymon Godynicki, Thelma Lee Gross, Renate Hämmerling, Rubert Judd, Miguel Angel Toro Ibáñez, Markus Maget, Kevin McElwee, Claudia Nett, Thierry Olivry, Ralf Paus, Eva M.J. Peters, Sylvia Ruefenacht, Neil Sargison, Rudolf Schwarz, David Steffen, Gudrun Wirth, Pat White, Stephen White, Yulie Yager, and the team from the Section of Clinical Dermatology and the Institute of Veterinary Pathology of the Vetsuisse Faculty, University of Berne.

Lars Mecklenburg
Monika Linek
Desmond J. Tobin
May 2008

Contributors

Lars Mecklenburg Dr med vet, PhD,
Fachtierarzt für Pathologie, Consultant in Veterinary Dermatopathology, Hamburg, Germany

Monika Linek Dr med vet, Dipl ECVD,
Director of Dermatology, Veterinary Specialists of Hamburg, Hamburg, Germany

Desmond J. Tobin PhD, FRCPath, FIBiol,
Professor of Cell Biology, Center for Skin Sciences, School of Life Sciences, University of Bradford, Bradford, West Yorkshire, Great Britain

Rosario Cerundolo DVM, Cert VD, Dipl ECVD, MRCVS,
Associate Professor of Veterinary Dermatology, School of Veterinary Medicine, University of Pennsylvania, Philadelphia, PA, USA

Linda Frank MS, DVM, Dipl ACVD,
Professor of Dermatology, Department of Small Animal Clinical Sciences, University of Tennessee, Knoxville, TN, USA

Wilfried Meyer Dr rer nat,
Professor of Anatomy, Anatomical Institute, Veterinary School of Hannover, Hannover, Germany

Manon Paradis DMV, MVSc, Dipl ACVD,
Professor of Dermatology, Department of Clinical Sciences, Faculty of Veterinary Medicine, University of Montreal, St-Hyacinthe, Quebec, Canada

Monika Welle Dr med vet, Dipl ECVP,
Fachtierärztin für Pathologie, Professor of Pathology, Institute of Animal Pathology, Vetsuisse Faculty, University of Berne, Berne, Switzerland

Part 1

Hair Follicle Biology

1.1

Ontogeny of the hair follicle

Desmond J. Tobin

Both humans and domestic animals communicate significantly via their physical appearance, and the hair fiber-producing mini organ called the hair follicle accounts for much of the variation in domestic mammal phenotype. Although commonly dismissed as being of superficial importance, the hair follicle is truly one of the nature's most fascinating structures (Chuong 1998). Hair growth, one of the only two uniquely mammalian traits (the other is the mammary gland), serves several important functions. These include thermal insulation, camouflage, social and sexual communication, sensory perception, and protection against trauma, noxious insults, insects, and so on. These features have clearly facilitated evolutionary success in animals.

The hair follicle or, as it is known in humans, the "pilosebaceous unit" encapsulates all the important physiologic processes found in mammalia, including controlled cell growth and death, interactions between cells of different histologic type, cell differentiation and migration, and hormone responsitivity. Thus, the value of the hair follicle as a model for biological scientific research goes way beyond its scope for cutaneous biology or dermatology alone. Indeed, the recent and dramatic upturn in interest in hair follicle biology has focused principally on the pursuit of two of biology's holy grails: post-embryonic morphogenesis and control of cyclical tissue activity.

If one first considers the role of the skin, arguably our body's largest organ, as the mammal's sensor at the periphery (a veritable "brain on the outside"), one can begin to appreciate some of the contributions its principal appendage, the hair follicle, can make. The skin incorporates all major support systems found in the body: blood, muscle, and innervation as well as its role in immunocompetence, psycho-emotion, ultraviolet radiation sensing, and endocrine function, among others. These participate in the homeostasis of the mammalian body. Not surprisingly, therefore, the skin contains several reservoirs of stem cells located in the epidermis, the hair follicle, and perhaps also the sebaceous gland.

The hair follicle is formed from a bewilderingly complex set of interactions involving ectodermal, mesodermal, and neuroectodermal components, which go to elaborate five or six concentric cylinders in humans of at least 15 distinct interacting cell subpopulations. These together provide a truly exceptional tissue that rivals the vertebrate limb bud as a model for studies of the genetic regulation of development. Much of the research on the regulation of hair follicle development or morphogenesis has been carried out in murine models, especially the mouse (Schmidt-Ullrich and Paus 2005). While some species-specific (and even intraspecies) differences are expected (Drögemüller et al. 2007), it is considered likely that broadly similar pathways and molecular regulators will operate in all mammals. Thus, the discussion below will largely refer to data that continues to emerge from studies in mice, given the ready availability of powerful mouse genetics.

The mysteries of the "creation" of the hair follicle in mammalian skin have only just recently begun to be unraveled. As with any highly complex multicellular structure that has experienced enormous evolutionary selective pressure, nature's master builder has designed the hair follicle with multiple levels of redundancy: with backup systems and with backup systems for these backup systems. A plethora of excellent reviews have appeared over the last 10 years that describe the exquisitely complex molecular mechanisms active during hair follicle development (Fuchs et al. 2001; Millar 2002; Botchkarev and Paus 2003; Schmidt-Ullrich and Paus 2005). It is attempted here to provide a comprehensive overview of some of the latest developments in this fascinating process. This is a rapidly developing field however, and new molecular regulators are being added to these pathways continually.

1.1.1 Skin development

The development of the forerunner of skin epithelium, the neuroectoderm, occurs after gastrulation in the embryo. Whether this neuroectodermal tissue develops into skin epithelium or continues to develop as neuronal tissue is determined by signaling via the Wnt pathway, which renders some of the ectoderm nonresponsive to fibroblast growth factors (FGFs). In the absence of FGFs the cells of the developing ectoderm can instead respond to another class of morphogens called bone morphogenetic proteins (BMPs), which help direct the ectodermal cells to form a layer of multipotential skin epithelium (cf. Botchkarev and Sharov 2004). The Wnt gene (named from the *Drosophila* gene "Wingless" and its vertebrate homologue "Int") was first identified in *Drosophila melanogaster* to function in embryogenesis and adult limb formation. Wnt is now known to represent a major class of secreted morphogens that are critical for the establishment of pattern development in all multicellular organisms.

The skin epithelium lies above a dermatome-derived mesenchymal or embryonic connective tissue primarily consisting of collagen-producing fibroblasts. Here, too, Wnt signaling determines the fate of dermis fibroblasts (Atit et al. 2006). A third major component of the developing skin is the neural crest-derived melanocyte, a cell that produces melanins. Primitive melanocytes (sometimes referred to as melanoblasts) migrate from the neural crest, through the dermis, and populate the basal layer of the epidermis.

Hair follicle formation in the developing skin requires communication between specialized mesenchymal cells of the dermis and epithelial cells of the epithelium above. This interaction is very complex and operates via pathways that direct specialized outcomes for both the epithelial (keratinocytes) and dermal cells (fibroblasts). Much debate in the literature remains centered on the hierarchy of the increasing numbers of factors implicated in hair follicle morphogenesis, and on the degree of their redundancy. Of particular interest has been the nature of the first signals that determine where along the overlying epidermis a hair follicle is likely to be produced (so-called 'patterning').

As an aid to conceptualizing the impact of these molecular signaling events, it may be useful to associate them directly with morphologically distinct stages in hair follicle development, as significant morphologic change is required to form a fully developed hair follicle. These changes can be broadly separated into the following phases: (a) induction/initiation, (b) organ downgrowth, and (c) cellular differentiation. A useful guide to aid recognition of these distinct stages has been prepared for C57Bl6 mice (Paus et al. 1999). Therein, the preplacode stage of hair follicle development is assigned as Stage 0, while the clustering of keratinocytes in the basal layer of the epidermis that lengthen and assume an altered "north–south" polarity to form the hair follicle placode stage is referred to as Stage 1 (Fig. 1.1.1).

1.1.2 Hair follicle placode formation

It is now considered most likely that the first signal(s) that trigger(s) the formation of the regularly spaced epithelial thickenings called hair follicle "placodes" emerge(s) from the mesenchyme (Olivera-Martinez et al. 2004). This is derived from the evidence of rather uniform β-catenin accumulation in dermal cells under the control of Wnt, effective only at short distances. Subsequently, β-catenin translocates to the nuclei of some of these dermal cells, where it can form complex with lymphoid enhancer factor (LEF) family members for DNA binding and subsequent gene activation (Noramly et al. 1999). It is of note that while LEF expression is required in the mesenchyme before initiation of vibrissae development is possible (Kratochwil et al. 1996), loss of LEF in pelage skin results in only a partial reduction in hair follicle development overall, suggesting the existence of hair follicle type-specific controls and also a degree of functional redundancy. In a similar way it has been suggested that BMP-associated inhibition may operate in several different ways, to specify the development of hair follicles of different types, and thereafter may additionally affect hair follicle density (Fuchs 2007). The BMPs, a subfamily with over 16 distinct secreted signaling protein members, belong to the transforming growth factor beta (TGF-β) superfamily of proteins.

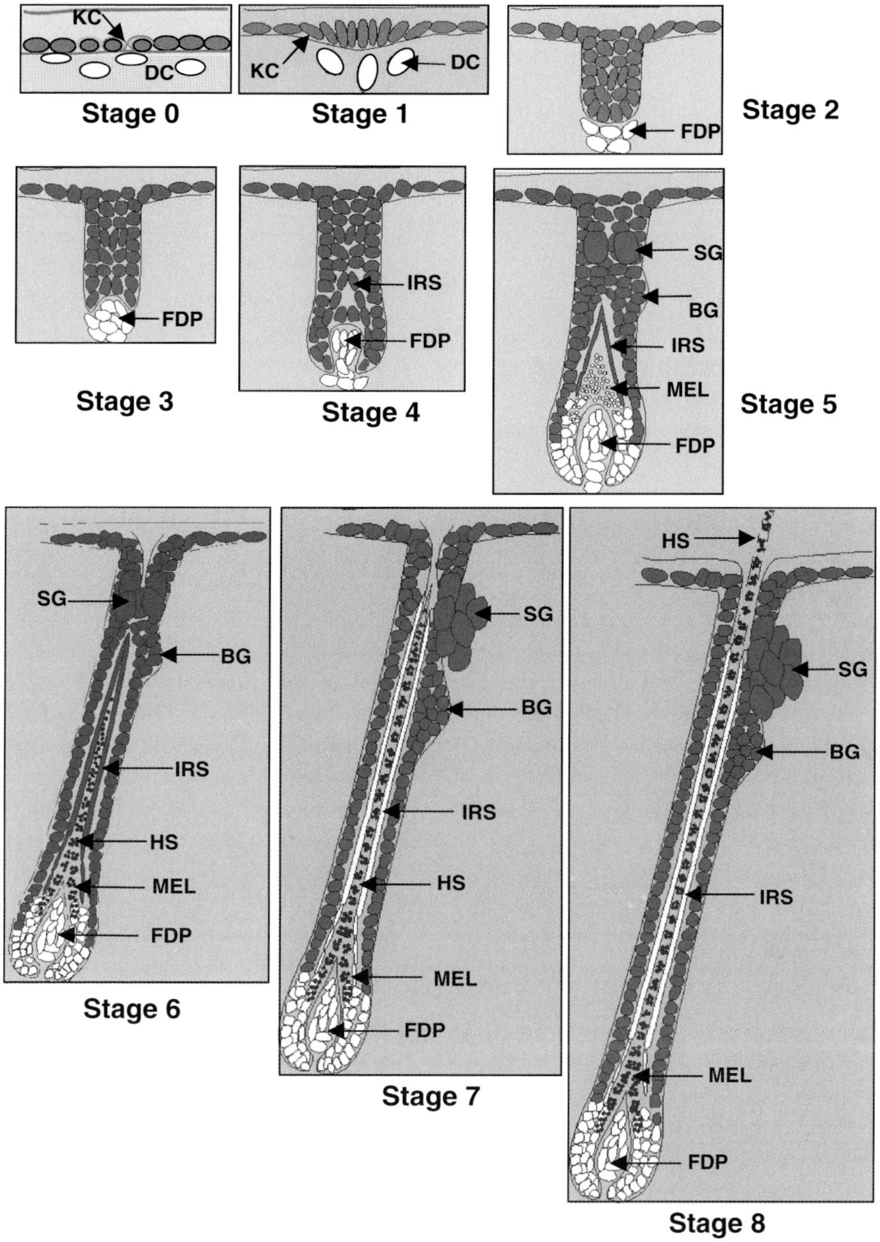

Fig. 1.1.1 Cartoon of hair follicle morphogenesis. Stages 0–8 according to Paus et al. 1999. KC, keratinocytes; FDP, follicular dermal papilla; DC, dermal mesenchymal cells; SG, sebaceous gland; BG, bulge; IRS, inner root sheath; HS, hair shaft; MEL, melanin. (Modified from Tobin (2005).)

Readers should also be aware that for any given species, and even within the same species, the skin can produce hair follicles of several different types that generate different types of hair fiber (Maderson 2003). The molecular regulation underlying this diversity is of significant interest. There is evidence in the mouse that the control of placode initiation to form any of the four different types of hair fiber involves different regulatory controls. For example, ectodysplasin signaling is required for guard hair development, while the development of secondary hairs (i.e., "awl" and "auchene" hairs in mice) involves ectodysplasin-independent signaling. The latter, however, is instead dependent on the Wnt/β-catenin and Noggin/LEF pathway (Schmidt-Ullrich and Paus 2005). NFκB signaling is required in early hair follicle induction downstream of ectodysplasin (Schmidt-Ullrich et al. 2001). NFκB transmits the ectodysplasin signal that activates sonic hedgehog (Shh) and cyclin D1 expression, responsible for postinitiation hair placode downgrowth (Schmidt-Ullrich et al. 2006).

As a consequence of the initial dermal signal, the epithelium is induced to initiate the expression of molecules that act as either promoters or repressors of placode formation. Molecular participants in this initial signaling to Wnt-responsive epithelial cells in mice include the FGFs (e.g., FGF10, FGF7), inhibitors of BMPs (e.g., noggin), and inhibitors of Wnt (e.g., Dickkopf) (Jung et al. 1998; Botchkarev et al. 1999; Sick et al. 2006). Indeed, hair follicle density is reduced where there is either an excess BMP production, a failure to inhibit BMP (e.g., via an absence of noggin), or via lack of FGF receptor (Petiot et al. 2003; Mou et al. 2006). Thus, hair follicle formation at a particular site in the epidermis results from a highly orchestrated interaction of mesenchyme with epithelium. This process responds to dynamic reaction–diffusion type gradients of stimulating/inhibiting signals generated from secreted factors and their cognate receptors. Also implicated in this complex process are transcription factors (proteins that work with other proteins to either promote or suppress the transcription of genes) and cell adhesion molecules.

The activation of the Wnt signaling pathway is an absolute requirement for the initiation of Stage 1 of hair follicle morphogenesis. Currently 19 distinct members of the Wnt family of ligands (and over 10 distinct receptors, named "frizzled") have been identified in humans and mice, and it is not yet clear which of these are involved in Stage 1 initiation. It has recently been shown that Wnt10b promotes the development of hair follicles in a mouse embryonic skin tissue model (Ouji et al. 2006). While Wnt10b is uniformly expressed in embryonic mouse skin, this molecule becomes strikingly upregulated in the hair follicle placode (St-Jacques et al. 1998; Reddy et al. 2001). Indeed, the expression of Wnt10b is abolished in ectodysplasin-mutant mice that exhibit a hypoplastic hair formation. Moreover, a mutation in the gene for the ectodysplasin receptor (EDAR) (named "downless" in mice) results in a similar phenotype (Headon and Overbeek 1999). Consequently, in the absence of EDAR, neither Shh nor BMP4 is expressed (Barsh 1999).

It is important to note that the Wnt pathway is active in both the epithelial and mesenchymal components of developing hair follicles (DasGupta and Fuchs 1999). Activation of the Wnt signaling pathway is sufficient for induction of hair follicle development. Similarly, if β-catenin (i.e., the mediator of Wnt signals) is lost from murine epidermis, no hair follicles will develop (Huelsken et al. 2001), and if β-catenin signaling is excessively stimulated, excess hair follicles will develop (Gat et al. 1998; Lo Celso et al. 2004). Moreover, BMP (i.e., BMP2, −4, and −7) as well as Shh expression (but not ectodysplasin) are dependent on β-catenin, suggesting that expression of ectodysplasin lies upstream of Wnt activation in the epithelium (Huelsken et al. 2001).

The reaction and diffusion model for biological patterning proposed originally by Alan Turning in the 1950s and recently demonstrated experimentally for Wnt and its antagonist "Dickkopf" in murine skin (Sick et al. 2006) permits an understanding of hair formation based on the control of these molecules by positive and negative regulators expressed either in the developing hair follicle itself or in the surrounding tissues. Examples of negative regulators for hair follicle development include the BMPs and activinαA. These inhibitors can in turn be inhibited by noggin and follistatin, respectively. Mice lacking noggin have slower hair follicle development and also fewer total hair follicles formed (Botchkarev et al. 1999). Moreover, these mice also exhibit a reduced expression of LEF and this may suggest that its expression is also controlled by BMP. BMPs appear to inhibit hair follicle initiation. Several other secreted molecules are expressed in developing hair follicles where they can inhibit BMP activity. These include follistatin, an inhibitor of activinαA. TGF-β2 (which belongs to the same family as activinαA) is expressed in the placode epithelium and, when administered to mesenchyme in the absence of overlying epithelium, can induce the formation of follicular papilla (Foitzik et al. 1999). In contrast, mice lacking the TGF-β2 gene exhibit retarded hair follicle morphogenesis and have fewer hair follicles.

Several other potential players that can either stimulate or inhibit hair follicle development have been suggested from recent research including the transcription factors Msx1 and Msx2 (Satokata et al. 2000); signaling via the epidermal growth factor receptor (Kashiwagi et al. 1997); extracellular matrix proteins including laminin-10 (Li et al. 2003); and neurotrophins and their receptors (Botchkarev and Paus 2003). Recently, a role for the chromatin remodeler Mi-2beta in hair follicle morphogenesis has been reported (Kashiwagi et al. 2007). This study showed that depletion of Mi-2beta blocked the induction of hair follicles in mice. While Mi-2beta appears to be dispensable for the maintenance of established repopulating epidermal stem cells, this transcription factor appears to be essential for reprogramming basal cells of the developing epidermis into follicular and, subsequently, hair matrix fates (Kashiwagi et al. 2007).

Exciting new research has demonstrated that hair follicle neogenesis may occur in adult wounded skin, if the wound site is of sufficient size and the wound is allowed to repair physiologically (Ito et al. 2007). This example of reported neofolliculogenesis occurred via an upregulation of Wnt expression, and was shown experimentally by either inducing high Wnt expression or by inhibiting its expression to reduce the hair follicle number (Ito et al. 2007). This study may be the first formal demonstration that hair follicle numbers may not be preset at the embryogenesis state but can be increased as a function of wound healing in the adult animal. There may be room, however, for contribution from stem cells from hair follicles located at the edge of the wound after migration into the wound center.

1.1.3 Formation of the hair follicle mesenchyme

While formation of the hair follicle placode is being initiated, increasing organization of dermal cells underlying this epithelium structure becomes evident. A signal from the placode is thought to determine and direct the clustering of the dermal fibroblasts to form the "dermal papilla." The dermal condensate fails to develop in the absence of β-catenin expression (Huelsken et al. 2001), indicating a crucial role for Wnt signaling in the development of the early dermal papilla (DasGupta and Fuchs 1999). Moreover, efficient development of the dermal papilla appears to be influenced by cross talk between the epidermal placode and the developing dermal papilla via signaling through the platelet-derived growth factor A (PDGF-A) expressed in the epithelial placode and its cognate receptor PDGF-R in the dermal condensate (Karlsson et al. 1999). This is suggested by the observation that mice deficient in PDGF generate hypoplastic hair fibers, characterized by dermal papilla of reduced size. Presumably these cells reduce secretion of hair growth inducing morphogens and mitogens. Recent work suggests that BMP6 may have a dermal papilla-associated regulatory control in the hair follicle (Rendl et al. 2008).

Another early gene involved in the organizing of the mesenchyme to form a dermal papilla is Shh (St-Jacques et al. 1998; Oro and Higgins 2003; Levy et al. 2005). Mice lacking Shh still exhibit placode initiation and formation of the dermal condensate (Iseki et al. 1996). Although these data indicate that Shh signaling lies downstream of Wnt/β-catenin signaling, Wnt5a is expressed in the developing dermal condensate of wild-type but not Shh−/− embryos, suggesting that this Wnt is a target of Shh in hair follicle morphogenesis. Thus, while Shh is not critical for the first epithelial signal, nor perhaps even for the initial gathering of the presumptive dermal papilla fibroblasts, it is required for subsequent hair follicle downgrowth and for subsequent papilla formation. Evidence for the latter can be gleaned from the coexpression in the forming papilla of Shh pathway-related molecules including Patched1 (i.e., the Shh receptor) and Gli1 (i.e., a Shh transcription factor) (Oro and Higgins 2003). Recent data from Gli1 knockout mice, however, suggest that some hair types can still develop in the absence of Gli1 (Mill et al. 2003). This finding suggests that different hair types have different requirements for Gli1 signaling. By contrast, the loss of smoothened (an obligate component of all Shh signaling) results in severely affected hair follicle morphogenesis (Gritli-Linde et al. 2007). The increasing inductive capacity of the developing dermal papilla may be indicated by upregulation of hepatocyte growth factor and versican at this stage (Kaplan and Holbrook 1994).

1.1.4 Hair follicle downgrowth

"Second" signals from the developing dermal papilla induce proliferation in the follicular epithelium to drive the initial downgrowth of the epidermal placode to form the Stage 2 hair follicle. These initial hair follicle "commitment" events presage subsequent active epithelial–mesenchymal cross talk that drives cytodifferentiation to determine which cells will go on to form keratinocytes of the hair fiber and follicular sheaths, and which fibroblasts form the growth-inducing follicular papilla versus the dermal sheaths. The cell fate-determining "signals" are mediated by intercellular signaling molecules secreted from specific subpopulations of skin cells and that have multiple receptors/targets to transduce their effects.

Of note here is the exquisite specificity of the signaling events occurring between different cell subpopulations. For example, recombination experiments have shown that dermis taken from one body region when combined with epidermis from another body site (even in another individual) will direct the formation of hair follicles that are characteristic of the dermis donor site. A test of this in humans was recently carried out whereby male follicular dermal tissue taken from the scalp directed the formation of terminal hairs when recombined with female arm epidermis (Reynolds et al. 1999).

One of the enigmas of hair follicle development is how a relatively undifferentiated cluster of epithelial and mesenchymal cells can give rise to such a large number of distinct cell lineages with variable different differentiated products (Fig. 1.1.2). It is clear from knockout mice that downgrowth will only occur in the presence of Shh (Chiang et al. 1999). Although Shh engages in highly significant signaling events between hair follicle epithelium and mesenchyme, the identification of the pathway activated by the Shh signal in this process remains unknown. ActivinαA and hepatocyte growth factor (HGF) may be possible candidates. ActivinαA not only is a secreted signaling molecule expressed by the early dermal papilla cells, but is also inhibited by follistatin (also a BMP inhibitor). Consequently, mice lacking either activinαA or follistatin produce defective vibrissa follicles (Millar 2002). On the other hand, mice that overexpress HGF not only exhibit accelerated hair follicle development, but also produce more hair follicles (Lindner et al. 2000). It is also likely that adhesion molecules and extracellular proteins are also important contributors to these developmental processes.

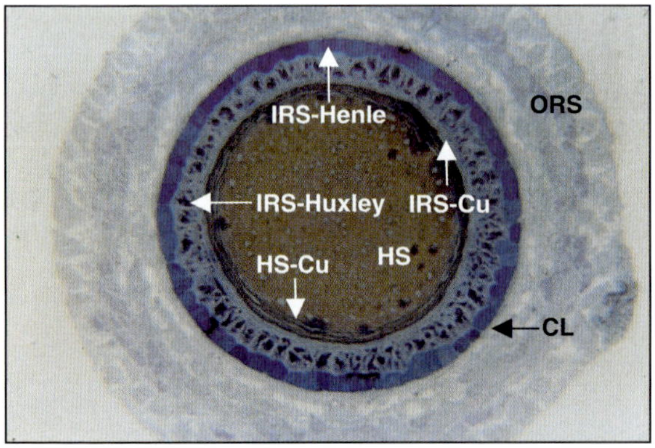

Fig. 1.1.2 High-resolution light microscopy image of a transverse section of a human hair follicle cut at the level where maximum cell lineage commitment occurs (suprabulbar level). IRS, inner root sheath; ORS, outer root sheath; HS, hair shaft; Cu, cuticle; CL, companion layer.

Hair follicle morphogenesis (Fig. 1.1.3) is morphologically appreciable only at Stage 3 when the forerunner of a hair follicle "bulb" becomes evident—a process reflecting the activation/induction of multiple keratinocyte differentiation pathways that lead to considerable structural change within the tissue (Fig. 1.1.3d). At Stage 3 the developing hair follicle appears as a "peg" of tissue consisting of an elongated column of concentrically layered keratinocytes—at least seven different layers of epithelium can be appreciated at this stage. A little later at Stage 4 (Fig. 1.1.3e) the mesenchymal component of the hair follicle, that is, the follicular dermal papilla, is now located within the cavity of the developing epithelial bulb. The hair peg continues to elongate into the dermis of the skin during this stage and there is evidence now of the formation of the inner root sheath (IRS), as it assumes a cone-shaped structure. The follicular papilla becomes progressively invaginated by the enlarging epithelial hair bulb.

1.1.5 Formation of the hair follicle inner root sheath

The emergence of such an impressive differentiation programming in the hair follicle epithelium at Stages 3–5 (Fig. 1.1.3d–f) is of course dependent on the spatiotemporal expression of relevant cell fate genes. Moreover, it is during this stage of hair follicle development that the additional processes that see the hair follicle's polarity and shape occur (see below). One of the first and most striking events of cytodifferentiation within the developing hair follicle is the emergence of the IRS layer of the hair follicle wall during late

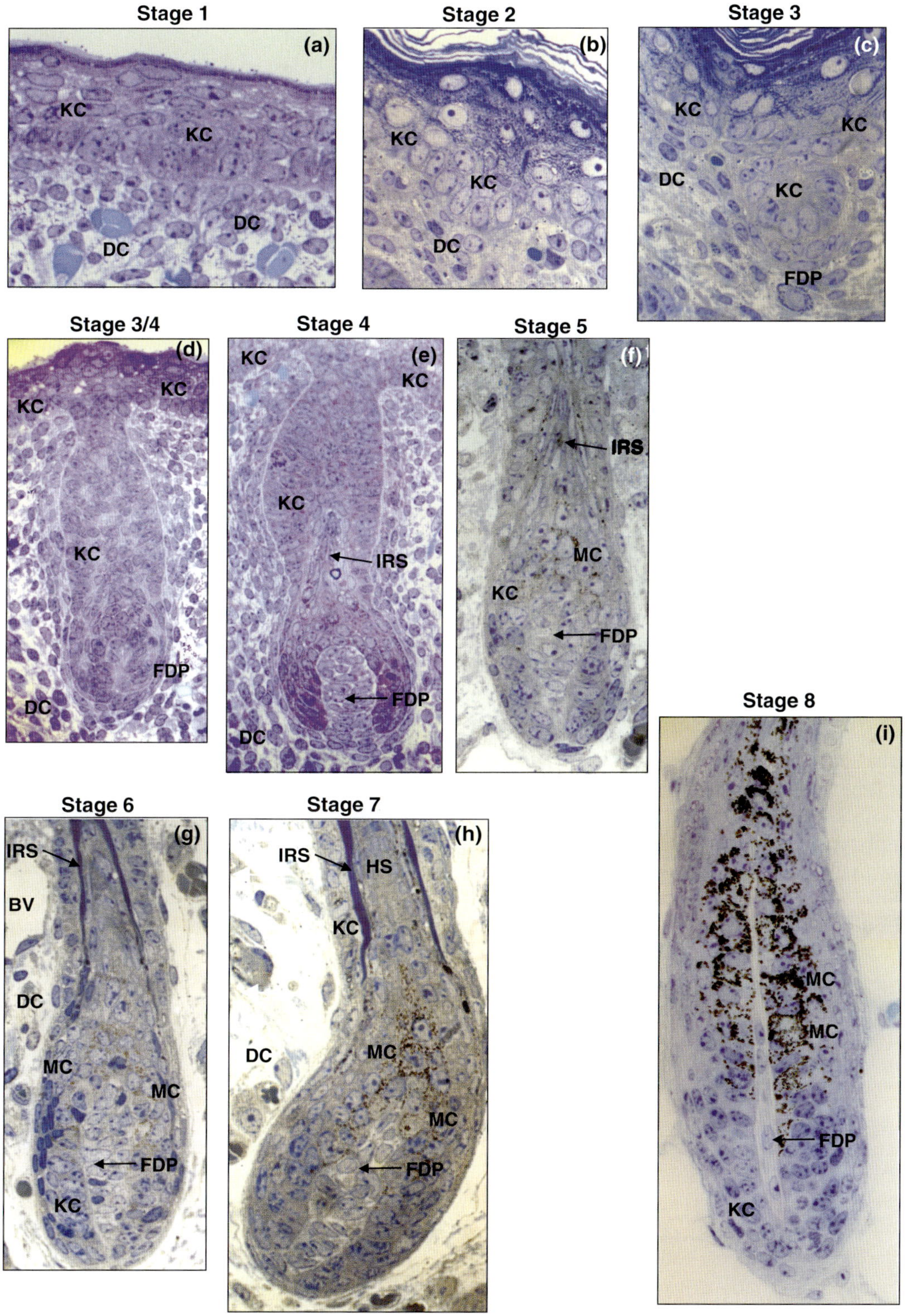

Fig. 1.1.3 High resolution light microscopy images of hair follicle development in mouse skin. Stages 0–8 according to Paus et al. 1999. KC, keratinocytes; FDP, follicular dermal papilla; DC, dermal mesenchymal cells; IRS, inner root sheath; HS, hair shaft; MC, melanocytes; BV, blood vessel. (Modified from Tobin (2005).)

Stage 3. Signaling via the BMP receptor is also important for the determination of matrix keratinocyte differentiation into both IRS and hair shaft keratinocytes (Ming Kwan et al. 2004). Indeed, if the BMP receptor R1A is lacking, matrix keratinocytes fail to differentiate and instead matrix cell tumors occur.

The cells of the hair bulb matrix that go on to develop into IRS and hair shaft begin to express genes encoding for Notch1. At this stage this membrane-associated receptor protein interacts with its ligands Jagged-1 and Jagged-2 (Favier et al. 2000), which is then cleaved by secretase to yield a nuclear intracellular cofactor. Interestingly, in hair follicles deficient in secretase, IRS cells fail to retain their IRS fate and the affected hair follicles appear to undergo a reversion to epidermal differentiation fate with resultant cyst formation (Blanpain et al. 2006). Transgenic mice expressing a constitutive activated form of Notch1 under the control of the involucrin promoter were reported to develop both skin and hair abnormalities. Here, hair follicle IRS differentiation is significantly delayed, resulting in a "Mohawk"-like alopecia associated with the anagen phase of the hair cycle (Uyttendaele et al. 2004). Furthermore, when overexpression of Notch1 was directed to precortical keratinocytes, the differentiation of hair shaft medullary cells was disrupted and yielded a wavy hair phenotype (Lin et al. 2000).

Cells that differentiate into IRS keratinocytes begin to express components of the cornified envelope (e.g., loricrin, involucrin, and transglutaminases) that make them similar to suprabasal keratinocytes. However, they also begin to express trichohyalin protein, a cross-linker of keratin filaments, in this layer. Trichohyalin is also found in cells forming the medulla (Alibardi 2004). Signaling via the epidermal growth factor receptor (EGFR) can cause defects in the keratinization of the IRS, loss of cohesion with the hair shaft within, and may also result in the production of wavy hair fibers (Luetteke et al. 1993; Hansen et al. 1997).

Another control of IRS cell fate is the transcriptional regulator "CCAAT displacement protein" (CDP, Cutl1), that is, a transcription factor involved in the regulation of cell growth and differentiation. Mice with a null mutation in Cutl1 develop an abnormal pelage due to disrupted hair follicle morphogenesis with reduced IRS formation. The recent observation of Cutl1 expression in cells of the so-called companion layer suggests that this mysterious layer is really the fourth and most external layer of the IRS (Ellis et al. 2001; Gu and Coulombe 2007). The transcription of Shh- and IRS-specific genes is deregulated in Cutl1 mutant hair follicles, suggesting that the progenitors and cell lineages of the IRS specifically express Cutl1 (Ellis et al. 2001). By contrast, it appears that progenitors of the nonkeratinizing outer root sheath are not derived from the differentiating matrix keratinocytes (as in the IRS and hair shaft lineages), but rather may derive from laterally migrating cells from the bulge (Panteleyev et al. 2001).

The expression of the winged-helix/forkhead transcription factor FOXN1 in the IRS and hair shaft is thought to function in the differentiation of these cell types (Lee et al. 1999). Moreover, mice overexpressing FOXN1 in the IRS exhibit disruptions of hair shaft formation (Prowse et al. 1999), whereas a spontaneous mutation in FOXN1 is associated with hair, nail, and immune defects (Frank et al. 1999; Mecklenburg et al. 2005).

1.1.6 Formation of the hair shaft

One of the main ways to distinguish each of the different cell layers of the developing hair follicle is by analyzing the expression of particular keratin genes (Schweizer et al. 2007). Indeed, some of these keratin genes are reported targets of the Wnt gene (Merrill et al. 2001). For example, Wnt/β-catenin/LEF signaling is considered to be very important for differentiation of matrix keratinocytes into precortical keratinocytes. Not only do the promoters of some hair keratin genes contain LEF binding sites and precortical keratinocytes express LEF, but also hair follicle development ceases before the formation of the hair shaft (i.e., Stage 5/6) (Fig. 1.1.3f and g) in LEF knockout mice (DasGupta and Fuchs 1999). This indicates that this stage of hair follicle development is in part regulated by Wnt signaling. As mentioned above, transcription regulators of hair shaft genes also include FOXN1 and HOXC13, which are expressed in hair shaft differentiation cell lineages. Mutating HOXC13 can result in brittle hair alopecia (Godwin and Capecchi 1998), while FOXN1 is mutated in the nude mouse (Mecklenburg et al. 2005) where it results in alopecia and in the absence of keratin K33 in truncal hair follicles (Meier et al. 1999).

The interrelated nature of signaling pathways in hair follicle development is further evidenced by the finding that the expression of both HOXC13 and FOXN1 can be regulated by BMP signaling (Kulessa et al. 2000). Cells in the hair bulb matrix that are destined to become hair shaft cortical keratinocytes also express BMP4. The expression of Noggin (i.e., the inhibitor of BMP4) can disrupt the differentiation of the cortical keratinocytes needed for hair shaft formation.

It has long been suspected that the IRS plays a significant role in modulating the phenotype of the initially pliant hair shaft within the lower hair follicle. Thus, defects in IRS development (e.g., caused by mutations in Gata-3) are likely to result in the impairment of the hair fiber phenotype (Kaufman et al. 2003). The conditional knockout of the Gata-3 gene from the hair follicle results in mice with a range of phenotypes. These include abnormal and delayed postnatal growth and development, aberrant hair follicle tissue organization, and irregular hair pigmentation. When the transcriptome of these mice was analyzed, the affected hair follicles exhibited upregulation of Notch, Wnt, and BMP signaling pathways (Kurek et al. 2007). Similarly, mice with a conditional knockout of the transcription factor gene Runx1 also display a hair shaft structural deformation in zigzag hairs (Raveh et al. 2006).

Finally, a role for the transmembrane desmosomal cadherin, desmoglein 4, in the development of the hair shaft has been suggested recently. This is supported by observations that mutations in this gene can cause hypotrichosis in humans, mice, and rats. In human hair follicles desmoglein 4 is expressed specifically in the hair cortex and in the cuticle of the IRS and hair shaft, suggesting that this molecule is very important for trichocyte adhesion of the hair shaft (Bazzi et al. 2006).

The events underlying Stage 0 to Stage 5 of hair follicle morphogenesis (Fig. 1.1.3a–f) is a rapidly growing field, and it is likely that we are only at the beginning of elucidating the full range of molecular players involved in hair follicle differentiation.

Significant additional morphologic features are apparent by Stage 5 of hair follicle morphogenesis (Fig. 1.1.3f). Not only does the IRS continue to develop and extend upward within the hair follicle, but several epithelial prominences or bulges also appear along the external wall of the developing hair follicle or outer root sheath (Fig. 1.1.1). One of these "bulges" will generate the future repository of the hair follicle stem cells (e.g., for both epithelial cells and melanocytes). A second more distal bulge will become a site of specialized lipid-forming epithelial cells that will form the holocrine sebaceous gland. Sebum flow from this gland coats and lubricates the hair shaft surface, and may also have antimicrobial function. Differentiation of immature keratinocytes to sebocytes is thought to be regulated in part by the product of the proto-oncogene c-Myc, as this occurs independently of the other cell lineages of the hair follicle. It is thought that c-Myc stimulates some epithelial cells to leave the stem cell compartment and differentiate into sebocytes rather than hair follicle lineages (Arnold and Watt 2001). The transcription factor peroxisome proliferator-activated receptor-γ (PPARγ) is a second transcription factor that specifically regulates the differentiation of sebocytes (Rosen et al. 1999).

1.1.7 Development of the hair follicle pigmentary unit

The developing hair follicle contains—in addition to epithelial keratinocytes and mesenchymal fibroblasts—cells of neuroectodermal origin, the melanocytes. Cutaneous melanocytes of both the epidermis and pilosebaceous unit originate from pluripotent cells that commit to the melanocyte lineage while in the embryonic neural crest. To reach the skin, so-called melanoblasts leave the neural tube and migrate dorsolaterally and differentiate along stereotypical routes from the closing neural tube, migrate between the dermamyotome of the somites and the overlying ectoderm, until they enter the dermis (Rawles 1947). Melanoblasts migrate under the control of specific growth factors (e.g., endothelin-1, stem cell factor/c-kit) through the dermis and subsequently to the epidermis, and distribute within the developing hair follicle. Disruption of the stem cell factor/c-Kit signaling pathway interferes with not only the survival and migration of these early melanocytes, but also their differentiation during this stage of hair follicle morphogenesis.

Much of our knowledge of the events involved in the development of melanocyte compartments within the skin and hair follicle derives from the analysis of gene mutations in mice that affect differentiation, proliferation, and migration of melanocyte precursors (Jackson 1994). There are over 100 genes shown so far to affect hair color in the mouse (Nakamura et al. 2002), and equivalents of many of these continue to be described in other mammals, where mutations range from total loss of all-over pigmentation (e.g., types of albinism) to loss of pigment from specific body sites (e.g., piebaldism) (Fleischman et al. 1996). Recently, a role for the Notch signaling pathway in the maintenance of melanoblasts and melanocyte stem cells was proposed, where severe coat color dilution resulted when the Notch pathway was disrupted. Loss of hair pigment was also seen when Notch1 and/or Notch2 receptors were ablated in melanocytes (Schouwey et al. 2007).

Even before the onset of hair bulb melanogenesis, that is, around morphogenesis Stage 4 (Fig. 1.1.3f and g), strongly c-Kit and S100 positive cells are visible in selected cells of the hair follicle placode and plug. Later these cells become increasingly dendritic and invade the hair bulb (Peters et al. 2002). There, they appear to distribute as either "dihydroxy-phenylalanine (DOPA)-positive" or "DOPA-negative" melanocytes (Chase et al. 1951), where DOPA positivity refers to their ability to produce the rate-limiting enzyme for melanin formation called tyrosinase or whether it can oxidize DOPA and produce the melanin precursor dopaquinone. As hair follicle morphogenesis progresses to the stage of synthesizing a hair fiber, DOPA-positive melanocytes cluster around the apex of the dermal papilla in the hair bulb. Other amelanotic DOPA-negative melanocytes occupy positions in the outer root sheath (Fig. 1.1.1). The first melanin granules are evident in precortical keratinocytes at this stage.

1.1.8 Final stages of hair follicle morphogenesis

The forming fiber now starts to pass through the hair follicle core in order to exit the skin surface. Its passage through intact follicular epithelium is facilitated by the formation of a "hair canal" (Robins and Breathnach 1970), which is constructed via focal cell death or apoptosis. The developing hair follicle continues to extend deeper and deeper into the skin until its proximal bulbar end is situated within the adipocyte-rich subcutis. Anatomic features characteristic of Stage 6 hair follicles include an increasing complexity of the now multilayered IRS (Fig. 1.1.3e–h). Furthermore, the hair shaft can now be visualized within the hair canal and melanin granules can be seen within its cortical keratinocytes. The final two stages of hair follicle development are characterized by the growth of the hair shaft through the IRS and hair canal until the tip of the fiber emerges from the surface of the skin (Figs. 1.1.1 and 1.1.3h). In addition, the aspect of the sebaceous gland changes relative to the hair follicle horizontal axis at this stage. Finally, the hair follicle attains its maximal length and bulk during Stage 8 when the distal hair shaft is positioned well, free of the skin surface (Figs. 1.1.1 and 1.1.3i).

The anatomy of the fully developed Stage 8 hair follicle is very similar to the anatomy of the growing/cycling anagen hair follicle in the adult (see Section 1.2.1). Epithelial and mesenchymal cells of the developing hair follicle therefore contrive to produce the mature hair follicle via massive cell proliferation and cell differentiation. However, considerable tissue sculpting is also required. Such sculpting events also require intermittent and highly localized programmed cell death (Magerl et al. 2001). Only in this way can this hair follicle assume its full hair shaft-forming status.

Cessation of hair fiber production (i.e., hair shaft growth) during Stage 8 of hair follicle development signals entry into the "hair growth cycle," from which the hair follicle usually does not escape during the life of the individual (see Section 1.2.1).

In summary, the development or morphogenesis of the hair follicle provides an exquisite example and model system to study the earliest communications involved in organ development. It is likely that this system will reveal much about how cells communicate to aid the development of treatments for developmental abnormalities in general and those affecting the hair follicle (e.g., congenital hyper/hypo/a/-trichosis) in particular.

References

Alibardi L. 2004. Fine structure of marsupial hairs, with emphasis on trichohyalin and the structure of the inner root sheath. *Journal of Morphology* 261(3):390–402.

Arnold I, Watt FM. 2001. c-Myc activation in transgenic mouse epidermis results in mobilization of stem cells and differentiation of their progeny. *Current Biology* 11(8):558–568.

Atit R, Sgaier SK, Mohamed OA, Taketo MM, Dufort D, Joyner AL, Niswander L, Conlon RA. 2006. Beta-catenin activation is necessary and sufficient to specify the dorsal dermal fate in the mouse. *Developmental Biology* 296(1):164–176.

Barsh G. 1999. Of ancient tales and hairless tails. *Nature Genetics* 22(4):315–316.

Bazzi H, Getz A, Mahoney MG, Ishida-Yamamoto A, Langbein L, Wahl JK III, Christiano AM. 2006. Desmoglein 4 is expressed in highly differentiated keratinocytes and trichocytes in human epidermis and hair follicle. *Differentiation* 74(2–3):129–140.

Blanpain C, Lowry WE, Pasolli HA, Fuchs E. 2006. Canonical notch signaling functions as a commitment switch in the epidermal lineage. *Genes and Development* 20(21):3022–3035.

Botchkarev VA, Botchkareva NV, Roth W, Nakamura M, Chen LH, Herzog W, Lindner G, McMahon JA, Peters C, Lauster R, McMahon AP, Paus R. 1999. Noggin is a mesenchymally derived stimulator of hair-follicle induction. *Nature Cell Biology* 1(3):158–164.

Botchkarev VA, Paus R. 2003. Molecular biology of hair morphogenesis: development and cycling. *Journal of Experimental Zoology Part B: Molecular and Developmental Evolution* 298(1):164–180.

Botchkarev VA, Sharov AA. 2004. BMP signaling in the control of skin development and hair follicle growth. *Differentiation* 72(9–10):512–526.

Chase HB, Rauch R, Smith VW. 1951. Critical stages of hair development and pigmentation in the mouse. *Physiology and Zoology* 24(1):1–8.

Chiang C, Swan RZ, Grachtchouk M, Bolinger M, Litingtung Y, Robertson EK, Cooper MK, Gaffield W, Westphal H, Beachy PA, Dlugosz AA. 1999. Essential role for sonic hedgehog during hair follicle morphogenesis. *Developmental Biology* 205(1):1–9.

Chuong C-M. 1998. *Molecular Basis of Epithelial Appendage Morphogenesis.* Austin, Texas: RG Landes.

DasGupta R, Fuchs E. 1999. Multiple roles for activated LEF/TCF transcription complexes during hair follicle development and differentiation. *Development* 126(20):4557–4568.

Drögemüller C, Rüfenacht S, Wichert B, Leeb T. 2007. Mutations within the FGF5 gene are associated with hair length in cats. *Animal Genetics* 38(3):218–221.

Ellis T, Gambardella L, Horcher M, Tschanz S, Capol J, Bertram P, Jochum W, Barrandon Y, Busslinger M. 2001. The transcriptional repressor CDP (Cutl1) is essential for epithelial cell differentiation of the lung and the hair follicle. *Genes and Development* 15(17):2307–2319.

Favier B, Fliniaux I, Thélu J, Viallet JP, Demarchez M, Jahoda CA, Dhouailly D. 2000. Localisation of members of the notch system and the differentiation of vibrissa hair follicles: receptors, ligands, and fringe modulators. *Developmental Dynamics* 218(3):426–437.

Fleischman RA, Gallardo T, Mi X. 1996. Mutations in the ligand-binding domain of the kit receptor: an uncommon site in human piebaldism. *Journal of Investigative Dermatology* 107(5):703–706.

Foitzik K, Paus R, Doetschman T, Dotto GP. 1999. The TGF-beta2 isoform is both a required and sufficient inducer of murine hair follicle morphogenesis. *Developmental Biology* 212(2):278–289.

Frank J, Pignata C, Panteleyev AA, Prowse DM, Baden H, Weiner L, Gaetaniello L, Ahmad W, Pozzi N, Cserhalmi-Friedman PB, Aita VM, Uyttendaele H, Gordon D, Ott J, Brissette JL, Christiano AM. 1999. Exposing the human nude phenotype. *Nature* 398(6727):473–474.

Fuchs E. 2007. Scratching the surface of skin development. *Nature* 445(7130):834–842.

Fuchs E, Merrill BJ, Jamora C, DasGupta R. 2001. At the roots of a never-ending cycle. *Developmental Cell* 1(1):13–25.

Gat U, DasGupta R, Degenstein L, Fuchs E. 1998. De novo hair follicle morphogenesis and hair tumors in mice expressing a truncated beta-catenin in skin. *Cell* 95(5):605–614.

Godwin AR, Capecchi MR. 1998. Hoxc13 mutant mice lack external hair. *Genes and Development* 12(1):11–20.

Gritli-Linde A, Hallberg K, Harfe BD, Reyahi A, Kannius-Janson M, Nilsson J, Cobourne MT, Sharpe PT, McMahon AP, Linde A. 2007. Abnormal hair development and apparent follicular transformation to mammary gland in the absence of hedgehog signaling. *Developmental Cell* 12(1):99–112.

Gu LH, Coulombe PA. 2007. Keratin expression provides novel insight into the morphogenesis and function of the companion layer in hair follicles. *Journal of Investigative Dermatology* 127(5):1061–1073.

Hansen LA, Alexander N, Hogan ME, Sundberg JP, Dlugosz A, Threadgill DW, Magnuson T, Yuspa SH. 1997. Genetically null mice reveal a central role for epidermal growth factor receptor in the differentiation of the hair follicle and normal hair development. *American Journal of Pathology* 150(6):1959–1975.

Headon DJ, Overbeek PA. 1999. Involvement of a novel TNF receptor homologue in hair follicle induction. *Nature Genetics* 22(4):370–374.

Huelsken J, Vogel R, Erdmann B, Cotsarelis G, Birchmeier W. 2001. Beta-catenin controls hair follicle morphogenesis and stem cell differentiation in the skin. *Cell* 105(4):533–545.

Iseki S, Araga A, Ohuchi H, Nohno T, Yoshioka H, Hayashi F, Noji S. 1996. Sonic hedgehog is expressed in epithelial cells during development of whisker, hair, and tooth. *Biochemical and Biophysical Research Communications* 218(3):688–693.

Ito M, Yang Z, Andl T, Cui C, Kim N, Millar SE, Cotsarelis G. 2007. Wnt-dependent de novo hair follicle regeneration in adult mouse skin after wounding. *Nature* 447(7142):316–320.

Jackson IJ. 1994. Molecular and developmental genetics of mouse coat color. *Annual Reviews in Genetics* 28:189–217.

Jung HS, Francis-West PH, Widelitz RB, Jiang TX, Ting-Berreth S, Tickle C, Wolpert L, Chuong CM. 1998. Local inhibitory action of BMPs and their relationships with activators in feather formation: implications for periodic patterning. *Developmental Biology* 196(1):11–23.

Kaplan ED, Holbrook KA. 1994. Dynamic expression patterns of tenascin, proteoglycans, and cell adhesion molecules during human hair follicle morphogenesis. *Developmental Dynamics* 199(2):141–155.

Karlsson L, Bondjers C, Betsholtz C. 1999. Roles for PDGF-A and sonic hedgehog in development of mesenchymal components of the hair follicle. *Development* 126(12):2611–2621.

Kashiwagi M, Kuroki T, Huh N. 1997. Specific inhibition of hair follicle formation by epidermal growth factor in an organ culture of developing mouse skin. *Developmental Biology* 189(1):22–32.

Kashiwagi M, Morgan BA, Georgopoulos K. 2007. The chromatin remodeler Mi-2beta is required for establishment of the basal epidermis and normal differentiation of its progeny. *Development* 34(8):1571–1582.

Kaufman CK, Zhou P, Pasolli HA, Rendl M, Bolotin D, Lim KC, Dai X, Alegre ML, Fuchs E. 2003. GATA-3: an unexpected regulator of cell lineage determination in skin. *Genes and Development* 17(17):2108–2122.

Kratochwil K, Dull M, Farinas I, Galceran J, Grosschedl R. 1996. Lef1 expression is activated by BMP-4 and regulates inductive tissue interactions in tooth and hair development. *Genes and Development* 10(11):1382–94.

Kulessa H, Turk G, Hogan BL. 2000. Inhibition of BMP signaling affects growth and differentiation in the anagen hair follicle. *EMBO Journal* 19(24):6664–6674.

Kurek D, Garinis GA, van Doorninck JH, Van Der Wees J, Grosveld FG. 2007. Transcriptome and phenotypic analysis reveals Gata3-dependent signalling pathways in murine hair follicles. *Development* 134(2):261–272.

Lee D, Prowse DM, Brissette JL. 1999. Association between mouse nude gene expression and the initiation of epithelial terminal differentiation. *Developmental Biology* 208(2):362–374.

Levy V, Lindon C, Harfe BD, Morgan BA. 2005. Distinct stem cell populations regenerate the follicle and interfollicular epidermis. *Developmental Cell* 9(6):855–861.

Li J, Tzu J, Chen Y, Zhang YP, Nguyen NT, Gao J, Bradley M, Keene DR, Oro AE, Miner JH, Marinkovich MP. 2003. Laminin-10 is crucial for hair morphogenesis. *EMBO Journal* 22(10):2400–2410.

Lin MH, Leimeister C, Gessler M, Kopan R. 2000. Activation of the Notch pathway in the hair cortex leads to aberrant differentiation of the adjacent hair-shaft layers. *Development* 127(11):2421–2432.

Lindner G, Menrad A, Gherardi E, Merlino G, Welker P, Handjiski B, Roloff B, Paus R. 2000. Involvement of hepatocyte growth factor/scatter factor and met receptor signaling in hair follicle morphogenesis and cycling. *FASEB Journal* 14(2):319–332.

Lo Celso C, Prowse DM, Watt FM. 2004. Transient activation of beta-catenin signalling in adult mouse epidermis is sufficient to induce new hair follicles but continuous activation is required to maintain hair follicle tumours. *Development* 131(8):1787–1799.

Luetteke NC, Qiu TH, Peiffer RL, Oliver P, Smithies O, Lee DC. 1993. TGF alpha deficiency results in hair follicle and eye abnormalities in targeted and waved-1 mice. *Cell* 73(2):263–278.

Maderson PF. 2003. Mammalian skin evolution: a reevaluation. *Experimental Dermatology* 12(3):233–236.

Magerl M, Tobin DJ, Müller-Röver S, Hagen E, Lindner G, McKay IA, Paus R. 2001. Patterns of proliferation and apoptosis during murine hair follicle morphogenesis. *Journal of Investigative Dermatology* 116(6):947–955.

Mecklenburg L, Tychsen B, Paus R. 2005. Learning from nudity: lessons from the nude phenotype. *Experimental Dermatology* 14(11):797–810.

Meier N, Dear TN, Boehm T. 1999. Whn and mHa3 are components of the genetic hierarchy controlling hair follicle differentiation. *Mechanisms of Development* 89(1–2):215–221.

Merrill BJ, Gat U, DasGupta R, Fuchs E. 2001. Tcf3 and Lef1 regulate lineage differentiation of multipotent stem cells in skin. *Genes and Development* 15(13):1688–1705.

Mill P, Mo R, Fu H, Grachtchouk M, Kim PC, Dlugosz AA, Hui CC. 2003. Sonic hedgehog-dependent activation of Gli2 is essential for embryonic hair follicle development. *Genes and Development* 17(2):282–294.

Millar SE. 2002. Molecular mechanisms regulating hair follicle development. *Journal of Investigative Dermatology* 118(2):216–225.

Ming Kwan K, Li AG, Wang XJ, Wurst W, Behringer RR. 2004. Essential roles of BMPR-IA signaling in differentiation and growth of hair follicles and in skin tumorigenesis. *Genesis* 39(1):10–25.

Mou C, Jackson B, Schneider P, Overbeek PA, Headon DJ. 2006. Generation of the primary hair follicle pattern. *Proceedings of the National Academy of Sciences of the United States of America* 103(24):9075–9080.

Nakamura M, Tobin DJ, Richards-Smith B, Sundberg JP, Paus R. 2002. Mutant laboratory mice with abnormalities in pigmentation: annotated tables. *Journal of Dermatological Science* 28(1):1–33.

Noramly S, Freeman A, Morgan BA. 1999. Beta-catenin signaling can initiate feather bud development. *Development* 126(16):3509–3521.

Olivera-Martinez I, Viallet JP, Michon F, Pearton DJ, Dhouailly D. 2004. The different steps of skin formation in vertebrates. *International Journal of Developmental Biology* 48(2–3):107–115.

Oro AE, Higgins K. 2003. Hair cycle regulation of hedgehog signal reception. *Developmental Biology* 255(2):238–248.

Ouji Y, Yoshikawa M, Shiroi A, Ishizaka S. 2006. Promotion of hair follicle development and trichogenesis by Wnt-10b in cultured embryonic skin and in reconstituted skin. *Biochemical and Biophysical Research Communications* 345(2):581–587.

Panteleyev AA, Jahoda CA, Christiano AM. 2001. Hair follicle predetermination. *Journal of Cell Science* 114(Pt 19):3419–3431.

Paus R, Müller-Röver S, Van Der Veen C, Maurer M, Eichmüller S, Ling G, Hofmann U, Foitzik K, Mecklenburg L, Handjiski B. 1999. A comprehensive guide for the recognition and classification of distinct stages of hair follicle morphogenesis. *Journal of Investigative Dermatology* 113(4):523–532.

Peters EM, Tobin DJ, Botchkareva N, Maurer M, Paus R. 2002. Migration of melanoblasts into the developing murine hair follicle is accompanied by transient c-Kit expression. *Journal of Histochemistry and Cytochemistry* 50(6):751–766.

Petiot A, Conti FJ, Grose R, Revest JM, Hodivala-Dilke KM, Dickson C. 2003. A crucial role for Fgfr2-IIIb signalling in epidermal development and hair follicle patterning. *Development* 130(22):5493–5501.

Prowse DM, Lee D, Weiner L, Jiang N, Magro CM, Baden HP, Brissette JL. 1999. Ectopic expression of the nude gene induces hyperproliferation and defects in differentiation: implications for the self-renewal of cutaneous epithelia. *Developmental Biology* 212(1):54–67.

Raveh E, Cohen S, Levanon D, Negreanu V, Groner Y, Gat U. 2006. Dynamic expression of Runx1 in skin affects hair structure. *Mechanisms of Development* 123(11):842–850.

Rawles ME. 1947. Origin of pigment cells from the neural crest in the mouse embryo. *Physiology and Zoology* 20:248–266.

Reddy S, Andl T, Bagasra A, Lu MM, Epstein DJ, Morrisey EE, Millar SE. 2001. Characterization of Wnt gene expression in developing and postnatal hair follicles and identification of Wnt5a as a target of sonic hedgehog in hair follicle morphogenesis. *Mechanisms of Development* 107(1–2):69–82.

Rendl M, Polak L, Fuchs E. 2008. BMP signaling in dermal papilla cells is required for their hair follicle-inductive properties. *Genes and Development* 22(4):543–557.

Reynolds AJ, Lawrence C, Cserhalmi-Friedman PB, Christiano AM, Jahoda CA. 1999. Trans-gender induction of hair follicles. *Nature* 402(6757):33–34.

Robins EJ, Breathnach AS. 1970. Fine structure of bulbar end of human foetal hair follicle at stage of differentiation of inner root sheath. *Journal of Anatomy* 107(Pt 1):131–146.

Rosen ED, Sarraf P, Troy AE, Bradwin G, Moore K, Milstone DS, Spiegelman BM, Mortensen RM. 1999. PPARγ is required for the differentiation of adipose tissue in vivo and in vitro. *Molecular Cell* 4(4):611–617.

Satokata I, Ma L, Ohshima H, Bei M, Woo I, Nishizawa K, Maeda T, Takano Y, Uchiyama M, Heaney S, Peters H, Tang Z, Maxson R, Maas R. 2000. Msx2 deficiency in mice causes pleiotropic defects in bone growth and ectodermal organ formation. *Nature Genetics* 24(4):391–395.

Schmidt-Ullrich R, Aebischer T, Hülsken J, Birchmeier W, Klemm U, Scheidereit C. 2001. Requirement of NF-kappaB/Rel for the development of hair follicles and other epidermal appendices. *Development* 128(19):3843–3853.

Schmidt-Ullrich R, Paus R. 2005. Molecular principles of hair follicle induction and morphogenesis. *Bioessays* 27(3):247–261.

Schmidt-Ullrich R, Tobin DJ, Lenhard D, Schneider P, Paus R, Scheidereit C. 2006. NF-kappaB transmits Eda A1/EdaR signalling to activate Shh and cyclin D1 expression, and controls post-initiation hair placode down growth. *Development* 133(6):1045–1057.

Schouwey K, Delmas V, Larue L, Zimber-Strobl U, Strobl LJ, Radtke F, Beermann F. 2007. Notch1 and Notch2 receptors influence

progressive hair graying in a dose-dependent manner. *Developmental Dynamics* 236(1):282–289.
Schweizer J, Langbein L, Rogers MA, Winter H. 2007. Hair follicle-specific keratins and their diseases. *Experimental Cell Research* 313(10):2010–2020.
Sick S, Reinker S, Timmer J, Schlake T. 2006. WNT and DKK determine hair follicle spacing through a reaction–diffusion mechanism. *Science* 314(5804):1447–1450.
St-Jacques B, Dassule HR, Karavanova I, Botchkarev VA, Li J, Danielian PS, McMahon JA, Lewis PM, Paus R, McMahon AP. 1998. Sonic hedgehog signaling is essential for hair development. *Current Biology* 8(19):1058–1068.
Tobin DJ (ed). 2005. *Hair in Toxicology: An Important Bio-monitor.* London: Royal Society of Chemistry.
Uyttendaele H, Panteleyev AA, de Berker D, Tobin DT, Christiano AM. 2004. Activation of Notch1 in the hair follicle leads to cell-fate switch and Mohawk alopecia. *Differentiation* 72(8):396–409.

1.2

Anatomy and physiology of the hair follicle

Desmond J. Tobin

The hair follicle is formed from a bewilderingly complex set of interactions involving ectodermal, mesodermal, and neuroectodermal components, which go to elaborate five or six concentric cellular cylinders of at least 15 distinct interacting cell subpopulations (Philpott and Paus 1998; Botchkarev and Paus 2003).

Much, if not most, of current hair research is conducted in murine models (after an extended period of time when this was dominated by research on wool for economic reasons), and particularly in black-haired mice strains like C57BL6 (Paus et al. 1990). While it is likely that there will be some important species-specific differences, the consensus is that the fundamentals of hair growth will be broadly similar in all mammals. Unlike many other mammals, humans have all but lost their ability to grow hair synchronously (i.e., as a wave). Instead, human hair grows in a mosaic pattern where significant autonomy for growth and pigmentation resides in individual hair follicle.

1.2.1 The hair growth cycle

As discussed earlier (see Section 1.1.8), the fully developed Stage 8 hair follicles actively produce hair fibers. Each follicle will continue to do so until it is induced to enter the first hair growth cycle. Thus, hair cycling paradoxically begins with a regression phase characterized by a massive cell death via apoptosis to yield the first catagen. Upon completion of this catagen phase, the hair follicle will have lost up to 70% of its original Stage 8 tissue mass, as it enters a period of relative rest during telogen. After some time the telogen follicle is reactivated to enter into the first anagen phase of the hair cycle. Thereafter, the hair follicle continues with lifelong cyclical activity (Fig. 1.2.1) until death of the individual (Fuchs et al. 2001; Stenn and Paus 2001).

1.2.1.1 First anagen

This first anagen of the hair growth cycle morphologically resembles several aspects of hair follicle development in utero. In this way the lifelong cyclical activity of the hair follicle recapitulates, at least in part, several embryologic events involved in hair follicle morphogenesis (Paus and Cotsarelis 1999; Botchkarev and Paus 2003). Remarkably, several signaling pathways that drive and follow mesenchymal–epithelial interactions during hair follicle morphogenesis are reused during the hair growth cycle (cf. Chuong 1998). While hair growth cycle dynamics vary somewhat between different mammalian species (see Section 1.3.3), between different body sites, and even between different hair follicle subtypes in the same body site, there exists an intrinsic rhythmic activity that can be modulated not only by systemic factors but more importantly also by the hair follicle's own locally directed activities.

1.2.1.2 Catagen

Catagen has been described by Ralf Paus as a "partial organ suicide" whereby the growing terminal hair follicle is reduced by more than two-thirds of its growing tissue mass (Figs 1.2.1 and 1.2.2). This massive cell death is both controlled and rapid (about 2–3 weeks on human scalp and 3–5 days in mice) and involves substantial remodeling not only of the hair follicle itself (Lindner et al. 1997), but also the surrounding dermis.

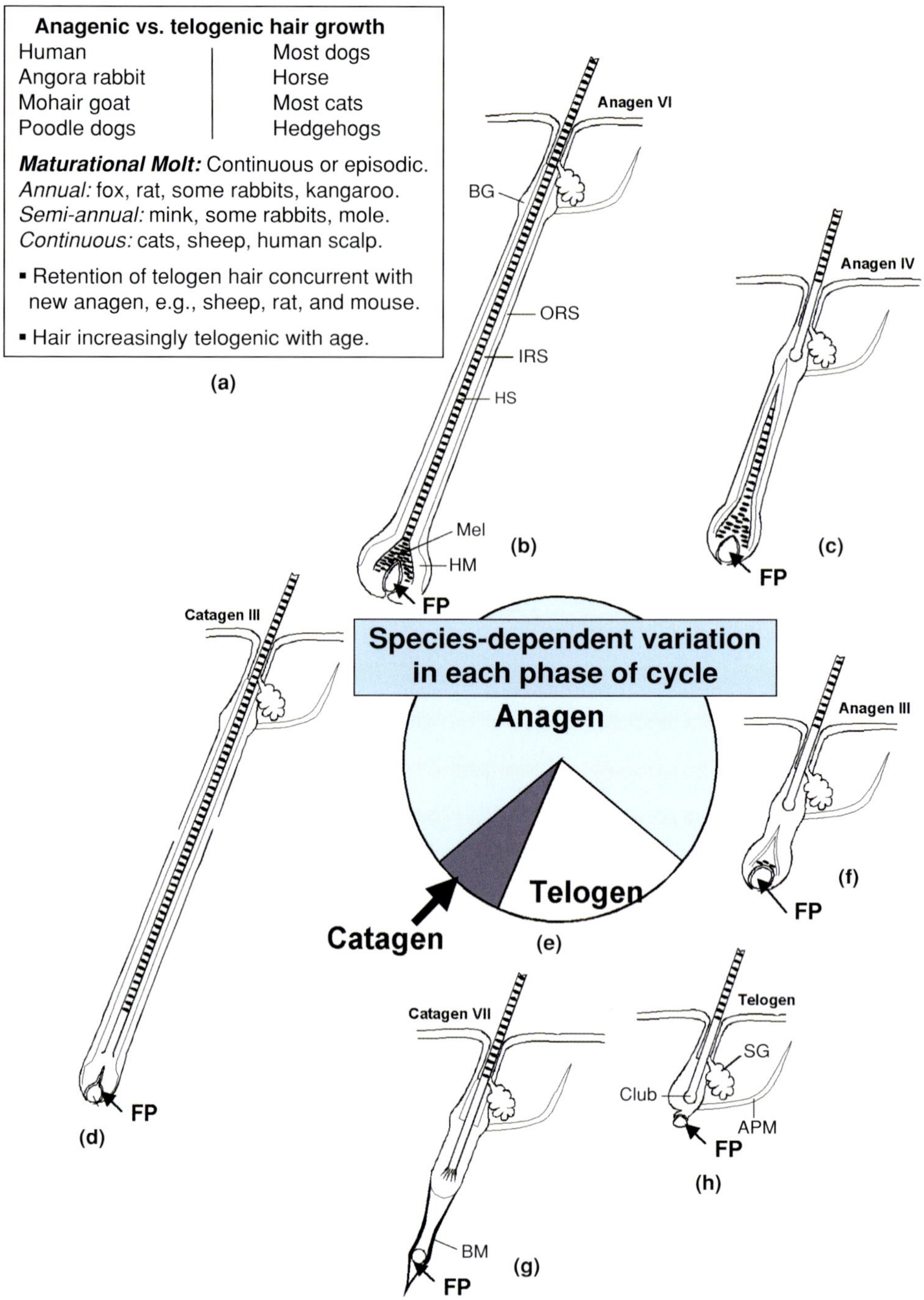

Fig. 1.2.1 Schematic representation of the hair growth cycle with staging according to Müller-Röver et al. (2001). BM, basement membrane; HS, hair shaft; FP, follicular dermal papilla; SG, sebaceous gland; IRS, inner root sheath; ORS, outer root sheath; BG, bulge; Mel, melanin; HM, hair matrix; APM, arrector pili muscle. (Modified from Tobin and Paus (2001).)

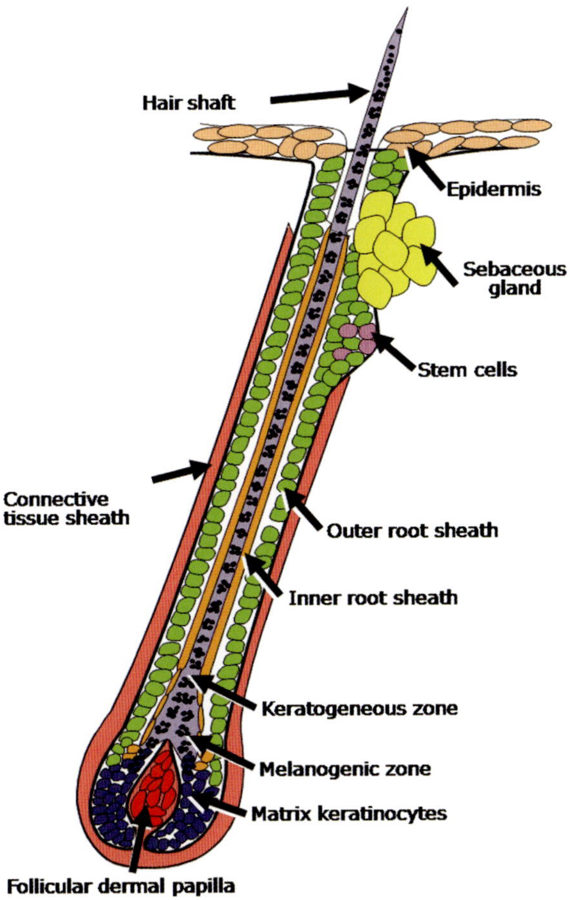

Fig. 1.2.2 Cartoon of an anagen hair follicle showing all lineages of hair follicle cells.

The nature of the catagen trigger(s) remains elusive, although interestingly it has recently been shown in mice that psychosocial stress can also precipitate anagen hair follicles into catagen (Arck et al. 2003). In addition, environmental factors including chemicals, trauma, and experimentally administered hormones (e.g., epidermal growth factor, EGF) can induce catagen. Entry into catagen may even be a default setting for most mammals, whereby the hair follicle is moved from the much more labile anagen stage to a more stable or resting "setting" in telogen during times of stress. Thus, it may be likely that catagen can be induced by changes in levels of cytokines/hormones required for anagen (e.g., inhibition of the receptor for insulin-like growth factor and altered levels of neurotrophins can induce catagen) (Stenn and Paus 2001).

The first morphologic clue that hair follicle regression is impending is the cessation of anagen-coupled hair follicle melanogenesis (Tobin et al. 1999). Interestingly, this too involves apoptosis (Tobin et al. 1998), so while keratinocyte proliferation slows down but continues for a short time, some of this latest hair shaft production lacks incorporation of melanin. As a result, the most proximal end of shed hair fibers is usually pigment free. Thereafter, a massive apoptosis of selected keratinocyte lineages occurs in the lower hair follicle, though there is evidence that some bulbar keratinocytes may survive to form part of the secondary germ of the telogen hair follicle (Panteleyev et al. 2001) (Figs 1.2.1 and 1.2.3).

While keratinocytes and melanocytes of the lower hair follicle are vulnerable to the catagen/apoptosis signal, fibroblasts of the follicular dermal papilla appear by contrast to be remarkably resistant (Tobin et al. 2003a,b). As the hair follicle epithelium shortens dramatically, the papilla is drawn upward toward the epidermis by maintaining direct association with the shrinking hair follicle epithelial strand until it comes to rest at the hair "bulge" (Fig. 1.2.1). Maintenance of close follicular dermal papilla/epithelium contact is critical for continued cycling (Panteleyev et al. 2000), without which hair growth and cycling will fail. Tissue change associated with the transition from full growth (anagen) to the relative resting stage (telogen) is conventionally divided into the characteristic morphologically defined stages catagen I–VIII (Müller-Röver et al. 2001).

1.2.1.3 Telogen

When hair follicle involution is complete at catagen VIII, the hair follicle enters a period of relative rest called telogen. Indeed, for many mammalian species this may be the preferred holding position of the hair cycle. Keratinocytes of the epithelial sac surrounding the telogen hair are specialized to moor the hair club/hair shaft tightly in the hair follicle. Although the telogen hair follicle may appear paltry by comparison to its former growing anagen state, it remains vascularized and innervated and contains all the cell types needed to produce the next fully developed anagen hair follicle. Indeed, there is enormous scientific interest in this region of the hair follicle, as it includes the so-called bulge that together with parts of the upper outer root sheath (ORS)

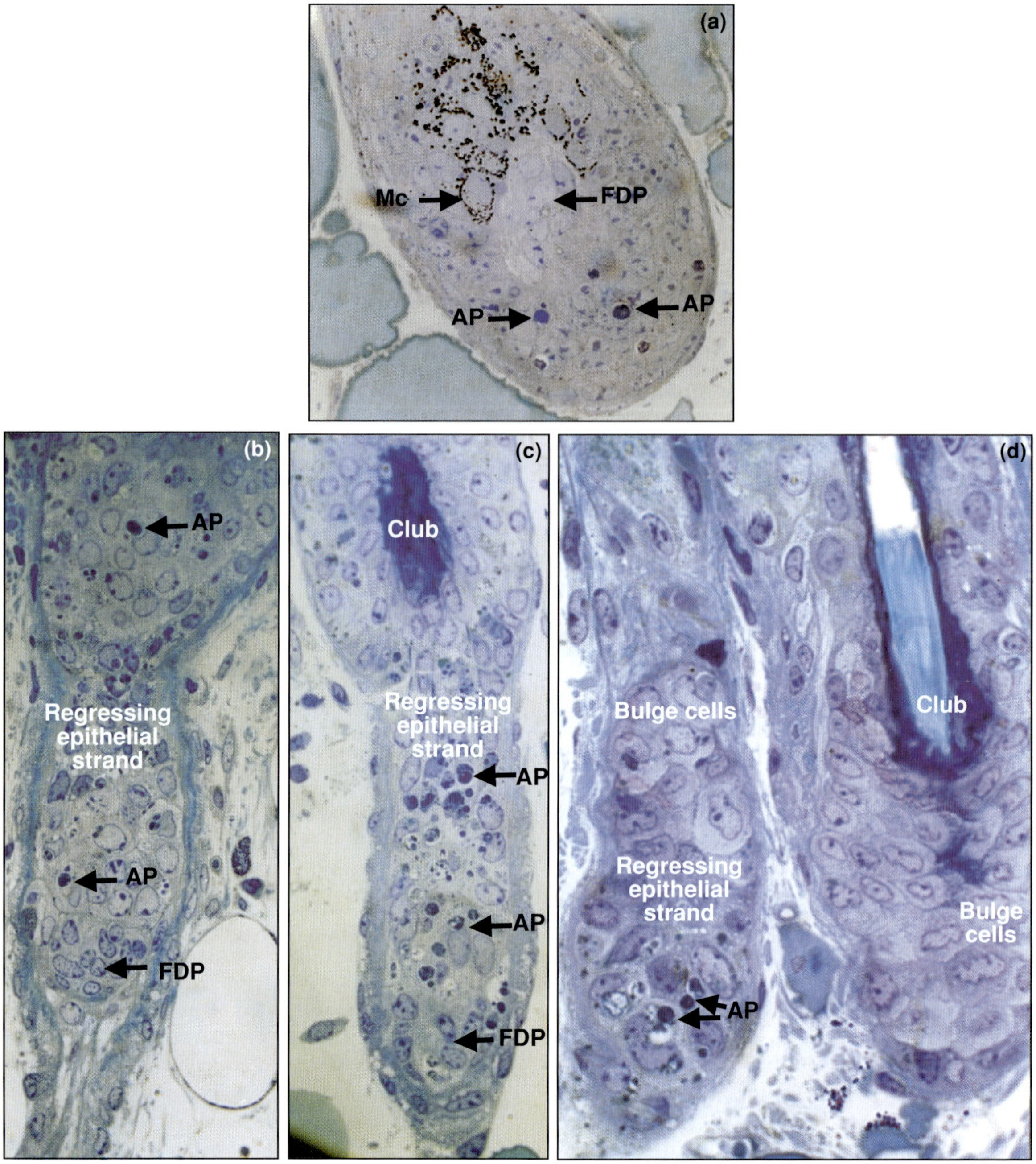

Fig. 1.2.3 High-resolution light microscopy views of longitudinal semithin sections of the C57BL/6 murine hair growth cycle. (a) Catagen I hair bulb showing earliest keratinocyte apoptosis (AP) in a pigmented hair follicle (Mc, melanocyte). (b,c) Advanced catagen VII exhibiting massive apoptosis of keratinocytes (AP) resulting in the generation of a regressing epithelial strand that draws the follicular dermal papilla (FDP) toward the developing club. (d) End stage catagen hair follicle and adjacent full telogen follicle. Note the location of the bulge stem cells with characteristic pleomorphic nuclei. *(Continues)*

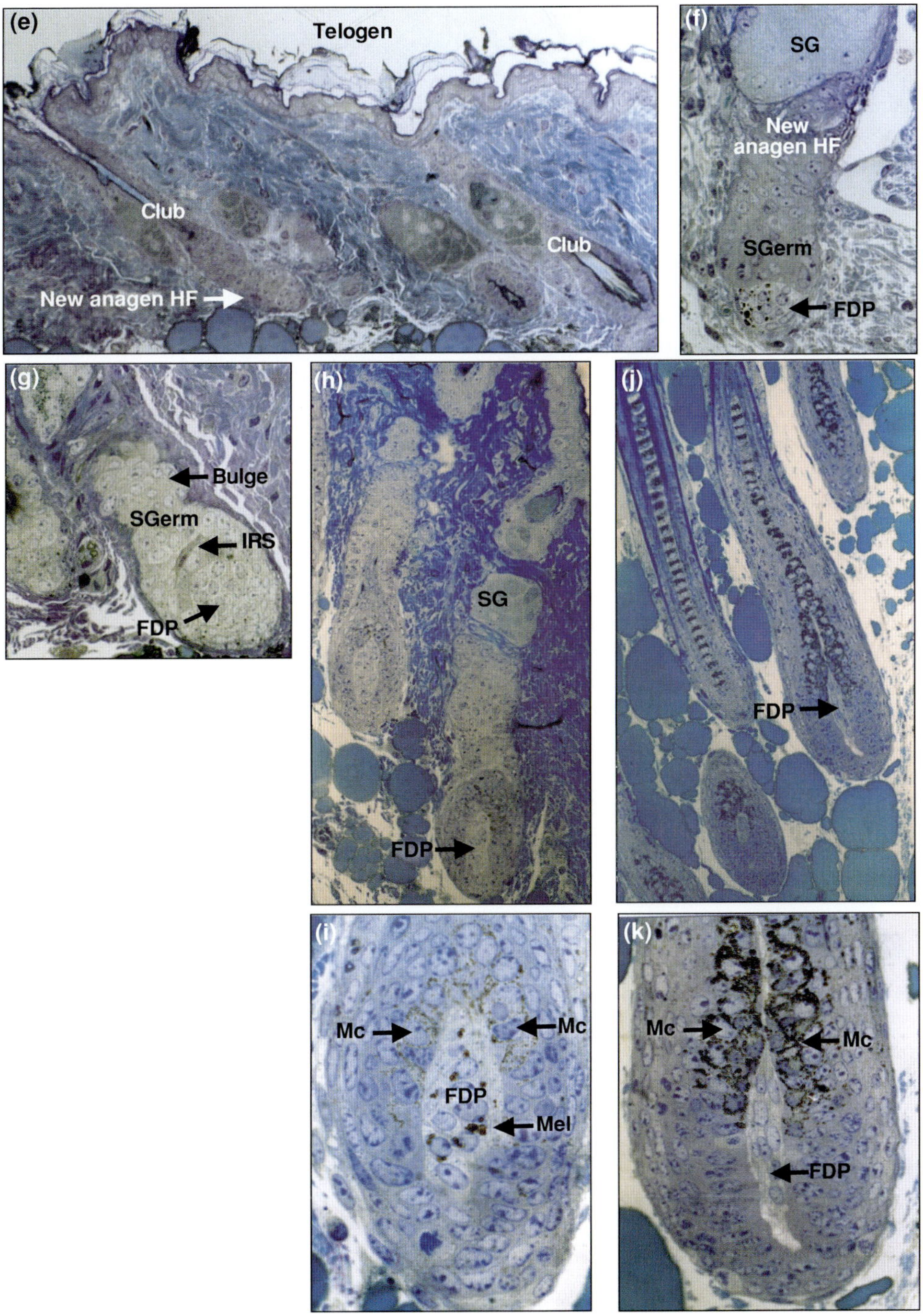

Fig. 1.2.3 *Continued* (e) Telogen skin showing a telogen club hair (right) and very early anagen I/II (left). (f) Early anagen I hair follicle with the FDP containing some melanin from the previous anagen. (g) Anagen III showing early differentiation of the inner root sheath (IRS, arrow). (h) Anagen IV showing commencement of hair bulb melanogenesis. (i) High-power view of anagen IV hair bulb with initiation of melanogenesis in hair bulb melanocytes (Mc). Note also some melanin (Mel) from the previous anagen deposited in the follicular papilla (FDP). (j) Anagen VI hair follicle engaged in full pigmented hair fiber production. (k) High-power view of anagen IV hair bulb with clear FDP and highly melanogenic Mc. SG, sebaceous gland; SGerm, secondary germ. (Modified from Tobin (2005).)

contains a range of different stem cell populations, including stem cells for epithelial cells (Cotsarelis et al. 1990), melanocytes/melanoblasts (Nishimura et al. 2002), and likely also mesenchymal stem cells needed for replenishment of the follicular dermal papilla and dermal sheath (Tobin et al. 2003a, b) (Figs 1.2.1d,e and 1.2.2).

The completion of the telogen phase has sometimes mistakenly been associated with the a priori shedding of the old hair shaft in humans. Instead the process of hair shedding, termed "exogen," appears to constitute an independent and active event (Milner et al. 2002). Unfortunately, this stage of the hair growth cycle has received little attention to date, perhaps surprisingly so given that hair shedding is the major concern for both affected humans and for owners of affected animals. Importantly, exogen does not appear to be due to any motive force exerted by the tip of the new anagen hair shaft below (as is seen with the extrusion of deciduous teeth by adult permanent teeth). Rather, exogen usually occurs when the new growing hair follicle has reached only anagen IV—before the stage of anagen that is associated with the emergence of the hair fiber tip at the base of the telogen club hair. Thus, the disengagement of the telogen club may instead result from an active release phase associated with altered protease/protease inhibitor levels/activity, perhaps also involving the lysosomal protease, cathepsin L (Tobin et al. 2002).

1.2.1.4 Subsequent anagen

The hair follicle remains in the "resting" telogen phase for a highly variable and often very long time. Moreover, the skin becomes increasingly telogenic with age, perhaps related to depletion or loss of activity of the stem cell population. However, under normal circumstances telogen is eventually broken by some, as yet unspecified, signal(s) that initiate(s) the new growth of hair. Several fundamental questions remain regarding the regulation of this critical transition point of the hair growth cycle. For example, it is not yet clear which cell type is responsible for initiating entry into anagen or what this stimulus is, or how it influences its target cell pathway. Moreover, there are many other biologic systems in the skin and the microenvironment of the hair follicle that are likely to influence the process. For example, the vascular (Mecklenburg et al. 2000), neural (Peters et al. 2001), pigmentary (Tobin et al. 1999), and extracellular matrix (Messenger 1991; Westgate et al. 1991a, b) systems among others exhibit a remarkably tight coupling to the hair growth cycle.

We can at least speculate, however, on the likely nature of these anagen growth-inducing cells. First, they must have stem cell-like characteristics, with the biologic capability to maintain a unique cellular rhythm or periodicity of activity that is intrinsic to the individual hair follicle itself. More importantly perhaps these cells must send and coordinate inductive signals to the surrounding epithelium and/or mesenchyme. Morphologically, the telogen-to-anagen transition can be viewed as the reconstruction of a hair fiber factory via the addition of significant new "cycling" epithelial tissue to the so-called permanent/noncycling portion of the hair follicle (Figs 1.2.2 and 1.2.3e–h).

The new anagen hair bulb emerges from the so-called secondary germ at the base of the telogen hair follicle. Researchers are particularly interested in dissecting the signals sent by the follicular dermal papilla to the epithelial stem cells located here (or vice versa), which may lead to both the initiation and regulation of the massive proliferation of hair bulb keratinocytes. There is stimulation also of proliferation of ORS keratinocytes and melanocytes. Together this highly proliferative region of the growing hair follicle also exhibits a rare example of immune privilege, which exists during anagen only (Westgate et al. 1991b; Paus 1997; Paus et al. 2005).

1.2.1.5 Molecular mechanisms of hair follicle cycling

As mentioned above, anagen development resembles several of the morphologic changes observed during hair follicle development. Thus, it is not surprising that many soluble growth factors associated with hair follicle morphogenesis have also been detected during anagen development. However, this process is not an exact recapitulation of hair follicle morphogenic events; some factors associated with tissue development during hair follicle morphogenesis (e.g., NT-3 and TGF-β2) can actually induce tissue involution in the cycling hair follicle (Botchkarev and Paus 2003). Levels of key regulatory molecules (e.g., WNT family members, Shh, and BMPs) also fluctuate during the hair growth cycle such that gradients/ratios of these stimulators and inhibitors can drive cell proliferation, differentiation, or involution. While sonic hedgehog is not a requirement for anagen onset (and so is similar in this context to morphogenesis), it is needed for subsequent epithelial cell proliferation to drive anagen hair follicle downgrowth into the dermis (Wang et al. 2000).

It is now known that the follicular dermal papilla is the principal regulator of the hair cycle "clock" (cf. Jahoda and Reynolds 1996). Convincing demonstration of the papilla's critical role was done in early tissue recombination and implantation studies (Oliver 1967). Surprisingly, the follicular dermal papilla appears to exhibit minimal postnatal change, and while there is some debate regarding its intrinsic proliferative capacity (Tobin et al. 2003a, b), it now appears that follicular dermal papilla cell numbers do indeed increase/decrease during normal cycling.

Although dermal papilla cell proliferation and cell death may be rare during the hair cycle, there are significant changes in the amount and nature of associated extracellular matrix (ECM) during the hair cycle. Specifically, ECM is markedly reduced at the end of hair growth; in fact, follicular dermal papilla ECM differs strikingly from that in the dermis (Westgate et al. 1991b) and it is likely that one or more of the papilla-associated proteoglycans may play a role in the control of the hair growth cycle. For example, chondroitin proteoglycan diminishes during catagen and is absent in telogen. It has been suggested that during anagen these ECM molecules may confer on the hair follicle a protective environment for maintenance and growth associated with maintaining immune privilege (Westgate et al. 1991a).

1.2.2 Hair follicle stem cells

The highly regenerative and highly differentiated hair follicle tissue has prompted several researchers to suggest that the hair follicle may be exploited as a repository of primitive cell populations for replacement in other tissues and organs. During catagen the follicular papilla is pulled up toward the "permanent" portion of the hair follicle and particularly to a region called the "bulge"—part of the permanent epithelium at the base of the telogen hair follicle (Figs 1.2.2 and 1.2.3f,g). Despite much recent progress in dissecting the main events driving the continual hair cycling that form the basis of a fairly robust hypothesis, we still are some way from explaining some critical aspects of the hair growth cycle including its intrinsic periodicity, how autonomy continues to reside in single hair follicles, and how cycling persists throughout adult life.

1.2.2.1 Epithelial stem cells

Of the hair cycle hypotheses, the "bulge-activation" hypothesis (Cotsarelis et al. 1990; Sun et al. 1991) is currently favored. This theory supports the view that the mesenchymal–epithelial interaction at the end of telogen involves the stimulation of stem cells in the "bulge" by the papilla fibroblasts. This event is then followed by epithelial stem cell proliferation. The progeny cells are termed "transit amplifying" (TA) cells and function to re-form the lower "temporary" part of the hair follicle in anagen (Cotsarelis et al. 1990). Unlike the stem cell, the TA cell has a limited mitotic potential before undergoing differentiation. The bulge-activation hypothesis also suggests that the loss of proliferative potential by TA cells may be the cue for impending catagen. However, recent studies have shown that catagen induction may originate elsewhere in the epithelium, for example, via the TGF-β family (Soma et al. 2002) in the follicular papilla itself, perhaps via molecules including FGF-5 (Suzuki et al. 1998). Underlining the main focus of this book, most hair follicle pathologies will have their origin in hair follicle cycle dysregulation, and thus some aspects of their pathology may be explained by the bulge-activation hypothesis. A reappraisal of hair follicle stem cells may be advised on the basis of new data showing a population of Lgr5+ actively dividing cells located in the hair follicle bulge and secondary germ that have multipotent stem cells characteristics, i.e., can give rise to new hair follicles, maintain all hair follicle cell lineages, and retain stem cell traits (Jaks et al. 2008).

1.2.2.2 Nonepithelial stem cells

In addition to the epithelium the hair follicle generates neuroectodermal melanocytes, as well as neural, vascular, and muscle components (i.e., arrector pili muscle). Stem cells for melanocytes have also been located in the bulge (Nishimura et al. 2002). It has been shown (at least for mouse) that some of these are recruited to proliferate at early anagen and can also be recruited to empty niches (like damaged epidermis). Moreover, immature cells also located in the bulge can be induced to express neural cell markers (e.g., nestin) and these may even be able to transdifferentiate to Schwann cells among others (Amoh et al. 2005). Epithelial stem cells of the hair follicle may also transdifferentiate into other histologic cell types (e.g., endothelial cells) and some cells associated with the anatomic region of the follicular papilla may transform into hematopoietic cells, adipocytes, or osteoblasts (Jahoda et al. 2003).

1.2.3 Systemic and intrinsic influences on hair growth

While the autonomy of individual hair follicles is frequently emphasized, they are still able to interconnect with multiple systemic regulatory networks of the body. Remarkably, the hair follicle can respond to most hormones known to biomedicine. Even more surprising is its capacity to produce a wide range of hormones via synthesis, conversions, and so on. Prominent examples include sex hormones, proopiomelanocortin (POMC) peptides, corticotropin-releasing factor, and prolactin (cf. Slominski and Wortsman 2000). Neuropeptides, neurotransmitters, and neurohormones are also increasingly been implicated in mediating hair follicle events particularly those that may be stress related (Paus et al. 1997; Arck et al. 2003).

Mass depilation of telogen hairs induces the rapid onset of anagen in these hair follicles. This is an excellent example of the effect of local factors on the regulation of the hair growth cycle, and can be ascribed to numerous causes including the reduction in the level of local growth inhibitors (chalones) (Paus et al. 1990). Further, there is increasing support for the involvement of local autocrine and paracrine factors, particularly cytokines, in the regulation of the hair growth cycle (Moore et al. 1991). Hair growth in mice, for example, is associated with the sequential expression of TGF-β and its receptors during the different phases of the cycle. TGF-βs are not only potent growth inhibitors for most cell types, but also regulate cell differentiation, migration, extracellular matrix production and modulate immune function. Interestingly, the administration of large doses of EGF induces a catagen-like state both in vivo (e.g., in sheep, where it was a failed strategy to provide a less labor-intensive form of wool shearing) and in vitro. By contrast, the addition of insulin growth factor (IGF-I or IGF-II) maintains in vivo anagen growth rates ex vivo, and the hair follicle can be precipitated into a premature catagen in their absence. Thus, the hair follicle represents a potent environmental responder and transducer of biologically relevant information. Perhaps we could have expected this, given the enormous evolutionary selective pressure for furred mammals to maintain an adequate coat at all costs.

1.2.3.1 Sex hormones and hair growth

All but the most casual observer of hair growth will be aware of links with hormones. In some mammals synchronicity of hair growth is observed as lifelong molt waves that are sensitive to environmental stimuli (e.g., photoperiod). It is here that the link between hair growth and endocrine systemic effects is especially clear (Ebling 1990). Hair growth is sensitive to the transduction of environmental signals that occur via the pineal gland. The level of circulating prolactin is another factor important in the regulation of the molting response in mammals. Modulation of the hair molt can also be seen as the result of multiple hormone effects peripherally. In rats, estradiol, testosterone, and adrenal steroids delay anagen onset, while thyroid hormones accelerate hair follicle activity (Safer et al. 2001). However, it is apparent that these hormones have different points of actions, for example, estradiol decreases anagen length, while tyroxine can have the opposite effect.

The nature of the effect of androgens on hair growth in humans is very complex, and is further compounded by their ability to undergo considerable conversions once in the target tissue (Randall et al. 2000). One such conversion that is highly significant for hair growth in man is the metabolism of testosterone to the more potent 5α-dihydro-testosterone by the enzyme 5α-reductase (type II). In the postpubertal human male, a deficiency in this enzyme results in female-distributed hair growth, poor beard growth, and retention of frontal hairline. Androgens can alter (both increase and decrease) hair follicle size and thus hair shaft caliber and pigment level. They also can modulate the hair growth cycle in some cases. This effect can be observed during hair miniaturization in androgenetic alopecia (i.e., "male pattern baldness"). It is likely that androgen-induced effects on hair growth are mediated in part through other growth factors for follicular epithelium (e.g., via IGF-1) in a paracrine fashion.

Pregnancy in humans is associated with a higher percentage of hair follicles in the anagen growth phase and this may be followed by the simultaneous entry postpartum of many hair follicles into telogen. Here, there appears to be a partial synchronization of hair follicle cycling stage due to increased estradiol levels during pregnancy, followed by hair loss possibly due to a reduction in estradiol and thyroxine levels postnatally.

1.2.4 Hair follicle immune privilege

The immune status of the growing hair follicle differs dramatically from the skin immune system in that the epithelium of the proximal anagen hair follicle lacks classical MHC class I (i.e., HLA-A, B, C) antigen expression (Paus et al. 2005). All other nucleated cells express MHC class I, with the rare exceptions of parts of the testis, eye, and brain and fetotrophoblasts. It has been proposed that, like these other sites, the hair follicle may enjoy immune privilege. Immune privilege appears to exist to prevent inappropriate recognition of antigens that may result in the attack of cells presenting these antigens in the context of MHC. This is important in preventing the induction of autoimmunity if immunogenic autoantigens were to be exposed. The proximal ORS, inner root sheath (IRS), and all hair bulb keratinocytes express no detectable MHC class I. Thus, for as long as they exist, the IRS and the hair bulb matrix remain MHC class I negative. By contrast, perifollicular dermal sheath fibroblasts and immune cells are MHC class I positive. The lower hair follicle also produces immunosuppressive peptides derived from POMC including α-melanocyte-stimulating hormone (MSH) and adrenocorticotropic hormone (ACTH) (Paus et al. 1999; Kauser et al. 2004, 2005). Furthermore, the extracellular matrix of the follicular papilla and that encapsulating the hair follicle in the dermal sheath may provide a further protective role to the lower hair follicle (Westgate et al. 1991b). Similar basement membrane matrix barriers surround other tissues with immune privilege.

There is also some evidence that the hair follicle uses a primitive epithelial defense system against bacteria (Paus 1997). Normally, the hair canals contain a resident microflora of nonpathogenic bacteria including *Propionibacterium acnes*, *Staphylococcus aureus*, *S. epidermidis*, *Demodex mites*, and *Malassezia* species. The hair follicle appears to have a very effective anti-infection capacity as can be seen by the comparatively rare occurrence of folliculitis in the skin of nonimmunocompromised individuals.

1.2.5 Aging of the hair follicle

All mammals are born with their full complement of hair follicles, with the notable exception of the minute antler "velvet" hair follicles. The latter are shed with the old antlers and are reborn again with the emergence of new antler buds in the subsequent season (Randall et al. 2003). However, for all mammals there is usually a striking difference, anatomically, between the skin coverage of the neonate and that of the fully grown adult. Thus, the density of hair follicles per unit area of skin is greatly reduced during our journey from neonate to mature adulthood (Giacometti 1965; Van Neste and Tobin 2004). There also appears to be a progressive loss of hair follicles with age, at least for humans. Although a bald human scalp may appear fully denuded, as many of 300 hair follicles/cm^2 can still be found. Alas, these hair follicles produce cosmetically unsatisfactory "vellus" hair fibers rather than robust and pigment "terminal" hairs.

Many animals, including humans, become increasingly telogenic with age. Indeed, telogen, with its non-growing hair shaft retained in situ, may even be the most energy-efficient hair follicle status for mammals as a group. This may appear a reasonable occurrence, given that telogen would be associated with a reduced risk of malignant transformation in hair follicle cells. Furthermore, anagen-associated hair bulb matrix keratinocytes display one of the highest rates of proliferation in the body (faster than many malignant tumors) and are exposed to melanogenesis-related reactive oxygen species generated only during active growth.

1.2.6 Pigmentation of hair

Of all mammalian phenotypic traits, skin and hair color communicate more immediate information to the observer than any other. Mammals display a rich and varied palette of surface color that not only highlights striking superficial variations between the genders and age groups, but also underscores how mammalian species differ from one another. Despite such variation, all hair color is derived from the pigment melanin, synthesized via a phylogenetically ancient biochemical process termed melanogenesis (Wood et al. 1999). Synthesis occurs within melanosomes, i.e., specialized organelles unique to highly dendritic, neural crest-derived cells called melanocytes (Slominski et al. 2004). Study of coat color in mice has contributed hugely to our elucidation of the regulatory factors involved in the continuous pigmentation in the mammalian epidermis and cyclically regulated pigmentation of the hair follicle.

The sheer variety of colors among mammals underscores the value of pigment to the mammal. Hair color provides camouflage (e.g., seasonal coat color change in the arctic hare) and social and sexual communication (e.g., silver-backed gorilla). While humans do not rely on such adaptations for their actual survival, these still play a significant role in our social and sexual communication.

However, the dramatic diversity of hair colors is one of the enduring enigmas of the mammalian phenotype. Molecular geneticists have started to unravel this enigma and have shown that skin and hair pigmentation phenotypes are linked to genetic variations (called polymorphisms) in several genes, most especially the gene encoding the melanocortin-1 receptor (MCR-1). The MCR-1 receptor acts as a "lock" that is activated or engaged via binding a small number of POMC-derived peptides including α-MSH and ACTH. More recently, a new locus (the K locus) has been identified in domestic dogs coding for beta-defensin 103 (CBD103) whose protein product can bind with high affinity to MCR-1 (Candille et al. 2007). This gene regulates pigment-type switching in domestic dogs.

1.2.6.1 Biology of the hair follicle pigmentary unit

While follicular melanocytes are derived from epidermal melanocytes during hair follicle development, these pigment cell subpopulations diverge in many important ways as they distribute to their respective though open distinct compartments. For example, hair bulb melanogenic melanocytes are larger, have longer and more extensive dendrites, contain more developed Golgi and rough endoplasmic reticulum, and produce melanosomes two to four times larger than those in epidermal melanocytes. While melanin degrades almost completely in the differentiating layers of the epidermis, melanin granules (especially eumelanin) transferred into hair cortical keratinocytes remain minimally digested (Tobin and Paus 2001). By far the most striking difference between these two melanocyte subpopulations, and one with significant implications for the regulation of hair pigmentation, is the observation that the activity of the hair bulb melanocyte is tightly coupled to the hair growth cycle (Slominski and Paus 1993). Constitutive melanogenesis in the epidermis, by contrast, appears to be continuous (Nordlund and Ortonne 1998), though this can be further upregulated (i.e., facultative) via a number of stimuli including UV radiation.

Although the murine and human hair follicle pigmentary units are clearly the best characterized, it is likely that a very similar situation exists in other mammalian species (Barsh 2007; Candille et al. 2007; Schmutz and Berryere 2007). Briefly, DOPA-positive melanotic melanocytes occur in three hair follicle locations, namely, the basal layer of the ORS of the infundibulum, the sebaceous gland, and in the hair bulb around the follicular papilla. DOPA-negative and amelanotic hair follicle melanocytes are distributed in the mid-to-lower ORS and also in the peripheral and most proximal hair bulb (Fig. 1.2.4). While DOPA-oxidase activity of tyrosinase may not be detectable in amelanotic hair follicle melanocytes, the protein itself may be detected in some of these cells (Tobin 2004). Moreover, amelanotic melanocytes may express c-Kit and Bcl-2 (Grichnik et al. 1996), though these cells do not tend to express the melanogenesis enzymes such as tyrosinase-related protein-1 (TRP-1) and tyrosinase-related protein-2 (TRP-2, also called dopachrome tautomerase) (Horikawa et al. 1996).

Although several melanocyte subpopulations are located in the hair follicle, the hair bulb is the only site of pigment production for the hair shaft. The melanogenically active melanocytes are restricted to the upper hair matrix of the anagen hair follicle, just below the precortical keratinocyte population (Tobin et al. 1995; Tobin and Bystryn 1996)(Figs 1.2.1–1.2.4). This location correlates with the fact that melanin is transferred during anagen to the hair shaft cortex, less so to the medulla, and very rarely to the hair cuticle in the human follicle. By contrast, melanin is predominant in the medulla of the murine hair follicle, where it forms the majority of the hair fiber's melanin.

In a manner analogous to the epidermal melanin unit of the skin, the melanogenically active melanocytes in the hair bulb form functional units with neighboring immature precortical keratinocytes. The follicular melanin unit resides in the proximal anagen bulb and, in man, consists of approximately one melanocyte to five keratinocytes in the hair bulb as a whole and a 1:1 ratio in the basal layer of the

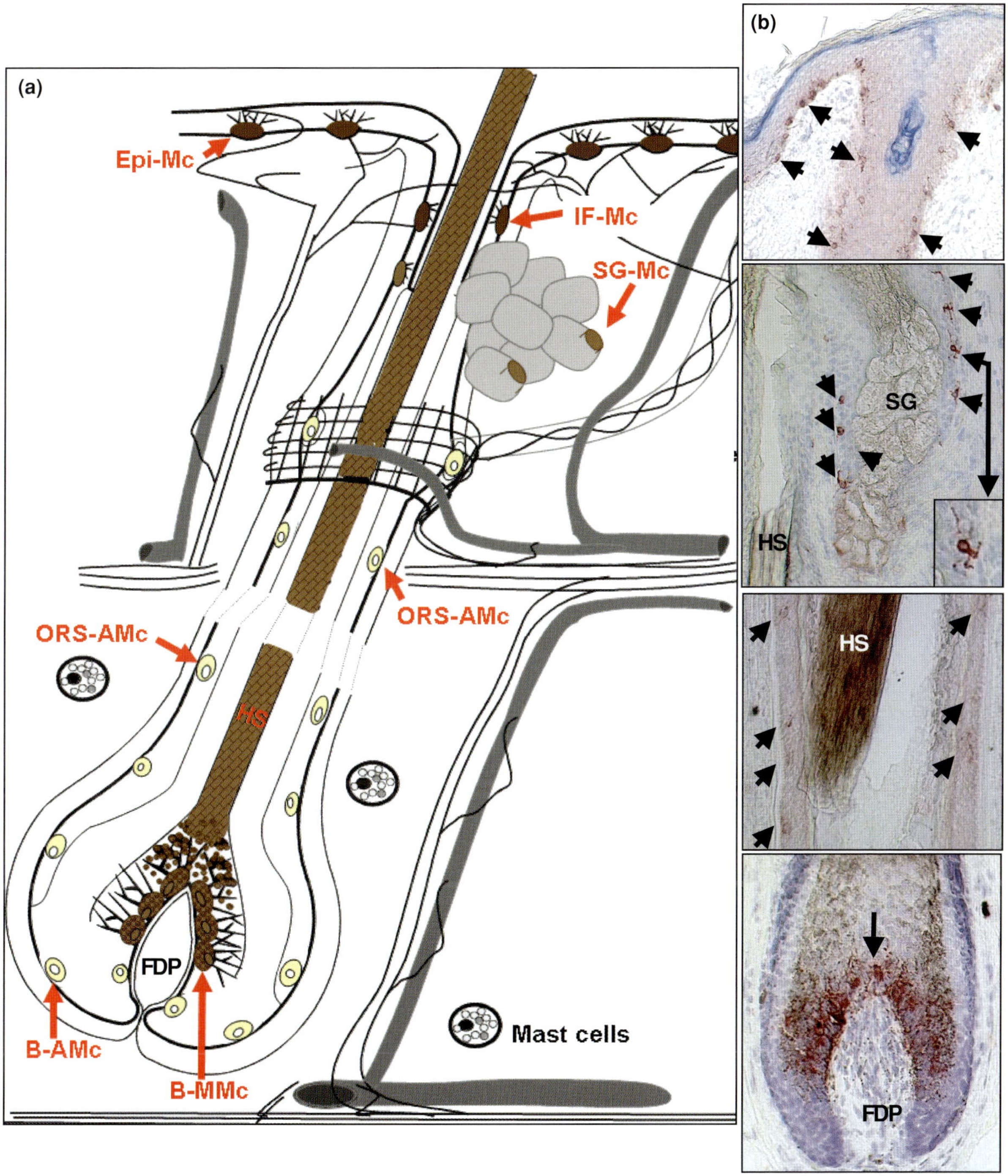

Fig. 1.2.4 Melanocytes in the anagen hair follicle. (a) Cartoon of the distribution of melanocytes in the anagen human hair follicle; (b) immunohistologic localization of melanocytes using an antibody against the melanocyte-lineage marker gp-100 in different regions of the human anagen scalp hair follicle. Epi-Mc, epidermal melanocyte; IF-Mc, infundibular melanocyte; SG, sebaceous gland; ORS-AMc, outer root sheath amelanogenic melanocyte; FDP, follicular dermal papilla; B-MMc, bulbar melanogenic melanocyte; B-AMc, bulbar amelanotic melanocyte; HS, hair shaft. The cartoon also depicts perifollicular blood vessels, nerves and mast cells. (Modified from Tobin (2003).)

hair bulb next to the follicular papilla. Melanogenic bulbar melanocytes interact closely with the follicular papilla via the thin basal lamina that separates them from the mesenchymal follicular papilla (Fig. 1.2.5). By contrast, each human epidermal melanocyte is associated with 36 "viable" keratinocytes in the epidermal melanin unit (Fitzpatrick and Breathnach 1963).

The cytoplasm of melanocytes in the hair bulb commonly contains a high proportion of fully mature, highly melanized (i.e., stage IV) melanosomes, in contrast to epidermal melanocytes that rarely collect significant numbers of mature melanosomes (Fig. 1.2.5b,c). Rather, in the latter these maturing melanosomes are swiftly transferred to surrounding epidermal keratinocytes. Melanocyte dendricity is an important phenotypic regulator of melanin transfer to keratinocytes. Notably, myosin Va (encoded by the "dilute" gene), Rab27a (encoded by the "ashen" gene), and melanophilin (encoded by the "leaden" gene) have all been proposed as molecular motors involved in dendrite outgrowth and melanosome movement in mammalian melanocytes (Wu et al. 1997; Lambert et al. 1999). When mutated they can be associated with dilution of hair color, for example, in Griscelli syndrome in humans (Menasche et al. 2003) or in black hair follicle dysplasia and coat color dilution in dogs (Philipp et al. 2005).

Transfer of melanin granules to cortical and medullary keratinocytes of the growing hair shaft is presumed to involve the same mechanism as that in the epidermis, although its ultimate fate (i.e., degradation) is strikingly different compared to its status in the epidermis. Eumelanin granules transferred into hair cortical keratinocytes remain minimally digested, contrasting with epidermis where melanin is almost completely degraded in the differentiating keratinocytes. A striking phenotypic verification of this differential tissue processing of melanin can be seen in eumelanic Caucasians with raven black hair coexpressed with very fair skin.

An evaluation of the biosynthetic pathway involved in the production of melanins (called melanogenesis) is beyond the scope of this chapter. However, the interested reader is directed to a recent and comprehensive review on the subject (Slominski et al. 2004). Briefly, melanins are the end products of multistep transformations of L-phenylalanine/L-tyrosine. These polymorphous and multifunctional biopolymers include the cutaneous melanins (eumelanin, pheomelanin, and mixed melanins) (Biliska 2001) and neuromelanin (Prota 1995). Despite the broad association of eumelanin with brown/black hair and pheomelanins with red/blonde hair, relatively minor differences in melanin content can have significant effects on the visible hair color. Moreover, melanocytes in the blackest of hair (in Caucasians best characterized by Indian hair fibers) can produce both eumelanins and pheomelanins within the same hair fiber and even within the same melanocyte.

1.2.6.2 Regulation of hair pigmentation

The pigmentation of hair fibers is affected by numerous intrinsic factors including species differences, hair cycle-dependent changes, body distribution, gender differences, variable hormone responsiveness, genetic defects, and age-associated change (Slominski et al. 2004). Study of hair pigmentation may be further complicated by the effects of extrinsic variables including climate and season, infestations, pollutants, toxins, and chemical exposure. Given that melanosome biogenesis and melanogenesis involves multiple steps, it is perhaps not surprising that positive and negative regulators of hair follicle melanogenesis will involve multiple biological factors that can target one or more of these checkpoints in the process. These include growth factors, cytokines, hormones, neuropeptides and neurotransmitters, cyclic nucleotides, nutrients microelements, and cations/anions (Nordlund and Ortonne 1998). These may act via autocrine, paracrine, and endocrine mechanisms (Nordlund and Ortonne 1998; Slominski et al. 2004).

In stark contrast to its primary regulatory role in epidermal pigmentation, UVB radiation does not penetrate to the melanogenic cells of the anagen hair bulb, commonly located deep in the subcutaneous fat layer of the skin. Thus, UV radiation is unlikely to influence the follicular melanin unit, at least directly. Examples of positive regulators of melanogenesis are α-MSH, ACTH, prostaglandin E, and endothelin-1 and -3 (Nordlund and Ortonne 1998; Hearing 1999; Slominski and Wortsman 2000; Slominski et al. 2004). By contrast, negative regulation is provided by melatonin, interleukin-1 and -6, TNF-α, and TGF-β (Swope et al. 1991; Slominski and Pruski 1993; Valverde et al. 1995a,b; Carroll et al. 1997; Martinez-Esparza et al. 1999).

Follicular pigmentation occurs only during the anagen hair growth phase (Figs 1.2.1 and 1.2.6). The

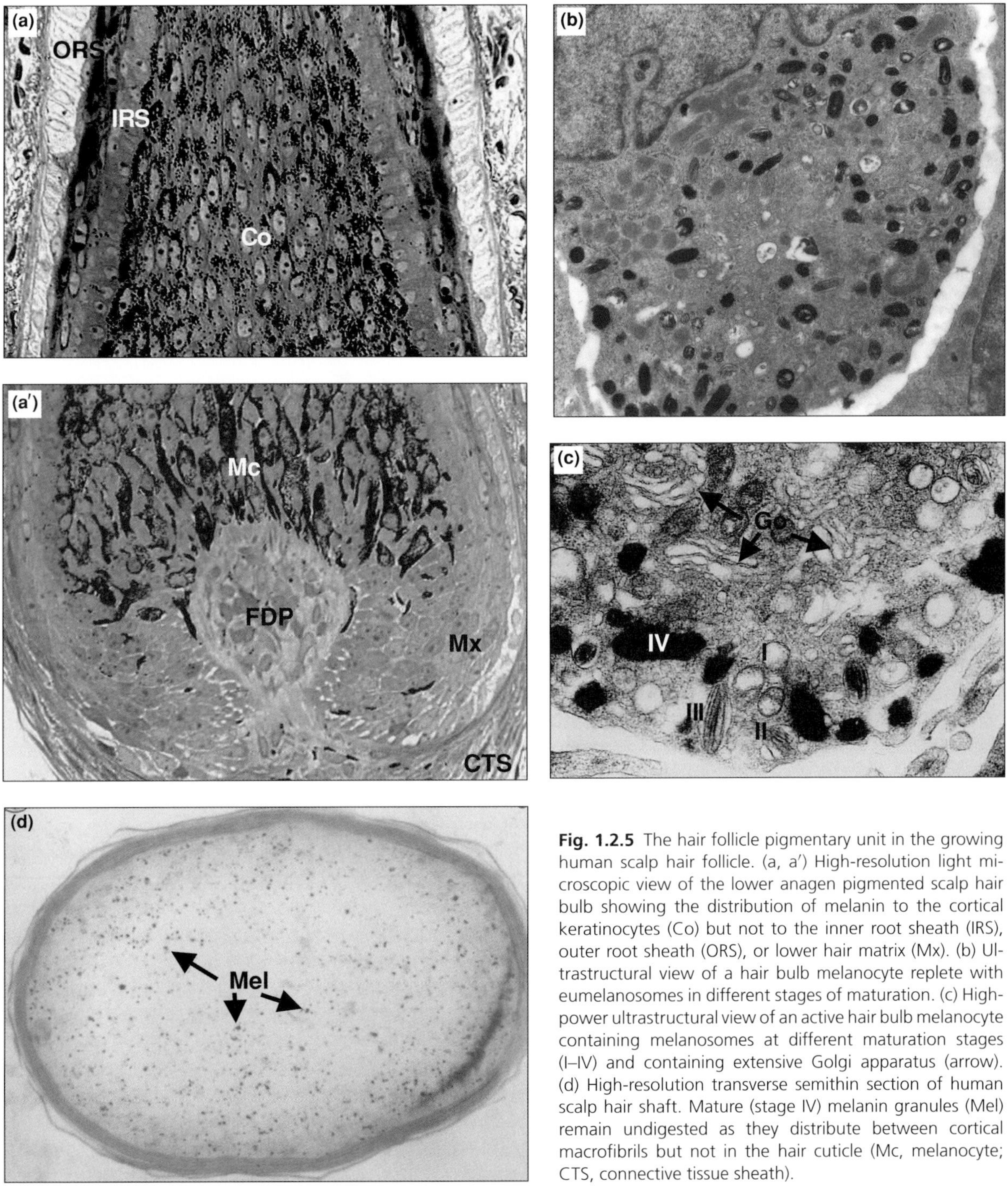

Fig. 1.2.5 The hair follicle pigmentary unit in the growing human scalp hair follicle. (a, a′) High-resolution light microscopic view of the lower anagen pigmented scalp hair bulb showing the distribution of melanin to the cortical keratinocytes (Co) but not to the inner root sheath (IRS), outer root sheath (ORS), or lower hair matrix (Mx). (b) Ultrastructural view of a hair bulb melanocyte replete with eumelanosomes in different stages of maturation. (c) High-power ultrastructural view of an active hair bulb melanocyte containing melanosomes at different maturation stages (I–IV) and containing extensive Golgi apparatus (arrow). (d) High-resolution transverse semithin section of human scalp hair shaft. Mature (stage IV) melanin granules (Mel) remain undigested as they distribute between cortical macrofibrils but not in the hair cuticle (Mc, melanocyte; CTS, connective tissue sheath).

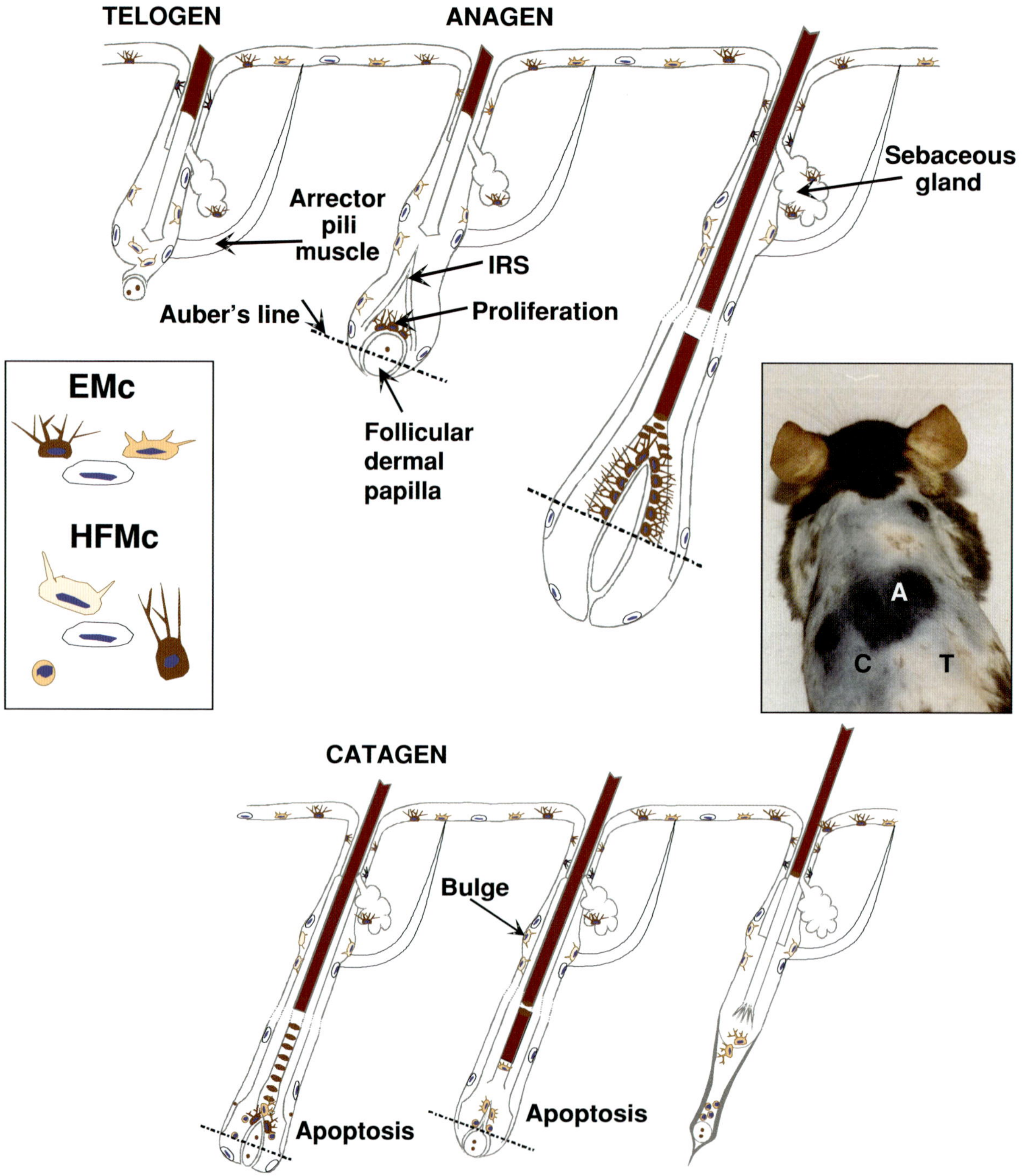

Fig. 1.2.6 Schematic representation of changes in hair bulb melanocyte status during the hair growth cycle. EMc, epidermal melanocyte; HFMc, hair follicle melanocyte. Inset: Dorsum pelage of C57BL/6 mouse at different stages after cycle initiation post depliation. A, anagen characterized by black skin; C, catagen characterized by gray skin; T, telogen skin characterized by pink skin. These color changes reflect relative activity of hair bulb melanocytes in these regions, with full melanogenesis in anagen skin, cessation of active melanogenesis in catagen skin, and telogen skin lacking any melanin. (Modified from Tobin (2008).)

extended anagen phase of human scalp hair, together with its mosaic pattern of hair growth, has hindered a systematic analysis of melanocyte dynamics during the human hair cycle. By contrast, the relatively short growth phase (15–17 days), synchronous hair growth pattern, and restriction of melanogenically active truncal melanocytes to the hair follicles (Reynolds 1954) all make black-haired mice an invaluable tool for hair pigmentation studies (Paus et al. 1990). The junctions of the hair cycle phases exhibit striking changes in the status of the follicular melanin unit (Fig. 1.2.6).

Briefly, the relatively quiescent telogen hair germ contains all cell precursors needed to reconstitute a fully developed anagen VI hair follicle, including the follicular melanin unit (Slominski and Paus 1993). Telogen murine truncal skin does not contain tyrosinase (either mRNA or protein), TRP-1 protein, and melanin (Silver and Chase 1970). During the first one or two days of anagen induction, tyrosinase mRNA and protein become just about detectable and occasional tyrosinase-positive premelanosomes can be detected in amelanotic melanocytes (Slominski et al. 1991). Interestingly, the follicular papilla pools high concentrations of L-phenylalanine (Schallreuter et al. 1998) at this stage, conditions that support the production of high amounts of L-tyrosine. In this way, the anagen-associated stimulation of undifferentiated telogen melanocytes (i.e., melanoblasts) predates the melanogenic stimulus delivered during anagen III. This is followed by active melanogenesis and the subsequent transfer of mature melanosomes into keratinocytes of the precortical matrix.

Melanocytes in the S-phase of the cell cycle have been reported as early as anagen II (Silver and Chase 1970, Sugiyama et al. 1995, Commo and Bernard 2000) and significant proliferation is clearly apparent in anagen III (Jimbow et al. 1975). Mitosis is also observed in melanogenically active cells, indicating that melanocyte differentiation does not in all cases preclude mitotic activity (Tobin et al. 1999). Bulbar melanocytes during the anagen III to anagen VI transition increase in their dendricity, develop more Golgi bodies and rough endoplasmic reticulum, increase the size and number of their melanosomes (Sugiyama and Kukita 1976), and begin to transfer mature melanosomes to precortical keratinocytes.

Even before catagen-associated structural changes are apparent in the hair bulb, the earliest signs of imminent hair follicle regression include the retraction of melanocyte dendrites and the attenuation of melanogenesis during late anagen VI (Sugiyama and Kukita 1976). Limited keratinocyte proliferation continues for a while, leaving the most proximal telogen hair shaft characteristically unpigmented. One can already detect a dramatic and rapid drop in levels of active tyrosinase beginning during late anagen VI itself. The termination of melanogenesis may reflect an induction of melanogenesis inhibitory factors (see below)(Slominski et al. 2004). Alternatively, the low supply of L-tyrosine in the now reducing hair bulb environment inhibits melanogenesis, until an increased production of GTP-cyclohydrolase-1,6-tetrahydrobiopterin and phenylalanine hydroxylase occurs again during telogen in preparation for optimal melanogenesis conditions during the subsequent anagen phase (Schallreuter et al. 1998).

An enduring enigma of both hair follicle and pigment biology concerns the fate of the pigmented hair bulb melanocytes during catagen (Figs 1.2.3a–d and 1.2.6). When follicular melanogenesis is resumed during the next anagen phase, the particularly relevant questions to be answered are, where do formerly melanogenically active melanocytes go during catagen and telogen? and Where do they originate from? Although melanogenically active melanocytes are no longer detectable in the proximal hair follicle during catagen, their “disappearance” is not unannounced and residual melanin generated during anagen can be seen “deposited” in the follicular papilla (cf. Tobin 2004). Our current view suggests that many of the melanocytes in early anagen, previously described as “redifferentiating” by earlier authors, actually correspond to newly recruited immature melanocytes derived from a melanocyte stem reservoir (Grichnik et al. 1996; Tobin et al. 1999) and are not reactivated from preexisting hair bulb melanocytes that were melanogenically active during the previous anagen phase. This is supported by the recent identification of a population of immature TRP-2-positive melanocytes (though these are apparently more mature than true stem melanocytes themselves) in the hair follicle “bulge” region—a site of epithelial stem cells.

It is possible that at least some of the “new generation” of melanogenically active melanocytes derive from a population of catagen-surviving postmelanogenically active cells. Indeed, low numbers of apparently dendritic melanocytes can be detectable in the retreating epithelial strand of catagen hair follicles undergoing active resorption via apoptosis (Commo and Bernard 2000; Tobin 2004). Alternatively, these weakly or nonmelanogenic cells, which lack tyrosinase and TRP-1 expression, may in fact represent the poorly differentiated melanocytes that codistribute with pigmented bulbar melanocytes in anagen hair matrix (Tobin et al. 1995), especially in the most peripheral and proximal matrix. Explaining most, if not all, of the aforementioned observed changes during catagen is perhaps the demonstration that the highly melanotic (presumably terminally differentiated) hair bulb melanocytes do not survive catagen (Tobin et al. 1998, 1999).

Curiously, not all the pigment formed during anagen-associated melanogenesis is actually incorporated into the hair shaft. The "excess" pigment appears to be removed from the hair follicle, though not immediately. Its origin appears to be related to melanocyte degeneration by apoptosis and the resultant pigment-containing apoptotic fragments enter the follicular papilla, epithelial strand, or connective tissue sheath of catagen. Pigment incontinence may also be detected in the epithelial sac of the telogen hair follicle. The precise mechanism of this pigment redistribution is unclear, although it is likely to involve phagocytosis, particularly by macrophages (Paus 1997; Christoph et al. 2000) and Langerhans cells (Tobin 1998), whose numbers increase during hair follicle regression (Paus 1997).

Among positive regulators of follicular melanogenesis are the POMC-derived peptides ACTH, α-MSH, β-MSH, and β-endorphin (Eberle 1988; Slominski and Paus 1993; Cone et al. 1996; Paus et al. 1999; Slominski and Wortsman 2000; Slominski et al. 2000; Kauser et al. 2003, 2004, 2005). A full discussion of the role of POMC peptides in pigmentation is beyond the scope of this chapter. Interested readers can learn more in Slominski et al. (2004). Briefly, these neuropeptides are also produced locally in anagen skin or can be released locally from nerve endings (Furkert et al. 1997; Paus et al. 1999; Mazurkiewicz et al. 2000; Slominski et al. 2000). Murine studies have underpinned much of our current knowledge on the regulation of skin pigmentation by POMC peptides. However, this species lacks functional melanocytes in the truncal epidermis and shows restricted distribution of melanogenic melanocytes to the hair follicle bulb in anagen. Thus, we need to interpret the rodent coat color literature very carefully before extrapolating to other mammals. For example, studies in guinea pigs have shown that α-MSH increased the proportion of black to gray hairs when administered intramuscularly (Snell 1972), while the injection of both α-MSH and a potent synthetic analogue ([Nle^4,D-Phe^7]-α-MSH) into human skin was observed to increase melanogenesis particularly of sun-exposed skin with no effect seen in hair follicles (Levine et al. 1991).

Recently, we have proposed a role for the β-endorphin/μ-opiate receptor system in the regulation of both epidermal and follicular melanocyte biology (Kauser et al. 2003, 2004), suggesting that POMC peptides may also modulate melanocyte biology in a non-MC1R-dependent manner. Moreover, the hormone corticotrophin-releasing factor can also induce phenotypic change in hair follicle melanocytes in vitro by upregulating cell dendricity and pigmentation levels (Kauser et al. 2006), though it is not yet clear if this activity operates via direct or indirect mechanisms.

Agouti signaling protein is likely to be an important negative regulator of nonhuman hair pigmentation. It can act as an antagonist to α-MSH and an inverse agonist at the MC1-R (Barsh 1999; Hearing 1999). Transient synthesis of agouti protein switches eumelanogenesis (brown/black) to pheomelanogenesis (red/yellow) (Silvers 1979), a change that can be associated with decreased tyrosinase activity overall. Moreover, the products of attractin (Atrn) and mahogunin (Mgrn1) may also act as modulators of pigmentation, as they appear to prevent hair follicle melanocytes from responding to the agouti protein (He et al. 2003). This system has so far been described most thoroughly in rodents, though a similar system is also thought to operate in other mammals (Schmutz and Berryere 2007).

Other negative regulators of hair pigmentation include melatonin, glucocorticoids, INF-γ, and dopaminergic and cholinergic agonists (Silvers 1979; Logan and Weatherhead 1980; Burchill and Thody 1986; Carroll et al. 1997; Ermak and Slominski 1997; Barsh 1999). Melatonin, albeit at pharmacological doses, inhibits tyrosinase activity (Slominski et al. 1994, 2008), and anagen epidermis and hair follicles express melatonin-binding sites (Slominski et al. 2003).

1.2.7 The hair fiber

The hair fiber is a truly amazing natural composite with unique physical and chemical properties. The product of millennia of evolutionary selective pressures, the hair fiber exhibits a wide variability in form – the scientific basis for the latter remains broadly enigmatic. Despite its robust nature, the hair shaft is not indestructible and lesions on/in the hair can provide us with a plethora of valuable information as a sensor of the external world we live in etc., and importantly, can be the most apparent diagnostic clue to intrinsic systemic biological disorders and deficiencies. It is the unique growth characteristics of hair that permits such enormous scope for examination, from study of interactions with topical modifications (personal care/cosmetic scientists) to assessment of individuals' medical status (dermatologists, trichologists) in humans to yielding medicolegal (forensic scientists), historical (bio-archeologists) aspects for both human and nonhuman hair as well as in conservation for endangered species (Jones 2001). As in most aspects of hair follicle biology research, we owe much to investigators of hair growth in particular nonhuman mammal systems, and for the hair fiber, the wool literature has been most informative.

The terminal hair shaft, as exemplified by human scalp hair, contains a significant water content (up to 30% by weight) with the remainder consisting of proteins. A hair fiber consists of an outer cuticle ensheathing an inner cortex. All hairs, irrespective of their caliber (i.e., diameter), length, color, or stage of growth within the hair follicle, are constructed of a bulk cortex surrounded by a protective covering of flattened cuticle cells. However, a third component, the medulla, is commonly located in the fiber center, especially of large terminal hair fibers. The relative size of each of these three components differs throughout the mammalian class (Figs 1.2.5d and 1.2.7b,e,f). This variation is, in large part, dependent on their associated requirements for thermoregulation.

Before examining each of these layers in detail, it is perhaps appropriate to review some general terminology used in descriptions of hair fiber morphology. The cylindrical hair fiber exhibits an elliptical transverse sectional shape, the extent of which can vary considerably between different mammals, so much so that hair cross section in specific groups may appear round, oval, or flattened. As a result, hair fibers have a major and minor axis. However, for ease of comparison, an average "equivalent circular diameter" (ECD) may be quoted. In humans, the average Caucasian ECD value for scalp hairs is approximately 70 μm (though it can be up to 180 μm) (cf. Robbins 2002). Specific structural traits can also generate hairs that vary between straight, wavy, and crimped.

In humans, fine hairs commonly average less than 30 μm and tend to be termed "vellus" if less than 1 mm in length, though vellus hairs can be as fine as just 4 μm across. It is important to emphasize that normal coats contain hairs throughout this caliber range. Furthermore, different types of hair fiber can be produced during mammalian life, even for the same hair follicle, as classically observed in this "vellus-to-terminal transformation" of hairs on the face of the postpubertal male and "terminal-to-vellus miniaturization" of hair on the balding human scalp.

1.2.7.1 The hair fiber cuticle

The surface of the hair fiber consists of the hair cuticle, which forms an overlapping cortex-encircling sheath of flattened cells (sometimes also called scales) arranged in a longitudinal–circumferential manner with free ends of the scales oriented in a root-to-tip direction. It should be remembered that the surface of the cuticle is likely to reflect the significant interactions experienced during its "molding" within the hair follicle's second cuticular layer provided by one of the three component layers of the IRS of the hair follicle. Indeed, the hair fiber remains tightly anchored in the skin via reciprocal hair cuticle to IRS cuticle interactions, deep within the growing hair follicle. Hair fibers of each mammal species exhibit their own peculiarities, which facilitate easy identification, and so is important for species conservation and protection issues.

Each cuticle cell is a multilaminated, translucent, and pigment-free structure measuring approximately 0.3–0.5 μm width and 60 μm long (Swift 1997). The cells are slightly overlapping and create a 4° angle with the long axis of the hair fiber (Fig. 1.2.7a). Cuticle cells are at their most intact as the hair fiber emerges from the follicle at the skin surface, and here there may be as many as 10 cuticle cells ensheathing the human terminal scalp hair cortex. However, as one

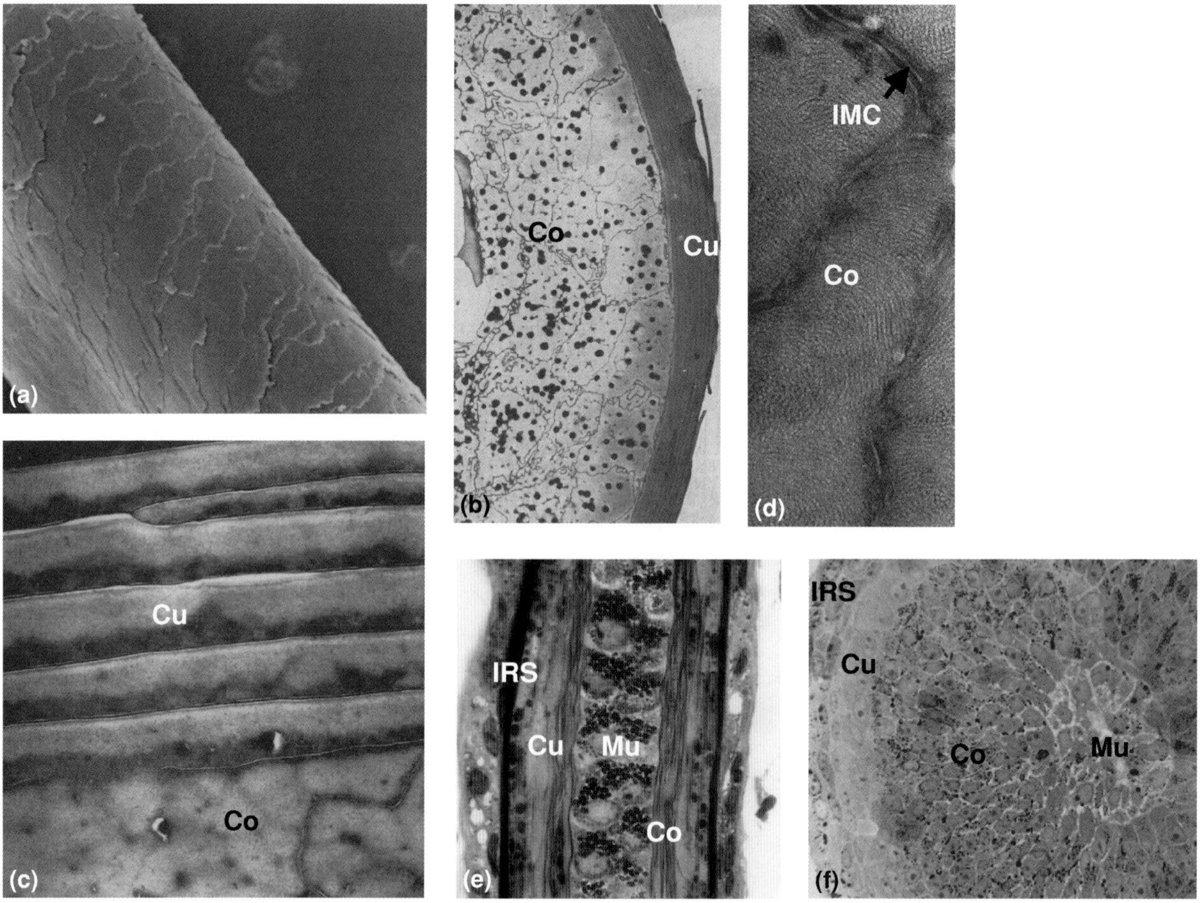

Fig. 1.2.7 Structure of the hair fiber. (a) Scanning electron microscopic view of the surface of a human scalp hair fiber showing the distally oriented and overlapping cuticular scales. (b) Low-power transmission electron microscopic view of a transverse section of a human scalp hair fiber showing the location of the cuticle (Cu) and the cortex (Co) containing numerous melanin granules. (c) High-power transmission electron microscopic view of a transverse section of a human scalp hair fiber showing the detailed structure of the cuticle (Cu) layers; (d) High-power ultrastructure view of the cortical macrofilbrils and the inter-cortical cell membrane complexes (IMC); (e) High-resolution light microscopy view of a longitudinal resin section of a C57BL/6 murine hair follicle showing the relative volume of the medula (Mu) replete with melanin, compared with the narrow cortex (Co). Other visible layers include the cuticular layers (Cu) and the inner root sheath (IRS). (f) High-resolution light microscopy view of a transverse resin section of a human scalp hair follicle showing the low volume of the medula (Mu) compared to the much greater of that of cortex (Co). Other visible layers include the cuticular layers (Cu) and the IRS.

moves distally along the hair fiber, especially on the human scalp, natural wear-and-tear forces reduce this number. Moreover, cuticle quality is further modified by chipping of small fragments at the scale edges. The multilaminated substructure of a cuticle cell can be best appreciated by transmission electron microscopy (Fig. 1.2.7b and c). Individual cuticle cells connect to one another at intercellular membrane complexes (approximately 25 nm across), which contain a trilaminar substructure of a central dense δ-band (approximately 18 nm), sandwiched between two lightly or nonstaining narrower β-bands (Leeder 1986) (Fig. 1.2.7c).

1.2.7.2 The hair fiber cortex

Without the cuticle, the hair fiber cortex would fray and fall apart. The cortex, which forms the bulk of the fiber mass, is composed of elongated (50–100 μm long) spindle-shaped (3–6 μm across) cortical keratinocytes with fine finger-like projections. In human scalp hair fibers, these high sulfur-containing cells are arranged symmetrically (unlike in sheep wool) and contain both fibrillar and nonfibrillar material arranged in a mostly orthocortical pattern (Robbins 2002; Wolfram 2003). The cortex cells next to the cuticle exhibit a more flattened morphology and contain lower levels of sulfur proteins than elsewhere in the cortex. Each cortical cell usually contains recognizable features of its prehardened life, for example, centrally located nuclear remnants and pigment (melanin) granules. In the absence of pigment granules (e.g., in senile white hair) the entire cortex appears translucent with a yellowish tinge—the intrinsic color of keratin. In transverse section, the packing of individual cortical cells can be seen to depend on the presence of intercellular membrane complexes, which appear tortuous due to incorporating the fluted intersections of the cells' finger-like projections. Nonkeratinaceous membrane complexes not only consist of the two cell membranes, but also contain a glue-like material that confers adhesion to the cortical cells.

The repeating structural unit of the hair cortex is the cysteine-rich macrofibril unit (40–200 μm across) that extends the full length of the cell. Hair cortex, where individual macrofibril units are positioned very close to one another (Fig. 1.2.7d), has been termed paracortex, while macrofibril units interspersed with nonkeratin inter-macrofibrillar matrix has been termed orthocortex (cf. Robbins 2002).

Under high-power transmission electron microscopy, individual keratinaceous macrofibrils can be seen to consist of a composite of spirally arranged α-keratin intermediate filaments (α-KIF) (Fig. 1.2.7d). These are 7.5 nm across, form a spiral 40 nm across, and are termed microfibrils and matrix, and consist of KIF-associated protein (KAP), in a ratio generally less than 1.0 (Wolfram 2003).

1.2.7.3 The hair fiber medulla

Hair fibers of a particular diameter contain this nonessential component of the hair fiber. In humans, all scalp hairs, except the most fine or miniaturized, contain a medulla (Fig. 1.2.7f). However, unlike in some nonhuman mammals with very coarse hairs (e.g., horse) this component contributes little to the overall mass of the hair fiber (Fig. 1.2.7e). The medulla may be continuous (especially in fibers of large caliber), discontinuous, or fragmented in finer hairs. The medullary cell is a relatively poorly described, spherical, and mostly hollow cell within the hair shaft core, which becomes highly vacuolated during its formation as a result of progressive dehydration. Both the presence of a medulla and also its degree of vacuolation influence the physical properties of the fiber, particularly with regard to reflection of incident light. In this way, this component can contribute the fiber's sheen and subtle color tone. For animals, the air-trapping characteristic of the medulla provides a degree of insulation to the pelage. During medulla cell formation, distinctive large electron-dense granules can be seen by ultrastructural analysis. These granules contain trichohyalin, a nonfilamentous material that lacks cysteine but contains citrulline residues with isopeptide cross-links of ε-(γ-glutamyl)-lysine, accounting for low solubility of this fiber component (Steinert et al. 2003).

1.2.7.4 Biochemical constituents of the hair fiber

The hair fiber is constructed as a highly integrated system of several components including, in order of decreasing amount, keratins, water, lipids, pigment, and trace elements. The biosynthesis of hair proteins begins in the bulb of the anagen hair follicle and ceases in the keratogeneous zone, approximately 500 μm above the level of the zone of maximal keratinocyte proliferation (so-called sub-Auber's matrix) in human scalp terminal hair follicles. This location will differ of course for hair follicles in other regions of the human body, and also for other mammalian species. Low-sulfur and high-sulfur proteins are synthesized simultaneously, though the synthesis of the latter peaks later. Despite the significant variability in hair form between humans of different ethnicities (e.g., with regard to environment, diet, and hair texture) the chemical composition of hair protein across the human ethnic groups is remarkably uniform (Wolfram 2003). Thus, there are no significant differences in amino acid composition of hair of different ethnicities.

1.2.7.4.1 Hair keratins

The highly complex field of hair or "hard" α-keratins in hair and nail (i.e., claw) has benefited much from recent advances in molecular cloning, yielding unexpected new information about keratin genes and their expression as a function to hair growth and cycling. Hair keratins are the products of several gene families, each with closely related family members and with structural similarities shared across different families. Recently, there have been attempts to simplify the rather confusing nomenclatures for classifying keratins within the KIF gene system and to apply a similar system to the one used in naming keratin-associated proteins (KAPs) (Schweizer et al. 2006). The reader is directed to the following excellent and comprehensive treatments of this topic (Powell and Rogers 1997; Langbein et al. 1999, 2001).

Hair keratins have been grouped into two major classes: (a) low-sulfur, high-molecular-weight α-helical keratins (45–58 kDa) and (b) high-sulfur, low-molecular-weight (10–20 kDa) random-coil keratins. The former, the fibrillar fraction, is termed "α-keratin intermediate filaments" and is embedded in the matrix protein of the latter. Thus, the hair fiber exhibits a very high sulfur content (5% in humans). KIF can be further subgrouped into Type I (acidic) and Type II (basic to neutral) keratins, with nine hair keratin Type I genes and six Type II genes currently recognized. Both gene families exhibit great similarities of physical organization. Type I hair keratin genes can be further subclassified by gene organization and sequence homology into subgroups A, B, C, where A and B are highly related and C keratins are less related. The six Type II genes are also organized into subgroups that are counterparts of subgroups A and C in Type I genes.

Broadly speaking, highly related Type I and II group A genes are all expressed in the cortex of terminal scalp hair, while unrelated Type I and II genes appear to be differentially expressed in hair matrix, cuticle or cortex. Remarkably, some specific keratin gene products are expressed in only singly scattered cortical keratinocytes (e.g., Type I group B keratin hHa8). Recently, an exceptional Type I group B hair keratin (hHa7), previously undetectable in terminal scalp hair, was found to be expressed in sexual hair (Jave-Suarez et al. 2004).

The keratin intermediate filament (8–10 nm across) unit differs from other intermediate filaments in that it is a heterodimeric unit formed as a pair of equimolar amounts of one Type I and one Type II keratin. Furthermore, these units are expressed in a highly tissue-specific and differentiation status-specific manner. Type I hair keratins are acidic and range in size from 392–416 amino acids, with mostly highly conserved N-terminal sequences. Type II hair keratins are basic to neutral and range in size from 479–506 amino acids. Both Type I and II hair keratins have similar levels of cysteine residues.

The "hard" hair keratins (7–8 nm across) can be distinguished from epidermal "soft" keratins by their lack of extended runs of glycine residues; instead "hard" hair keratins contain many cysteine residues (particularly at the N- and C-terminal domains) that enable them to form extensive disulfide bond cross-linking with other cysteine-rich proteins. Due to the presence of nonpolar amino acid residues (e.g., leucine and valine) within a repeating heptad sequence, the filaments take up a coiled-coil conformation whereby right-handed α-helices coil around each other in a left-handed coil to form a rod structure (Jones 2001). A pair of these (heterodimer α-helices) coiled rods align in an anti-parallel manner to form a tetrameric unit—the KIF subunit.

The dynamics of assembly of keratin intermediate filaments in epidermis and in hair fibers are very different. Whereas these can disassemble during mitosis in epidermal keratinocytes, they are the product of nonviable keratin-producing cortical keratinocytes in the keratogeneous zone of the hair follicle.

1.2.7.4.2 Keratin-associated proteins

Keratin-associated proteins (KAPs) are essential for the formation of a rigid and resistant hair shaft because they form extensive disulfide bonds that cross-link with the abundant cysteine residues of the hair keratins. Hair proteins have been fractionated to reveal an increasingly complex group of proteins. Rogers and Powell described eight families of KAPs and classified these on the basis of their amino acid composition as (a) high sulfur (16–30 mol% cysteine), (b) ultra-high sulfur (>30 mol% cysteine), and (c) high glycine/tyrosine proteins (Powell and Rogers 1997). These were described mostly in wool, but also in rabbit fur.

Since then there has been considerable growth in this field with at least 23 KAP families now known (Shimomura et al. 2002). These have been grouped as follows: high sulfur KAPs—family 1–3, 10–16, and 23; ultra-high sulfur—family 4, 5, 9, and 17; and high glycine/tyrosine KAPs—6–8 and 18–22. However, research from the last couple of years has led to even greater complexity, with large clusters of novel human KAP genes now defined (Rogers et al. 2001; Shimomura et al. 2002, 2003).

KIFs and the interfilamentous matrix of the cortex composed of KAPs form a complex group of interactive proteins in the hair cortex and cuticle. As alluded to above (hair) keratins contain many cysteine residues (particularly at the N- and C-terminal domains) that enable them to form extensive disulfide bond cross-linking (both intra-chain and inter-chain) with other cysteine-rich proteins of the matrix. Indeed, some KAP families may contain up to 70 cysteine residues (out of approximately 180 amino acids) that would facilitate many covalent interactions within and between proteins.

Thus, there is a potential for a bewilderingly complex set of interactions given the sheer numbers of proteins involved and their potential for interaction. It is of some relief to note from in situ hybridization studies that genes for different KIFs and KAPs are sequentially activated as a function of hair growth. For example, Type II KIF genes are expressed sequentially in precortical keratinocytes in separate stages. Moreover, expression of hard hair and soft epidermal KIF genes is usually mutually exclusive during hair growth. These observations may suggest a degree of order for sets of preferential protein interactions during hair fiber formation. There is good evidence for linkage between KIFs and the keratinocyte plasma membrane via desmosomes (Smith and Fuchs 1998), suggesting that desmosomes play an important role in hair keratinocyte differentiation.

Unlike the precortical keratinocyte, cuticle cells contain a very different protein composition of mostly cysteine-rich proteins that form cytoplasmic granules. While these cells do contain some KIFs, only very rarely are filamentous structures detectable. Thus, protein–protein interactions here are mostly to permit the formation of lamellar structures—the product of fusion between these granules. This difference is reflective of the cuticle's greater protective function.

The medulla of the hair fiber contains a major arginine-rich multirepeat matrix protein called trichohyalin of 200–220 kDa, seen most dramatically as a differentiation-associated protein in the IRS. Indeed, trichohyalin serves as an excellent marker of hair follicle differentiation as it is expressed earlier than KIF mRNA. However, the formation and functionality of trichohyalin in the IRS and medulla are very different, perhaps reflective of the nonobligatory involvement of the medulla in hair growth. In IRS cells, trichohyalin forms as granules of matrix protein with the role of linking arrays of KIF. These then fuse to form multiple trichohyalin–KIF granules in citrulline-rich lamellar arrays. By contrast, medullary cells synthesize small granules of trichohyalin that later fuse to form large mature medullary granules, though without any apparent involvement of KIFs. The unusual conversion of arginine to citrulline with IRS and medullary cell differentiation is catalyzed, at least in part, by a peptidylarginine deaminase (Rogers et al. 1977).

1.2.7.4.3 Genetic variation in hair fiber proteins

Several mouse mutations have been described that map to KIF or KAP genes (Sundberg 1994). For example, the nude phenotype in mice is due to reduced content of cysteine-rich proteins, resulting in weakened hair fibers. A similar mutation in the winged-helix nude (WHN) gene is associated with a hairless phenotype in humans (Frank et al. 1999). The congenital hair disorder monilethrix is caused by mutations in the hair keratin hHb1 or hHb6 genes (Winter et al. 1997), while copper deficiency in Menkes' syndrome results in kinked hair with defective oxidation of sulfhydryl groups in disulfide bonds (Price 1990). Reduction in sulfur content leads to increased fiber fragility as seen in some trichomalacias (see Chapter 3.2).

Evidence that hair fibers are coated with surface lipids is inferred from data showing that increasing hair fiber diameter is associated with a decrease in total bound fatty acid. Thus, it is now well-appreciated that hair fibers have approximately a 3 nm or greater coating of long chain fatty acids covalently bonded to the protein membrane of the epicuticle. Recent technological advances have allowed exceptionally high observational power views of the surface of the hair fiber surface, and how this is altered by changes in temperature, hydration, pH, lipid layer removers, topically applied cosmetic products, and so on. The main function of the branched methyleicosanoic acid found on the fiber surface "F-layer" is currently unknown, but it may be involved with increasing the degree of hydrophobicity over straight-chain fatty acids and/or altering the frictional quality of the fiber (Wertz and Downing 1989). Small amounts of cholesterol sulfate, cholesterol, and fatty alcohol are also associated with the F-layer, though the nature of bonding (e.g., via thioester linkages) is unclear.

1.2.7.5 Mechanical properties of the hair fiber

What our eyes see when we look at hair or fur is the interplay of several physical characteristics including the hair fiber's geometry/curvature, its color/shade, and its shine/luster. These attributes, however, can be subcategorized further to include fiber diameter, tensile strength, torsion, swelling, and friction (Wolfram 2003).

While the cuticle is most important for protecting the hair fiber, the actual strength and elasticity of the hair fiber is very much derived from the nature of the KIFs and KAPs and their interactions within the hair cortex. Thus, stretching the hair fiber can cause the cuticle, particularly the endocuticle and cell membrane complexes, to split. Although keratin biosynthesis occurs in an aqueous environment within the hair follicle, the process of hydration–dehydration of the hair fiber reveals an anisotropism (nonuniform hardness) when wet. However, despite the relatively high affinity of hair keratin for water and the relative ease of water to permeate the hair fiber, this process is highly selective whereby water molecules are variably excluded from certain molecular structures within the hair. Whereas the matrix material of the hair cortex absorbs water and then softens, the microfibrilar components themselves remain water-impenetrable (Wolfram 2003). Keratin fibers are significantly weakened when wet. The remarkable ability of hair to extend by almost a third is due to the properties of the KIFs rather than reflecting any contribution of the KAPs.

The radial swelling of hair fibers, which occurs when it is wet, results from an uptake of water by the KAP matrix material. Several models have been proposed to explain the remarkable stress–strain curve of hair fibers in terms of either the KIFs alone or KIF–KAP combined (Wolfram 2003). However, matrix proteins do have the effect of excluding water from the intercortical KIF space, so the higher the content of KAPs the stiffer (and less swellable) the fiber is likely to be.

Torsional properties of the hair fiber rely on mechanical properties of hair fiber components that are very different from those for tensile strength. Whereas the matrix material confers little to the tensile strength of the hair fiber, there is a 15-fold corresponding decrease in the torsion or rigidity modulus when the fiber is wet.

There appear to be some important differences in the mechanical properties of different hair fibers. However, little work has been conducted on this subject. There is some evidence that axial twisting of African hair can provide zones of weakness to breaking stresses upon extension. Other interesting differences include the dramatic variation in comb ability stress in African hair. While combing of Caucasian and Asian dry hair induces hair shaft parallelism, this does not occur in curly African hair. Moreover, a surprising reversal occurs when the comb ability/combing stress of wet hair is compared. Here, African hair becomes much more easily combed when wet than does wet hair in Asians and Caucasians. This difference is largely due to the significant configuration change of hair from Asians and Caucasians when wet compared to when dry, whereas little configuration change accompanies the wetting of African hair fibers. Similar considerations are likely to be relevant in mammals with coats of different crimp levels.

1.2.7.6 Hair fiber curvature

It is well known that hair fibers can assume noncircular profiles via twists, curls, crimps, and indentations in all mammalian species. For some mammals seasonality in the level of crimp may be apparent, usually with the summer coat exhibiting less crimp. The presumption here is that the additional volume of air trapped in highly crimped hair acts as a thermal insulator. Despite our familiarity with these phenotypes and our ability to technically induce these forms chemically (in humans), little is known of the actual physical explanations for natural curl and crimp. One possibility is that the IRS may "guide" or "mould" the still malleable hair fiber as it grows through the follicular wall. Any such molding influence is likely to be greatest at the keratogeneous zone of the hair follicle.

In this manner, a curved follicular wall of IRS should cause the emerging and hardening hair fiber to assume the corresponding shape. Perhaps more convincingly, variations in hair curl and crimp may reflect a variable degree of asymmetry in the hair fiber itself. For example, keratinization itself can occur asymmetrically on one side of the fiber causing it to exhibit short and long longitudinal axes. Asymmetrical keratinization could also affect how the hair shaft responds with variable levels of moisture. There is ample evidence from the sheep wool literature for asymmetry in cortical keratinocyte differentiation, such that different types of cells are formed (Jones et al. 1988; Franbourg et al. 2003).

When high-crimp and low-crimp merino wool were compared, cells on one side of the crimp expressed KIFs in a whorled pattern (so-called orthocortex) while cells on the opposite side of the fiber lacked this whorled pattern called paracortex in high-crimp fibers and mesocortex in low-crimp fibers. Furthermore, as hair fiber diameter increases so also does the amount of orthocortex. The above description applies particularly to ovine wool hair fibers. Indeed, this bi-/trilateral structure of hair cortex has been difficult to detect in human hair follicles. However, when Mongolian-type straight hair (consisting of paracortex) was compared with curly Caucasian hair, a small amount of orthocortex was found in the latter. This orthocortex was distributed preferentially at the cuticle–cortex junction (Swift 1997).

In the high-crimp hair of some people of African origin, an asymmetrical arrangement of ortho- and paracortex has been reported. It should be noted, however, that significant curvature of the hair follicle itself could be observed in some of these individuals. In any event it appears that the composition of the intermacrofibrillar matrix will be very important in determining the curve of the hair fiber.

1.2.7.7 Hair fiber abnormalities

Extreme trauma or protracted mechanical stress can result in damage to the normal hair shaft (trichomalacia, see Chapter 3.2), and this cause needs to be distinguished from hair shaft abnormalities due to intrinsic defects, either genetic or nutritional. In humans particularly, the location of the damage along the fiber is also highly relevant, as the "oldest" fractions (i.e., distal sections toward and at the tip) will have been "weathered" by repeated washings, cosmetic treatments, brushings, and other manipulations that cause splitting and cuticular damage. Conversely, these features when observed in short hair lengths suggests the presence of more traumatic damage, an underlying nutritional deficiency, or some intrinsic defect. Another source of structural damage to normal hair can be due to extreme heat stress. Cosmetic practices, for example, those associated with straightening (e.g., of human African hair), may induce the so-called "bubble" hair where extreme heat induces bubble formation under the cuticle within the hair cortex.

In summary, the hair follicle, as one of two mammal-specific traits, is a near-perfect biological universe through which nature provides this class of animals with significant survival advantage. The manner of its development, its lifelong cyclical activity, and its production of a unique biochemical composite material, that is, its fiber, makes the study and care of mammals such a joy and responsibility.

References

Amoh Y, Li L, Katsuoka K, Penman S, Hoffman RM. 2005. Multipotent nestin-positive, keratin-negative hair-follicle bulge stem cells can form neurons. *Proceedings of the National Academy of Sciences of the United States of America* 102(15):5530–5534.

Arck PC, Handjiski B, Peters EM, Peter AS, Hagen E, Fischer A, Klapp BF, Paus R. 2003. Stress inhibits hair growth in mice by induction of premature catagen development and deleterious perifollicular inflammatory events via neuropeptide substance P-dependent pathways. *American Journal of Pathology* 162(3):803–814.

Barsh G. 1999. From Agouti to Pomc—100 years of fat blonde mice. *Nature Medicine* 5(9):984–985.

Barsh GS. 2007. How the dog got its spots. *Nature Genetics* 39(11): 1304–1306.

Biliska B. 2001. On the structure of human hair melanins from an infrared spectroscopy analysis of their interactions with Cu^{2+} ions. *Spectrochimica Acta Part A: Molecular and Biomolecular Spectroscopy* 57(12):2525–2533.

Botchkarev VA, Paus R. 2003. Molecular biology of hair morphogenesis: development and cycling. *Journal of Experimental Zoology Part B: Molecular and Developmental Evolution* 298(1):164–180.

Burchill SA, Thody AJ. 1986. Dopaminergic inhibition of tyrosinase activity in hair follicular melanocytes of the mouse. *Journal of Endocrinology* 111:233–237

Candille SI, Kaelin CB, Cattanach BM, Yu B, Thompson DA, Nix MA, Kerns JA, Schmutz SM, Millhauser GL, Barsh GS. 2007. A beta-defensin mutation causes black coat color in domestic dogs. *Science* 318(5855):1418–1423.

Carroll JM, Crompton T, Seery JP, Watt FM. 1997. Transgenic mice expressing IFN-gamma in the epidermis have eczema, hair hypopigmentation, and hair loss. *Journal of Investigative Dermatology* 108(4):412–422.

Christoph T, Muller-Rover S, Audring H, Tobin DJ, Hermes B, Cotsarelis G, Ruckert R, Paus R. 2000. The human hair follicle immune system: cellular composition and immune privilege. *British Journal Dermatology* 142:862–873.

Chuong C-M. 1998. *Molecular Basis of Epithelial Appendage Morphogenesis*. Austin, Texas: RG Landes.

Commo S, Bernard BA. 2000. Melanocyte subpopulation turnover during the human hair cycle: an immuno-histochemical study. *Pigment Cell Research* 13:253–259.

Cone RD, Lu D, Koppula S, Vage DI, Klungland H, Boston B, Chen W, Orth DN, Pouton C, Kesterson RA. 1996. The melanocortin receptors: agonists, antagonists, and the hormonal control of pigmentation. *Recent Progress in Hormone Research* 51:287–317.

Cotsarelis G, Sun T-T, Lavker RM. 1990. Label-retaining cells reside in the bulge area of pilosebaceous unit: implications for follicular stem cells, hair cycle, and skin carcinogenesis. *Cell* 61: 1329–1337.

Eberle AN. 1988. *The Melanotropins: Chemistry, Physiology and Mechanism of Action*. New York: Karger.

Ebling FJG. 1990. The hormonal control of hair growth. In: Orfanos CE, Happle R (eds), *Hair and Hair Diseases*, pp. 267–299. Berlin: Springer-Verlag.

Ermak G, Slominski A. 1997. Production of POMC, CRH-R1, MC1, and MC2 receptor mRNA and expression of tyrosinase gene in relation to hair cycle and dexamethasone treatment in the C57BL/6 mouse skin. *Journal of Investigative Dermatology* 108(2):160–165.

Fitzpatrick TB, Breathnach AS. 1963. The epidermal melanin unit system. *Dermatologische Wochenschrift* 147:481–489.

Franbourg A, Hallegot P, Baltenneck F, Toutain C, Leroy F. 2003. Current research on ethnic hair. *Journal of the American Academy of Dermatology* 48(6 Suppl):S115–S119

Frank J, Pignata C, Panteleyev AA, Prowse DM, Baden H, Weiner L, Gaetaniello L, Ahmad W, Pozzi N, Cserhalmi-Friedman PB, Aita VM, Uyttendaele H, Gordon D, Ott J, Brissette JL, Christiano AM. 1999. Exposing the human nude phenotype. *Nature* 398(6727):473–474.

Fuchs E, Merrill BJ, Jamora C, DasGupta R. 2001. At the roots of a never-ending cycle. *Developmental Cell* 1(1):13–15.

Furkert J, Klug U, Slominski A, Eichmuller S, Mehlis B, Kertscher U, Paus R. 1997. Identification and measurement of beta-endorphin levels in the skin during induced hair growth in mice. *Biochimica et Biophysica Acta* 1336(2):315–322.

Giacometti L. 1965. The anatomy of the human scalp. In: Montagna W (ed), *Aging*, pp. 97–120. London: Pergamon.

Grichnik JM, Ali WN, Burch JA, Byers JD, Garcia CA, Clark RE, Shea CR. 1996. KIT expression reveals a population of precursor melanocytes in human skin. *Journal of Investigative Dermatology* 106:967–971.

He L, Eldridge AG, Jackson PK, Gunn TM, Barsh GS. 2003. Accessory proteins for melanocortin signaling: attractin and mahogunin. *Annals of the New York Academy of Sciences* 994:288–298.

Hearing VJ. 1999. Biochemical control of melanogenesis and melanosomal organization. *Journal of Investigative Dermatology Symposium Proceedings* 4(1):24–28

Horikawa T, Norris DA, Johnson TW, Zekman T, Dunscomb N, Bennion SD, Jackson RL, Morelli JG. 1996. DOPA-negative melanocytes in the outer root sheath of human hair follicles express premelanosomal antigens but not a melanosomal antigen or the melanosome-associated glycoproteins tyrosinase, TRP-1, and TRP-2. *Journal of Investigative Dermatology* 106:28–35.

Jahoda CA, Reynolds AJ. 1996. Dermal–epidermal interactions. Adult follicle-derived cell populations and hair growth. *Dermatologic Clinics* 4(4):573–583.

Jahoda CA, Whitehouse J, Reynolds AJ, Hole N. 2003. Hair follicle dermal cells differentiate into adipogenic and osteogenic lineages. *Experimental Dermatology* 12(6):849–859.

Jaks V, Barker N, Kasper M, van Es JH, Snippert HJ, Clevers H, Toftgard R. 2008. Lgr5 marks cycling, yet long-lived, hair follicle stem cells. *Nature Genetics* 40(11):1291–1299.

Jave-Suarez LF, Langbein L, Winter H, Praetzel S, Rogers MA, Schweizer JJ. 2004. Androgen regulation of the human hair follicle: the type I hair keratin hHa7 is a direct target gene in trichocytes. *Journal of Investigative Dermatology* 122(3):555–564.

Jimbow K, Roth SI, Fitzpatrick TB, Szabo G. 1975. Mitotic activity in non-neoplastic melanocytes in vivo as determined by histochemical, autoradiographic, and electron microscope studies. *Journal of Cell Biology* 66: 663–670.

Jones LN. 2001. Hair structure anatomy and comparative anatomy. *Clinics in Dermatology* 19:95–103.

Jones LN, Rivett DE, Tucker DJ. 1988. Wool and related mammalian fibers. In: Lewin M, Pearce EM (eds), *Handbook of Fiber Chemistry*, pp. 355-414, New York: Marcel Dekker.

Kauser S, Schallreuter KU, Thody AJ, Gummer C, Tobin DJ. 2003. Regulation of human epidermal melanocyte biology by beta-endorphin. *Journal of Investigative Dermatology* 120(6):1073–1080.

Kauser S, Slominski A, Wei ET, Tobin DJ. 2006. Modulation of the human hair follicle pigmentary unit by corticotropin-releasing hormone and urocortin peptides. *FASEB Journal* 20(7):882–895.

Kauser S, Thody AJ, Schallreuter KU, Gummer CL, Tobin DJ. 2004. Beta-endorphin as a regulator of human hair follicle melanocyte biology. *Journal of Investigative Dermatology* 123(1):184–195.

Kauser S, Thody AJ, Schallreuter KU, Gummer CL, Tobin DJ. 2005. A fully functional proopiomelanocortin/melanocortin-1 receptor system regulates the differentiation of human scalp hair follicle melanocytes. *Endocrinology* 146(2):532–543.

Langbein L, Rogers MA, Winter H, Praetzel S, Beckhaus U, Rackwitz HR, Schweizer J. 1999. The catalog of human hair keratins. I. Expression of the nine type I members in the hair follicle. *Journal of Biological Chemistry* 274(28):19874–19884.

Langbein L, Rogers MA, Winter H, Praetzel S, Schweizer J. 2001. The catalog of human hair keratins. II. Expression of the six type II members in the hair follicle and the combined catalog of human type I and II keratins. *Journal of Biological Chemistry* 276(37):35123–35132.

Lambert J, Vancoillie G, Naeyaert JM. 1999. Molecular motors and their role in pigmentation. *Cellular and Molecular Biology (Noisy-le-Grand, France)* 45(7):905–918.

Leeder JD. 1986. The cell membrane complex and its influence on the wool fibre. *Wool Science Review* 63:3–35.

Levine N, Sheftel SN, Eytan T, Dorr RT, Hadley ME, Weinrach JC, Ertl GA, Toth K, McGee DL, Hruby VJ. 1991. Induction of skin tanning by subcutaneous administration of a potent synthetic melanotropin. *Journal of the American Medical Association* 266:2730–2736.

Lindner G, Botchkarev VA, Botchkareva NV, Ling G, Van Der Veen C, Paus R. 1997. Analysis of apoptosis during hair follicle regression (catagen). *American Journal of Pathology* 151(6):1601–1617.

Logan A, Weatherhead B. 1980. Post-tyrosinase inhibition of melanogenesis by melatonin in hair follicles in vitro. *Journal of Investigative Dermatology* 74(1):47–50.

Martinez-Esparza M, Solano F, Garcia-Borron JC. 1999. Independent regulation of tyrosinase by the hypopigmenting cytokines TGF beta1 and TNF alpha and the melanogenic hormone alpha-MSH in B16 mouse melanocytes. *Cellular and Molecular Biology (Noisy-le-Grand, France)* 45(7):991–1000.

Mazurkiewicz JE, Corliss D, Slominski A. 2000. Spatiotemporal expression, distribution, and processing of POMC and POMC-derived peptides in murine skin. *Journal of Histochemistry and Cytochemistry* 48(7):905–914.

Mecklenburg L, Tobin DJ, Müller-Röver S, Handjiski B, Wendt G, Peters EM, Pohl S, Moll I, Paus R. 2000. Active hair growth (anagen) is associated with angiogenesis. *Journal of Investigative Dermatology* 114(5):909–916.

Menasche G, Ho CH, Sanal O, Feldmann J, Tezcan I, Ersoy F, Houdusse A, Fischer A, de Saint Basile G. 2003. Griscelli syndrome restricted to hypopigmentation results from a melanophilin defect (GS3) or a MYO5A F-exon deletion (GS1). *Journal of Clinical Investigations* 112(3):450–456.

Messenger AG. 1991. Extracellular matrix and the hair growth cycle. *Journal of Investigative Dermatology* 96(5):75S.

Milner Y, Sudnik J, Filippi M, Kizoulis M, Kashgarian M, Stenn K. 2002. Exogen, shedding phase of the hair growth cycle: characterization of a mouse model. *Journal of Investigative Dermatology* 119(3):639–644.

Moore GP, Du Cross DL, Issacs K, Pisansarakit P, Wynn PC. 1991. Hair growth induction: roles of growth factors. *Annals of the New York Academy of Sciences* 642:308–325.

Müller-Röver S, Handjiski B, van der Veen C, Eichmuller S, Foitzik K, McKay IA, Stenn KS, Paus R. 2001. A comprehensive guide for the accurate classification of murine hair follicles in distinct hair cycle stages. *Journal of Investigative Dermatology* 117(1):3–15.

Nishimura EK, Jordan SA, Oshima H, Yoshida H, Osawa M, Moriyama M, Jackson IJ, Barrandon Y, Miyachi Y, Nishikawa

S. 2002. Dominant role of the niche in melanocyte stem-cell fate determination. *Nature* 416(6883):854–860.

Nordlund JJ, Ortonne J-P. 1998. The normal color of human skin. In: Nordlund JJ, Boissy RE, Hearing VJ, King RA, Ortonne J-P (eds), *The Pigmentary System: Physiology and Pathophysiology*, pp. 475–535. New York: Oxford University Press.

Oliver RF. 1967. The experimental induction of whisker growth in the hooded rat by implantation of dermal papillae. *Journal of Embryology and Experimental Morphology* 18:43–51.

Panteleyev AA, Jahoda CA, Christiano AM. 2001. Hair follicle predetermination. *Journal of Cell Science* 114(Pt 19):3419–3431.

Panteleyev AA, Paus R, Christiano AM. 2000. Patterns of hairless (hr) gene expression in mouse hair follicle morphogenesis and cycling. *American Journal of Pathology* 157(4):1071–1079.

Paus R. 1997. Immunology of the hair follicle. In: Bos JD (ed), *Skin Immune System*, pp. 377–398. Boca Raton: CRC Press.

Paus R, Botchkarev VA, Botchkareva NV, Mecklenburg L, Luger T, Slominski A. 1999. The skin POMC system (SPS). Leads and lessons from the hair follicle. *Annals of New York Academy of Sciences* 885:350–363.

Paus R, Cotsarelis G. 1999. Biology of hair follicles. *New England Journal of Medicine* 341(7):491–497.

Paus R, Nickoloff BJ, Ito T. 2005. A "hairy" privilege. *Trends in Immunology* 26(1):32–40.

Paus R, Peters EM, Eichmuller S, Botchkarev VA. 1997. Neural mechanisms of hair growth control. *Journal of Investigative Dermatology Symposium Proceedings* 2(1):61–68.

Paus R, Stenn KS, Link RE. 1990. Telogen skin contains an inhibitor of hair growth. *British Journal of Dermatology* 122(6):777–784.

Peters EM, Botchkarev VA, Botchkareva NV, Tobin DJ, Paus R. 2001. Hair-cycle-associated remodeling of the peptidergic innervation of murine skin, and hair growth modulation by neuropeptides. *Journal of Investigative Dermatology* 116(2):236–245.

Philipp U, Quignon P, Scott A, André C, Breen M, Leeb T. 2005. Chromosomal assignment of the canine melanophilin gene (MLPH): a candidate gene for coat color dilution in Pinschers. *Journal of Heredity* 96(7):774–776.

Philpott M, Paus R. 1998. Principles of hair follicle morphogenesis. In: Chuong C-M (ed), *Molecular Basis of Epithelial Appendage Morphogenesis*, pp. 75–110. Austin, Texas: RG Landes.

Powell BC, Rogers GE. 1997. The role of keratin proteins and their genes in the growth, structure and properties of hair. In: Jolles P, Zahn H, Hocker H (eds), *Formation and Structure of Human Hair*, pp. 59–149. Basel: Birkhauser Verlag.

Price VH. 1990. Structural abnormalities of the hair shaft. In: Orfanos CE, Happle R (eds), *Hair and Hair Disease*, pp. 363–423. New York: Springer-Verlag.

Prota G. 1995. The chemistry of melanins and melanogenesis. *Fortschritte der Chemie Organischer Naturstoffe* 64:93–148.

Randall VA, Hibberts NA, Thornton MJ, Hamada K, Merrick AE, Kato S, Jenner TJ, De Oliveira I, Messenger AG. 2000. The hair follicle: a paradoxical androgen target organ. *Hormone Research* 54:243–250.

Randall VA, Sundberg JP, Philpott MP. 2003. Animal and in vitro models for the study of hair follicles. *Journal of Investigative Dermatology Symposium Proceedings* 8(1):39–45.

Reynolds J. 1954. The epidermal melanocytes of mice. *Journal of Anatomy* 88:45–58.

Robbins CR. 2002. Morphological and macromolecular structure. In: Robbins CR (ed), *Chemical and Physical Behavior of Human Hair*, pp. 1–58. New York: Springer.

Rogers GE, Harding HW, Llewellyn-Smith IJ. 1977. The origin of citrulline-containing proteins in the hair follicle and the chemical nature of trichohyalin, an intracellular precursor. *Biochimica et Biophysica Acta* 495(1):159–175.

Rogers MA, Langbein L, Winter H, Ehmann C, Praetzel S, Korn B, Schweizer J. 2001. Characterization of a cluster of human high/ultrahigh sulfur keratin-associated protein genes embedded in the type I keratin gene domain on chromosome 17q12–21. *Journal of Biological Chemistry* 276(22):19440–19451.

Safer JD, Fraser LM, Ray S, Holick MF. 2001. Topical triiodothyronine stimulates epidermal proliferation, dermal thickening, and hair growth in mice and rats. *Thyroid* 11(8):717–724.

Schallreuter KU, Beazley WD, Hibberts NA, Tobin DJ, Paus R, Wood JM. 1998. Pterins in human hair follicle cells and in the synchronized murine hair cycle. *Journal of Investigative Dermatology* 111(4):545–550.

Schmutz SM, Berryere TG. 2007. Genes affecting coat colour and pattern in domestic dogs: a review. *Animal Genetics* 38(6):539–549.

Schweizer J, Bowden PE, Coulombe PA, Langbein L, Lane EB, Magin TM, Maltais L, Omary MB, Parry DA, Rogers MA, Wright MW. 2006. New consensus nomenclature for mammalian keratins. *Journal of Cell Biology* 17;174(2):169–174.

Shimomura Y, Aoki N, Rogers MA, Langbein L, Schweizer J, Ito M. 2003. Characterization of human keratin-associated protein 1 family members. *Journal of Investigative Dermatology Symposium Proceedings* 8:96–99.

Shimomura Y, Aoki N, Schweizer J, Langbein L, Rogers MA, Winter H, Ito M. 2002. Polymorphisms in the human high sulfur hair keratin-associated protein 1, KAP1, gene family. *Journal of Biological Chemistry* 277:45493–45501.

Silver AF, Chase HB. 1970. DNA synthesis in the adult hair germ during dormancy (telogen) and activation (early anagen). *Developmental Biology* 21:440–451.

Silvers WK. 1979. *The Coat Colors of Mice: A Model for Mammalian Gene Action and Interaction*. New York: Springer.

Slominski A, Chassalevris N, Mazurkiewicz J, Maurer M, Paus R. 1994. Murine skin as a target for melatonin bioregulation. *Experimental Dermatology* 3(1):45–50.

Slominski A, Paus R. 1993. Melanogenesis is coupled to murine anagen: toward new concepts for the role of melanocytes and the regulation of melanogenesis in hair growth. *Journal of Investigative Dermatology* 101(1 Suppl):90S-97S.

Slominski A, Paus R, Constantino R. 1991. Differential expression and activity of melanogenesis-related proteins during induced hair growth in mice. *Journal of Investigative Dermatology* 96:172–179.

Slominski A, Pisarchik A, Zbytek B, Tobin DJ, Kauser S, Wortsman J. 2003. Functional activity of serotoninergic and melatoninergic systems expressed in the skin. *Journal of Cellular Physiology* 196(1):144–153.

Slominski A, Pruski D. 1993. Melatonin inhibits proliferation and melanogenesis in rodent melanoma cells. *Experimental Cell Research* 206(2):189–194.

Slominski A, Tobin DJ, Shibahara S, Wortsman J. 2004. Melanin pigmentation in mammalian skin and its hormonal regulation. *Physiological Reviews* 84(4):1155–1228.

Slominski A, Tobin DJ, Zmijewski MA, Wortsman J, Paus R. 2008. Melatonin in the skin: synthesis, metabolism and functions. *Trends in Endocrinology and Metabolism* 19(1):17–24.

Slominski A, Wortsman J. 2000. Neuroendocrinology of the skin. *Endocrine Reviews* 21(5):457–487.

Slominski A, Wortsman J, Luger T, Paus R, Solomon S. 2000. Corticotropin releasing hormone and proopiomelanocortin involvement in the cutaneous response to stress. *Physiological Reviews* 80(3):979–1020.

Smith EA, Fuchs E. 1998. Defining the interactions between intermediate filaments and desmosomes. *Journal of Cell Biology* 141(5):1229–1241.

Snell RS. 1972. Hormonal control of hair color. In: Riley V (ed), *Pigmentation: Its Genesis and Biologic Control*, pp. 193–210. New York: Meredith.

Soma T, Tsuji Y, Hibino T. 2002. Involvement of transforming growth factor-beta2 in catagen induction during the human hair cycle. *Journal of Investigative Dermatology* 118(6):993–997.

Steinert PM, Parry DA, Marekov LN. 2003. Trichohyalin mechanically strengthens the hair follicle: multiple cross-bridging roles in the inner root shealth. *Journal of Biological Chemistry* 278(42):41409–41419.

Stenn KS, Paus R. 2001. Controls of hair follicle cycling. *Physiological Reviews* 81(1):449–494.

Sugiyama S, Kukita A. 1976. Melanocyte reservoir in the hair follicles during the hair growth cycle: an electron microscopic study. In: Hori Y, Morikawa F (eds), *Biology and Disease of the Hair*, pp. 81–92. Tokyo: University of Tokyo Press.

Sugiyama S, Saga K, Morimoto Y, Takahashi M. 1995. Proliferating activity of the hair follicular melanocytes at the early and anagen III stages in the hair growth cycle: detection by immunocytochemistry for bromodeoxyuridine combined with DOPA reaction cytochemistry. *Journal of Dermatology* 22:396–402.

Sun TT, Cotsarelis G, Lavker RM. 1991. Hair follicular stem cells: the bulge-activation hypothesis. *Journal of Investigative Dermatology* 96(5):77S-78S.

Sundberg JP. 1994. The nude (*nu*) and streaker (nu^{str}) mutations, chromosome 11. In: Sundberg JP (ed), *Handbook of Mouse Mutations with Skin and Hair Abnormalities: Animal Models and Biomedical Tools*, pp. 379–391. Boca Raton: CRC Press.

Suzuki S, Kato T, Takimoto H, Masui S, Oshima H, Ozawa K, Suzuki S, Imamura T. 1998. Localization of rat FGF-5 protein in skin macrophage-like cells and FGF-5S protein in hair follicle: possible involvement of two Fgf-5 gene products in hair growth cycle regulation. *Journal of Investigative Dermatology* 111:963–972.

Swift JA. 1997. Morphology and histochemistry of human hair. In: Jolles P, Zahn H, Hocker H (eds), *Formation and Structure of Human Hair*, pp. 149–177. Basel: Birkhauser Verlag.

Swope VB, Abdel-Malek Z, Kassem LM, Nordlund JJ. 1991. Interleukins 1 alpha and 6 and tumor necrosis factor-alpha are paracrine inhibitors of human melanocyte proliferation and melanogenesis. *Journal of Investigative Dermatology* 96(2): 180–185.

Tobin DJ. 1998. A possible role for Langerhans cells in the removal of melanin from early catagen hair follicles. *British Journal of Dermatology* 138:795–798.

Tobin DJ. 2003. The aging hair follicle pigmentary unit. In: Van Neste (ed), *Hair Science and Technology*, pp. 155–168. Tournai, Belgium: Skinterface srl.

Tobin DJ. 2004. Biology of hair pigmentation. In: Forslind B, Lindberg M (eds), *Skin, Hair, and Nails—Structure and Function*, pp. 319–365. New York: Marcel Dekker.

Tobin DJ. 2005. Pigmentation of human hair. In: Tobin DJ (ed), *Hair in Toxicology: An Important Biomonitor*, pp. 57–88. Cambridge: The Royal Society of Chemistry.

Tobin DJ. 2008. Human hair pigmentation-biological aspects. *International Journal of Cosmetic Science.* 30(4):233–257.

Tobin DJ, Bystryn JC. 1996. Different populations of melanocytes are present in hair follicles and epidermis. *Pigment Cell Research* 9:304–310.

Tobin DJ, Colen SR, Bystryn JC. 1995. Isolation and long-term culture of human hair-follicle melanocytes. *Journal of Investigative Dermatology* 104:86–89.

Tobin DJ, Foitzik K, Reinheckel T, Mecklenburg L, Botchkarev VA, Peters C, Paus R. 2002. The lysosomal protease cathepsin L is an important regulator of keratinocyte and melanocyte differentiation during hair follicle morphogenesis and cycling. *American Journal of Pathology* 160(5):1807–1821.

Tobin DJ, Gunin A, Magerl M, Handijski B, Paus R. 2003a. Plasticity and cytokinetic dynamics of the hair follicle mesenchyme: implications for hair growth control. *Journal of Investigative Dermatology* 120(6):895–904.

Tobin DJ, Gunin A, Magerl M, Paus R. 2003b. Plasticity and cytokinetic dynamics of the hair follicle mesenchyme during the hair growth cycle: implications for growth control and hair follicle transformations. *Journal of Investigative Dermatology Symposium Proceedings* 8(1):80–86.

Tobin DJ, Hagen E, Botchkarev VA, Paus R. 1998. Do hair bulb melanocytes undergo apoptosis during hair follicle regression (catagen)? *Journal of Investigative Dermatology* 111(6):941–947.

Tobin DJ, Paus R. 2001. Graying: gerontobiology of the hair follicle pigmentary unit. *Experimental Gerontology* 36:29–54.

Tobin DJ, Slominski A, Botchkarev V, Paus R. 1999. The fate of hair follicle melanocytes during the hair growth cycle. *Journal of Investigative Dermatology Symposium Proceedings* 4(3):323–332.

Valverde P, Benedito E, Solano F, Oaknin S, Lozano JA, Garcia-Borron JC. 1995a. Melatonin antagonizes alpha-melanocyte-stimulating hormone enhancement of melanogenesis in mouse melanoma cells by blocking the hormone-induced accumulation of the c locus tyrosinase. *European Journal of Biochemistry* 232(1):257–263.

Valverde P, Healy E, Jackson I, Rees JL, Thody AJ. 1995b. Variants of the melanocyte-stimulating hormone receptor gene are associated with red hair and fair skin in humans. *Nature Genetics* 11:328–330.

Van Neste D, Tobin DJ. 2004. Hair cycle and hair pigmentation: dynamic interactions and changes associated with aging. *Micron* 35(3):193–200.

Wang LC, Liu ZY, Gambardella L, Delacour A, Shapiro R, Yang J, Sizing I, Rayhorn P, Garber EA, Benjamin CD, Williams KP, Taylor FR, Barrandon Y, Ling L, Burkly LC. 2000. Conditional disruption of hedgehog signaling pathway defines its critical role in hair development and regeneration. *Journal of Investigative Dermatology* 114(5):901–908.

Wertz PW, Downing DT. 1989. Integral lipids of mammalian hair. *Comparative Biochemistry and Physiology. Part B: Comparative Biochemistry* 92(4):759–761.

Westgate GE, Craggs RI, Gibson WT. 1991a. Immune privilege in hair growth. *Journal of Investigative Dermatology* 97:417–420.

Westgate GE, Messenger AG, Watson LP, Gibson WT. 1991b. Distribution of proteoglycans during the hair growth cycle in human skin. *Journal of Investigative Dermatology* 96:191–195.

Winter H, Rogers MA, Langbein L, Stevens HP, Leigh IM, Labreze C, Roul S, Taieb A, Krieg T, Schweizer J. 1997. Mutations in the hair cortex keratin hHb6 cause the inherited hair disease monilethrix. *Nature Genetics* 16:372.

Wolfram LJ. 2003. Human hair: a unique physicochemical composite. *Journal of American Academy of Dermatology* 48(6 Suppl):S106–S114.

Wood JM, Jimbow K, Boissy RE, Slominski A, Plonka, PM, Slawinski J, Wortsman J, Tosk J. 1999. What's the use of generating melanin? *Experimental Dermatology* 8:153–164.

Wu X, Bowers B, Wei Q, Kocher B, Hammer JA. 1997. Myosin V associates with melanosomes in mouse melanocytes: evidence that myosin V is an organelle motor. *Journal of Cell Science* 110(Pt 7): 847–859.

1.3 Hair follicles in domesticated mammals with comparison to laboratory animals and humans

Wilfried Meyer

The biology of the hair follicle has been extensively studied in humans, laboratory animals, and fine wool-producing sheep. However, information from a comparative point of view regarding all important groups of domesticated mammals is still rather scarce. Nevertheless, the wool hair follicle of sheep (for the correct definition of a "wool hair follicle" see Section 1.3.1.1) has become a particularly unique model for hair follicle research. This includes studies on the molecular controls involved in the development of epithelial–mesenchymal appendages, photoperiodic influences on these interacting systems, the origin of wool fiber curliness, the origin of hair growth wave patterns, and the effect of alterations in nutrient supply on epithelial growth and wool fiber structure.

1.3.1 General principles of hair follicle anatomy and physiology

The hair follicle is a very complex biological unit and shows the same basic structure and function in all recent groups of mammals, including rather primitive ones such as the egg-laying monotremes or the marsupials and the placental mammals (Figs 1.3.1 and 1.3.2). Depending on hair type and body region, hair follicles are more or less deeply, and with different angles, located in the skin. In most parts of the haired skin, the angle of insertion is rather large (i.e., steep), but in specific body areas it is very low (i.e., flat). In this way, the hair follicles are not only very effectively anchored within the dermis, but can also completely penetrate the latter, if necessary, for close contact to the energy supplying fat cells of the hypodermis. In all mammals, the hair follicle is covered along its total length by two epithelial root sheaths and one outer sheath of connective tissue. It is linked to the dermal connective tissue by a dense network of elastic fibers within a mesh of loosely or tightly interwoven collagen fiber bundles (Chapman 1979; Meyer 2009).

1.3.1.1 The different types of hair follicles

According to their fetal developmental course and in view of the fact that they are equipped with specific glands, three types of hair follicles can be clearly determined: central primary hair follicles which emerge first during ontogenesis, and subsequently appearing lateral primary hair follicles. Both primary hair follicles produce heavy and light guard hairs, respectively. Only these two primary hair follicle types are equipped, besides sebaceous glands, with an apocrine tubular gland, and are covered by an extensive network of blood capillaries and nerve fibers. The last follicle type during the ontogenetic time course, the secondary hair follicle that produces wool hairs, shows sebaceous glands only but no apocrine tubular gland. In addition, secondary follicles have a rather thin inner root sheath (Fig. 1.3.3). In small mammals, wool hair follicles are arranged in dense groups, whereas in large mammals, they appear as single follicles between primary follicles.

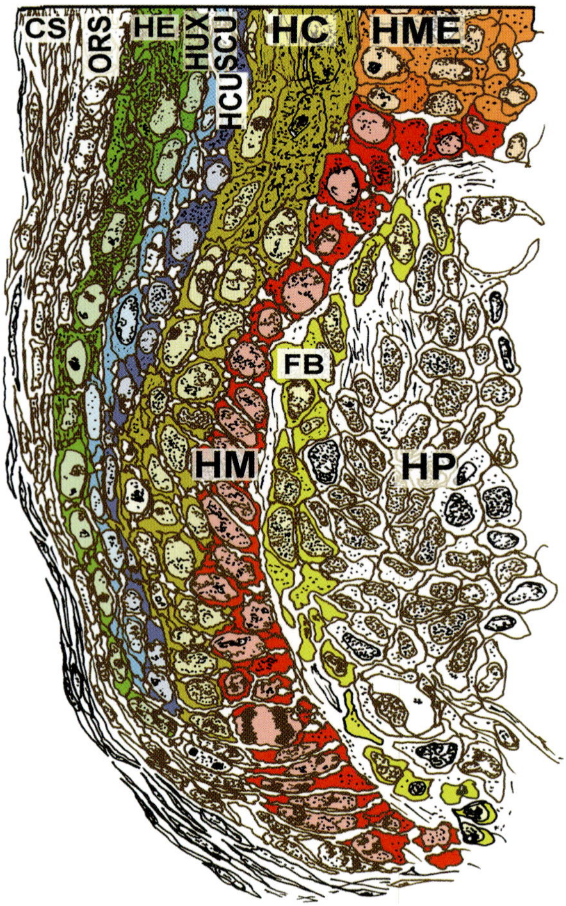

Fig. 1.3.1 Histological organization of the hair bulb. Semischematic drawing from a longitudinal semithin section. CS, connective tissue sheath; ORS, outer root sheath; HE, Henley's layer; HUX, Huxley's layer; SCU, sheath cuticle; HCU, hair cuticle; HC, hair cortex; HME, hair medulla; HM, hair matrix; FB, fibroblasts; HP, hair papilla (W. Meyer).

All primary hair follicles exhibit relatively thick bulbs (diameters: 150–600 μm), whereas secondary hair follicles show smaller bulbs (diameters: 70–200 μm). Moreover, each primary hair follicle has a strong arrector pili muscle composed of smooth muscle cells (the muscle thickness varies according to the size of the hair follicle thickness and is in the range of 10–140 μm). On one side, these muscles connect to the basement membrane of the epidermis by a bundle of fine elastic fibers, and on the other side they are linked to the hair follicle to which they are attached elastically below the sebaceous gland. The arrector pili muscle specifically functions to erect the primary hair follicles with their guard hairs. Indirectly, wool hairs surrounding the guard hairs are also erected. In this way, the insulation of the hair coat is optimized by producing and maintaining an air-containing layer. The connective tissue sheath of the hair follicle is typically composed of thin collagen fiber bundles and a dense and fine elastic fiber net that anchors the hair follicles in a movable system, as clearly visible in thin dermis types of densely haired species and likewise in thick skin of sparsely haired mammals such as the horse (Fig. 1.3.4a–c). This allows the hair follicle to passively regain its former position in the dermis after erection by activity of the arrector pili muscle (Meyer and Neurand 1987; Meyer et al. 1994). Embedded in the connective tissue sheath is a network of cholinergic and adrenergic nerve fibers and free nerve endings and also is a network composed of capillaries supplied by relatively large blood vessels. The capillary network is very distinct in both small (e.g., cat) and large hair follicles (e.g., pig) (Fig. 1.3.5) (Meyer et al. 2008a).

1.3.1.2 The pattern of hair follicle arrangement

The hair-producing unit and the accessory glands (sebaceous glands and apocrine tubular glands) form the hair follicle complex (Fig. 1.3.6a), also known in humans as the pilosebaceous unit. In the latter case, however, the hair follicle complex only shows sebaceous glands, whereas eccrine tubular glands are present that develop independent of the hair follicle.

The primary hair follicles are arranged in groups of three, whereby the central primary hair follicle represents the center and the two lateral primary hair follicles are situated on each side of the group (Fig. 1.3.6b). This group formation is a phylogenetically old characteristic of the mammalian integument, and is still present in most domesticated species. The group arrangement is completed by varying numbers of secondary (wool) hair follicles, particularly in densely haired species such as rodents, cats, or sheep.

1.3.1.3 Hair follicle cycling

One of the most important features of hair follicle biology is the fact that this unique, highly regenerative mammalian skin structure undergoes lifelong cycles of rapid growth (anagen), short regression

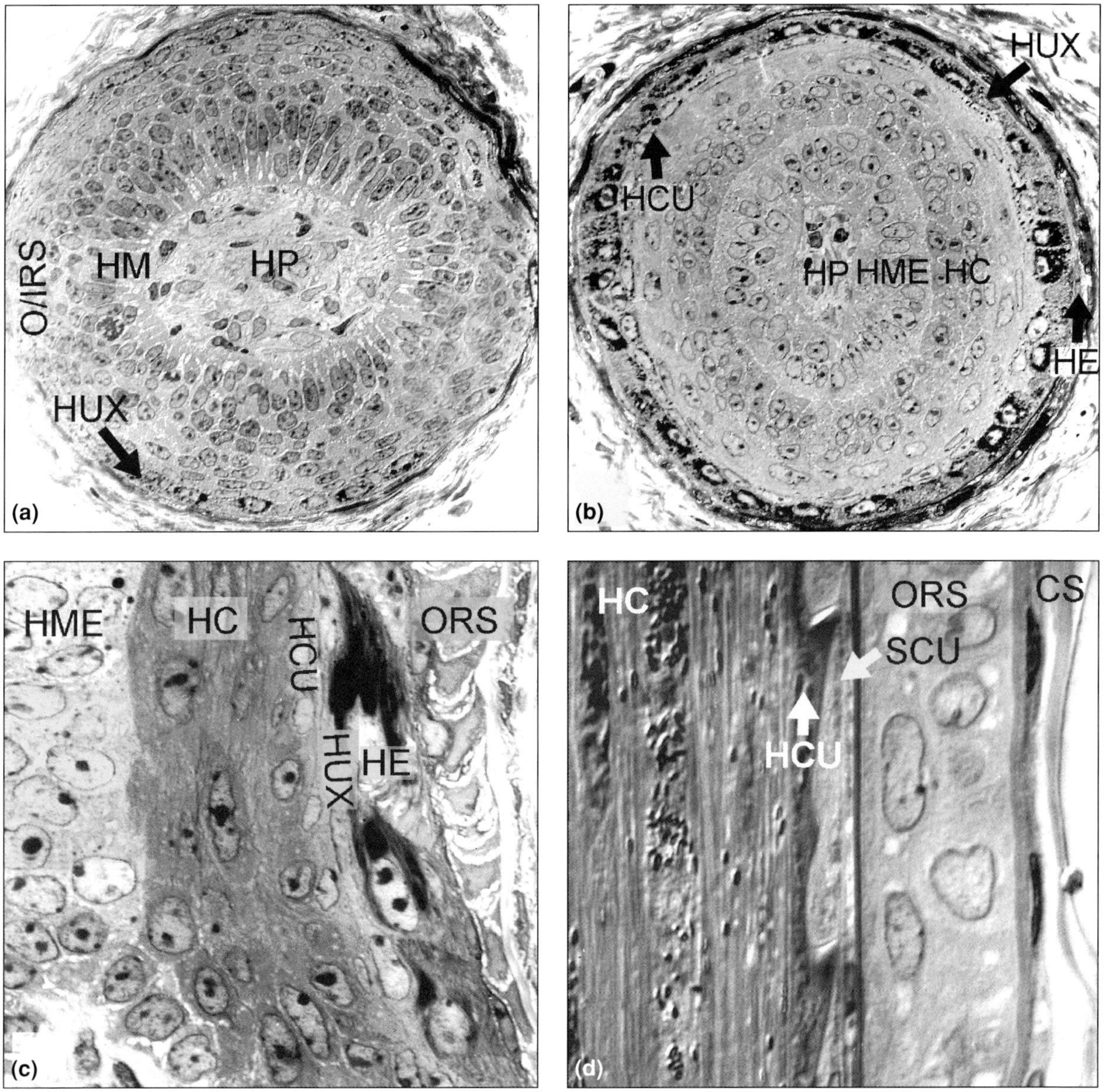

Fig. 1.3.2 Basic histology of the primary hair follicle. (a) Lower bulb region, goat, transverse semithin section, ×500; (b) upper bulb region, goat, transverse semithin section, ×500; (c) upper bulb region, goat, longitudinal semithin section, ×1,000; (d) wall of bulge region, goat, longitudinal semithin section, ×1,400; (*Continues*)

(catagen), and long resting periods (telogen). This is known as the "hair growth cycle" (see Section 1.2.1). These typical structural transformations of the lower third of the hair follicle are recognizable in both primary and secondary follicle types (Fig. 1.3.7). They are controlled by changes in the local signaling milieu, in particular regarding the natural light environment (day length), based on changes in expression and activity of a high number of substances such as cytokines, hormones, neurotransmitters, and their

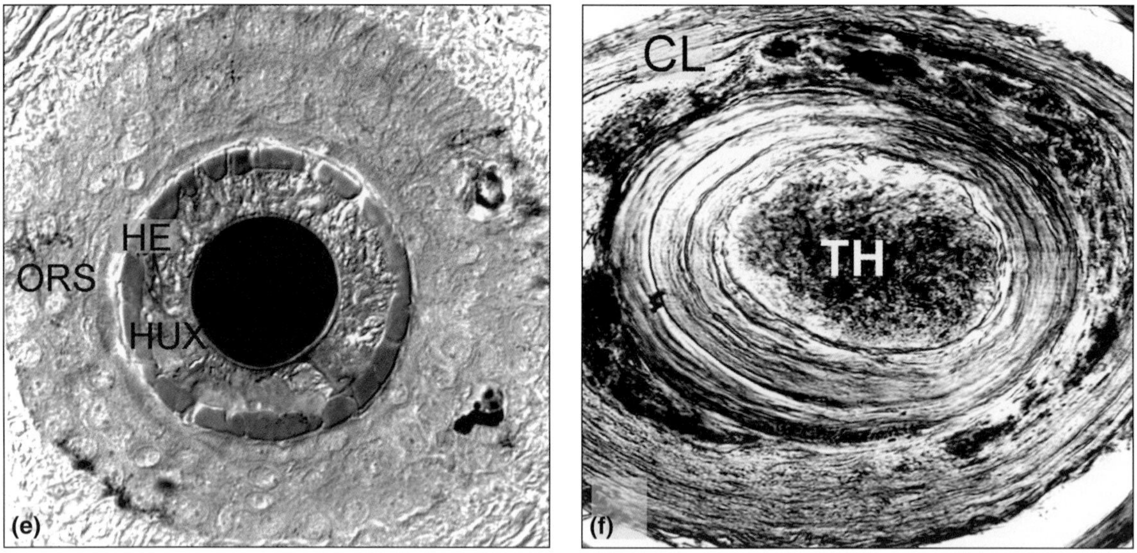

Fig. 1.3.2 (*Continued*) (e) outer hair follicle part with weakly keratinized hair fiber, pig, transverse semithin section, ×500; (f) outer opening of hair canal with numerous corneal lamellae and inclusions, pig, transverse paraffin section, hematoxylin and eosin (HE) staining, ×250. CL, corneal lamellae; TH, telogen hair; CS, connective tissue sheath; ORS, outer root sheath; HE, Henley's layer; HUX, Huxley's layer; SCU, sheath cuticle; HCU, hair cuticle; HC, hair cortex; HME, hair medulla; HM, hair matrix; HP, hair papilla.

cognate receptors as well as transcription factors and enzymes that have been recognized as key mediators (see Section 1.2.1.5). In view of all these intriguing control possibilities, it seems clear that any influence coming from numerous domestication effects can deeply and nonbiologically vary normal hair follicle cycling and thus hair coat qualities, as is discussed also below (Meyer et al. 1980a; Hardy 1992; Cotsarelis 1997; Lindner et al. 1997; Paus et al. 1997; Botchkarev et al. 1999; Meyer et al. 2002; Krause and Foitzik 2006; Pascucci et al. 2006; Rogers 2006; Fischer et al. 2008; Meyer 2009).

The identification of stem cells for hair follicle regeneration has been an important topic during the last years (see Section 1.2.2). Stem cell populations often occupy specific locations or niches where they can reside indefinitely and undergo self-renewal or differentiation into specific cell lineages, as is also required for hair follicle regrowth after the telogen stage. Although the discovery of stem cells in the bulge/isthmic region of the outer root sheath of hair follicles in humans, mice, and dogs has encouraged research to find more mutual basics of mammalian hair follicle biology, recent findings have emphasized that not only the hair follicle itself but also its environment contains unipotent, multipotent, and possibly even pluripotent stem cell populations of different developmental origin (Braun and Prowse 2006; Cotsarelis 2006; Cianferotti et al. 2007; Tiede et al. 2007).

1.3.1.4 Influences of domestication

It has been emphasized already that the basic hair follicle system described beforehand has undergone more or less severe structural and functional changes during domestication. Influences of domestication, however, show a high variability when the different domesticated species and their manifold breeds are compared. Changes induced by domestication have very rarely affected the basic follicular anatomy, but have mainly influenced the hair fibers, that is, the heavy and light guard hairs, and the wool hairs (Fig. 1.3.8). Domestication can be associated with changes in hair density, hair length, hair thickness, hair structure, and hair color, eventually resulting in a hair coat that no longer can fulfill all its functions necessary for a typical life under normal outdoor conditions. These changes have been caused by genetic alterations, particularly appearing in intensely bred and thoroughbred species such as the cat and the dog or small and large ruminants (sheep, goats, cattle), and even in the pig and the horse.

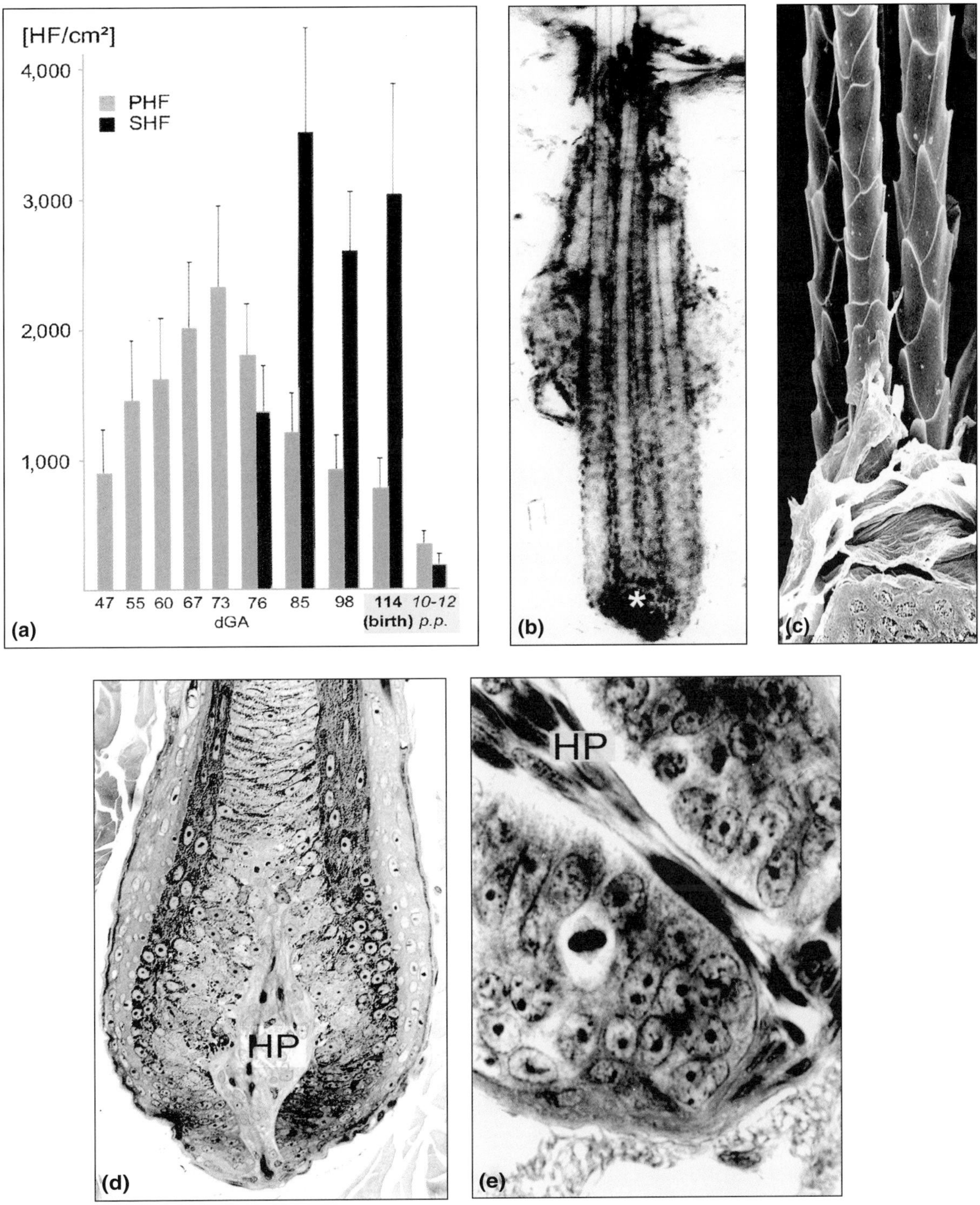

Fig. 1.3.3 Developmental and histological aspects of the secondary hair follicle. (a) Prenatal loss of secondary follicles in the pig, modified from Meyer and Görgen (1986); PHF, primary hair follicle; SHF, secondary hair follicle; dGA, gestation day; pp, post partum; (b) bundle of secondary follicles with complex bulb region (asterisk), cat, paraffin section, HE staining, ×200; (c) bundle of secondary hair shafts, dog, scanning electron microscopy, ×400; (d) typical small secondary hair follicle showing strong pigmentation of hair cortex and medulla, cat, longitudinal semithin section, toluidine blue, ×500; (e) bulb region with cell division near hair matrix, cat, longitudinal paraffin section, HE staining, ×1,450. HP, hair papilla.

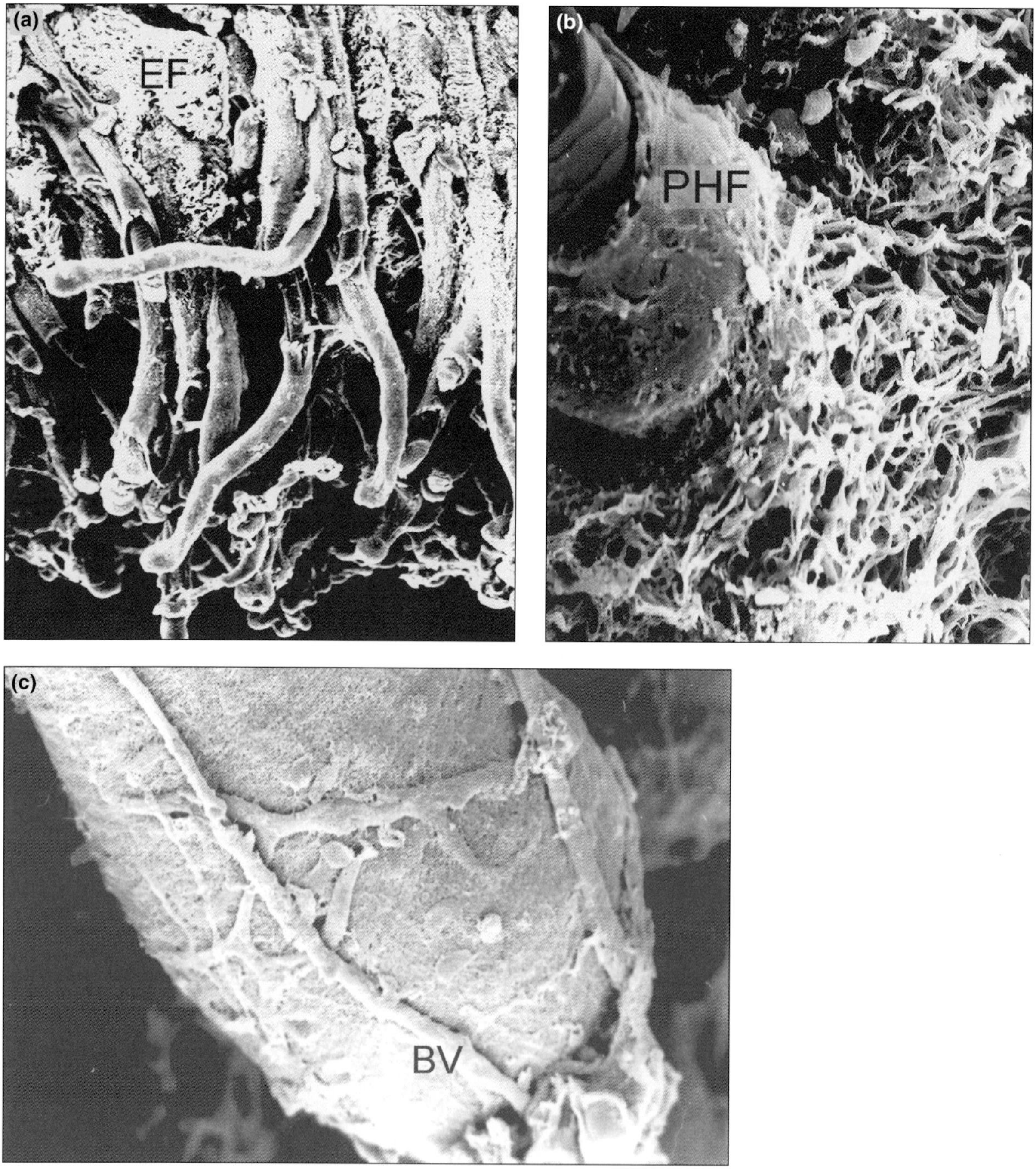

Fig. 1.3.4 Importance of elastic fibers for hair follicle anchoring and sheathing. (a) Elastic anchoring (EF) of curved primary hair follicles (HF) (adapted in thickness to secondaries), merino sheep, scanning electron microscopy, $\times 170$; (b) anchoring of thick primary HFs in a dense elastic fiber network, horse, SEM, $\times 160$; (c) sheathing of primary HF by a fine elastic mesh with small overlying blood vessels, cat, SEM, $\times 1{,}700$; for elastic fiber demonstration technique see Meyer et al. (1994). PHF, primary hair follicle; BV, blood vessel.

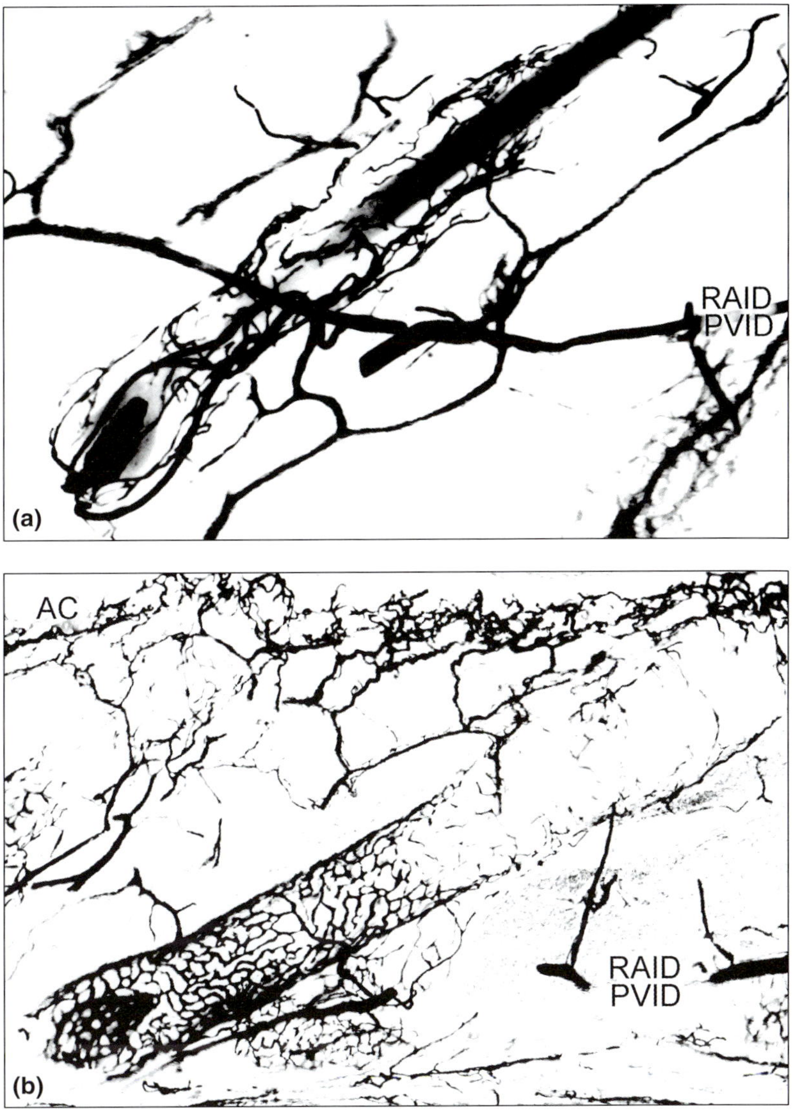

Fig. 1.3.5 Blood supply of the primary hair follicle. (a) Typical vessel pattern for thin hair follicles of densely haired mammals, cat, ×250; (b) typical vessel pattern for thick HF of sparsely haired mammals, pig, ×150; ink injection technique (courtesy of S. Godynicki). RAID, rete arteriosum intradermale; PVID, plexus venosus intradermale (Meyer et al. 2008a).

1.3.2 Variations in hair coat and hair follicle structure

1.3.2.1 Hair density and hair coat

Hair density varies clearly when the carnivores and the small ruminants (mean density between 1,500 and 6,000 hairs/cm^2) are compared with the large species like cattle or the horse (mean density between 500 and 2,500 hairs/cm^2). A sparse hair coat in domesticated mammals is often caused by a reduced number of wool hair follicles. The development of such reduction starts long before birth and the number of this follicle type even declines prenatally (Fig. 1.3.3a), as is particularly prominent in pigs, dogs, and sheep. In domesticated pigs, the number of secondary follicles is reduced up to 30% of the original number in wild pigs. In the domesticated dog, between 10 and 80% of the original amount of wool follicles are present when compared to its wild predecessors (Brunsch 1956; Ryder 1958, 1962; Meyer 1986, 1991; Meyer and Görgen 1986; Herre and Röhrs 1990; Meyer and Schwarz 1992; Meyer et al. 1992, 2000; Edwards 1999).

In addition to the rather sparse wool hair coat, the diameter of primary hair follicles and their primary

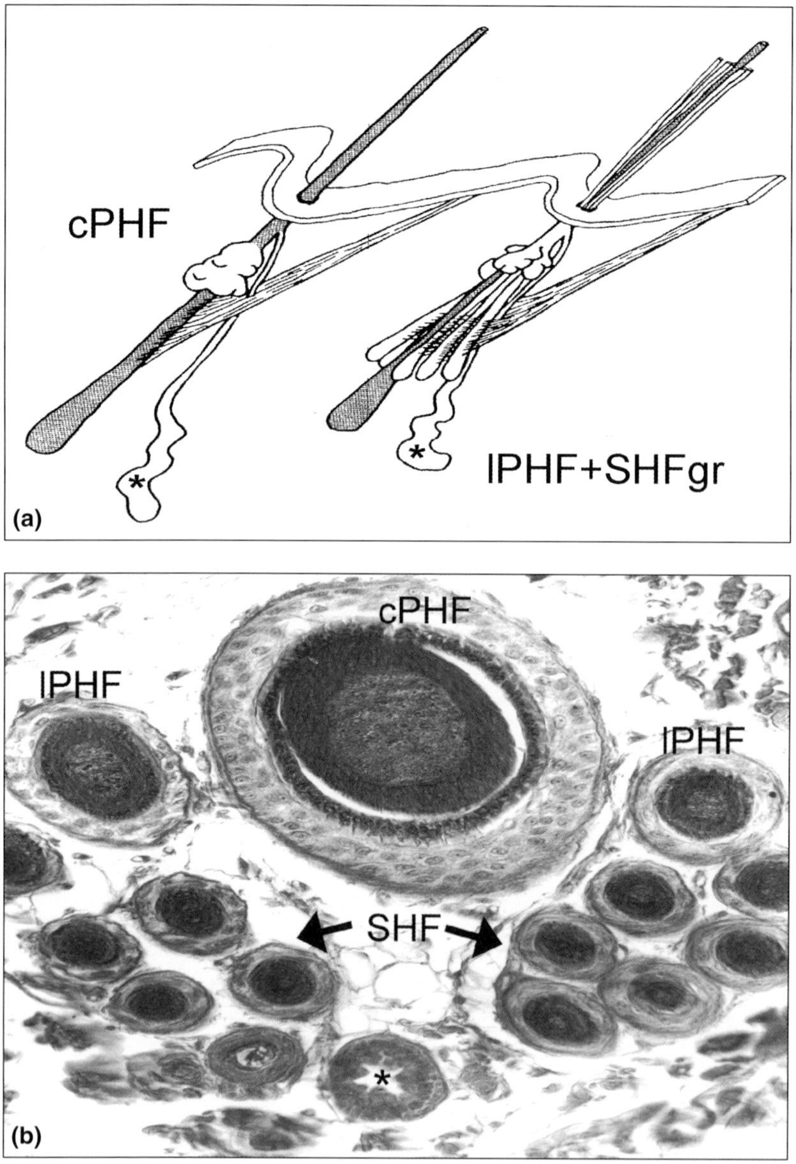

Fig. 1.3.6 Organization of the hair follicle complex and of hair grouping. (a) Hair follicle complex with central primary hair follicles (cPHF) and lateral primary hair follicles (lPHF), both primary types showing not only sebaceous glands but also one apocrine tubular gland each: the lateral PHFs form a small hair group with several secondary hair follicles (SHF); (b) typical hair group, cat, transverse paraffin section, HE staining, ×500, asterisk marks excretory duct of apocrine tubular gland. gr, group.

hairs may also decline with domestication, which results in an overall finer hair coat. This is particularly obvious in wool-producing species such as sheep and goats, but can also be found in the cat (e.g., Persian breeds) and the dog (e.g., poodle). Hair thinning is frequently associated with a loss of the hair fiber medulla, whereas a medulla is regularly found in wild mammals, even in wool hairs of densely haired species (Meyer et al. 1982). In this context it has to be emphasized that studies of fine-woolled sheep often incorrectly refer to thin primary hairs as "wool follicles," although these have the typical apocrine tubular glands and as such are distinct from the true secondary wool hair follicles (see Section 1.3.1.1).

1.3.2.2 Hair follicle structure

In principle, hair follicles of all mammalian species show the same histological structure (Figs 1.3.1 and 1.3.2). Nevertheless, in some cases structural variations have been observed that can clearly be explained as domestication-related effects, for example, in some

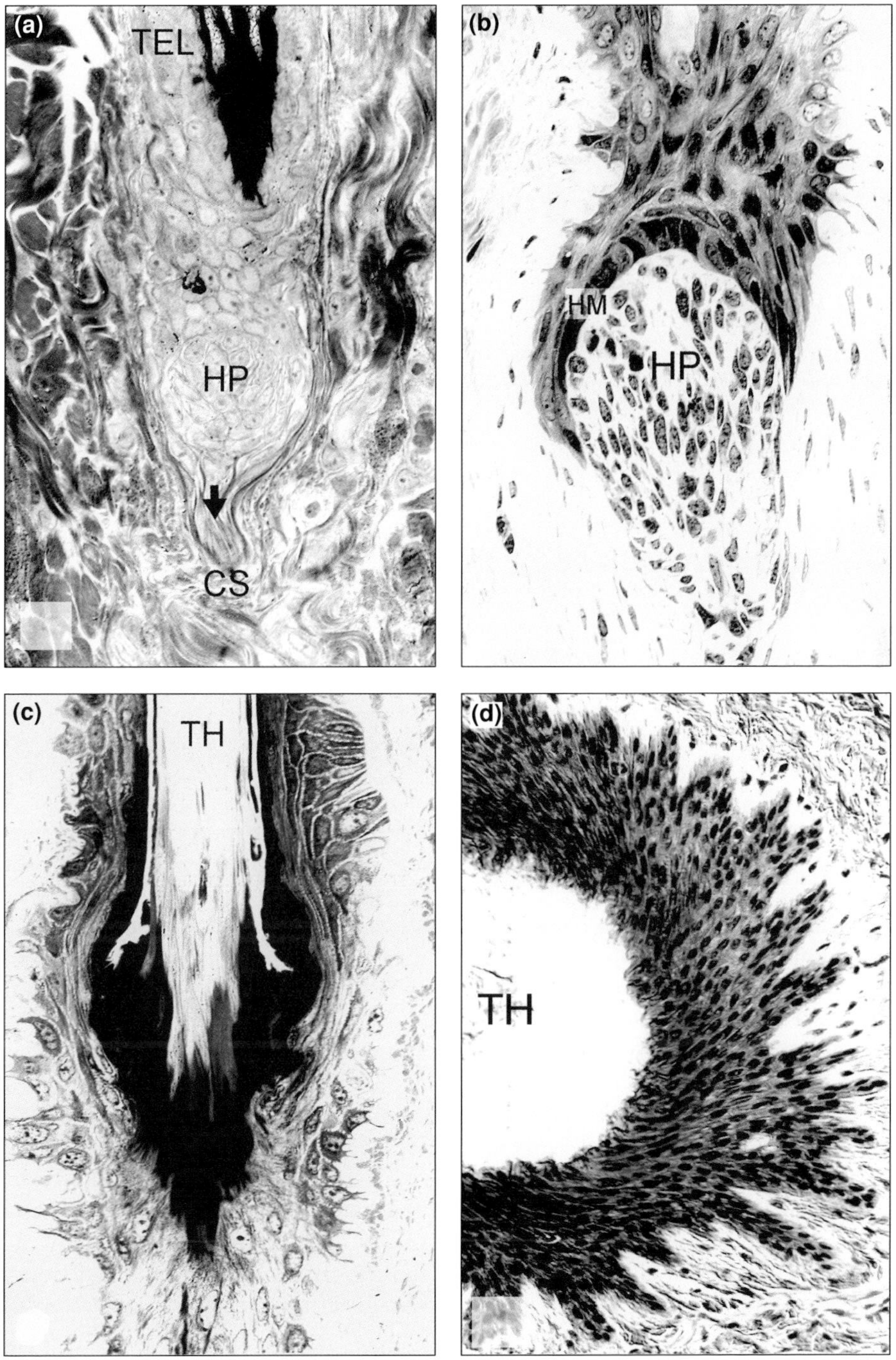

Fig. 1.3.7 Examples of important hair cycle stages. (a) Early anagen together with late telogen, dog, longitudinal semithin section, toluidine blue, ×600; (b) hair bulb regeneration during early anagen with new hair matrix (HM) and hair papilla (HP), Angora goat, longitudinal semithin section, toluidine blue, ×550; (c) telogen with typical club hair (TH) showing anchoring of the hair fiber by brush-like keratin cells forming helical ridges around the club, merino sheep, longitudinal semithin section, toluidine blue, ×660; (d) telogen primary HF showing helical ridge formation also in the outer root sheath, pig, transverse paraffin section, HE staining, ×330.

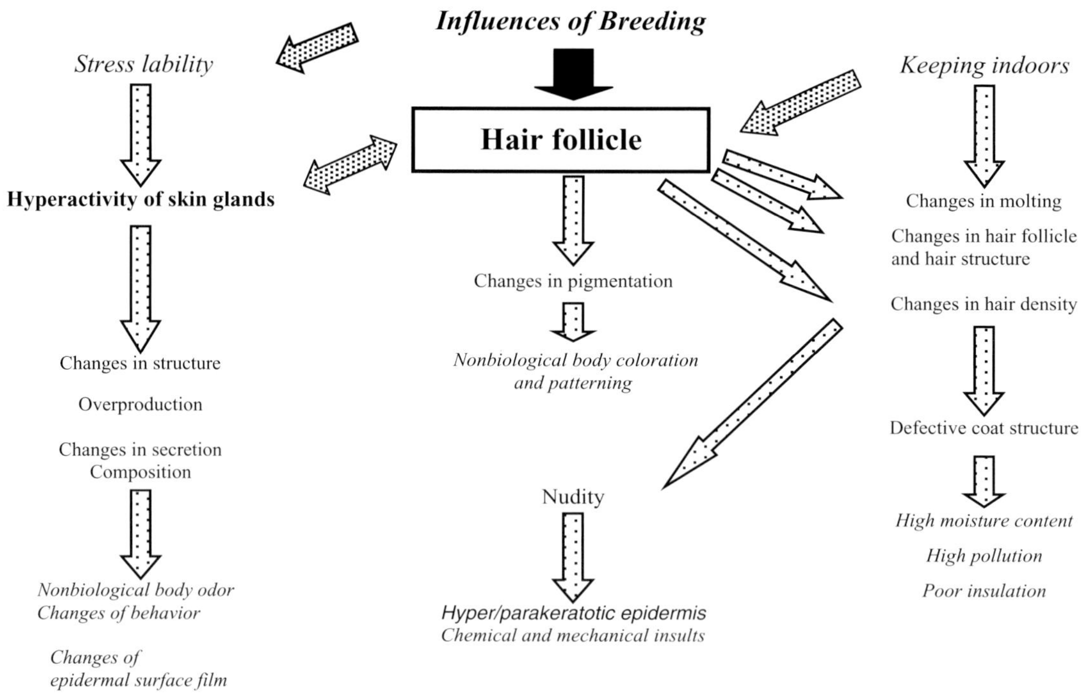

Fig. 1.3.8 Variations of structure and function of the primary hair follicle as caused by domestication influences (defects). (Modified from Meyer (1991); Meyer and Schwarz (1992).)

breeds of pigs (Meyer 1986; Schwarz and Meyer 1994; Cotsarelis 1997).

1.3.2.2.1 Hair matrix and dermal papilla

The hair bulb is composed of the one-layered epithelial hair matrix surrounding the onion-like hair papilla of mesodermal origin. The cells of the hair matrix show a periodical mitotic activity and produce all cell types of the hair follicle and the hair fiber. In contrast to the connective tissue that surrounds the entire hair follicle, the follicular dermal papilla contains an extracellular matrix, the composition of which is similar to that of the epidermal basement membrane, thus enabling communication between the ectodermal and the mesodermal compartment. This is particularly relevant during the anagen phase of the hair growth cycle and is associated with high contents of proteoglycans (heparan sulfate, papilla-specific chondroitin sulfate) or fibronectin. The dermal papilla lacks collagen I and (to some extent) collagen III. The basement membrane-separating matrix cells and dermal papilla fibroblasts are typically trilaminar, but all three layers are thinner than found in the epidermal basement membrane. Furthermore, it lacks any hemidesmosomes or distinct anchoring structures (Nutbrown and Randall 1995; Jahoda and Reynolds 1996; Meyer et al. 2002; Frase 2007). In support of the high metabolic activity in anagen hair follicles (as indicated by glycogen contents of papilla fibroblasts and strong activities of pentose phosphate pathway enzymes and β-glucuronidase in this region), the hair papilla may contain a very dense anastomosing network of nutritive blood capillaries. These capillaries are often accompanied by nerve fibers, representing one part of the sensory mechanoreceptive properties of the primary hair follicle. More networks of blood vessels and sensory and autonomic nerve fibers are found surrounding the follicular isthmus and the arrector pili muscle (Meyer and Neurand 1976; Meyer 1986; Meyer et al. 2002). The dermal papilla has the same structure in both wild and domesticated mammals, including humans (Fig. 1.3.1). However, in particularly large primary hair follicles such as the bristles of pigs, the dermal papilla may show a ridged shape, in this way offering a very large surface area to support a high metabolic activity (Meyer 1986).

1.3.2.2.2 Inner root sheath and hair fiber

Hair matrix cells produce all cell types of the hair shaft (i.e., medulla, cortex, and cuticle) and the inner root sheath (Fig. 1.3.1). Cells forming the inner root sheath are distinct from those forming the hair cortex and medulla (Meyer and Neurand 1987). The inner root sheath, that is, inwards Huxley's layer and outwards Henle's layer, is of specific relevance for the shape of the hair fiber (Fig. 1.3.2). Inner root sheath cells contain large numbers of trichohyalin granules that are essential for the keratinization process within the inner root sheath. Sheep trichohyalin is particularly well characterized and demonstrates a high proportion of glutamate, arginine, glutamine, and leucine residues, making more than 75% of the total amino acids. Besides trichohyalin, cells of the inner root sheath contain numerous keratin filaments and free sugar residues (α-D-mannose, α-D-glucose, α-L-fucose). Keratinization of the inner root sheath seems to result in a loss of sialyl residues from the plasma membrane, particularly in Huxley's and Henle's layers. This is in contrast to keratinization in the hair cortex, and supports the observation that Huxley's and Henle's layers differentiate much earlier than the hair cortex, since they most likely are essential for guiding the growing hair fiber (Tsukise and Meyer 1983; Meyer 1986; Meyer and Neurand 1987; Fietz et al. 1992, 1993; Bates et al. 1999; Pena et al. 1999; Hynd 2000; Ishii et al. 2001; Frase 2007). It is of basic hair biological interest that a unique type I keratin group (IRSa keratin), comprising three highly related proteins, has been identified in both sheep and humans (Bawden et al. 2001). A phylogenetic analysis suggests that the origin of this group precedes the origin of most of the epidermal cytokeratins and all hair keratins during emergence of the keratin intermediate filament genes, indicating a very early development of the hair follicle system during mammalian evolution (Alibardi 2004). There is most likely a close correlation between the formation of the inner root sheath and the development of the epidermis that finally allowed penetration of internally produced hair fibers through the skin.

In some breeds of the pig (Mangalicza pig, Göttingen miniature pig), and in some goats and sheep, the hair fiber has an oval to triangular rather than a round shape (Fig. 1.3.9c). Likewise, a slightly tortuous rather than straight tube is formed by Huxley's layer. This can be associated with an excentric hair canal in the upper follicle segment (Fig. 1.3.9d) and most likely explains the production of curly hairs, although other theories are still not ruled out (see below). Excentric hair canals can best be seen in sheep and Angora goats, whereby the wool follicles of merino sheep usually show retrocurvature, that is, the flexure of the bulb is opposite to the curvature of the shaft. The curliness of hair most likely results from selective breeding and is presumably established during early embryonic development. Curliness is found in some old dog breeds (e.g., Poodle, Curly-coated Retriever, Frisian Water Dog, Water Spaniels, and Puli), but is also present in rather sparsely haired species such as the pig (Mangalicza race), cattle (French Salers cattle), and horse (Curly horses, a robust North American breed that shows a very fine and smooth but unusually fatty hair coat because of hyperactive sebaceous glands). In Mangalicza pigs, the primary hair follicles show a curved appearance in the dermis and an oval-shaped inner root sheath (Herre and Langlet 1936; Herre and Wigger 1939; Auber 1951; Fraser 1964; Priestley and Rudall 1965; Straile 1965; Meyer 1986; Rogers 2006).

The innermost layer of the inner root sheath, the monolayered cuticle, also has an important function. Its strongly cornified cells are oppositely interlocked with the cells of the hair cuticle (Fig. 1.3.2d), and in this way the newly growing hair fiber is efficiently guided during its upward transport. Shape and size of the hair cuticle cells also demonstrate large interspecies and even interrace variations (Fig. 1.3.2d), and can therefore not be used to identify domesticated species in contrast to wild species (Meyer et al. 2000).

1.3.2.2.3 Outer root sheath

The outer root sheath does not keratinize below the level of the isthmus (in contrast to the inner root sheath). However, at the level of the isthmus where the inner root sheath disintegrates, the outer root sheath keratinizes without forming granules (trichilemmal keratinization), which is similar to the keratinization process of the hair cortex (Figs 1.3.2a,c–e and 1.3.10c). As is known from studies in sheep, the intermediate filament keratin 15 (K15) is expressed throughout the hair cycle in the basal (i.e., outer) layer of the outer root sheath. In the hair bulb, K15 is expressed in cells next to the dermal papilla but not in the inner bulb cells. Thus, K15 expression appears to signal an early stage in the pathway of keratinocyte differentiation. The bulge region of the basal outer root

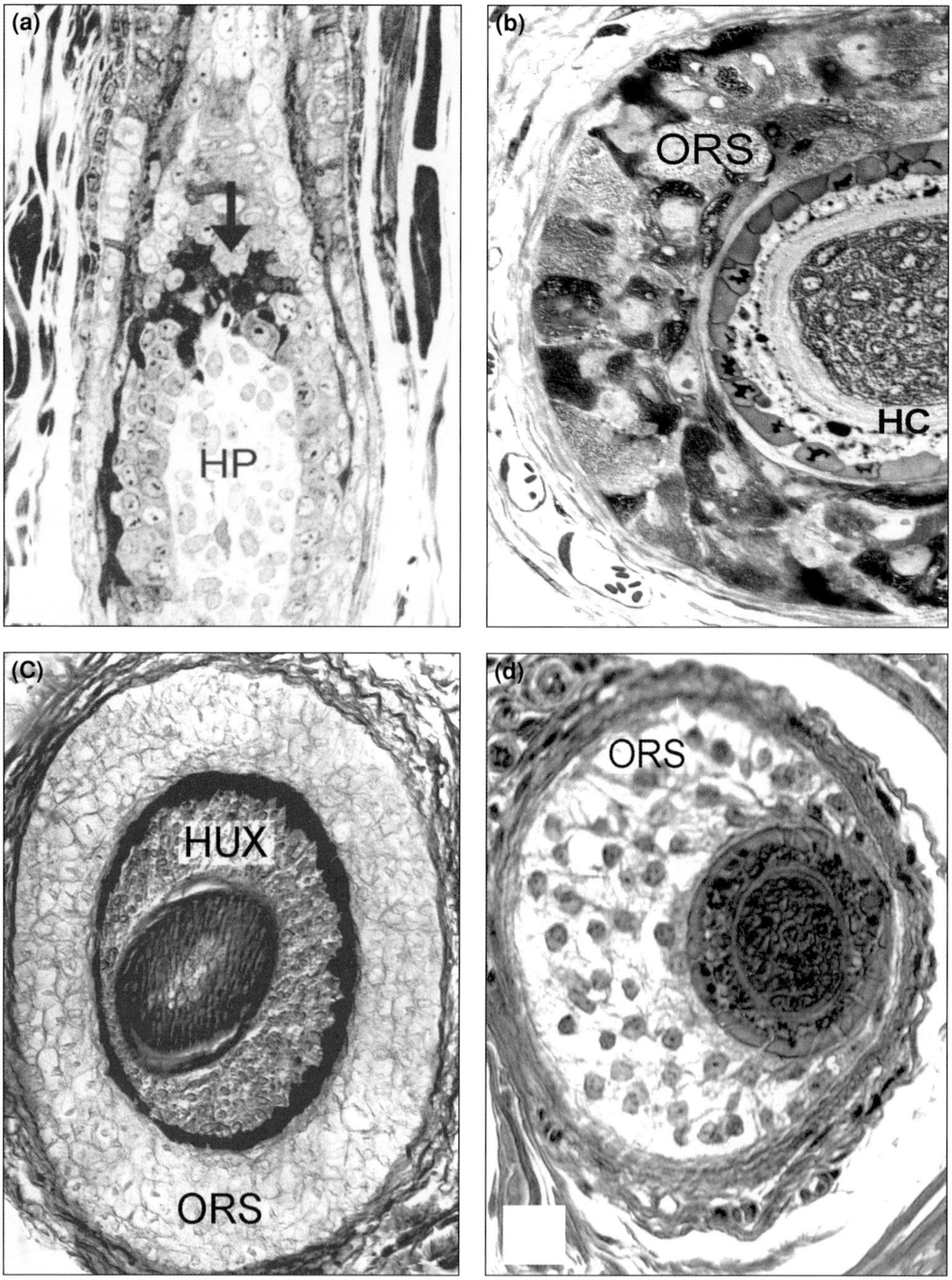

Fig. 1.3.9 Examples of domestication related defects of hair follicle structure. (a) Loss of hair medulla by degeneration of hair matrix cells and early medulla trichocytes, merino sheep, longitudinal semithin section, toluidine blue, ×620; (b) thinning of hair follicle and hair fiber by loss of hair medulla with the center of the hair fiber filled with cortex cells, Angora goat, transverse semithin section, toluidine blue, ×830; HC, hair cuticle; ORS, outer root sheath; (c) variations of hair fiber shape caused by thickness variations of Huxley's layer (HUX), pig, transverse paraffin section, histochemical S-S staining, ×400; (d) variations of hair shape by formation of a tortuous hair canal by the outer root sheath (ORS), secondary HF, dog, transverse paraffin section, HE staining, ×500. HP, hair follicle papilla.

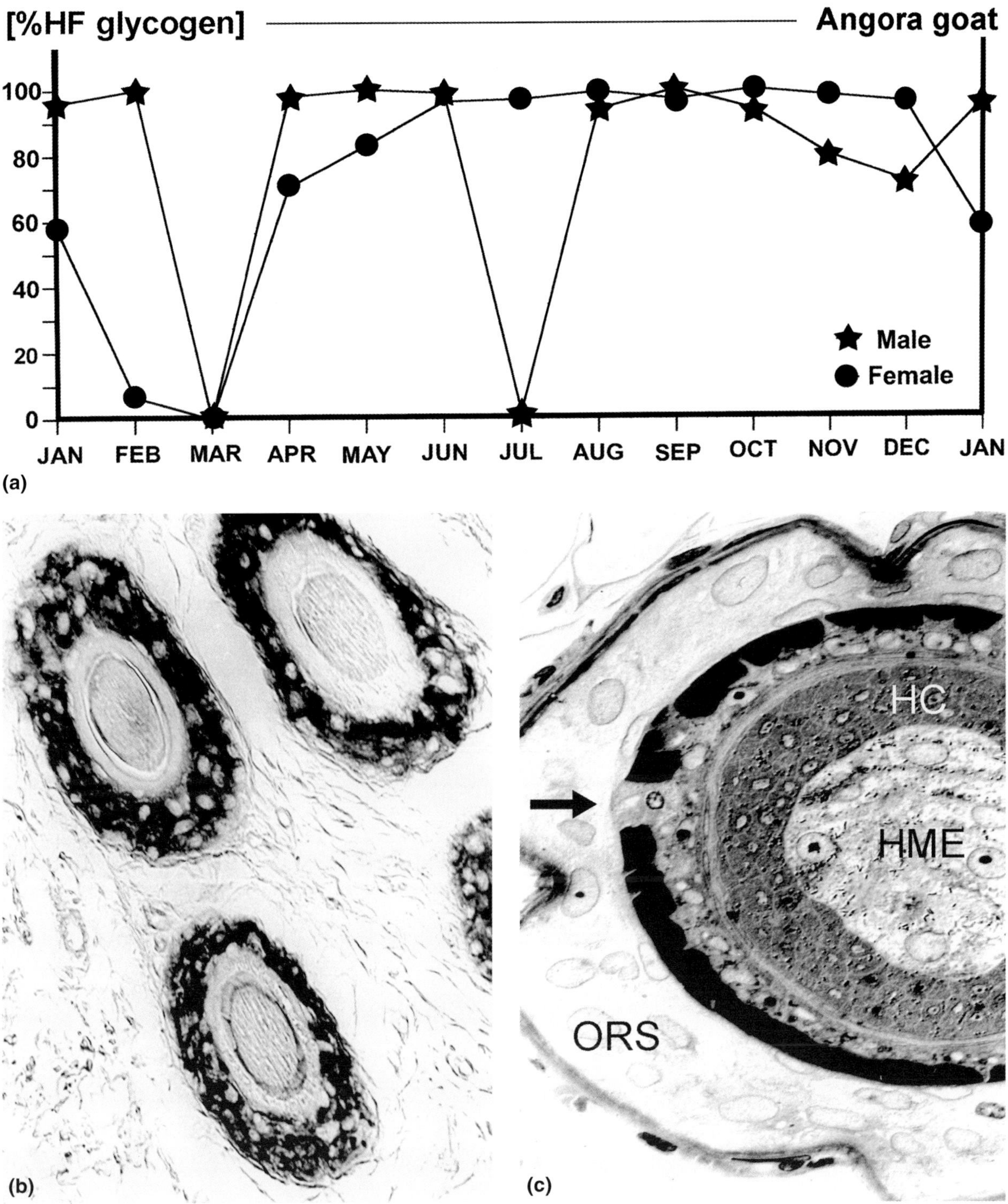

Fig. 1.3.10 Glycogen in the hair follicle of domesticated mammals. (a) Demonstration of indistinct hair cycle according to more or less constant glycogen deposition in the outer root sheath (ORS), typical for constantly growing hair fibers in the Angora goat (modified from Meyer et al. (1997)); (b) strong deposition of glycogen in outer root sheath cells of primary hair follicles, Angora goat, transverse paraffin section, PAS staining, ×330; (c) demonstration of a transit cell (arrow) for glucose transport in Henley's layer to reach Huxley's layer, cat, transverse semithin section, toluidine blue, ×500. HC, hair shaft cuticle; HME, hair shaft medulla.

sheath, thought to contain the hair follicle stem cells, is K15 negative but expresses the intermediate filament keratin 19 (K19), supposed to be a stem cell marker. This is the case in canine hair follicles but not in human hair follicles. Several studies have further corroborated the view that keratin expression in carnivore hair follicles differs from that in humans and laboratory rodents. The expression of steroid hormone receptors in the hair follicle and the content of glycogen appear to be susceptible to domestication influences. While in most domesticated mammals and in humans relevant glycogen storage in keratinocytes of the lower part of the outer root sheath varies with the season, in female Angora-haired mammals such as the Angora goat the cells of the outer root sheath often contain high glycogen amounts throughout the year (Fig. 1.3.10a,b) (Nutbrown and Randall 1995; Jahoda and Reynolds 1996; Cotsarelis 1997; Meyer et al. 1997; Whitbread and Powell 1998; Bates et al. 1999; Pena et al. 1999; Kozaki et al. 2001; Bratka-Robia et al. 2002; Meyer et al. 2002; Frase 2007).

1.3.2.3 Hair pigmentation

Melanocytes within the hair bulb transfer melanosomes into matrix keratinocytes by means of their long cellular processes (see Section 1.2.6), with follicular melanogenesis being strongly coupled to the anagen phase. From a comparative point of view, the number of melanocytes both within the hair bulb and the outer root sheath varies considerably in the different domesticated mammals. It can be very low with rather blonde types of hairs, and can be extremely high with black or dark hairs. This is best visualized in different dog breeds, but can also be found in cats (Fig. 1.3.3d), goats, cattle, or even horses. Such domestication-related variations in color can be explained by the very complex regulation of hair follicle pigmentation (see Section 1.2.6.2). In view of the manifold influences on hair pigmentation, even slight genetic alterations (likely to occur during intense breeding in several groups of domesticated animals, such as dogs or sheep and cattle) can lead to changes in hair shaft coloration (Meyer 1986, 2009; Slominski et al. 2005).

1.3.2.4 Hair cycling

Not all domestication-induced changes affect the hair structure. The hair growth cycle and its sensitivity to respond to extrinsic influences can be affected as well. In most wild mammals and in many free-ranging traditionally reared small ruminants, two annual hair growth cycles are recognized as the spring and autumn molt. This seasonality is also expressed in other physiological functions such as food intake and reproduction. Many studies have demonstrated that, among others, thyroid hormones play a crucial role in mediating this seasonality, not only with regard to hair growth but also in terms of reproductive performance. Variations in thyroid hormone activity allow the animals to adapt their metabolic balance to different environmental conditions, changes in nutrient availability, and homeorhetic changes during different physiological stages. Consequently, many endogenous (breed, age, gender, physiological state) and environmental factors (climate, season, nutrition) are able to affect thyroid hormone activity (Todini 2007). However, the strong influence of thyroid hormones in the onset of molting, as demonstrated for the cashmere goat, emphasizes that basic principles of hair cycle control are not completely lost during domestication (Villar et al. 2000; Pascucci et al. 2005).

In the process of domestication, humans created artificial environments for the animals that has considerably weakened the selection pressure directed to develop specific adaptations to different climatic zones. As a consequence of this, many breeds have lost their seasonal changes of hair. Studies have shown that in cattle breeds such as black spotted, Simmenthal, Schwitz, Jersey, or Red Dane, there is almost no seasonal change in hair density, even if bred in different climatic zones, whereas the ability to adapt is still present in other breeds (e.g., shorthorn). In sheep, the intensity of seasonal molting decreases from coarse-woolen breeds (e.g., Soay, Scottish Blackface, Limousine, Awasi, and Kazakh) via medium-woolen breeds (e.g., Suffolk, Southdown, Wiltshire horn, German Blackface) to fine-woolen animals (merino breeds of different origin), in which it is practically lost, especially in secondary hair follicles (Yeates 1955; Ryders 1962, 1976; Raushenbach 1972; Raushenbach and Prasolova 1973; Herre and Röhrs 1990; Meyer 1991; Meyer and Schwarz 1992; Meyer et al. 1997, 1998; Villar et al. 2000; Rogers 2006). Some breeds of cats, dogs, and pigs have also lost their molting seasonality, particularly if kept indoors. Mane and tail hairs in horses are no longer molted seasonally but grow continuously over years. Angorism as in the Turkish Angora goat or the Angora rabbit is characterized by a growth period of at least 9 months. Finally, a hair growth cycle of about 8 years' duration is found in the merino sheep, and nonshedding sheep breeds such as Romney sheep even remain in the anagen stage for life, although with seasonal variation in the rate of wool growth. All these observations illustrate consequences of very intense breeding, since ancestral sheep breeds such as the Wiltshire sheep still exhibit hair growth cycles that classically respond to the photoperiod (Meyer et al. 1980b; Neurand et al. 1980; Rogers 2006). Nevertheless, domestication does not exclude that dogs living outdoors under varying daylight can still show a typical molt with production of some sort of lighter summer coat and a denser winter coat (Favarato and Conceicao 2008). This underlines the general importance of a diurnal rhythm for hair cycling.

The regional or topographical course of the hair molt may also be influenced by domestication. The molt normally begins at the head and proceeds dorsoventrally and caudally. A synchronized wave-like pattern of hair follicle cycling is found in young mice, rats, rabbits, and in few domesticated mammalian species, whereas some small and several medium-sized and large mammals such as guinea pigs, pigs, dogs, and cats mostly show a nonsynchronized mosaic pattern of hair follicle cycling, as is also present in the scalp region of humans (Yeates 1955; Brunsch 1956; Raushenbach 1972; Raushenbach and Prasalova 1973; Ryder 1976; Meyer et al. 1980b; Neurand et al. 1980; Diaz et al. 2004).

1.3.2.5 Activity of hair follicle glands

Influences of domestication may also affect the activity of the sebaceous glands and the apocrine tubular glands of the hair follicle complex. Whereas under natural conditions, glandular activity shows seasonal activity (i.e., increased secretion during late anagen stages in spring), many intensely bred animals exhibit continuously increased glandular secretion rates and distinct changes in the composition of the sebum with subsequent changes in the spectrum and activities of the microbial flora on the epidermal surface (Meyer et al. 2001, 2008b).

1.3.3 Species-specific aspects of hair follicle anatomy and physiology

The integument of most domesticated mammals, in particular of carnivores and small ruminants, has structural and functional features that are very distinct from the hair coat of humans. The most important differences between domesticated animal species and man are related to hair density. However, there are also differences in the hair follicles themselves. Although the general hair follicle structure is very similar between humans and domesticated animals, variations occur in the size of hair follicles and the quality of the hair fiber produced. In addition, one needs to be aware of regional differences, with head, anogenital regions, parts of the abdominal region, or mediolateral surfaces of the extremities, axillar, and inguinal regions exhibiting several structural peculiarities. In general, the dorsolateral region is most homogeneous with regard to hair follicle structure.

1.3.3.1 Dog and cat

Dog and cat show the typical structure of primary and secondary hair follicles. The former hair follicle type often projects into the hypodermal fat reservoir, whereby the skin is relatively thin. The insertion depth varies between 0.40 and 1.20 mm in both species. Hair follicles are arranged in groups and display a higher density in the cat (800–1,600 groups/cm^2, each group with about 8–20 individual hairs; 6,000–10,000 hairs/cm^2) than in the dog (100–600 groups/cm^2, each group with 2–15 hairs; 1,500–4,000 hairs/cm^2). The number of hair follicles per group not only varies between the different body regions (particularly in the cat), but also within one body region. The largest (central) primary hair follicle is typically placed in the center of a group and is flanked by several lateral primary or secondary hair follicles. Primary hair follicles are surrounded by a distinct arrector pili muscle. The diameter of hair bulbs varies between 150 and 450 μm in primary hair follicles (thickest in the dog), and between 70 and 120 μm in secondary hair follicles. Up to 85% (cat) and 75% (dog) of follicles are wool follicles, if animals are kept outside in the winter. Hair shaft quality varies markedly between breeds, particularly in highbred animals. The numerous holocrine sebaceous glands are arranged in groups around the follicles. The tubular apocrine glands have straight secretory ducts and only slightly coiled secretory portions. Hair follicles and associated glands are remarkably well supplied with blood vessels, the latter deriving from the rete arteriosum intradermale/plexus venosus intradermale (Brunsch 1956; Schwarz et al. 1976; Meyer et al. 1978, 1982; Meyer and Neurand 1987; Schwarz and Meyer 1994; Ishii et al. 2001).

1.3.3.2 Small ruminants

The rather densely haired sheep and goat demonstrate a similar hair follicle grouping as carnivores. Three primary hair follicles form groups with 15–16 (sheep) or 3–6 (goat) secondary follicles, whereby 5,000–7,000 hairs/cm^2 can be found in sheep and 1,200–1,800 hairs/cm^2 in the goat. There is a great variation in the number of secondary (wool) hair follicles per group, particularly in medium-woolen and fine-woolen animals. In sheep, the extremely fine-woolen merino breed shows a maximum of 40–60 secondary hair follicles per hair group similar to (the Angora goat or the cashmere goat), whereby the number of secondary hair follicles is significantly higher in Angora goats (15–40) than in cashmere goats (8–22). Comparing the different breeds in sheep and goats, it seems that there has been a movement of secondaries from between the primaries accompanied by a tendency for the primaries to move closer together and to lie on an arc. As more secondaries are found in medium- and finer-woolen breeds, this hair follicle type has spread away from the primaries, so that in view of the development of a more and more homogeneous hair coat, as is typical for fine-woolen sheep, the number of branched hair follicles increased to become the dominating structure of the common integument. The diameter of the hair bulbs in fine-woolen sheep and goats measures 180–300 μm in primary hair follicles, and 80–130 μm in secondary hair follicles. Insertion depths of primary and secondary hair follicles varies between 0.50 and 0.85 mm. The sebaceous glands have no structural peculiarities. The apocrine tubular glands form a typical layer with their secretory portions below the hair bulbs of the primary follicles. The hair follicle complex is supplied from the rete arteriosum intradermale/plexus venosus intradermale, and, additionally, the rete arteriosum dermidis/plexus venosus dermidis. In sheep, blood vessels arising from the deep vascular network do not directly penetrate into the deepest part of the hair follicle but enter laterally between the hair bulb and the upper border of the prekeratinizating zone; this is in contrast, for example, to hair follicle vascularization in humans.

With regard to hair follicle biology both medium to fine-woolen sheep and goats undergo significant morphological changes throughout the year. These changes differ from the normal sequence of events associated with the hair cycle and appear to be associated with relevant changes in dietary quality and quantity. The continuous production of hair fibers despite fluctuations in the supply of oxygen and nutrients (including biotin, riboflavin, pyridoxine, folate, pantothenic acid, vitamin D, vitamin A, copper, zinc, and amino acids) may be responsible for a minor coat quality in autumn and winter, which is a typical consequence of purebred animals with high wool production rates (see Section 3.2.1) (Meyer et al. 1978, 1997, 1998, 2008a; Meyer and Neurand 1987; Schwarz et al. 1991; Jonen et al. 1994; Hynd et al. 1997; Nagorcka et al. 1998; Hynd 2000).

1.3.3.3 Large ruminants

The rather sparsely haired cattle generally show single primary and secondary hair follicles, so that a grouping can hardly be detected, although the triple primary follicle pattern is still present. Hair follicle density varies according to the different body regions and breeds between 600 and 2,500 hairs/cm^2. About 70% of hair follicles are secondary follicles. Glands are similar to the small ruminants with a typical subfollicular layer of the secretory portions of the apocrine glands. Data on hair follicle density, even from animals in the same environment sampled at the same age, are of little comparative value because of differences in body weight or body size (e.g., in Herefords, shorthorns, or Brahman and Afrikander breeds). Hair follicle diameters are between 200 and 450 μm in primary follicles, and 100–180 μm in secondary follicles. Insertion depth varies between 0.85 and 1.65 mm, whereby there seems to be a negative correlation between hair follicle density and follicle depth. From a comparative point of view, African, Asian, and South American cattle have a more shallow insertion than European breeds (Turner et al. 1962; Jenkinson and Nay 1973; Amakiri and Hill 1975; Meyer et al. 1978; Meyer and Neurand 1987).

1.3.3.4 Pig

In the pig, single primary and secondary hair follicles are forming a rather sparse hair coat, with a density between 10 and 40 hairs/cm^2. Strong bristles are very obvious and dominate as typical primary follicles, whereas the short secondary hairs are inconspicuous and often are not found in modern breeds such as the Yorkshire or German landrace. Hair bulb diameters between 200 and 600 μm for primary follicles and

100–180 μm for secondary hair follicles are normal in the pig. The primary hair follicles are deeply inserted (3.00–5.30 mm), with the hair roots crossing the whole dermis and bulbs that normally anchor in the hypodermis between fat cells. Secondary follicles show a rather constant insertion depth of about 1.20 mm. Primary hair follicles possess large sebaceous glands with sebum reservoirs in the excretory duct (as in humans) and distinct apocrine tubular glands with a secretory unit lying near or below the hair bulb. In this species, the base of primary follicles is surrounded by a unique but distinct horizontally arranged interfollicular muscle that is independent of the arrector pili muscle (thickness 40–80 μm) (Meyer and Neurand 1976; Meyer et al. 1978; Tsukise and Meyer 1983; Meyer 1986; Meyer and Görgen 1986; Meyer and Neurand 1987).

1.3.3.5 Horse

The horse very clearly exhibits the single hair follicle system, with a hair density varying at the trunk between 1,000 and 1,500 hairs/cm^2. There are high breed-related regional variations in hair density. About 60% of hair follicles are secondary wool follicles. Relatively large (hair bulb diameter: 200–500 μm) and rather steeply and deeply (0.80–1.00 mm) inserted primary follicles are found, particularly in the mane and anogenital regions (3.00–4.00 mm). Secondary follicles are particularly deep and comparatively strong (hair bulb diameter: 100–200 μm) and insert with depths of 0.30–0.50 mm more or less in the superficial part of the medium dermis (Meyer et al. 1978; Meyer and Neurand 1987; Cook et al. 2005; Meyer 2009).

1.3.3.6 Laboratory rodents

Laboratory rodents (mice and rats) with their rather thin skin have 5,000 up to 8,000 hairs/cm^2 in the common integument, and show a typical mixture and grouping of primary and secondary (wool) hair follicles. A typical summer hair coat, as developed for example by animals kept constantly in the laboratory under indoor conditions, will show about 70% wool hairs. Apocrine tubular glands related to primary hair follicles are only present in specific body regions.

1.3.3.7 Humans

Humans exhibit a hair density of only 20–35 hairs/cm^2. Each hair fiber grows at the rate of 5–10 mm per month, with one hair cycle lasting for about three years. Only very delicate primary hair follicles are present in the common integument, whereas larger primary hairs are restricted to specific body regions, for example, the scalp and anogenital regions. Humans do not have secondary (wool) hair follicles. Eccrine tubular glands are independent of the primary hair follicles and distributed in the hairy skin, whereas apocrine tubular glands are only found in specific body regions, for example, axillar and anogenital regions. The latter feature is typical for the great apes (hominids) and in contrast to all the other mammalian groups (Meyer 2002).

1.3.4 Domestic animals in hair follicle research

Although laboratory rodents are specifically bred for various research purposes, they are not generally best suited to research human skin, particularly because of the above-mentioned large differences in skin anatomy and physiology. Normally, only hair follicles of the dorsolateral body region are studied in laboratory rodents. However, it is primarily this body region where hair follicles are synchronized opposed to the non-synchronized mosaic hair cycle in humans. In addition, intense breeding may have influenced the ability of hair follicles to respond to external stimuli such as photoperiod and temperature. In view of the great differences between rodent and human hair follicles (Cotsarelis 2006), research would best be performed on human hair follicles or on scalp hair follicles from large apes kept under controlled indoors conditions.

Because of the above-mentioned limitations, the integument of domesticated mammals has developed increasing biomedical relevance as a model for experimental skin research. In contrast to laboratory rodents, the integument of domesticated animals has been subjected to many structural and functional modifications during domestication, which resulted in a number of similarities to man (e.g., paucity of hair, hairlessness, hair curling, thickness of skin layers, and variations in pigmentation). This suggests that some of the oldest domesticated species (e.g., pig, cattle, and horse) are ideally suited for comparative dermatological research. Yet differences in the microstructure and the specific functions of all parts of the skin must still be fully appreciated, before the most relevant experimental animal species is selected.

In summary, every scientist needs to be aware of the species-specific differences in skin anatomy and physiology before an extrapolation can be made to hair follicle diseases in humans. Studies in healthy and diseased domestic animals can further contribute to the understanding of hair follicle diseases in humans, since they have undergone similar domestication changes as humans and, opposed to laboratory rodents, share the same environment with them.

References

Alibardi L. 2004. Comparative aspects of the inner root sheath in adult and developing hairs of mammals in relation to the evolution of hairs. *Journal of Anatomy (London)* 205:179–200.

Amakiri SF, Hill DH. 1975. Hair follicle measurements in some tropical and temperate breeds of cattle in Nigeria. *International Journal of Biometeorology* 19:115–121.

Auber L. 1951. The anatomy of follicles producing wool fibres with special reference to keratinization. *Transactions of the Royal Society of Edinburgh* 62(Pt I):191–254.

Bates EJ, Penno NM, Hynd PI. 1999. Wool follicle matrix cells: culture conditions and keratin expression in vitro. *British Journal of Dermatology* 140:216–225.

Bawden CS, McLaughlan C, Nesci A, Rogers G. 2001. A unique type I keratin intermediate filament gene family is abundantly expressed in the inner root sheath of sheep and human hair follicles. *Journal of Investigative Dermatology* 116:157–166.

Botchkarev VA, Botchkareva NV, Welker P, Metz M, Lewin GR, Subramaniam A, Bulfone-Paus S, Hagen E, Braun A, Lommatzsch M, Renz H, Paus R. 1999. A new role for neurotrophins: involvement of brain-derived neurotrophic factor and neurotrophin-4 in hair cycle control. *FASEB Journal* 13:395–410.

Bratka-Robia CB, Egerbacher M, Helmreich M, Mitteregger G, Benesch M, Bamberg E. 2002. Immunohistochemical localization of androgen and oestrogen receptors in canine hair follicles. *Veterinary Dermatology* 13:113–118.

Braun KM, Prowse DM. 2006. Distinct epidermal stem cell compartments are maintained by independent niche microenvironments. *Stem Cell Reviews* 2(3):221–231.

Brunsch A. 1956. Vergleichende Untersuchungen am Haarkleid von Wildcaniden und Haushunden. *Zeitschrift für Tierzüchtung und Züchtungsbiologie* 67:205–240.

Chapman RE. 1979. Das Tierhaar. In: Orfanos CE (ed), *Haar und Haarkrankheiten*, pp. 167–195. Stuttgart: Springer.

Cianferotti L, Cox M, Skorija K, Demay MB. 2007. Vitamin D receptor is essential for normal keratinocyte stem cell function. *Proceedings of the National Academy of Sciences of The United States of America* 104:9428–9433.

Cook CP, Scott DW, Erb HN, Miller WH. 2005. Bacteria and fungi on the surface and within noninflamed hair-follicles of skin biopsy specimens from horses with healthy skin or inflammatory dermatoses. *Veterinary Dermatology* 16:47–51.

Cotsarelis G. 1997. The hair follicle. *American Journal of Pathology* 151:1505–1509.

Cotsarelis G. 2006. Gene expression profiling gets to the root of human hair follicle stem cells. *Journal of Clinical Investigation* 116:19–22.

Diaz SF, Torres SMF, Dunstan RW, Lekcharoensuk C. 2004. An analysis of canine hair re-growth after clipping for a surgical procedure. *Veterinary Dermatology* 15:25–30.

Edwards JEH. 1999. Reduction in wool follicles prior to birth in Merino sheep. *Reproduction, Fertility and Development* 11:229–234.

Favarato ES, Conceicao LG. 2008. Hair cycle in dogs with different hair types in a tropical region of Brazil. *Veterinary Dermatology* 19:15–20.

Fietz MJ, McLaughlan CJ, Campbell MT, Rogers GE. 1993. Analysis of the sheep trichohyalin gene—potential structural and calcium-binding roles of trichohyalin in the hair follicle. *Journal of Cell Biology* 121:855–865.

Fietz MJ, Rogers GE, Eyre HJ, Baker E, Callen DF, Sutherland GR. 1992. Mapping of the trichohyalin gene—colocalization with the profilaggrin, involucrin, and loricrin genes. *Journal of Investigative Dermatology* 99:542–544.

Fischer TW, Slominski A, Tobin DJ, Paus R. 2008. Melatonin and the hair follicle. *Journal of Pineal Research* 44:1–15.

Frase R. 2007. Immunhistochemische und biochemische Untersuchungen zur Expression von epithelialen Keratinen in klinisch unveränderter Pferdehaut und Fußhaut vonKaltblutpferden mit Warzenmauke-Syndrom. Dissertation Thesis, University of Veterinary Medicine, Hannover.

Fraser IEB. 1964. Studies on the follicle bulbs of fibres. I. Mitotic and cellular segmentation in the wool follicle with references to ortho- and parasegmentation. *Australian Journal of Biological Sciences* 17:521–531.

Hardy MH. 1992. The secret life of the hair follicle. *Trends in Genetics* 8:55–61.

Herre W, Langlet J. 1936. Untersuchungen über Haut, Haar- und Lockenbildung des Karakulschafes. *Zeitschrift für Tierzüchtung und Züchtungsbiologie* 35:401–412.

Herre W, Röhrs M. 1990. *Haustiere—zoologisch gesehen,* 2nd edn. Stuttgart: Fischer.

Herre W, Wigger H. 1939. Die Lockenbildung der Säugetiere. *Kühn Archiv* 52:233–254.

Hynd PI. 2000. The nutritional biochemistry of wool and hair follicles. *Animal Science* 70:181–195.

Hynd PI, Hughes A, Earl CR, Penno NM. 1997. Seasonal changes in the morphology of wool follicles in finewool and strongwool Merino strains grazing at different stocking rates in southern Australia. *Australian Journal of Agricultural Research* 48:1089–1097.

Ishii M, Tsukise A, Meyer W. 2001. Lectin histochemistry of glycoconjugates in the feline hair follicle and hair. *Annals of Anatomy* 183:449–458.

Jahoda CA, Reynolds AJ. 1996. Dermal-epidermal interactions. Adult follicle-derived cell populations and hair growth. *Dermatologic Clinics* 14:573–583.

Jenkinson DM, Nay T. 1973. The sweat glands and hair follicles of Asian, African, and South American cattle. *Australian Journal of Biological Sciences* 26:259–275.

Jonen M, Meyer W, Schwarz R, Davies AS. 1994. Vergleichende Untersuchungen zur Struktur der Haarfollikelgruppen bei neuseeländischen Cashmere-, Angora- und Cashgoraziegen. *Journal of Animal Breeding and Genetics* 111:391–403.

Kozaki M, Nakamura Y, Iquchi M, Kano R, Watanabe S, Fujiwara K, Hasegawa A. 2001. Immunohistochemical analysis of cytokeratin expression in dog skin. *Journal of Veterinary Medical Science* 63:1–4.

Krause K, Foitzik K. 2006. Biology of the hair follicle: The basics. *Seminars in Cutaneous Medicine and Surgery* 25:2–10.

Lindner G, Botchkarev VA. Botchkareva NV, Ling G, van der Veen C, Paus R. 1997. Analysis of apoptosis during hair follicle regression (catagen). *American Journal of Pathology* 151:1601–1617.

Meyer W. 1986. *Die Haut des Schweines.* Hannover: Schlütersche.

Meyer W. 1991. Bemerkungen zu domestikationsbedingten Veränderungen des Säugetier-Integuments. *Zeitschrift für Säugetierkunde* 56(Sh):33–34.

Meyer W. 2002. Die tubulären Hantdrüsen in der allgemeinen Körperdecke von Primaten, mit einer Kennzeichnung phylogenetischer und biologischer Zusammenhänge. *Der Zoologische Garten* NF72:107–123.

Meyer W. 2009. Haut und Hautorgane. In: Wissdorf H, Gerhards H, Huskamp B, Deegen E (eds), *Praxisorientierte Anatomie des Pferdes*, 3rd edn. Hannover: Schlütersche, in press.

Meyer W, Godynicki S, Tsukise A. 2008a. Lectin histochemistry of the endothelium of blood vessels in the mammalian integument, with remarks on the endothelial glycocalyx and blood vessel system nomenclature. *Annals of Anatomy* 190:264–276.

Meyer W, Görgen S. 1986. Development of hair coat and skin glands in fetal porcine integument. *Journal of Anatomy (London)* 144:201–220.

Meyer W, Hülmann G, Seger H. 2002. *REM Atlas on the Hair Cuticle Pattern of Central European Mammals.* Alfeld-Hannover: Schaper.

Meyer W, Neurand K. 1976. The distribution of enzymes in the skin of the domestic pig. *Laboratory Animals* 10:237–247.

Meyer W, Neurand K. 1987. A comparative scanning electron microscopic view of the integument of domestic mammals. *Scanning Microscopy* 1:169–180.

Meyer W, Neurand K, Müller K. 1992. Integumental structure in a Friesian calf with congenital hypo- or atrichosis combined with prognathia inferior. *Veterinary Dermatology* 3:43–46.

Meyer W, Neurand K, Schwarz R. 1980a. Der Haarwechsel der Haussäugetiere. II. Topographischer Ablauf, Vergleich Haustier-Wildtier und Steuerungsmechanismen. *Deutsche Tierärztliche Wochenschrift* 87:96–102.

Meyer W, Neurand K, Schwarz R. 1980b. Der Haarwechsel der Haussäugetiere. III. Der Haarwechsel von Schaf und Ziege. *Deutsche Tierärztliche Wochenschrift* 87:346–353.

Meyer W, Neurand K, Schwarz R, Bartels T, Althoff A. 1994. Arrangement of elastic fibres in the integument of domesticated mammals. *Scanning Microscopy* 8:375–391.

Meyer W, Neurand K, Tanyolaç A. 2001. General antimicrobial properties of the integument in fleece producing sheep and goats. *Small Ruminant Research* 41:181–190.

Meyer W, Sağlam M, Schwarz R, Tanyolaç A. 1998. Der Energiestoffwechsel der Türkischen Angoraziege unter saisonaler Sicht. *Deutsch-Türkische Agrarforschung, 5. Symposium (Antalya 1997)*, 339–344.

Meyer W, Sağlam M, Tanyolaç A, Schwarz R, Hetzel U. 1997. Histochemische und biochemische Untersuchungen zu jahreszyklischen Aspekten des Kohlenhydrat-abhängigen Energiestoffwechsels der Haarfollikel von Türkischen Angoraziegen. *Schweizer Archiv für Tierheilkunde* 139:78–83.

Meyer W, Schnapper A, Hülmann G, Seger H. 2000. Domestication-related variations of the hair cuticula pattern in mammals. *Journal of Animal Breeding and Genetics* 117:281–283.

Meyer W, Schwarz R. 1992. Zu Bau und Funktion der Haut von Hund und Katze—mit Bemerkungen zu Domestikationseffekten. *Jahresberichte der Deutschen Veterinärmedizinischen Gesellschaft, Fachgruppe Kleintierkrankheiten* 37:93–99.

Meyer W, Schwarz R, Neurand K. 1978. The skin of domestic mammals as a model for the human skin, with special reference to the domestic pig. *Current Problems in Dermatology* 7:39–52.

Meyer W, Seegers U, Bock M. 2008b. Annual secretory activity of the skin glands in the Southern pudu (*Pudu puda* MOLINA 1782, Cervidae). *Mammalian Biology* 74:392–395.

Meyer W, Uhr G, Schwarz R, Radke B. 1982. Untersuchungen an der Haut der Europäischen Wildkatze (*Felis silvestris* Schreber). II. Haarkleid. *Zoologische Jahrbücher, Abteilung für Anatomie und Ontogenie der Tiere* 107:205–234.

Nagorcka BN, Dollin AE, Ringrose-Voase AJ. 1998. Measurement of fibre density and fibre bundles in the skin of sheep from different breeds. *Australian Journal of Agricultural Research* 49:113–126.

Neurand K, Meyer W, Schwarz R. 1980. Der Haarwechsel der Haussäugetiere. I. Allgemeine Problematik und zeitlicher Ablauf. *Deutsche Tierärztliche Wochenschrift* 87:27–31.

Nutbrown M, Randall VA. 1995. Differences between connective tissue-epithelial junctions in human skin and the anagen hair follicle. *Journal of Investigative Dermatology* 104:90–94.

Pascucci L, Mercati F, Gargiulo AM, Pedini V, Sorbolini S, Ceccarelli P. 2006. CD34 glycoprotein identifies putative stem cells located in the isthmic region of canine hair follicles. *Veterinary Dermatology* 17:244–251.

Pascucci L, Pedini V, Parillo F, Gargiulo AM. 2005. Apoptotic cell death in canine hair follicle. *Histology and Histopathology* 20:1–9.

Paus R, Peters EMJ, Eichmüller S, Botchkarev VA. 1997. Neural mechanisms of hair growth control. *Journal of Investigative Dermatology Symposium Proceedings* 2:61–68.

Pena JC, Kelekar A, Fuchs EV, Thompson CB. 1999. Manipulation of outer root sheath cell survival perturbs the hair growth cycle. *EMBO Journal* 18:3596–3603.

Priestley GC, Rudall KM. 1965. Modifications in the Huxley layer associated with changes in fibre diameter and output. In: Lyne AG, Short BF (eds), *Biology of the Skin and Hair Growth*, pp. 165–170. Sidney: Angus & Robertson.

Raushenbach YO. 1972. Disturbances of seasonal rhythm of adaptive changes in animals under domestication. *Journal of Interdisciplinary Cycle Research* 3:166.

Raushenbach YO, Prasalova LA. 1973. The disturbance of adaptive rhythm of seasonal changes during domestication of animals in the U.S.S.R. *Journal of Interdisciplinary Cycle Research* 4:369–377.

Rogers GE. 2006. Biology of the wool follicle: an excursion into a unique tissue interaction system waiting to be re-discovered. *Experimental Dermatology* 15:931–940.

Ryder ML. 1958. Follicle arrangement in skin from wild sheep, primitive domestic sheep and in parchment. *Nature* 182:781–783.

Ryder ML. 1962. The histological examination of skin in the study of the domestication of sheep. *Zeitschrift für Tierzüchtung und Züchtungsbiologie* 77:168–171.

Ryder ML. 1976. Seasonal changes in the coat of the cat. *Research in Veterinary Science* 21:280–283.

Schwarz R, Le Roux JMW, Neurand K. 1976. Lichtmikroskopische Untersuchungen an der Haut der Katze. Verteilung, Anordnung und Morphologie der Haare bzw. Haarfollikel. *Zentralblatt für Veterinärmedizin Reihe C* 5:325–341.

Schwarz R, Meyer W. 1994. Haut und Hautorgane. In: Frewein J, Vollmerhaus B (eds), *Anatomie von Hund und Katze*, pp. 316–340. Berlin: Blackwell.

Schwarz R, Sağlam M, Tanyolaç A, Asti R, Özcan Z, Meyer W. 1991. Mikroskopische Untersuchungen an der Haut der Türkischen Angoraziege. II. Funktionelle Morphologie der Haarfollikel. *Deutsche Tierärztliche Wochenschrift* 98:297–303.

Slominski A, Wortsman J, Plonka PM, Schallreuter KU, Paus R, Tobin DJ. 2005. Hair follicle pigmentation. *Journal of Investigative Dermatology* 124:13–21.

Straile WE. 1965. Root sheath—dermal papilla relationships and the control of hair growth. In: Lyne AG, Short BF (eds),

Biology of the Skin and Hair Growth, pp. 35–57. Sidney: Angus & Robertson.

Tiede S, Kloepper JE, Bodò E, Tiwari S, Kruse C, Paus R. 2007. Hair follicle stem cells: walking the maze. *European Journal of Cell Biology* 86:355–376.

Todini L. 2007. Thyroid hormones in small ruminants: effects of endogenous environmental and nutritional factors. *Animal* 1:997–1008.

Tsukise A, Meyer W. 1983. Histochemistry of complex carbohydrates in the hairy skin of the domestic pig. *Histochemical Journal* 15:845–860.

Turner HG, Nay T, French GT. 1962. The hair follicle population of cattle in relation to breed and body weight. *Australian Journal of Agricultural Research* 13:960–973.

Villar D, McMillen SR, Dicks P, Rhind SM. 2000. The roles of thyroid hormones and prolactin in the control of fibre moult and associated changes in hair follicle activities in cashmere goats. *Australian Journal of Agricultural Research* 51:407–414.

Whitbread LA, Powell BC. 1998. Expression of the intermediate filament keratin gene, K15, in the basal cell layers of epithelia and the hair follicle. *Experimental Cell Research* 244:448–459.

Yeates TM. 1955. Photoperiodicity in cattle. I. Seasonal changes in coat character and their importance in heat regulation. *Australian Journal of Agricultural Research* 6:891–902.

Part 2

How to approach alopecic diseases

2.1

Clinical aspects

Monika Linek

Abnormalities of the hair coat are usually recognized by the owners of an animal early in the course of the disease. Alopecia (i.e., absence of hair in an area, where it is normally present) or hypotrichosis (i.e., a partial hair loss or abnormal thinning of the hair coat) may represent a mere cosmetic problem with no risk to the patient, or it may be a manifestation of an internal disease with potentially serious consequences. Therefore, a methodical approach and accurate diagnosis are prerequisites for successful management of these cases.

The diagnostic approach to alopecia in general is similar in all species and species specificities will only be mentioned where necessary. An overview on the most important alopecic diseases in dogs and cats can be found in Tables 2.1.1–2.1.3.

2.1.1 Breed

Many alopecic diseases have only been observed in a subset of breeds. It is therefore crucial to consider breed-specific diseases when dealing with alopecia.

Breeds with congenital or hereditary alopecia syndromes in cats are Sphinx and Canadian Hairless (see Section 3.1.2.2.5), Burmese, Birman, Devon Rex, and Siamese. Hairless dog breeds are Chinese Crested, Mexican Hairless, Inca, and Peruvian Hairless (see Section 3.1.2.1). In cattle, congenital alopecia has been described to occur in various breeds, with some forms being associated with early postnatal mortality (see Section 3.1.2).

Follicular lipidosis has so far only been described in Rottweilers (see Section 3.1.2.4.5), whereas color dilution alopecia and its subtype black hair follicular dysplasia have been observed in various breeds (see Section 3.1.2). Color dilution alopecia has a particularly high incidence in the Doberman Pinscher, whereas black hair follicle dysplasia occurs commonly in Yorkshire Terriers. Other breed-specific canine alopecias that are not color-linked have been described in breeds such as Curly-Coated Retrievers (see Section 3.3.9.4), Irish Water Spaniels (see Section 3.3.9.1), Portuguese Water Dogs (see Section 3.3.9.2), Siberian Huskies and Alaskan Malamutes (see Section 3.3.9.7), Greyhounds (see Section 3.3.9.5), and Chesapeake Bay Retrievers (see Section 3.3.9.3).

In small breeds such as Poodles, Dachshunds, and Terriers, hyperadrenocorticism is the most often seen endocrinopathy (see Section 3.3.2), whereas hypothyroidism (see Section 3.3.1) is more common in various large breed dogs. Alopecia X has been reported in plush-coated dogs such as Pomeranian and Chow Chow, in Miniature Poodles, and in some of the Nordic breeds like the Samoyed, Alaskan Malamute, and Keeshond (see Section 3.3.4.). Acquired pattern alopecia is most common in Manchester Terriers, Miniature Pinschers, Dachshund, Whippet, Italian Greyhound, and Greyhound, as well as the Boston Terrier (see Section 3.3.8). Cyclic recurrent flank alopecia is seen in the Doberman Pinscher, Boxer, Airedale Terrier, and Rhodesian Rigdgeback (see Section 3.3.5).

Even some inflammatory alopecias show breed predilections like demodicosis (see Section 4.1.3) in the short-coated dog breeds (Pugs, Boxers, Terriers) or sebaceous adenitis in Akita Inus, Poodles, Vizslas, and Hovawarts.

2.1.2 History

Taking a profound patient history before the clinical examination is a vital step in the diagnostic process. Important points to consider are breed, age of onset,

Table 2.1.1 Diseases with inflammatory alopecia in the dog, their incidence, and their most important diagnostic procedure

Disease	Incidence	Diagnostic procedures
Alopecia areata	Rare	Biopsy, trichogram
Demodicosis	Common	Deep skin scraping, trichogram
Dermatomyositis	Rare, most common in Collies and Shelties	Biopsy
Dermatophytosis	Common in rural areas	Wood's lamp, trichogram, culture
Drug reaction	Rare	Cytology, biopsy
Eosinophilic folliculitis	Rare	Cytology, biopsy
Epitheliotropic lymphoma	Rare	Cytology, biopsy
Granulomatous mural folliculitis	Very rare	Biopsy
Leishmaniasis	Common in endemic areas	Cytology, FNA LN/BM, serology, PCR, biopsy
Pemphigus foliaceus	Rare	Cytology, biopsy
Post rabies alopecia	Quite rare	Clinical presentation and history, biopsy
Pyoderma	Common	Cytology, microbiology
Scaring alopecia	Very rare	Biopsy
Sebaceous adenitis	Rare	Biopsy, trichogram
Traction alopecia	Rare	History, biopsy

FNA LN/BM, fine needle aspiration of lymph nodes or bone marrow; PCR, polymerase chain reaction.

Table 2.1.2 Diseases with noninflammatory alopecia in the dog, their incidence, and their most important diagnostic procedure

Disease	Incidence	Diagnostic procedures
Alopecia X	Common in certain breeds	Exclusion of any endocrinopathy, biopsy
Anagen effluvium	Very rare	History, biopsy
Black hair follicular dysplasia	Common in certain breeds	Biopsy
Color dilution alopecia	Common in certain breeds	Trichogram, biopsy
Corticosteroid-induced alopecia	Common	ACTH stimulation test
Cyclic recurrent flank alopecia	Certain breeds	History, biopsy
Ectodermal dysplasia	Very rare	History, age, biopsy
Follicular lipidosis	Very rare, only in Rottweilers	Biopsy
Hyperadrenocorticism	Common in old dogs	Urin C/C, ACTH stimulation test, LDDST, ultrasound, CT/MRI,
Hypothyroidism	Common only in certain breeds	tT4/TSH, rhTSH stimulation test, TgAA, T4/T3 autoantibodies, ultrasound
Other breed-specific non-color-linked alopecias	In certain breeds only	Biopsy
Pattern baldness	Certain breeds	History, clinical features, biopsy
Post-clipping alopecia	Rare	History, clinical features, biopsy
Hyperestrogenism	Rare	Ultrasound estradiol/testosterone ratio
Telogen effluvium	Rare	History, clinical features

Urine C/C, urine cortisol/creatinin ratio; LDDST, low-dose dexamethasone suppression test; CT/MRI, computed tomography/magnetic resonance imaging; tT4, total T4; TSH, thyroid-stimulation hormone; rhTSH, recombinant human TSH; TgAA, thyroglobulin autoantibodies.

sex, environment, previous illnesses, progression of alopecia, response to treatment, and transmission to other animals or owners (Table 2.1.4).

2.1.2.1 Age of onset

The age when alopecia first occurred can be helpful for the diagnosis. Symmetrical noninflammatory alopecia during the first year of life is suggestive of ectodermal or follicular dysplasia, dysplasia of the hair follicle pigmentary unit (see Chapter 3.1) or a congenital endocrinopathy such as congenital hypothyroidism (see Section 3.3.1). Acquired hypothyroidism (see Section 3.3.1) is a disease of the young to middle-aged dog, whereas hyperadrenocorticism (see Section 3.3.2) occurs in the middle-aged to old dog. In contrast,

Table 2.1.3 Alopecic diseases in the cat, their incidence, and their most important diagnostic procedure

Disease	Incidence	Diagnostic procedure
Alopecia areata*	Very rare	Biopsy
Congenital alopecia	Very rare	Age, history, biopsy
Demodicosis	Rare	Deep skin scraping
Dermatophytosis	Very common	Wood's lamp, trichogram, dermatophyte culture
Ectoparasites/fleas	Very common	Combing, skin scraping, trial therapy
Exfoliative dermatitis	Rare	Biopsy
Follicular mucinosis	Very rare	Biopsy
Hyperadrenocorticism, iatrogenic	Rare	History, blood chemistry, ACTH stimulation test
Hyperadrenocorticism, spontaneous	Rare	Urin C/C, HDDT, ACTH stimulation test
Hypersensitivity	Common	Exclusion of other skin diseases, biopsy
Hypothyroidism	Rare	fT4, tT4, TSH
Lymphocytic mural folliculitis	Very rare	Biopsy
Paraneoplastic alopecia	Very rare	Biopsy
Pemphigus foliaceus	Rare	Cytology, biopsy
Pseudopelade (isthmic folliculitis)	Very rare	Biopsy
Pyoderma	Common	Cytology, microbiology
Psychogenic alopecia	Rare	Exclusion of other skin diseases, biopsy
Self-induced alopecia	Very common	Trichogram, history
Telogen effluvium	Rare	History, clinical examination

Urine C/C, urine cortisol/creatinin ratio; HDDT, high-dose dexamethasone suppression test; tT4, total T4; fT4, free T4; TSH, thyroid-stimulation hormone.
*, a disease with similarities to alopecia areata but without known pathogenesis.

inflammatory alopecia (see Part 4) with marked pruritus can occur at any age.

2.1.2.2 Sex and reproductive history

Male dogs with estrogen-producing testicular tumors and subsequent hyperestrogenism (see Section 3.3.3) may have a history of signs suggesting feminization (attractiveness to male dogs, gynecomastia, pendulous prepuce). Prolonged estrus has been reported in bitches with ovarian disorders and hyperestrogenism, whereas anestrus has been reported in bitches with hyperadrenocorticism (see Section 3.3.2) and hypothyroidism (see Section 3.3.1). Except for the dog, sex hormone-related alopecias are rare or do not exist. Although symmetrical alopecia of the trunk in cats has been associated with a sex hormone imbalance (since it responds to progesterone), most of these cases are in fact self-induced alopecias, and the response is likely explained by the immunomodulating effect of progesterone.

2.1.2.3 Signs of internal disease

Many endocrine diseases that affect the skin are associated with clinical signs that suggest interference with other organ systems. For example, owners of dogs with hyperadrenocorticism often report polyuria, polydipsia, and polyphagia (see Section 3.3.2.1). Cats with hyperadrenocorticism may develop diabetes mellitus (see Section 3.3.2.3). In canine hypothyroidism, the owner may describe signs that reflect the slowing of cellular metabolism, such as lethargy and weight gain. Most paraneoplastic syndromes will also be associated with signs of internal disease.

Table 2.1.4 Important anamnestic questions for alopecic skin diseases in domestic animals

At what age has hair loss started?
Are siblings or parents affected?
Are other animals or humans affected?
Does your pet scratch, lick, chew, or rub at the alopecic area?
Is progression of alopecia waxing and waning or does it progress continuously?
Is the severity of alopecia changing with the season?
Are there any other physical complaints, previous illnesses or signs of systemic illness?
Has there been a recent surgical intervention, blood loss or pregnancy?
What medications are currently being given or have recently been given?

2.1.2.4 *Progression of alopecia*

Seasonal or cyclic episodes of noninflammatory symmetrical truncal alopecia followed by spontaneous hair regrowth are typical of canine recurrent flank alopecia (see Section 3.3.5). Spontaneous regrowth, however, can also be seen in alopecia of the Portuguese Water Dog (see Section 3.3.9.2). Alopecia areata may spontaneously resolve and regrow white hair (see Chapter 4.7), whereas most endocrinopathies and inflammatory disorders tend to be progressive without intermittent remission.

2.1.2.5 *Stressful events*

Telogen effluvium is a transient disorder of excessive hair shedding, resulting from a synchronous cessation of hair growth. It usually follows pregnancy, lactation, severe illness, or a similar stressful event that has occurred 1–3 months earlier. Burns or scalds can be followed by alopecia developing only days after the insult.

2.1.2.6 *Drug administration and response to treatment*

The clinician confronted with an alopecic patient should enquire about previous drug administration. Long-term glucocorticoid therapy may cause iatrogenic hyperadrenocorticism and hair cycle arrest in most animals and is very well known in the dog (see Section 3.3.2.2). Estrogens (see Section 3.3.3) and cytotoxic drugs, such as cyclophosphamide (see Section 3.4.1), may as well interfere with hair growth. In horses and large animals, acaricides and chemicals are often used as topicals and may induce irritant alopecia. Focal alopecia may develop as a response to injections, especially rabies vaccines (see Section 3.4.3). In addition, the response or the lack of response to previous therapy is helpful in the diagnostic process; for example, failure of hair regrowth after 3–5 months of thyroxin supplementation at an appropriate dosage excludes hypothyroidism as the cause of alopecia.

2.1.2.7 *Nutrition*

In small-animal practice, alopecia due to nutritional deficiencies is uncommon nowadays in most countries, but in horses and cattle copper, selenium and zinc deficiencies can change hair quality and quantity (see Section 3.2.1).

2.1.3 Clinical examination of hair coat and skin

After taking a history, the close examination of the whole integument is the next step. Alopecia may be a feature of a myriad of skin diseases, if infectious diseases and alopecia caused by marked pruritus are included. Therefore, the clinical examination should first focus on signs of follicular inflammation and infection and should differentiate them from noninflammatory diseases. In addition, the clinician should watch out for signs that are specific for some dermatoses: erythema, papules, pustules, thickening of the skin or lichenification, self-traumatizing recognized by broken hairs, excoriations, erosions, and ulcerations are all suggestive of an inflammatory process with pruritus (see Section 3.5.2). Thinning of the skin with prominent subcutaneous vessels or calcium deposits along dermal collagen fibers known as calcinosis cutis are pathognomonic in hyperadrenocorticism (see Section 3.3.2), whereas hypothyroidism is often accompanied by thickened and hyperpigmented skin without inflammation (see Section 3.3.1). In canine recurrent flank alopecia the affected area of skin is well demarcated, hyperpigmented, and feels cold (see Section 3.3.5).

2.1.3.1 *Coat color change*

Color dilution alopecia should be strongly suspected if the dog has a dilute coat color (Fig. 3.1.20). Black hair follicular dysplasia should be considered if the alopecia is confined to black (or dark)-haired areas (see Section 3.1.2.4.1); these two diseases usually develop during the first year of life. A color-linked alopecia has also been described in the Appaloosa horse. A lightening of the coat color (leukotrichia) is not uncommon in dogs with hyperadrenocorticism. Changes in coat color and coat quality are also seen in many of the canine breed-specific hair cycle abnormalities. In Dalmatians the formerly called Bronzing Syndrome due to multiple brown spots over the rump is now recognized as folliculitis and furunculosis. A regrowth of white hair where the hair coat has formerly been

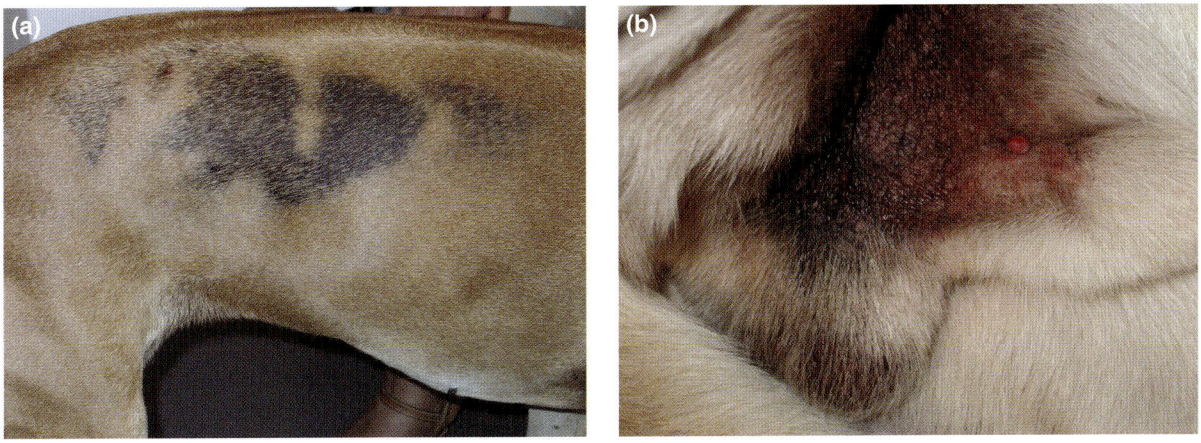

Fig. 2.1.1 Hyperpigmentation versus lichenification. (a) Hyperpigmentation without lichenification as a consequence of chronic alopecia in a dog with recurrent flank alopecia; (b) hyperpigmentation with lichenification of the skin due to chronic inflammation.

pigmented is suggestive for alopecia areata (see Chapter 4.7). The presence of miniaturized fine hairs in dogs is a key feature in pattern alopecia (see Section 3.3.8). Coat color change to brown is a hallmark of licking, especially in white dogs.

2.1.3.2 *Skin color change*

Intense hyperpigmentation of the alopecic areas is most commonly seen in dogs with recurrent cyclic flank alopecia (Fig. 3.3.21) and alopecia X (Fig. 3.3.16). However, hyperpigmentation is also seen in response to chronic inflammation often accompanied by lichenification. A careful examination should be able to distinguish inflammatory from noninflammatory hyperpigmentation (Fig. 2.1.1). Depigmentation will occur in scars.

2.1.3.3 *Pattern of hair loss*

The pattern of the hair loss such as focal, multifocal, moth-eaten, symmetric or asymmetric should be noticed, and is best recorded in a scheme. Schemes allow to document the progress of the disease (improvement or progression). Although the pattern only allows for a crude differentiation, infectious alopecias generally develop a more asymmetric, multifocal, sometimes moth-eaten pattern, whereas endocrine alopecias and other hair cycle abnormalities are more symmetric in pattern. Allergies may however also present with bilaterally symmetric alopecia.

2.1.4 Laboratory examination

Laboratory tests are required for a definitive diagnosis in most cases of alopecia.

2.1.4.1 *Forced combing*

Forced combing and subsequent microscopic examination of the collected hairs is a simple procedure to determine increased shedding, but it is not a very sensitive test as most animals shed more intensively under stressful conditions. Under physiologic conditions, the hair is shed in telogen only, that is the resting stage of the follicle. Shedding of anagen hair is always considered a pathologic finding because anagen presents the often together with proliferating stage of the follicle. Superficial parasites such as lice and fur mites are also easily detected with this examination technique.

2.1.4.2 *Hair plucking*

Hair plucking can evaluate if hairs are easily epilated. Microscopic examination of plucked hairs mounted onto a glass slide with mineral oil (Fig. 2.1.2) can be used to search for *Demodex* mites (Fig. 2.1.3) and arthospores of dermatophytes within or along the hair shaft (Fig. 2.1.4). Abnormal cycling of hair follicles can be detected by an altered ratio of anagen to telogen hairs. If keratinous debris is complicating the examination, the plucked hairs can be premixed with

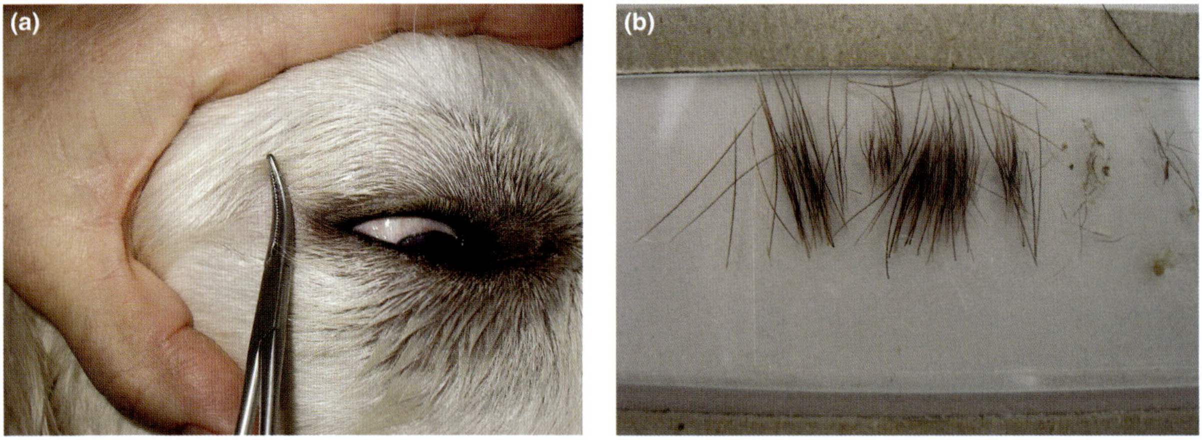

Fig. 2.1.2 Hair pull test. (a) Hairs are harvested using a surgical hemostat; (b) pulled hair shafts are mounted onto a glass slide with mineral oil.

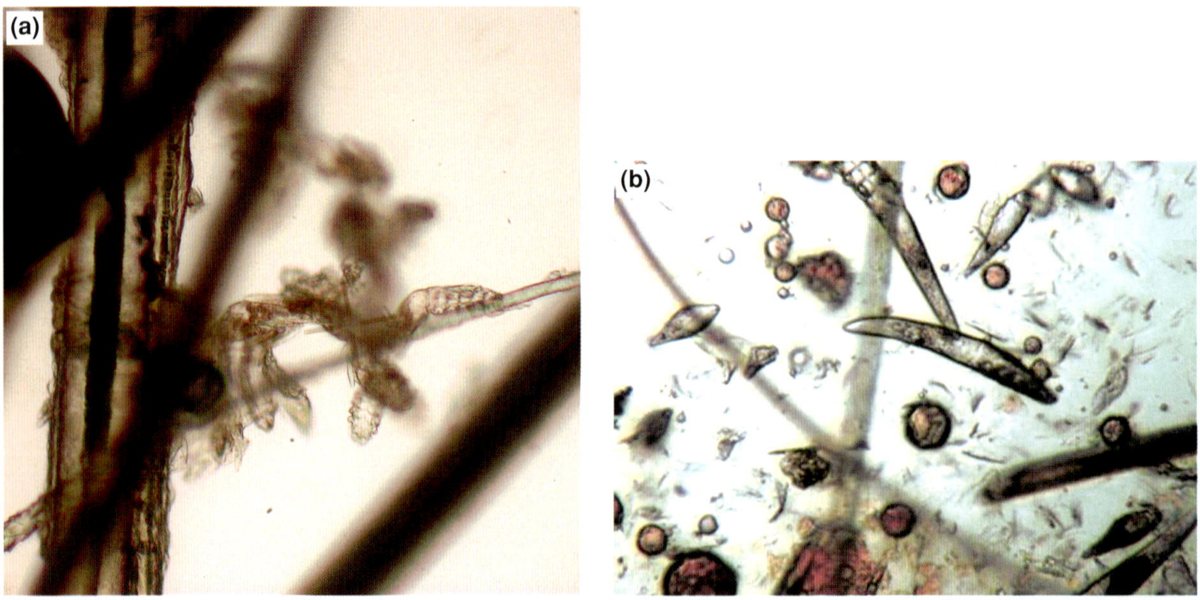

Fig. 2.1.3 Hair pluck test in canine demodicosis. (a) numerous *Demodex* mites along with hair shafts; (b) higher magnification demonstrates morphological characteristics of eggs, larvae, nymphs and adult *Demodex* mites (Courtesy of C. Nett)

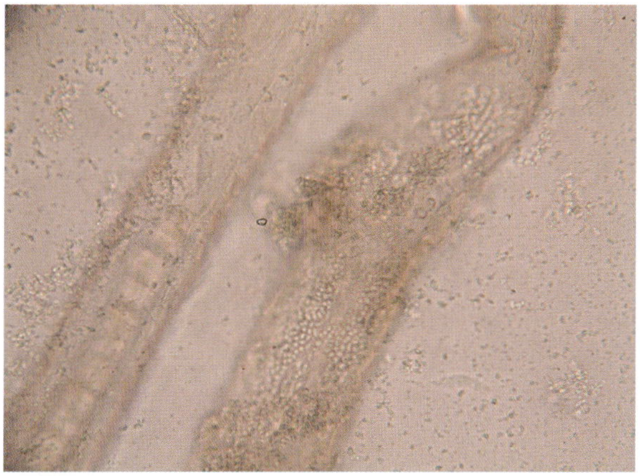

Fig. 2.1.4 Trichogram of canine dermatophytosis with numerous arthrospores along the hair shaft. (Courtesy of C. Nett.)

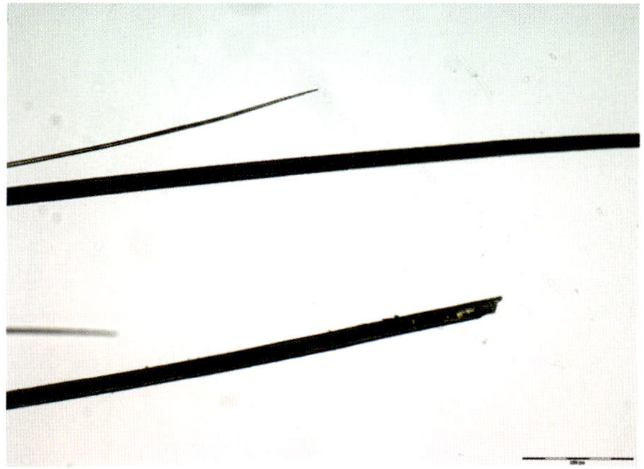

Fig. 2.1.6 Trichogram from a dog with broken hair shafts. Note the split ends.

potassium hydroxide. It is important to wait for 20 min or warm the slide up to clear the debris before examining the slide under a microscope.

2.1.4.3 Trichogram

Under physiologic conditions a trichogram will reveal hair shafts in anagen and in telogen. Some dog breeds, however, will show very high numbers of telogen hair follicles. In telogen effluvium (see Section 3.3.6.) or other hair cycle arrests there is a remarkable shift toward telogen follicles. A hair pluck will show a disproportional increase of telogen fibers with club-shaped proximal ends (Fig. 2.1.5). In dermatophytosis the hair shaft may reveal hyphae or arthroconidia, but their absence does not exclude dermatophytosis (see Section 4.1.2) (Fig. 2.1.4).

Looking microscopically at the hair tips of plucked hairs may help to differentiate broken hair shafts or split ends from the fine-peaked ends of normal hairs (Fig. 2.1.6). This is often the best way to diagnose alopecia due to licking especially in the cat (see Section 3.5.1). Furthermore, the hair shaft and hair bulb can reveal clumped melanin and thus will draw attention toward color dilution alopecia or black hair follicular dysplasia (see Section 3.1.2.4) (Fig. 2.1.7). Pili torti, trichoptilosis, and other trichomalacias are detected during this step of examination. There are anecdotal

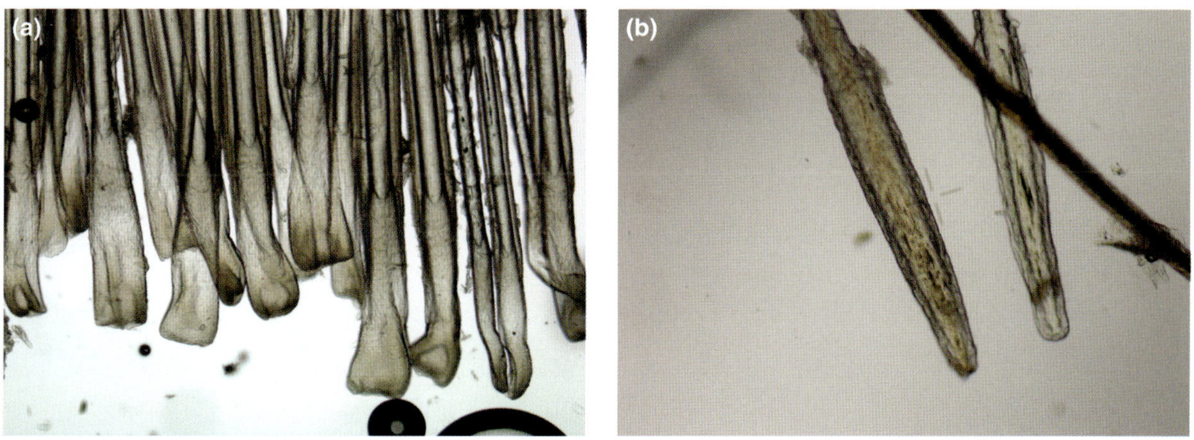

Fig. 2.1.5 Trichogram from a dog. (a) Anagen hair shafts; (b) telogen hair shafts.

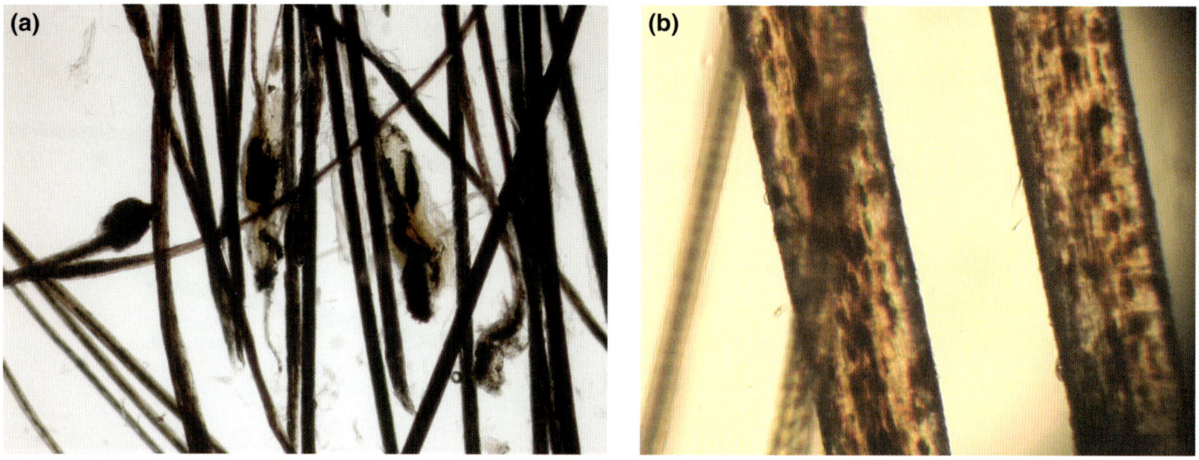

Fig. 2.1.7 Trichograms of canine black hair follicle dysplasia. (a) Melanin clumping and distortion of the hair bulb; (b) irregular pigmentation within the hair shafts.

reports that in alopecia areata the plucked hair bulbs have the shape of an exclamation point (see Chapter 4.7) (Fig. 2.1.4).

2.1.4.4 Wood's light examination

Wood's light examination is opportune, whenever dermatophytosis is on the list of differentials. The lamp has to be warmed up for at least 5–10 min before examination. The patient should be examined with the lamp in a dark room for at least 5 min. Hairs invaded by *Microsporum canis* may show a yellow-green fluorescence running along the hair shafts (Fig. 2.1.8). These hairs should be collected for culture and microscopic examination. It is important that a lack of fluorescence does not rule out dermatophytosis. The interpretation is sometimes difficult, and false-positive fluorescence due to creams or bacterial crusts is common. *M. canis* is the only fluorescing dermatophyte that is relevant in veterinary medicine.

2.1.4.5 Dermatophyte culture

A fungal culture on selective dermatophyte test medium (DTM) and Sabouraud's dextrose agar is necessary for the final diagnosis of dermatophytosis (see Section 4.1.2). Hairs and scales from the edge of a lesion should be collected and slightly pressed onto the culture medium. If the lesions are more widespread, the McKenzie toothbrush method is advisable, in which scales and loose hairs are caught by brushing the entire body with a sterile toothbrush. Cultures should be incubated between 25 and 30°C at 30% humidity in a dark environment and must be

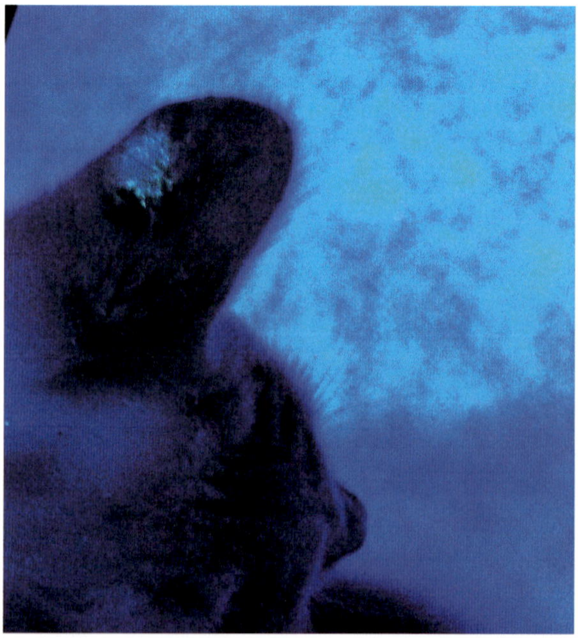

Fig. 2.1.8 Wood's lamp examination with fluorescent hair shafts in *Microsporum canis* infection of a cat.

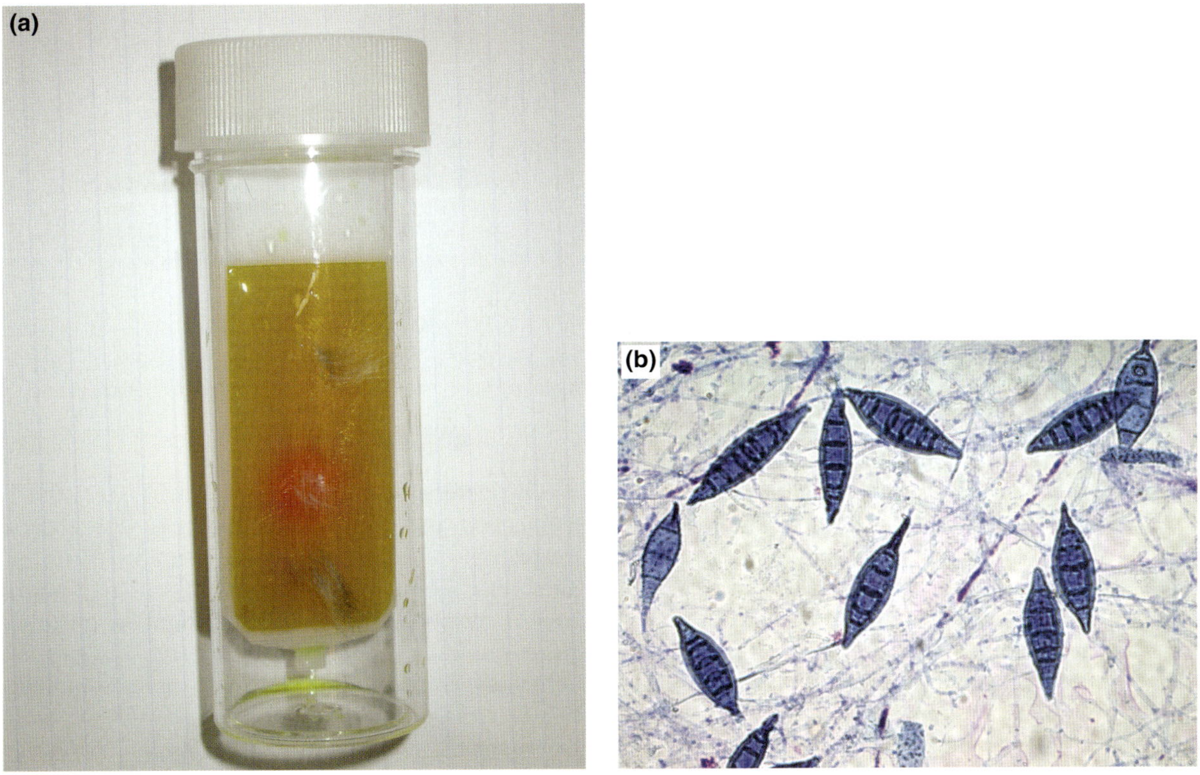

Fig. 2.1.9 Dermatophyte colony growing on a DTM agar. (a) Red discoloration around the colony; (b) cytology of the colony shows macroconidia of *Microsporum canis*.

evaluated daily. The DTM medium has to be checked for color change, which occurs before the growth of the colony. After a colony has grown, a tape strip is pressed onto the colony and mounted onto a slide. The colony is stained with lactophenol blue or methylene blue and examined microscopically for characteristic macroconidia (Fig. 2.1.9). Due to common false-positive and false-negative results with in-house cultures, it is recommend to send samples for dermatophyte culture to a specialized laboratory.

2.1.4.6 Deep skin scraping

In the dog, a deep skin scraping is warranted in most cases of alopecia to rule out demodicosis. The skin at different areas is squeezed thoroughly and then scraped with a scalpel blade covered with mineral oil until some blood is appearing in the orifices of hair follicles. The scraped material is mounted onto a slide with mineral oil and examined under the microscope (×100). *Demodex* mites and their eggs are easily detected (see Section 4.1.3).

2.1.4.7 Superficial skin scraping

Superficial skin scrapings for mite infestation as *Sarcoptes*, *Notoedres*, *Otodectes*, *Cheyletiella*, *Chorioptes*, and *Psoroptes* species are necessary if alopecia is a sequela to severe pruritus. Superficial skin scrapings have to be carried out over a large area of the skin. The mineral oil is applied directly to the skin, scraped off with a scalpel blade, and transferred to glass slides. The samples have to be systematically examined under low power (×40).

2.1.4.8 Cytology

Cytology will be needed in any alopecia with signs of inflammation. The sampling technique varies according to the lesion and is only briefly explained here.

Skin scrapings for cytology are done without oil. The gently sampled material is spread out on a slide and might need heat fixation before staining. This technique is especially useful for very dry skin or for material that is collected from around the nails.

The most commonly used technique is the impression smear, where a slide is gently pressed onto the affected skin. It might be necessary to either remove the overlying crust with the edge of the slide or to open the pustle or bulla before sampling.

Tape preparations are direct impressions using a clear sticky tape to collect debris from the surface of the skin. This technique is useful for a quick examination for *Malassezia* or infectious agents, but remains a crude technique for the evaluation of cells.

Fine-needle aspirations are used in nodular lesions. Cells are collected by a 22-gauge needle with or without an attached 10-mL syringe (the negative pressure of the syringe may increase the yield of cells). The skin is preferably disinfected before the procedure. The gathered material is placed on a glass slide and a smear is made by laying another glass slide on top of the material and pulling the slides apart to spread it. All cytology preparations have to be air-dried and stained. Modified Wright's stains such as DiffQuick® or Hemacolor® are fast and easy to apply stains that allow sufficient evaluation of most cytology samples.

Cytology can reveal definite signs of pyoderma such as neutrophils with intracellular bacteria (Fig. 2.1.10) or *Malassezia* (Fig. 2.1.11). Some cells are suggestive for specific skin diseases. Acantholytic keratinocytes

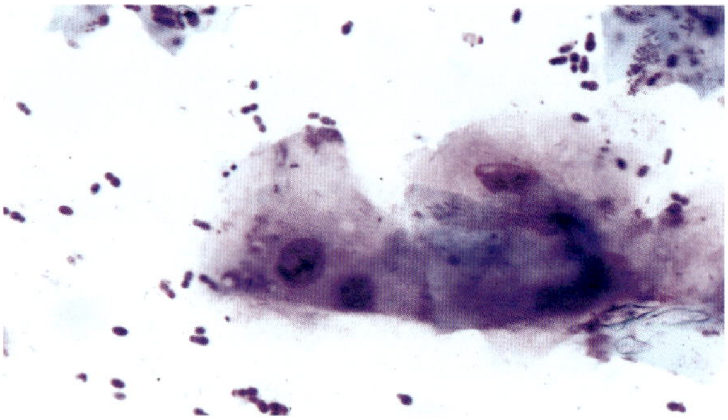

Fig. 2.1.11 Cytology of canine *Malassezia* dermatitis. Nucleated keratinocytes surrounded by numerous budding yeasts.

are keratinocytes, that have lost their intercellular connection and present as round cells with a dark purple central nucleus. They are encountered in the pemphigus complex (see Chapter 4.3). Large numbers of eosinophils are seen in eosinophilic pustulosis, eosinophilic folliculits/furunculosis, allergies, or with ectoparasites (Fig. 2.1.12). In noneosinophilic furunculosis, a more mixed type of infiltrate with macrophages, neutrophils and eosinophils is found. Giant cells suggest dermatophytes, mycobacteria, or foreign bodies (Fig. 2.1.13). Further examinations such as biopsies and cultures are warranted for definitive diagnosis in these cases.

Alopecias caused by marked pruritus after exclusion or effective treatment of infectious diseases will need the approach of pruritic skin diseases, which is

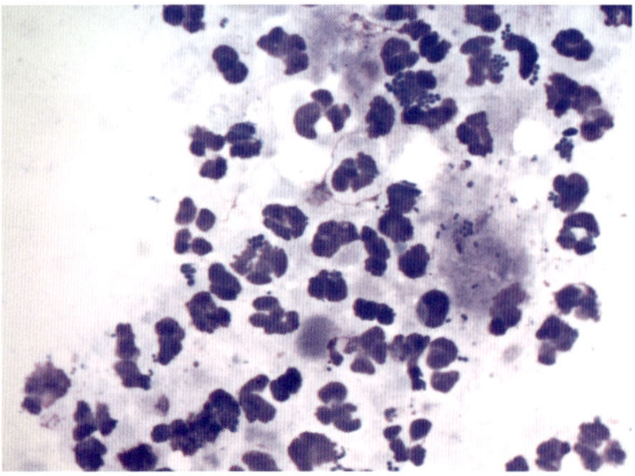

Fig. 2.1.10 Cytology of canine pyoderma with neutrophils, macrophages, and intracellular cocci.

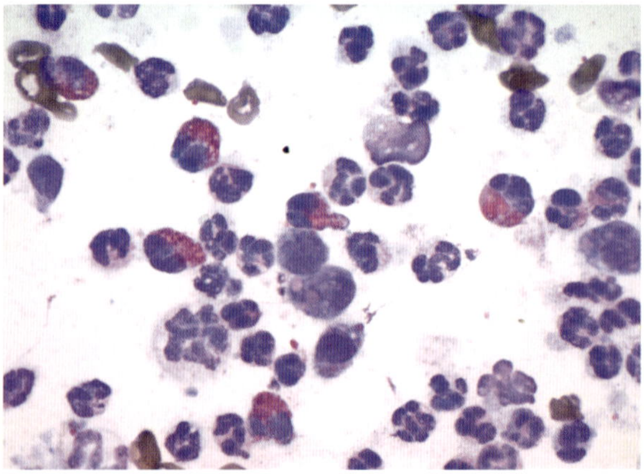

Fig. 2.1.12 Cytology of eosinophilic folliculitis in a dog. Numerous eosinophils admixed with neutrophils and lymphocytes.

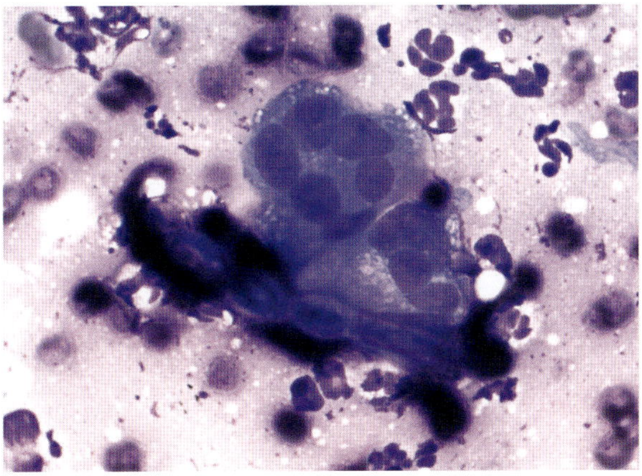

Fig. 2.1.13 Cytology of a dermatomycosis. Multinucleated giant cells surrounding fungal hyphae.

explained in many textbooks on veterinary dermatology.

2.1.4.9 Hematology, clinical chemistry and urinalysis

Further laboratory tests such as a complete hematology profile, a biochemical screen and urinalysis should be obtained, if internal or endocrine diseases are suspected. The laboratory findings may support a diagnosis of a particular endocrine disease, and specific hormone assays can then be performed as indicated. For most of the relevant hormones special assays are available but in many cases dynamic tests of endocrine function are required, as basal hormone levels may fluctuate widely in response to physiologic and pathologic factors (Table 2.1.5).

2.1.4.10 Skin biopsy

Biopsies offer the most valuable information in alopecic diseases, if the clinical findings are not sufficient to pinpoint the disease (see Chapter 2.2). It is important to form a differential list before taking the biopsy, as this will enable the clinician to choose the correct location and primary lesions to get the most specific histopathologic result. A thorough differential list will additionally help the pathologist to interpret the morphological findings.

Punch biopsies for alopecia should have a minimum size of 8 mm. With the exception of nodules, no surgical preparation is needed. General anesthesia

Table 2.1.5 Clinical pathology abnormalities in canine endocrinopathies

Disease	Hemogram	Serum biochemistry	Urinalysis	Hormone assays
Hypothyroidism	Normocytic, normochromic, nonregenerative anemia	Hypercholesterolemia Hypertriglyceridemia Slight ALT elevation Elevated fructosamine	Normal	tT4, TSH, fT4 (dialysis) TgAA rhTSH stimulation test TRH stimulation test
Hyperadrenocorticism	Leukocytosis Neutrophilia Lymphopenia Eosinopenia Thrombocytosis	Elevated ALP Moderately elevated ALT Hypercholesterolemia Hyperlipemia Decreased BUN	Specific gravity < 1.015 Elevated urine C/C Bacteriuria	LDDST ACTH stimulation test
Hyperestrogenism (males)	Nonregenerative anemia Leukopenia with lymphocytosis thrombocytopenia	Normal	Normal	Normal estrogens Elevated estrogen/ testosterone ratio
Alopecia X	Normal	Normal	Mostly normal, elevated long-term urine C/C	Mostly normal High concentrations of 17OH-progesterone before and/or post ACTH

Urine C/C, urine cortisol/creatinin ratio; tT4, total T4; fT4, free T4; TgAA, thyroglobulin autoantibodies; TSH, thyroid stimulating hormone; rhTSH, recombinant human; TRH, thyreotropin releasing hormone; BUN, blood urea nitrogen; LDDST, low-dose dexamethasone suppression test.

is rarely indicated except for biopsies of the nose, footpads, ears, or digits. Local anesthesia with 1 mL lidocain, xylocain, or prilocain for each biopsy location is sufficient in most cases. To avoid disturbance of morphological findings in the biopsy, it is important to enter the needle outside the proposed biopsy area and to administer the agent subcutaneously. Allow 3–5 min for the local anesthetic to have effect.

Before fixation, biopsies should be handled with great care in order to avoid squeezing defects or artifacts. A biopsy is most valuable before treatment and as long as the disease is in an acute phase. In later stages of the disease morphological findings are often less specific, and the original cause of hair loss might not be evaluated. Corticoids should be discontinued for at least 4 weeks before biopsies are taken.

2.1.4.11 Microbiological culture

If a deep inflammatory process is suggested, sterile biopsies for tissue culture should be obtained. Surgical preparation of the biopsy site as well as sterile collection of the biopsy is mandatory. The biopsy is then cut in half. One half is fixed in formalin for histopathology. The other half is sent to a laboratory for microbiological culture. The epidermis is best cut off to avoid further contamination from superficial bacteria. For shipping, the sample is then pressed either into a culture medium or is put into a small sterile bottle where it is placed on a cotton wool drenched with saline. The samples should be examined for aerobic and anaerobic bacteria. Further special cultures have to be discussed with the laboratory depending on the suggested type of infection.

Further reading

Campbell GA, Sauber L. 2007. Getting the most from dermatopathology. *Veterinary Clinics of North America Small Animal Practice* 37(2):393–402.

Frank LA. 2006. Comparative dermatology—canine endocrine dermatoses. *Clinics in Dermatology* 24(4):317–325.

Gross TL, Ihrke PJ, Walder EJ, Affolter VK. 2005. *Skin Diseases of the Dog and Cat: Clinical and Histopathologic Diagnosis*, 2nd edn. Oxford: Blackwell Science.

Linder KE. 2001. Skin biopsy site selection in small animal dermatology with an introduction to histologic pattern-analysis of inflammatory skin lesions. *Clinical Techniques in Small Animal Practice* 16(4):207–213.

Mecklenburg L. 2006. An overview on congenital alopecia in domestic animals. *Veterinary Dermatology* 17(6):393–410.

Mendelsohn C, Rosenkrantz W, Griffin CE. 2006. Practical cytology for inflammatory skin diseases. *Clinical Techniques in Small Animal Practice* 21(3):117–127.

Noxon JO. 1995. Diagnostic procedures in feline dermatology. *Veterinary Clinics of North America Small Animal Practice* 25(4):779–799.

Scott DW, Miller WH, Griffin CE. 2000. *Muller and Kirk's Small Animal Dermatology*, 6th edn. Philadelphia: WB Saunders.

Shelly SM. 2003. Cutaneous lesions. *Veterinary Clinics of North America Small Animal Practice* 33(1):1–46.

2.2

Histopathological aspects

Lars Mecklenburg

The purpose of doing a biopsy is to aid the patient by having a histopathologist render a precise, accurate diagnosis prior to the clinician's embarking upon appropriate management (Ackerman 1999). However, unless a biopsy specimen is taken properly, processed well technically, and analyzed skillfully, histopathology will not deliver a correct diagnosis and, even worse, may deliver a wrong one. Performance of histopathology depends on (i) the careful selection of the lesions to be biopsied and optimal removal of the specimen by the clinician, (ii) the proper processing of the fixed specimen by the pathologists technician, (iii) the accurate analysis of the submitted specimens by the histopathologist, and (iv) the proper interpretation of the histopathology report by the clinician. The clinician and the histopathologist are a team, one that only performs superbly if each member is informed about the discipline of the other. In that spirit, clinicians should read and be able to understand the morphologic description in the pathology report, and histopathologists should have a detailed understanding of the gross lesions prior to evaluating biopsies.

2.2.1 Selection of the lesions to be biopsied and sampling technique

Alopecic skin samples should be taken by excision using a punch or a scalpel. All sampling techniques should deliver subcutaneous fat, as it is there where follicles are rooted (Mondragon and Di Leonardo 1995). Instruments for biopsies need to be sharp and used properly to avoid "crush artifacts" that distort cells and patterns formed by them (Fig. 2.2.1). Skin samples need to be of sufficient size in order to allow analysis of numerous hair follicles. This means a punch biopsy should measure at least 6 mm in diameter, ideally 8 mm, and an excisional biopsy should measure at least 15 mm in length and 10 mm in width.

A big challenge for the sampling clinician is the identification of the lesions most likely to enable the histopathologist to come to a specific, accurate diagnosis. If a lesion is biopsied too early in the course of its development, histopathologic findings may be too scant to permit a reasonable diagnosis to be made. In contrast, a lesion sampled too late in its course may only reveal unspecific secondary findings. These common rules in surgical pathology also apply to the diagnosis of alopecia. Ideally, samples from early, florid, and late stages of the disease process should be sampled. It is recommended to fix and ship specimens in different containers, as to allow the histopathologist to analyze them separately. Although samples from the periphery of an alopecic patch will most likely reveal an active inflammatory process targeting the hair follicles, the chance of secondary inflammatory lesions that interfere with a primarily noninflammatory disease of hair follicles is also highest in the periphery. Therefore, it is recommended to sample both the center and the periphery of a lesion. Three to four biopsies are sufficient material for most cases: a single punch biopsy specimen rarely provides information sufficient to enable a precise diagnosis to be made. In specimens from completely alopecic skin, the direction of hair growth should be indicated by a line in the middle of the biopsy, using a waterproof marker (Fig. 2.2.2).

2.2.2 Processing of biopsies from alopecic skin

The likelihood of accomplishing a correct histopathologic diagnosis of an alopecic disease will be enhanced, if biopsies are performed correctly and specimens

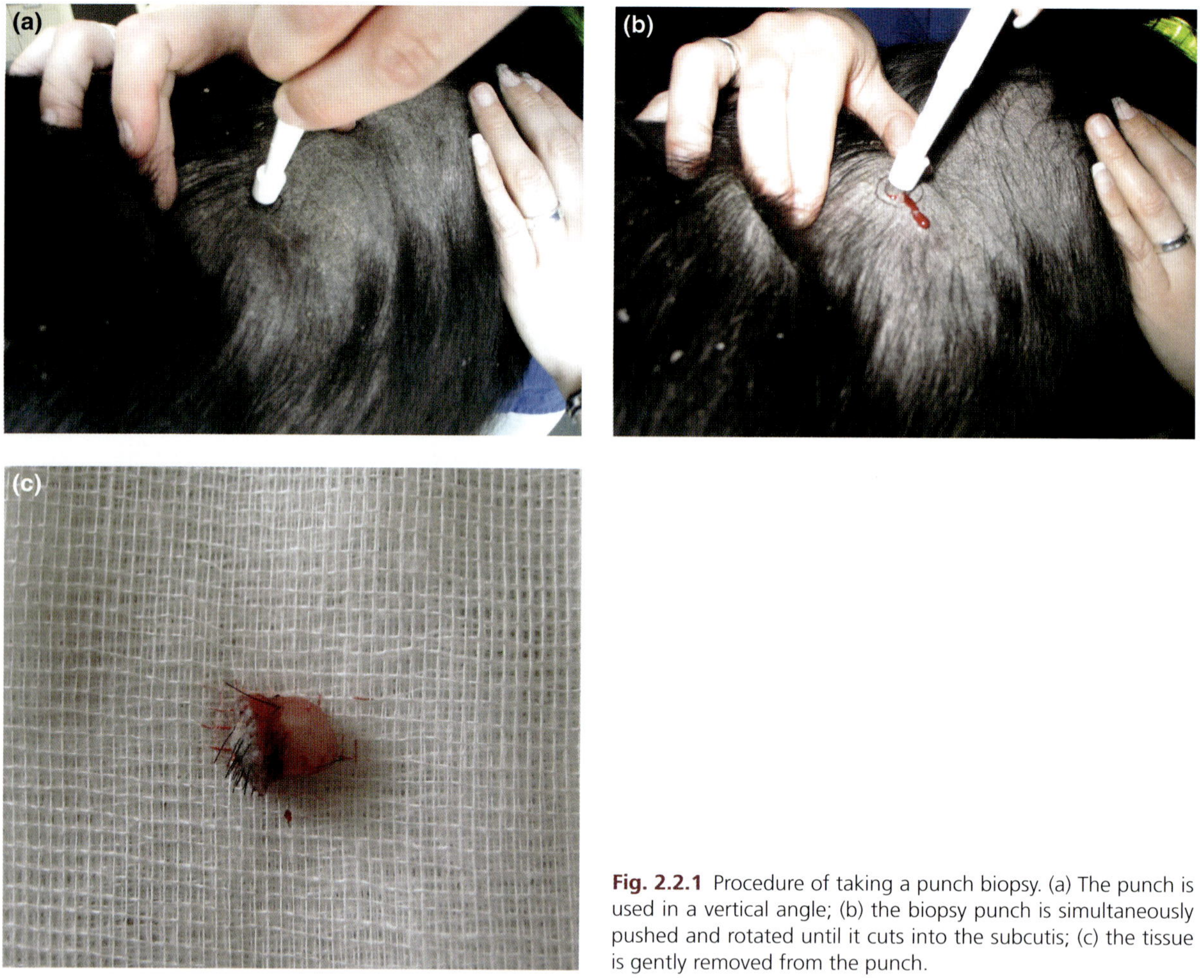

Fig. 2.2.1 Procedure of taking a punch biopsy. (a) The punch is used in a vertical angle; (b) the biopsy punch is simultaneously pushed and rotated until it cuts into the subcutis; (c) the tissue is gently removed from the punch.

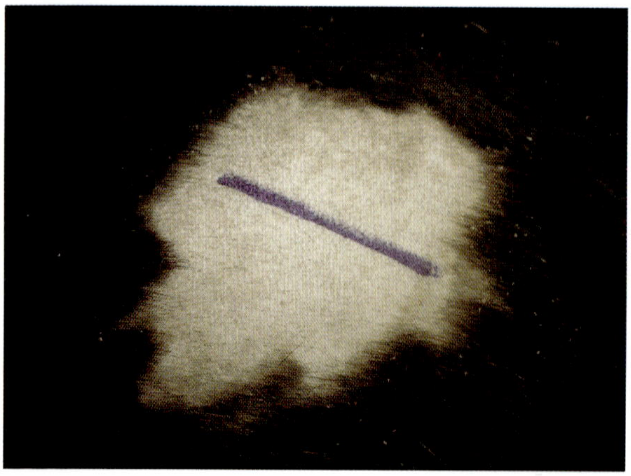

Fig. 2.2.2 Marking the direction of expected hair growth in alopecic skin enables the pathologist to make longitudinal sections of hair follicles.

are processed properly. Grossing of punch biopsy specimens, regardless of size, requires manual skill, precision, and the use of a very sharp blade (Yager and Wilcock 1994). Punches that measure 6 mm or more in diameter and excisional biopsies should be bisected parallel to the direction in which the hairs are growing. This enables the histopathologist to examine complete longitudinal sections of a maximum number of hair follicles. In specimens from completely alopecic skin, the direction of hair is ideally indicated by a line the clinician has drawn on the skin before sampling (Fig. 2.2.2). Punch biopsies of less than 6 mm diameter should be processed in their entirety, but need to be propped and rotated properly in order to allow longitudinal sectioning. Special care must be taken to orient them properly during embedding. Embedding should

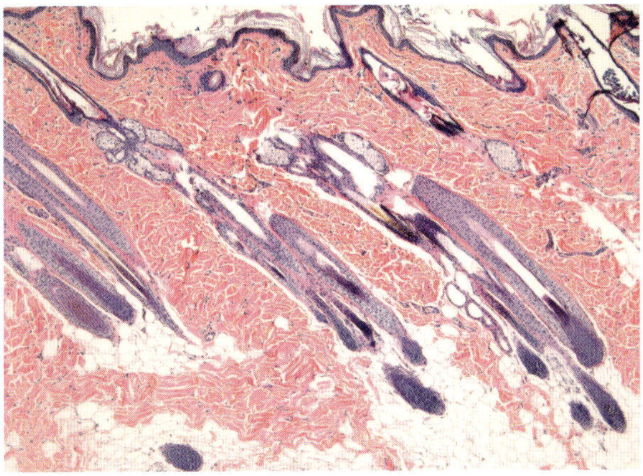

Fig. 2.2.3 Skin biopsy from a dog with numerous longitudinal sections of hair follicles. Note the compound nature of hair follicles.

allow longitudinal sectioning of hair follicles, and sections should ideally display the entire hair follicle from the ostium to the bulb (Fig. 2.2.3). Sections should be cut at different levels throughout the specimen housed in the paraffin block.

Transverse horizontal sections of alopecic skin are frequently promoted for the diagnosis of scarring alopecia in human medicine (Headington 1884; Sperling 2001). The main advantage is the higher yield of sectioned hair follicles, which is indeed an important aspect in human medicine where a diagnosis of an alopecic disease is usually made from a single 4-mm punch biopsy of the scalp. The limitation to a single biopsy is understandable considering the anatomy of the human scalp. In veterinary medicine, however, a diagnosis does not have to be based on a single biopsy. Most owners will allow sampling of at least three biopsies of 6 mm diameter or more. Therefore, the veterinary pathologist does not need to increase the yield of hair follicle numbers by cutting a biopsy horizontally instead of longitudinally. In addition, there is a large variety in domestic animal species with regard to the size and number of hair follicles that are normal in a biopsy of a given skin region. Interpretation of horizontal sections depends on comparing the number and size of hair follicles of the patients with a normal standard. As long as this standard has not been elaborated for each animal species, breed, and skin area, horizontal sections are of no benefit over longitudinal sections in veterinary pathology.

2.2.3 Light microscopical analysis of alopecic skin specimens

Histopathologists are well advised to confront abnormalities in sections with an open mind and a commitment to being thoroughly unbiased by not knowing anything beforehand about the patient from whom the biopsy specimen came (Ackerman 1999). Once a histopathologist has come to a tentative diagnosis, however, it is mandatory to learn as much clinical information as is useful for confirming or rejecting that diagnosis. This asks for accurate, concise clinical information to be submitted with the biopsy specimen.

The majority of skin diseases can be diagnosed with specificity using a scanning objective, that is, up to 2.5×. At that magnification, a histopathologist obtains a vantage of patterns formed by alterations in tissues as well as those formed by infiltrates of cells. The method of pattern analysis applies to all kinds of pathological processes in the skin, including the vast amount of alopecic diseases. Before assessing the general pattern in a biopsy, however, the pathologist should make a methodical judgment about the adequateness of the biopsy specimen, the quality of the tissue section, and the anatomic site in the skin from which the biopsy specimen was obtained.

The histopathologist should first evaluate whether any inflammatory infiltrate is present in the skin sample. If there is inflammation, it needs to be characterized and it needs to be evaluated whether inflammatory cells target hair follicles or whether they are a secondary phenomenon, independent of the hair follicle disease. Next, hair follicles are evaluated morphologically. This begins with an examination of hair follicle ostia and infundibula, and whether or not hair shafts penetrate them. If numerous hair shafts penetrate the follicular ostia although the biopsy is supposed to derive from an alopecic skin area, alopecia can only be explained by breaking of hair shafts once these have penetrated the skin. This points to either a self-induced alopecia or may indicate that hair shaft structure is altered, resulting in an increased fragility of hair shafts.

Using a higher magnification, hair follicles are evaluated in more detail. The morphologic evaluation of hair follicles requires a thorough understanding of their normal anatomy in general and of the changes that occur during the normal hair growth cycle in particular.

2.2.3.1 Hair follicle subtypes

Hair follicles can be divided into several subtypes. Whiskers or vibrissae hair follicles are differentiated from pelage hair follicles by their large vascular sinuses that surround the hair bulb. Whisker hair follicles have small sebaceous glands and lack apocrine glands. They occur on upper and lower lip, chin, cheeks, and around eyes. They function as tactile sensors. Pelage hair follicles represent the magnitude of hair follicles on the body. Their size and shape are very variable as are the arrangement and the density with which they occur in different skin regions (see Section 1.3.3). Some domestic animals (e.g., horse, some pig breeds) have single hair follicles, whereas dogs and cats have many compound hair follicles (Fig. 2.2.3). Compound hair follicles have the largest hair cranial and progressively smaller hairs caudal. However, the diameter of hair shafts represents a continuum, and there are no two clearly defined populations of follicles based on the hair shaft diameter. Calling the cranial follicle in each compound follicle a "primary" follicle and all others "secondary" follicles is the easiest and most consistent approach (Dunstan et al. 2001).

2.2.3.2 Morphology of hair follicle cycling

Regardless of the hair follicle subtype, all hair follicles undergo significant morphologic changes during the hair growth cycle (Al-Bagdadi et al. 1979).

2.2.3.2.1 Anagen

Hair follicles in the growing (anagen) stage of the growth cycle can be subdivided into the following compartments (Fig. 2.2.4): The follicular *ostium* is the opening of the hair follicle infundibulum into the epidermis. The *infundibulum* is the uppermost follicular compartment. It is lined by a cornifying epithelium with a stratum granulosum that is morphologically similar to the epidermis. The follicular infundibulum contains one (single follicles) or more (compound follicles) hair shafts. It also contains small amounts of desquamating fully keratinized keratinocytes similar to the epidermal stratum corneum (Fig. 2.2.5). In contrast to all other follicular compartments, the infundibulum does not change during the hair growth cycle. Opposite of the follicular ostium, the infundibulum merges into the follicular *isthmus*. The isthmic region is very complex, since it is the zone where upper and lower compartments merge into each other and where significant morphological changes occur during hair follicle cycling. The isthmus is characterized by (i) entry of the short duct that connects the hair

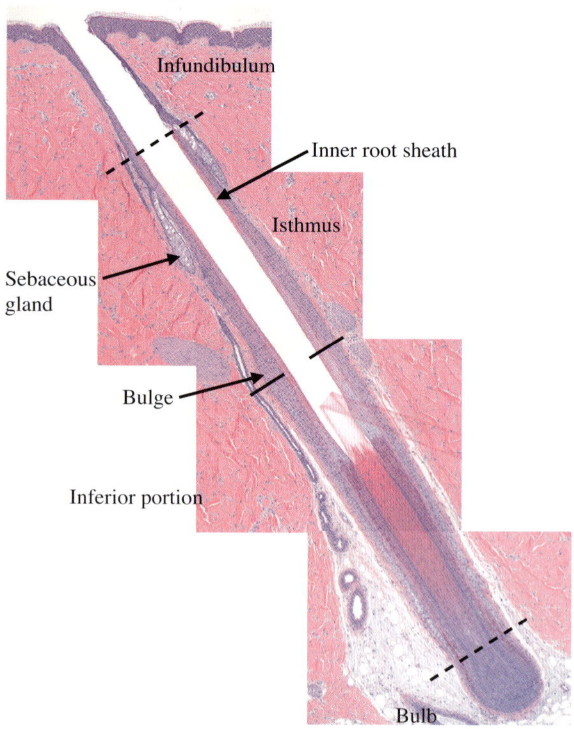

Fig. 2.2.4 Skin from a pig indicating the different compartments of an anagen hair follicle. Note the single hair follicle compared to compound hair follicles in dogs and cats.

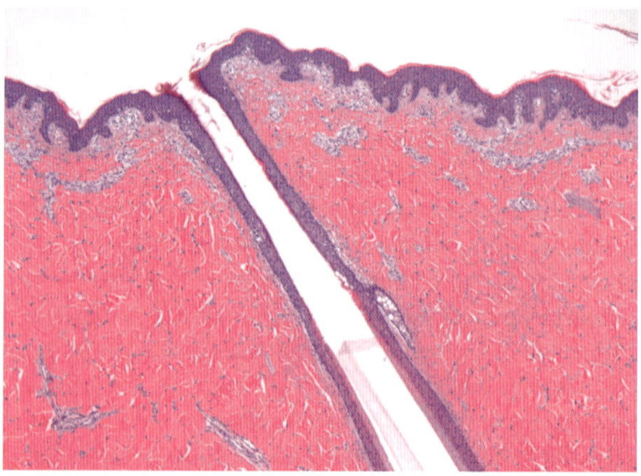

Fig. 2.2.5 Histology of the follicular infudibulum and isthmus (Goettingen minipig). Note disintegration of the inner root sheath at the level of the sebaceous gland.

canal to the holocrine sebaceous gland, (ii) disintegration of the highly eosinophilic inner root sheath, and (iii) a *bulge* region of the outer root sheath, which can be more or less distinct and which represents the attaching site of the arrector pili muscle (Fig. 2.2.5). Below the isthmus is a region that is known as the *inferior segment*. The inferior segment is rather long and is composed of a cylindrical arrangement of cells which build from outside in (Fig. 2.2.4): the *fibrous connective tissue sheath*, *basement membrane* (also known as glassy membrane), *outer root sheath* (with basal and suprabasal cell layers), *inner root sheath* (separated into Huxley layer, Henle layer, and cuticula), and finally the hair shaft (with cuticula, cortex, and medulla). Opposed to the infundibulum and the isthmus, the hair shaft is closely apposed to the inner and outer root sheath. The inferior segment merges into the *hair bulb*. The bulb is again a very complex region of the hair follicle (Fig. 2.2.6). It is characterized by a centrally located dermal papilla that is composed of mesenchymal cells, all separated by abundant extracellular matrix. The dermal papilla is tightly enclosed by keratinocytes and melanocytes. Keratinocytes of the bulb can be separated into different morphological and functional zones, that is, those below the line of Auber (i.e., a line through the dermal papilla at its largest diameter) that show the highest proliferative activity, and those above the line of Auber that are less proliferatively active but undergo early differentiation. The anatomical structures mentioned above characterize each anagen hair follicle, independent of its subtype. However, not all features may be histologically identifiable in each section since most hair follicles are cut obliquely. Therefore, the histopathologist needs to become familiar with oblique and transversal cuts of hair follicles as well.

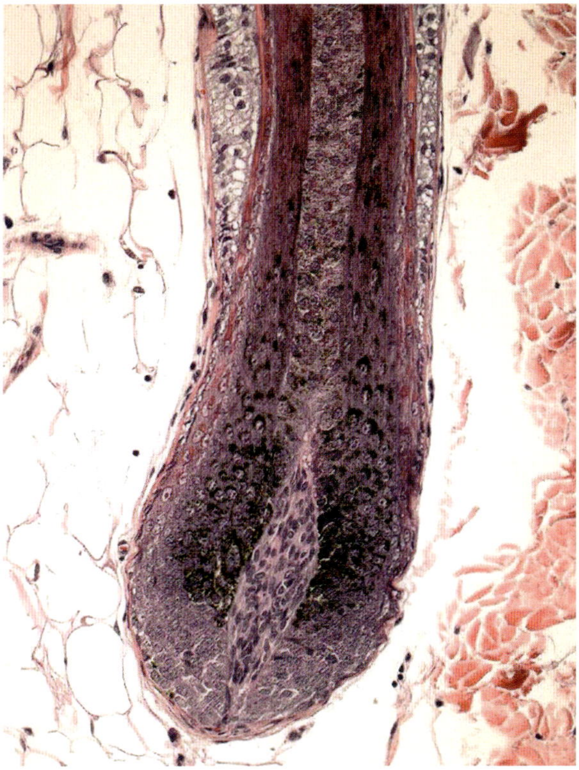

Fig. 2.2.6 Anatomy of the hair follicle bulb. Dog: note dermal papilla, matrix with proliferating keratinocytes, precortical matrix with melanocytes and differentiating keratinocytes, hair shaft medulla, hair shaft cortex, inner root sheath, and outer root sheath.

2.2.3.2.2 Catagen

The regression phase of the hair growth cycle is associated with very characteristic morphological changes. These changes are best studied in rodents where hair follicles cycle synchronously and therefore allow a more precise morphological evaluation (Muller-Rover et al. 2001). However, they are identical in nonrodent mammals, where they are less well described, because hair follicles cycle independent of one another. Catagen is a very short phase of the hair growth cycle and therefore only very few (less than 3%) catagen hair follicles can be examined in normal skin. The first event of catagen development is cessation of melanization and cessation of keratinocyte proliferation in the hair matrix. This leads to thinning of the entire hair bulb. As precortical matrix cells still undergo differentiation into hair shaft and inner root sheath, the matrix zone becomes thinner and keratinocytes no longer completely enclose the dermal papilla (Fig. 2.2.7). Further regression of the matrix zone separates it completely from the dermal papilla. A very distinct basement membrane occurs that separates a bunch of closely apposed mesenchymal cells from the epithelial remnants of the hair bulb (Fig. 2.2.8). As keratinocytes that derive from the precortical matrix continue to differentiate and since no further daughter cells are produced in the bulb, the inferior segment changes as well. It is transformed into an undulating *epithelial strand*, composed of largely similar small keratinocytes that frequently show morphologic features of apoptosis. The epithelial strand is surrounded by a markedly

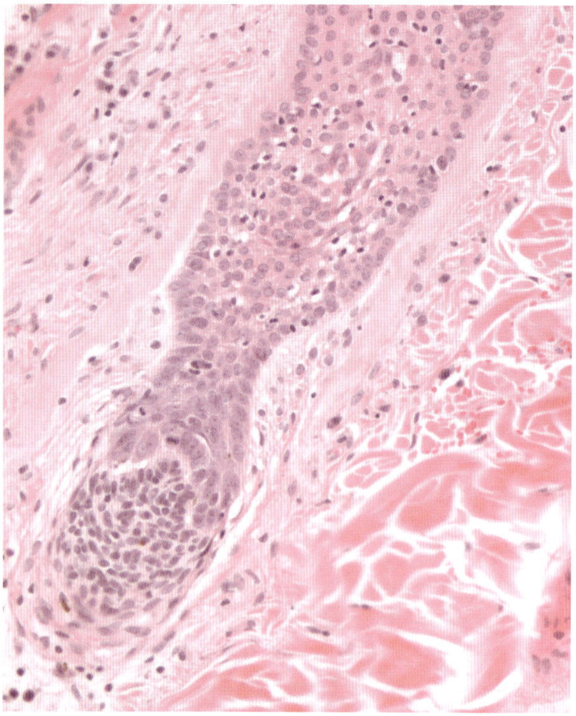

Fig. 2.2.7 Anatomy of the early catagen hair bulb. Dog: note dermal papilla, retracted matrix, prominent basement membrane, irregular epithelial strand, and prominent perifollicular connective tissue sheath.

thickened basement membrane that stains positively with PAS and is a very distinctive feature of catagen. During further catagen development, the epithelial strand shortens and the dermal papilla, still firmly attached but separated by a distinct basement membrane, moves upward, that is, toward the follicular isthmus. In the later stages of catagen development, the isthmus region undergoes characteristic changes too. Due to terminal differentiation of inner root sheath keratinocytes, a club hair forms, which is characterized by a highly eosinophilic material, known as trichilemmal keratinization. The keratinization forms a brush-like zone that separates the actual hair shaft from the surrounding keratinocytes of the isthmus region.

2.2.3.2.3 Telogen

Catagen finally merges into the resting stage called telogen. In telogen, regression of the inferior portion is completed and no further keratinocyte apoptosis is detected. The trichilemmal keratinization has now formed a distinct *club hair* that demarcates the isthmus region of the hair follicle. Directly below the isthmus is an accumulation of immature epithelial cells, called the "secondary hair germ." It is these cells that will proliferate and produce a new hair follicle upon initiation of a new anagen phase. Directly below the secondary hair germ is a small and condensed dermal papilla. It shows very little extracellular matrix. Its nuclei stain intensively for estrogen receptors (Fig. 2.2.9).

2.2.3.2.4 New anagen

The first morphological sign of a new anagen development is proliferation of keratinocytes in the secondary hair germ that start to form a new hair bulb where dermal papilla cells become enclosed by keratinocytes. This newly formed hair bulb will then be "pushed" downward into the dermis by the new formation of an inferior segment. Mid anagen stages are recognized by a remaining club hair of the previous telogen phase. Later anagen stages are morphologically indistinguishable from a mature anagen hair follicle that can persist for several months or even years.

When evaluating biopsies from alopecic diseases, the histopathologist needs to determine the hair cycle stage of each follicle and thus should be able to determine the ratio between early anagen, mature anagen, catagen, and telogen hair follicles. Most biopsies from normal skin should reveal a majority of anagen hair follicles. Simultaneous presence of telogen hair follicles is normal with a percentage as high as 50% in some breeds of dogs. Catagen should not be observed in any biopsy from any animal species in a significant level (less than 3% of all hair follicles). A larger percentage of catagen hair follicles always points to abnormalities in the hair growth cycle (see Chapter 3.3).

2.2.3.3 Hair follicle dysplasia

Dysplasia is an abnormality in the development or in the organization of cells. Keratinocyte proliferation is mandatory for the development of most forms of hair follicle dysplasia. Consequently, dysplasia of hair follicles usually occurs during morphogenesis (dysplastic morphogenesis). Most forms of dysplastic morphogenesis are congenital and most of these are hereditary (see Chapter 3.1). The variety of dysplastic changes during morphogenesis is huge and ranges from rudimentary hair follicle anlagen to almost normal hair follicles with very subtle changes of the hair shaft (Fig. 2.2.10).

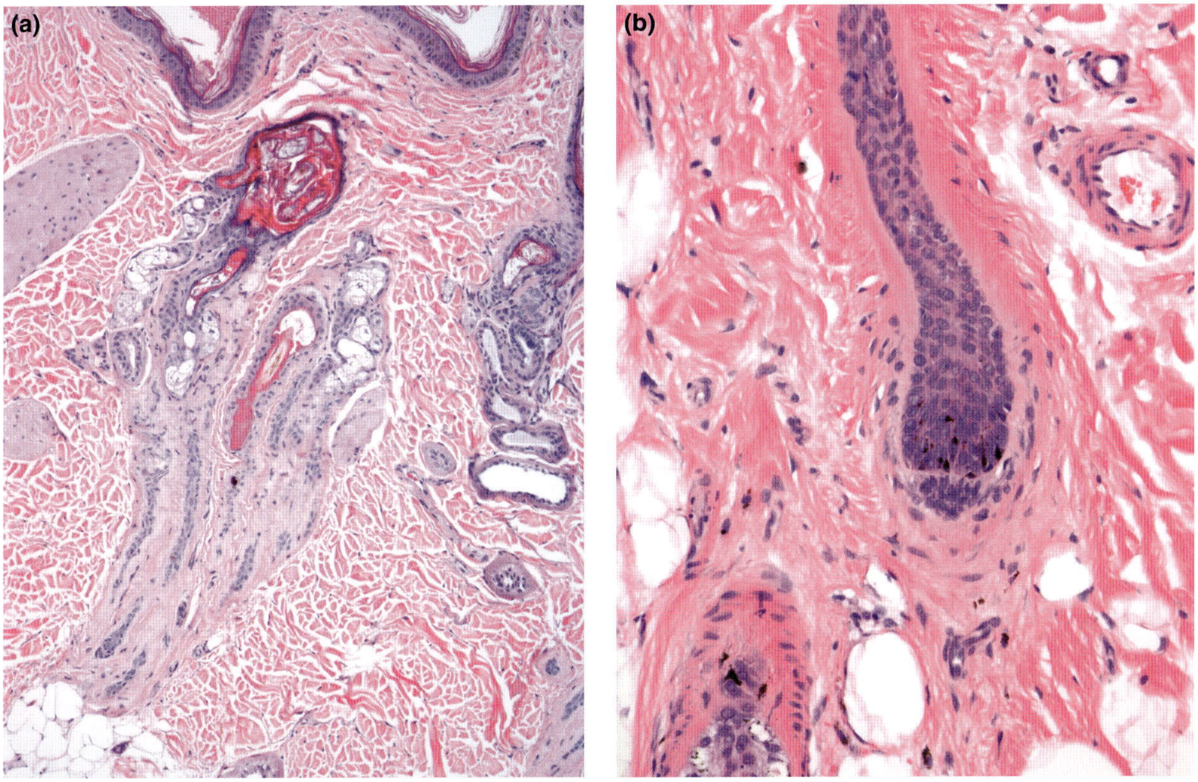

Fig. 2.2.8 Anatomy of the mid catagen hair follicle. Dog: (a) irregular epithelial strands connecting follicular isthmus and dermal papilla; note prominent perifollicular connective tissue sheath; (b) higher magnification of mid catagen hair bulb with dermal papilla, prominent basement membrane, and epithelial strand.

Since hair follicles undergo repeated regression (catagen) and reformation (anagen), abnormalities in the organization of hair follicle cells can also occur beyond morphogenesis. Malformations during the anagen phase should be termed "anagen dysplasia" opposed to those that occur during catagen development (i.e., "catagen dysplasia"). Anagen dysplasia refers to those malformations of hair follicles that occur spontaneously during hair follicle cycling. The prototypic example of anagen dysplasia is the dilated follicular infundibulum of hair follicles in canine recurrent flank alopecia before they undergo catagen development (Fig. 3.3.23). However, since this disease represents an abnormality of hair follicle cycling with increased catagen hair follicles, it is still under debate whether this disease should be classified as a dysplasia or a hair cycle abnormality (see Section 3.3.5).

The prototypic (and the only diagnostically relevant) form of catagen dysplasia described so far is hair follicles with excessive trichilemmal keratinization. Such hair follicles are also known as "flame follicles," since the highly eosinophilic trichilemmal keratin adopts the shape of a flame. The term flame follicle was originally used to describe an abnormal catagen hair follicle that shows an excessive amount of brightly eosinophilic homogenous material that surrounds the club hair and that projects radially and irregularly into the surrounding outer root sheath (Scott 1989; Yager and Wilcock 1994). The problem with this term is that brightly eosinophilic trichilemmal keratin is a normal feature of any late catagen and telogen hair follicle (Fig. 2.2.9). Therefore, the term flame follicle has also been used to describe normal telogen hair follicles (Ordeix et al. 2002). In order to avoid confusion, the pathologist needs to be familiar with the normal amount of trichilemmal keratin in catagen and telogen hair follicles of a given breed and species. In the disease "alopecia X" of plush-coated dogs, many hair follicles with an increased amount of trichilemmal keratin occur (see Section 3.3.4).

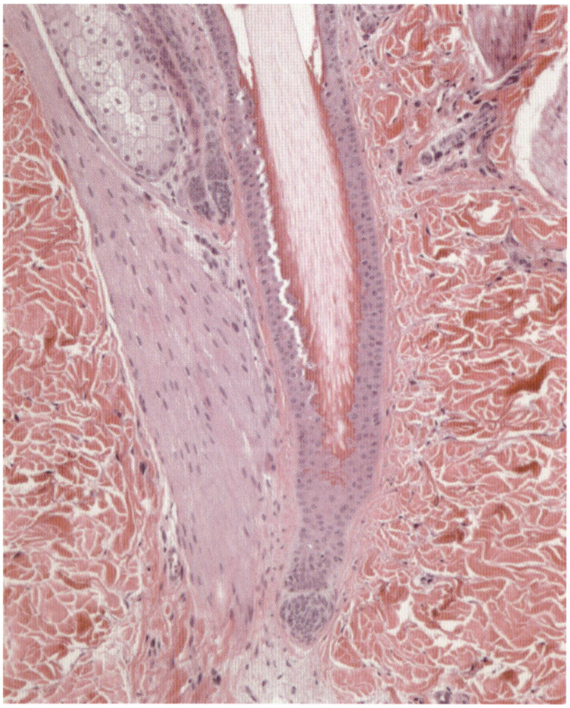

Fig. 2.2.9 Anatomy of a canine telogen hair follicle. Note arrector pili muscle, telogen hair shaft (club hair) with trichilemmal keratinization, and the prominent basement membrane separating secondary hair germ and dermal papilla.

2.2.3.4 Hair follicle dystrophy

The term dystrophy is used to describe a degenerative process that is due to "malnutrition" of an organ. There are rare hair follicle diseases in domestic animals that can be correctly addressed as dystrophy, since first they represent a degenerative process and, second, they are associated with the "malnutrition" of hair follicle cells in the wider sense (see Chapter 3.4). Morphological signs of hair follicle dystrophy are uncoordinated vacuolar degeneration or apoptosis of keratinocytes. It is important to differentiate dystrophic apoptosis in hair follicle keratinocytes from apoptosis occurring during catagen. Whereas in catagen, apoptosis follows a highly coordinated process that begins with cessation of follicular pigmentation and ends with complete disappearance of the lower follicular portion, dystrophy is uncoordinated. Uncoordinated keratinocyte degeneration without previous cessation of follicular pigmentation results in uneven distribution of melanin within the hair shafts. Melanin may spill out of the hair follicle and will be taken up by perifollicular melanophages (pigmentary incontinence). Therefore, perifollicular melanophages are very good evidence of hair follicle dystrophy. Other parameters of hair follicle dystrophy that may or may not be present are a wide-open hair canal, distortion of the entire follicle, and an irregular diameter of hair follicles (Hendrix et al. 2005) (Fig. 2.2.11). Dystrophic changes can occur in anagen or in catagen hair follicles. Therefore, terms such as "dystrophic anagen" and "dystrophic catagen" can and should be used to describe dystrophic hair follicles more precisely (Hendrix et al. 2005). Hair follicle dystrophy may be reversible if stem cells remain and if a new anagen phase is initiated after the follicle has reached telogen. However, if the insult is too severe, hair follicles may become terminally damaged and may undergo atrophy.

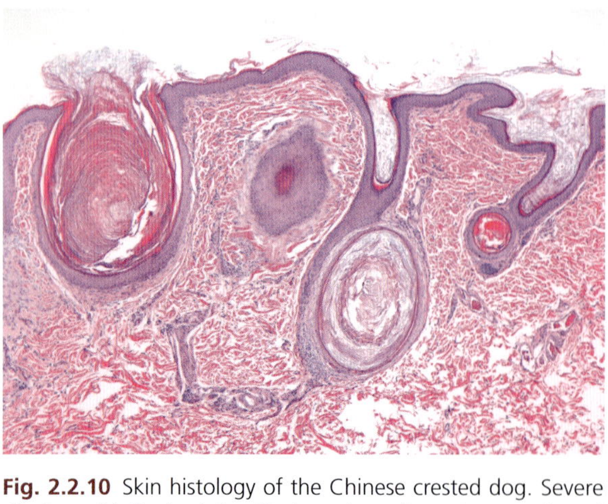

Fig. 2.2.10 Skin histology of the Chinese crested dog. Severe dilation of follicular infundibula and condensed mesenchymal cells, likely representing dermal papilla fibroblasts.

2.2.3.5 Hair follicle atrophy

Although cyclic hair follicle regression (catagen) and hair follicle rest (telogen) are associated with a loss of follicular cells, these physiological stages of hair growth cycling should not be termed "atrophy" since they do not necessarily represent a pathological change. Hair follicle atrophy is represented by a loss of hair follicle cells beyond the physiological telogen phase (see Chapter 3.4). Atrophic hair follicles have also been named "fading follicles," emphasizing their small size compared to the overall size of dermis and other cutaneous adnexa. Atrophic hair follicles are histopathologically characterized by small remnants of keratinocyte strands that are surrounded by a markedly thickened connective tissue sheath

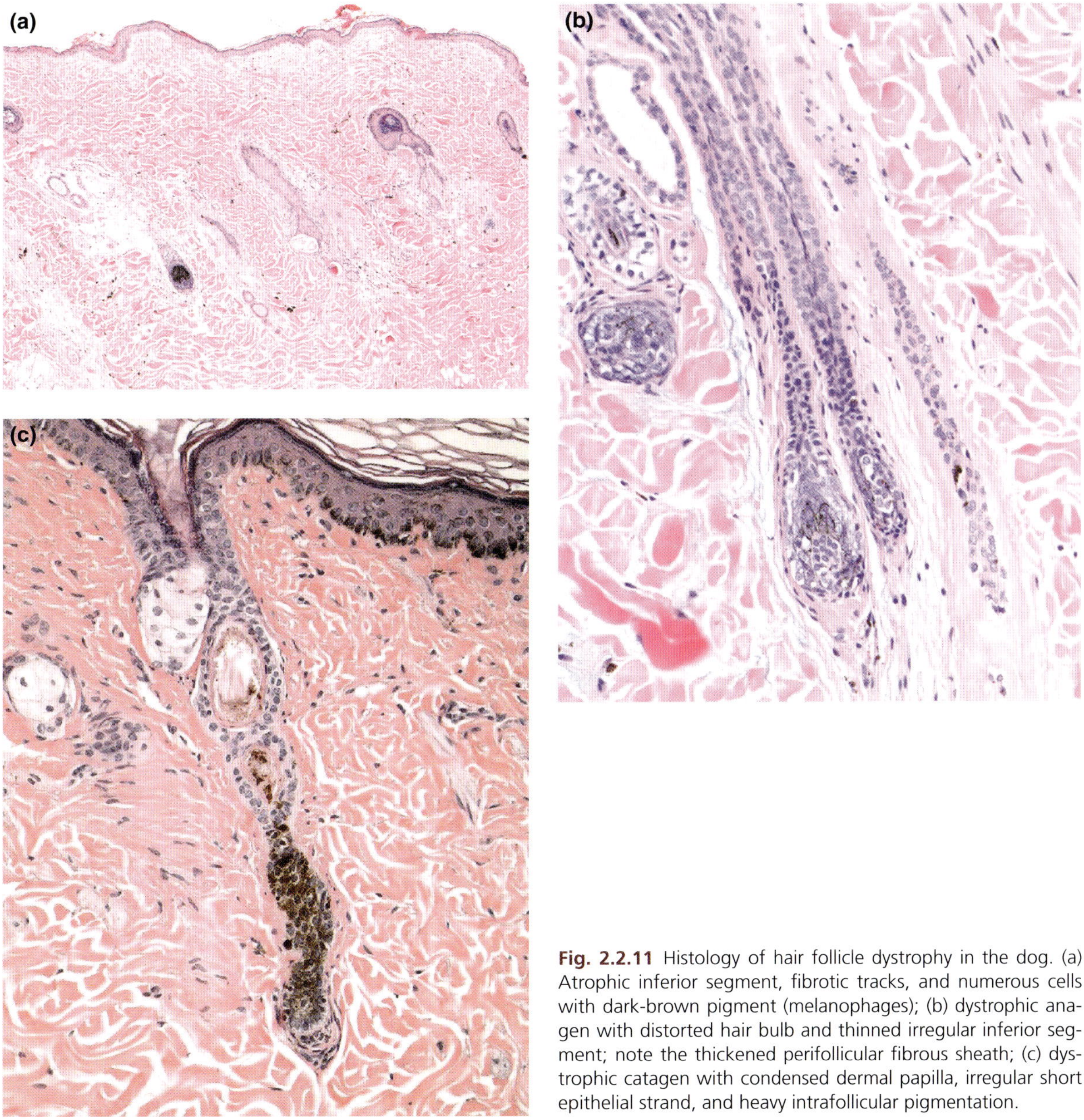

Fig. 2.2.11 Histology of hair follicle dystrophy in the dog. (a) Atrophic inferior segment, fibrotic tracks, and numerous cells with dark-brown pigment (melanophages); (b) dystrophic anagen with distorted hair bulb and thinned irregular inferior segment; note the thickened perifollicular fibrous sheath; (c) dystrophic catagen with condensed dermal papilla, irregular short epithelial strand, and heavy intrafollicular pigmentation.

(Fig. 2.2.12). Occasionally, dystrophic changes may be present as well, characterized by vacuolar degeneration or apoptosis of keratinocytes, and clumping of follicular melanin and perifollicular melanophages.

2.2.3.6 Infundibular hyperkeratosis

Hyperkeratosis within the follicular infundibulum is a common finding in hair follicle pathology. As in the epidermis, hyperkeratosis can be orthokeratotic or parakeratotic with the clear majority being orthokeratotic (Fig. 2.2.13). Marked infundibular hyperkeratosis is seen in diseases such as canine idiopathic seborrhea, demodicosis, canine sebaceous adenitis, canine idiopathic comedo formation, canine hyperestrogenism, canine hyperadrenocorticism, canine recurrent flank alopecia, and various other forms of hair cycle abnormalities. In canine sebaceous adenitis,

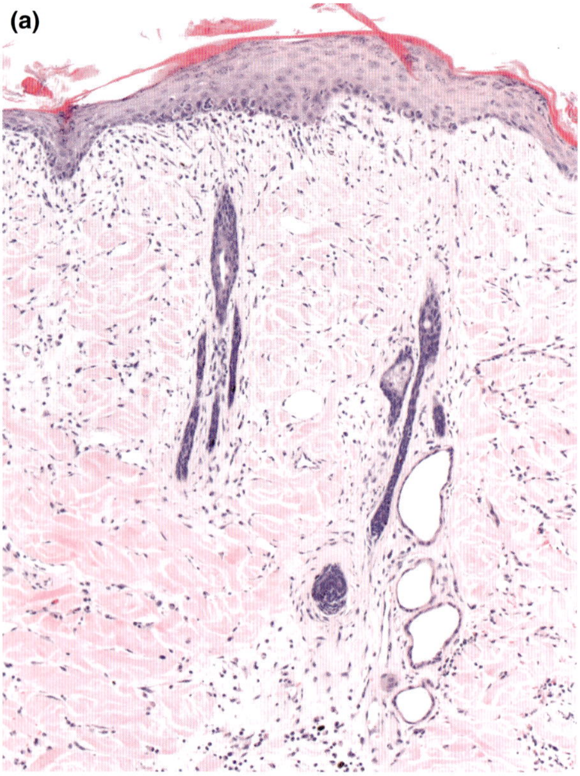

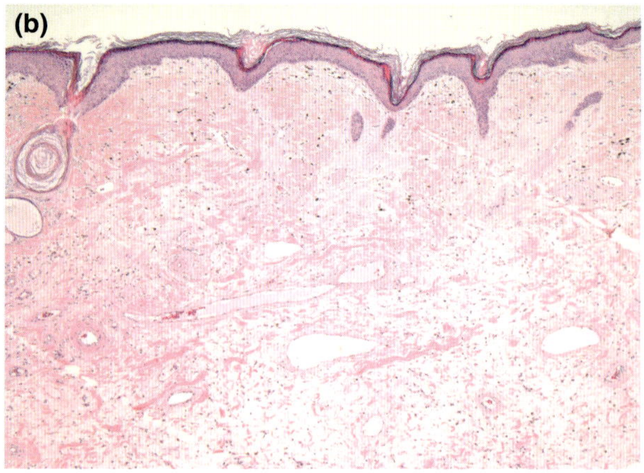

Fig. 2.2.12 Histology of hair follicle atrophy in the dog. (a) Hair follicles with thin inferior segment; (b) loss of hair follicles and replacement by fibrous tissue. Some follicular epithelial cells remain.

hyperkeratosis within the follicular infundibulum is due to the lack of sebum and impaired desquamation. In endocrine diseases and other hair cycle abnormalities, infundibular hyperkeratosis is likely caused by a lack of hair shaft elongation. Whereas normally the infundibular keratin is extruded with the elongating hair shaft, it accumulates within the infundibulum when the hair shafts do not grow properly or if they are lost entirely. In diseases such as idiopathic seborrhea, infundibular hyperkeratosis is associated with epidermal hyperkeratosis and simply reflects a yet unexplained abnormality in epithelial keratinization. A very severe form of infundibular hyperkeratosis with intralesional bacteria is termed "comedo" according to similar morphologies in human acne vulgaris. A closed comedo has an obstructed follicular ostium and may rupture to cause a foreign body inflammatory reaction, whereas an open comedo has a wide ostium and is capped with a crust composed of debris (Elder et al. 1997).

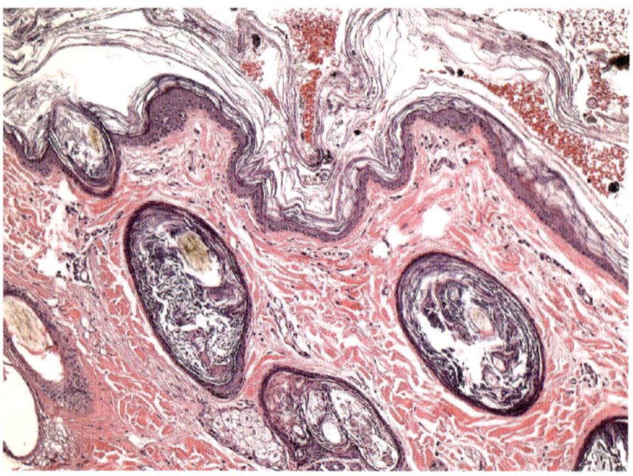

Fig. 2.2.13 Histology of infundibular orthokeratotic hyperkeratosis in the dog.

2.2.3.7 Hair follicle inflammation

Inflammation of the hair follicle is called "folliculitis," a term that is used both clinically and histopathologically. Whereas folliculitis is classified clinically by its etiology, hair follicle inflammation can be classified anatomically based on the character and distribution of inflammatory cells (see Part 4).

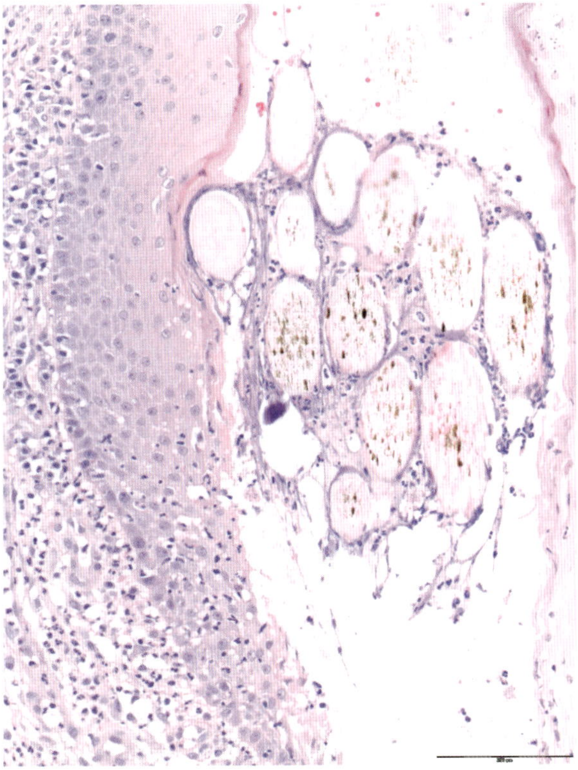

Fig. 2.2.14 Histology of luminal folliculitis in the dog. Perifollicular inflammatory cells that penetrate the follicular wall and accumulate in the follicular lumen.

Any inflammation that occurs outside of the hair follicle, that is, that strikingly surrounds hair follicles without inflammatory cells invading the glassy membrane, is called "perifolliculitis." Diagnostic specificity of this pattern is low since many nonfollicular inflammatory processes of the dermis will fit into this pattern.

Luminal folliculitis describes inflammation of the hair follicle wall and its periphery with simultaneous presence of inflammatory cells in the hair canal (Fig. 2.2.14). This is a frequent but not diagnostic finding in diseases such as bacterial folliculitis, dermatophytosis, or demodicosis (see Chapter 4.1). It is mostly associated with pathogens (i.e., bacteria, dermatophytes, or parasites) that are localized within the hair canal.

Mural folliculitis is used to describe inflammatory processes where inflammatory cells invade the glassy membrane and the outer root sheath, but where inflammatory cells do not reach the lumen. "Mural folliculitis" is a descriptive term in anatomic pathology and does not refer to a specific clinical diagnosis, even though it may be contained in a very descriptive disease name such as "lymphocytic mural folliculitis of the isthmus" (see Section 4.4.2.2). Mural folliculitis will occur in many different conditions and refers to all levels of the hair follicle wall unless otherwise specified. It can be purely lymphocytic as in lymphocytic mural foliculitis (see Chapter 4.4), can be dominated by eosinophils (see Chapter 4.2), or may even be histiocytic and granulomatous in nature (see Chapter 4.5). Mural folliculitis is a frequent finding in various diseases and its severity can range from cell poor to cell rich. Mural folliculitis can be further subdivided into an interface type, an infiltrative type, a pustular type, and a necrotizing type (Gross et al. 1997).

Interface mural folliculitis is associated with individual cell necrosis (apoptosis) or vacuolar degeneration of outer root sheath keratinocytes (Fig. 2.2.15). It has therefore some similarities to hair follicle dystrophy with the difference that dystrophy is a noninflammatory degenerative process. The inflammatory infiltrate may obscure the glassy membrane. Interface mural folliculitis can be associated with pigmentary incontinence and perifollicular accumulation of melanophages. It is usually dominated by lymphocytes with some plasma cells and histiocytes being associated with them. It occurs in association with similar epidermal changes in diseases such as erythema multiforme, lupus erythematosus, or cutaneous drug reactions (see Section 4.4.1), or without similar epidermal changes in diseases such as follicular mucinosis, dermatophytosis, or demodicosis.

Infiltrative mural folliculitis describes those inflammatory lesions where mural inflammation is not associated with degeneration of hair follicle keratinocytes. Infiltrative mural folliculitis can be subdivided according to the predominant type of inflammatory cells. Lymphocytic infiltrative mural folliculitis occurs in diseases such as equine linear alopecia, feline exfoliative dermatitis, or canine pseudopelade-like disease (see Section 4.4.2.2). Eosinophilic infiltrative mural folliculitis occurs in diseases such as canine eosinophilic pustular folliculitis and feline mosquito-bite hypersensitivity (see Chapter 4.2). Eosinophilic infiltrative mural follicuitis is often very destructive, and will frequently result in furunculosis. Histiocytic infiltrative mural folliculitis is a very rare variant of mural hair follicle inflammation. It can comprise large numbers of giant cells and is usually associated with marked destruction of the follicular wall (see Chapter 4.5).

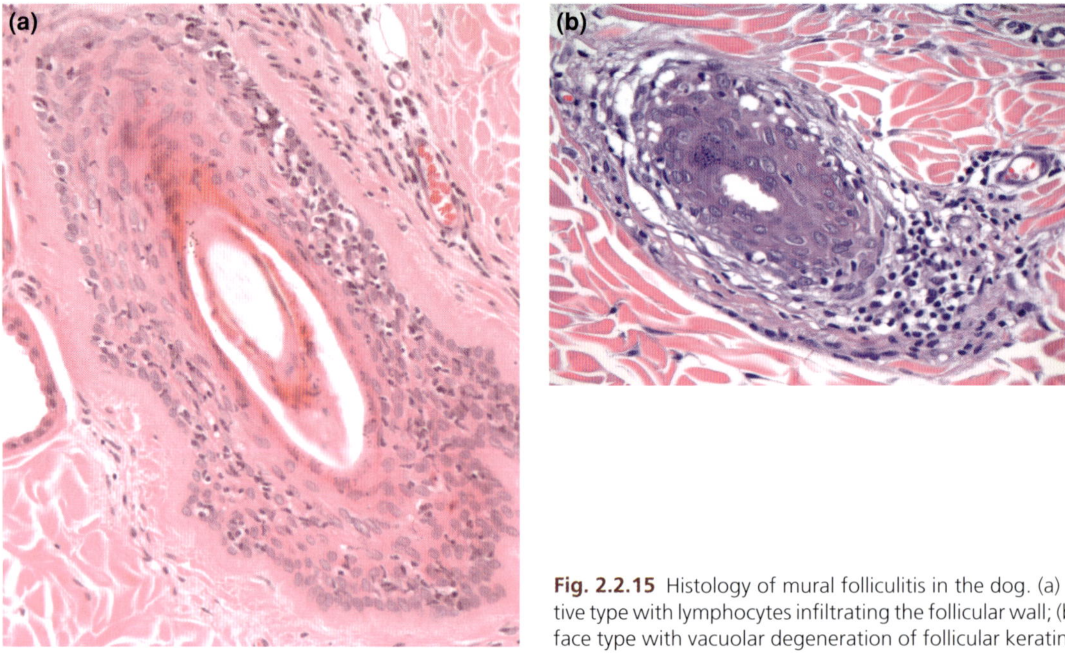

Fig. 2.2.15 Histology of mural folliculitis in the dog. (a) Infiltrative type with lymphocytes infiltrating the follicular wall; (b) interface type with vacuolar degeneration of follicular keratinocytes.

Necrotizing mural folliculitis summarizes diseases where there is severe degeneration of hair follicle keratinocytes with a secondary inflammatory response. This is the case in feline poxvirus infections or feline herpesvirus dermatitis (see Chapter 4.6).

Pustular mural folliculitis is used to describe pustule formation within the infundibular epithelium. This is usually associated with a pustular dermatitis, where epidermal lesions merge into the follicular infundibulum (see Chapter 4.3).

Finally, *bulbitis* describes a characteristic lymphocytic infiltrative folliculitis that targets the hair follicle bulb. Lymphocytes may also be found within the inferior segment. Bulbitis is characteristic for alopecia areata (see Chapter 4.7).

Furunculosis is a penetrating or perforating follicular inflammation, meaning that the follicular wall is destroyed by the inflammatory process. Furunculosis is associated with fragmented hair shafts that are no longer surrounded by an intact follicular wall. Inflammatory infiltrates are composed of neutrophils, eosinophils, and macrophages, often with some giant cells. These are surrounded by lymphocytes and plasma cells and often merge into a demarcation by fibrovascular granulation tissue (Fig. 2.2.16).

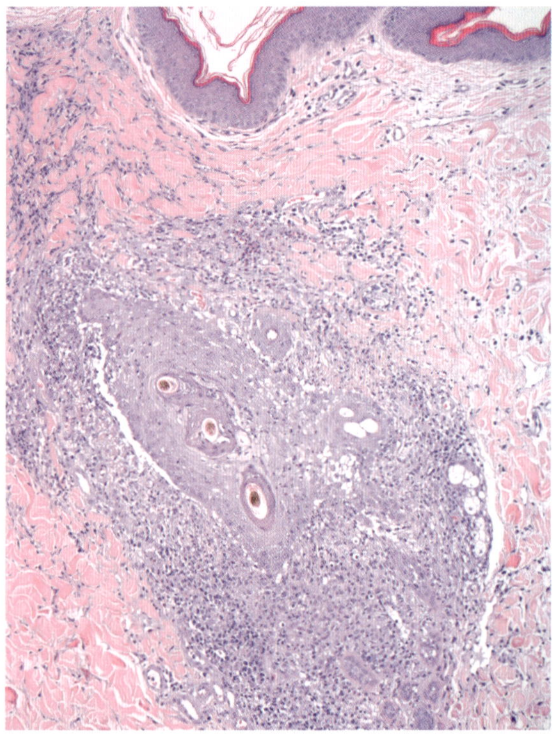

Fig. 2.2.16 Histology of furunculosis in the dog. Perifollicular inflammatory cells, infiltrating the follicular wall and surrounding hair shafts, associated with destruction of the follicular wall.

2.2.4 Interpretation of the histopathology report

As was mentioned before, the clinician and the histopathologist are a team that only works if both supply accurate information to each other. The clinician who has submitted skin biopsies should read the full histopathology report. No report without a morphological description should be accepted, since such a report does not allow to understand how the conclusion was drawn. An adequate pathology report mentions the tissue that was submitted, gives a thorough morphological description of lesions resulting in a morphological diagnosis, and ends with a conclusion that comments on correlation to gross lesions, etiology, and pathogenesis of the disease, exclusion of differential diagnoses, and the prognosis for the patient (Yager and Wilcock 1994).

References

Ackerman AB. 1999. *A Philosophy of Practice of Surgical Pathology: Dermatopathology as Model.* Philadelphia: Ardor Sribendi.

Al-Bagdadi FK, Titkemeyer CW, Lovell JE. 1979. Histology of the hair cycle in male beagle dogs. *American Journal of Veterinary Research* 40:1734–1741.

Dunstan RW, Credille KM, Mansell J, Tucker KA, Bloom PJ, Petersen AJ, Nachreiner RF, Davenport GM, Lupton CJ. 2001. A common sense approach to the morphology of alopecia: addressing 10 points of follicular confusion. *ISVD Meeting*, Norfolk, VA.

Elder D, Elenitsas R, Jaworsky C, Johnson B (eds). 1997. *Lever's Histopathology of the Skin*, 8th edn. Philadelphia: Lippincott-Raven Publishers.

Gross TL, Stannard AA, Yager JA. 1997. An anatomical classification of folliculitis. *Veterinary Dermatology* 8:147–156.

Headington J. 1884. Transverse microscopic anatomy of the human scalp. *Archives of Dermatology* 120:449.

Hendrix S, Handjiski B, Peters EM, Paus R. 2005. A guide to assessing damage response pathways of the hair follicle: lessons from cyclophosphamide-induced alopecia in mice. *Journal of Investigative Dermatology* 125(1):42–51.

Mondragon G, Di Leonardo M. 1995. Punch biopsy of alopecias: methods and implications. *American Journal of Dermatopathology* 1(2):138.

Muller-Rover S, Handjiski B, Van Der Veen C, Eichmuller S, Foitzik K, McKay IA, Stenn KS, Paus R. 2001. A comprehensive guide for the accurate classification of murine hair follicles in distinct hair cycle stages. *Journal of Investigative Dermatology* 117(1):3–15.

Ordeix L, Fondevila D, Ferrer L, Fondati A. 2002. Quantitative study of "flame follicles" in skin sections of Shar-pei dogs. *Veterinary Dermatology* 13:261–265.

Scott DW. 1989. Excessive trichilemmal keratinization (flame follicles) in endocrine skin disorders of the dog. *Veterinary Dermatology* 1:37–40.

Sperling LC. 2001. Scarring alopecia and the dermatopathologist. *Journal of Cutaneous Pathology* 28:333–342.

Yager JA, Wilcock BP. 1994. *Color Atlas and Text of Surgical Pathology of the Dog and Cat: Dermatopathology and Skin Tumors.* London: Wolfe Publishing.

Part 3

Non-inflammatory alopecias

3.1

Congenital alopecia

Lars Mecklenburg

Clinically, alopecia can be classified as either congenital or tardive. Congenital alopecia is present at birth or develops soon after birth, when normal individuals develop a hair coat. Since hair follicle development continues after birth, a congenital defect in hair follicle development does not necessarily present immediately at or shortly after birth. Even months after birth, when the first hair cycle is initiated, alopecia may develop due to a defect that has been present congenitally. Therefore, congenital alopecia should always be considered if lack of hair develops within the first year of life, but does not progress beyond that point of time.

Congenital alopecia is a result of defects in hair follicle morphogenesis that can be subdivided into an organogenesis and a differentiation phase (Fig. 3.1.1). The term "dysplasia" is defined as an abnormal development of tissues or organs, associated with alterations in size, shape, and organization of cells. It is therefore correctly and frequently used to describe morphological abnormalities associated with congenital alopecia. However, it must not be confused with "dysplastic" hair follicle diseases that occur later in life (such as canine recurrent flank alopecia) (see Section 3.3.5).

Congenital alopecia does not necessarily imply a genetic basis, although in most cases the disease is based on genetic abnormalities and thus is hereditary. In most cases, genetic abnormalities arise spontaneously, although rare cases of teratogenicity associated with alopecia have been described in domestic animal species. Congenital defects can occur in a single differentiated cell population, or can affect undifferentiated cells that transmit the defect to their daughter cells. A defect within the ectoderm can therefore be restricted to the hair follicle (i.e., follicular dysplasia) or can be associated with abnormalities in other ectoderm-derived cutaneous appendages such as apocrine and eccrine glands, nails/claws, and teeth (i.e., ectodermal dysplasia). More than 190 different forms of ectodermal dysplasia have been described in humans, and a huge amount of mouse models with ectodermal dysplasia exist (Freire-Maia et al. 2001). Data on ectodermal dysplasia in domestic animals, however, is very sparse.

3.1.1 Hair follicle aplasia

Hair follicles arise from an ectodermal thickening overlying a mesenchymal condensation (hair placode). The mechanisms that regulate placode formation in the mammalian ectoderm are extremely complex and still insufficiently understood. There are different subsets of hair follicles in most species that supposedly recruit different molecular mechanisms of placode formation, further complicating the mechanisms of early hair follicle development.

3.1.1.1 X-linked hair follicle aplasia and dental dysplasia (analogous to anhidrotic ectodermal dysplasia in humans)

Until now, only one molecular pathway has been discovered that is clearly linked to the very early stages of hair placode formation and that results in a lack of hair follicle development if one of its genes is mutated. This pathway involves the signaling molecule ectodysplasin (Eda, analogous to the mouse tabby gene) and its receptors (analogous of the mouse downless and crinkled gene). Mice with a defect in either tabby, downless, or crinkled gene show multifocal alopecia, based on a complete lack of primary (tylotrich) hair follicles in affected skin regions. As ectodysplasin signaling is

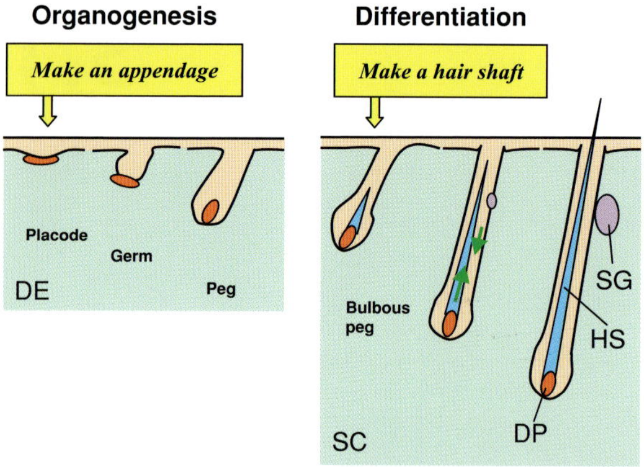

Fig. 3.1.1 Scheme on hair follicle morphogenesis that can be subdivided into organogenesis and differentiation. A first mesenchymal signal ("make an appendage") induces placode formation. This placode consists of an epidermal ingrowth and an underlying condensed mesenchyme (red). The condensed mesenchyme later builds the dermal papilla. The placode elongates and grows into the dermis (DE). Once a hair peg is formed (dermal papilla is completely enclosed by keratinocytes), hair shaft (HS) formation is induced by a second mesenchymal message ("make a hair shaft"). The hair shaft grows towards the skin surface, whereas the hair follicle simultaneously grows into the opposite direction by elongation of the outer root sheath (indicated by the green arrows). In the later stages of morphogenesis, the sebaceous gland (SG) is formed and the lower portion of the hair shaft grows into the subcutis (SC). (Reprinted with permission from Mecklenburg 2006.)

also involved in the development of other cutaneous appendages such as teeth, alopecia is associated with dental dysplasia, characterizing the disease as a true ectodermal dysplasia. In both mice and humans, the disease is X-linked and is inherited in a recessive pattern. In humans, the disease is called anhidrotic (or hypohydrotic) ectodermal dysplasia, emphasizing its most crucial effect, which is a complete lack of sweat glands and a resulting insufficient thermoregulation.

3.1.1.1.1 Canine X-linked hair follicle aplasia and dental dysplasia

A disease analogous to anhidrotic ectodermal dysplasia in humans has repeatedly been described in various breeds of dogs (Thomsett 1961; Kral and Schwartzman 1964; Selmanowitz et al. 1970a,b, 1977a,b; Muller and Kirk 1976; Kunkle 1984; Chastain and Swayne 1985; Grieshaber et al. 1986; Casal et al. 1997; Moura and Cirio 2004). Comparable to mice and humans, this form of ectodermal dysplasia in dogs is a recessive X-linked trait and as such primarily occurs in males, although very rare cases in females are possible because of inactivation (lyonization) of the unaffected allele (Moura and Cirio 2004). X-linked ectodermal dysplasia in dogs is characterized by multifocal alopecia, affecting the frontotemporal region, the sacral region, the abdomen, and the proximal limbs (Moura and Cirio 2004) (Fig. 3.1.2). The expressivity of alopecia varies, mostly affecting about two-third of the body. This variable expressivity is possibly due to allelic heterogeneity (Moura and Cirio 2004). Alopecia is caused by complete absence of hair follicles, associated with a lack of arrector pili muscles, sebaceous glands, and apocrine glands (Fig. 3.1.3). In contrast, biopsies from normally haired skin regions show normal pilosebaceous units (Casal et al. 1997). Dogs with X-linked ectodermal dysplasia also show a lack of eccrine glands in the footpads and dental alterations affecting both deciduous and permanent teeth. Claws are normal, as is the immune system. Frequent respiratory tract infections have been reported (Casal et al. 2005) and may be due to a lack of mucous glands as has been observed in ectodermal dysplasia in humans and cattle (Seeliger et al. 2005).

3.1.1.1.2 Bovine X-linked hair follicle aplasia and dental dysplasia

In cattle, congenital X-linked hypotrichosis associated with severe dental abnormalities (also called "hypotrichosis and anodontia defect" or "anhidrotic ectodermal dysplasia in cattle") has been described in several breeds (Drieux et al. 1950; Rieck 1985; Braun et al. 1988; Wijeratne et al. 1988; Distl et al. 2000; Drögemüller et al. 2002a, 2003). Other reports of hypotrichosis and dental dysplasia in cattle are probably also variants of this disease (Cole 1919; Ojo 1987). As in humans, mice, and dogs, this form of congenital hair follicle aplasia shows an X-linked monogenetic recessive inheritance and primarily occurs in male calves. Affected animals show a variable degree of alopecia, with head, ear pinnae, neck, back, and tail being most prominently affected. Eyelashes and vibrissae may be absent too (Fig. 3.1.4). Histologically, the number of hair follicles is greatly reduced (aplasia), as is the number of apocrine glands and eccrine nasolabial glands (Fig. 3.1.5). The disease is associated with incomplete dentition, resulting in the lack of several teeth and a lack of secondary tooth development. Mucous glands in the respiratory tract are reduced as well (Seeliger

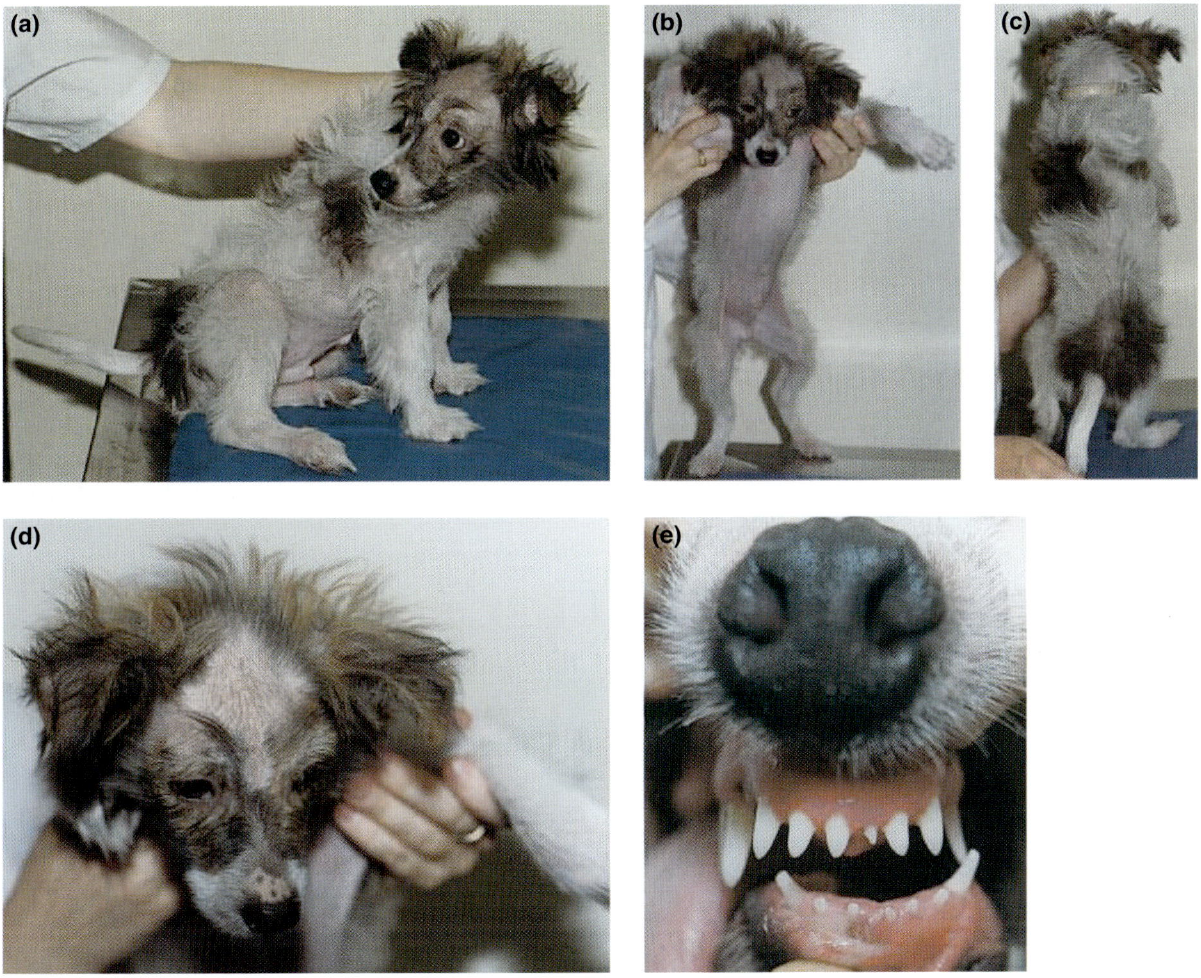

Fig. 3.1.2 X-linked ectodermal dysplasia in an 8-month-old dog. (a–d) Extensive alopecia on head and abdomen; (e) dental dysplasia. (Reprinted with permission from Moura and Cirio (2004).)

et al. 2005). Anhidrotic X-linked ectodermal dysplasia in cattle is linked to the bovine Ed1 gene, with various mutations leading to a defective Eda protein (Drögemüller et al. 2001, 2002b; Kuiper et al. 2001).

3.1.1.2 Aplasia of hair follicles without dental dysplasia

Except for the aforementioned X-linked aplasia of hair follicles with dental dysplasia that is analogous to anhidrotic ectodermal dysplasia in humans and that is associated with defects in ectodysplasin signaling, reports on hair follicle aplasia in domestic animals are very rare. A significant reduction in the number of hair follicles, with other ectodermal tissues not being affected, has been reported in swine (Roberts and Carroll 1931; Meyer and Drommer 1968). One report describes piglets that lack hair except for eye lashes and sparse hair on the bridge of the nose and the base of the ear pinnae. Hypotrichosis was inherited in a dominant autosomal trait (gene symbol: Hy) and was associated with a 70% reduction in the hair follicles in homozygous individuals. The affected piglets showed intolerance for cold temperatures and usually died within 10 days after birth. Another variant of congenital alopecia in swine (that appears to be distinct from X-linked hair follicle aplasia with dental dysplasia) involves *Iberian pigs* (Fig. 3.1.6). These are an ancient population of Mediterranean pigs that are differentiated into several subtypes, one of them being hairless (black Iberian

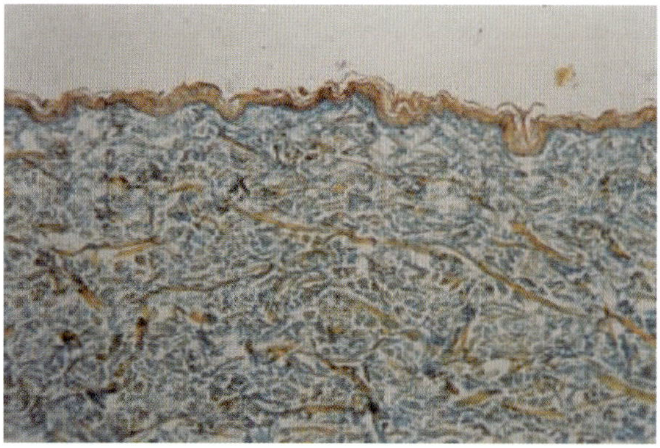

Fig. 3.1.3 Cutaneous histopathology in canine X-linked epidermal dysplasia. Absence of hair follicles, arrector pili muscles, sweat glands, and sebaceous glands. Note also orthokeratotic hyperkeratosis and normal dermal collagen fibers. Mallory stain, ×40. (Reprinted with permission from Moura and Cirio (2004).)

hairless pig) (Lemus-Flores et al. 2001). The responsible gene has been mapped to chromosome 14 but has not been further analyzed (Fernandez et al. 2003). Hairless Iberian pigs are probably the founders of the Mexican hairless pig breed that still exists in Mexico (also known as the Mexican Creole pig). Mexican hairless pigs have a reduced number of hair follicles and apocrine glands (David 1932). Remaining hair follicles are normal, except for rudimentary sebaceous glands associated with them. Dental dysplasia is not reported.

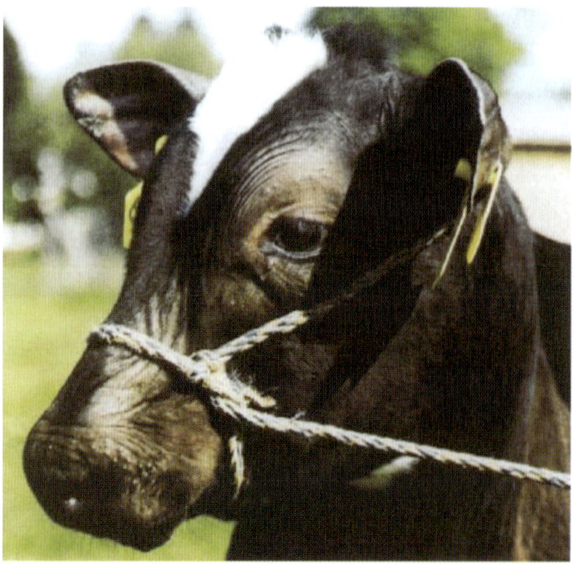

Fig. 3.1.4 X-linked ectodermal dysplasia (hypotrichosis and oligodontia) in a black and white German Holstein calf. Note the sparse haircoat, which is most obvious around the eyes, and the completely dry muzzle. (Reprinted with permission from Drögemüller et al. (2002a).)

3.1.2 Hair follicle dysplasia

Forms of congenital alopecia that are associated with malformed hair follicles are best described as "hair follicle dysplasia." In these diseases, hair follicle morphogenesis has progressed beyond the placode stage (differentiating them from mere hair follicle aplasia as discussed before). As mentioned earlier, dysplasia refers to a change in size, shape, and organization of cells. The severity of those structural changes can vary widely. For the ease of classification, hair follicle dysplasia can be separated into those forms where hair shafts are formed by dyslastic hair follicles and those where hair follicle dysplasia is so severe that no hair shaft formation is seen at all.

3.1.2.1 Hair follicle dysplasia without hair shaft formation

There are several dog breeds that per definition are supposed to lack fur and that are promoted for their "hypoallergenic" nature. Several extinct hairless breeds have been reported from Africa. It is assumed that Spanish traders introduced hairless dogs to the New World and four of those hairless breeds are still known today: the Chinese Crested Dog, the Mexican Hairless Dog, the Inca Hairless Dog, and the Peruvian Inca Orchid Dog.

Due to the phenotypic similarity, congenital alopecia in these breeds is assumed to be related to a similar genetic deficit. Indeed a recent publication reports a frameshift mutation within the FOX13 coding sequence in Mexican and Peruvian Hairless Dogs and Chinese Crested Dogs. FOX13 is a member of a transcription factor family encoded on dog chromosome 17. It appears to be involved in hair and tooth development, although its precise function has not been elucidated yet (Drögemüller et al. 2008).

3.1.2.1.1 Chinese Crested Dog

The Chinese Crested Dog is known since the late nineteenth century and is now the most popular breed of hairless dogs. Hairlessness is inherited as an autosomal dominant trait, symbolized as "hr." The hr allele is prenatally lethal when homozygous; hence, the hairless Chinese Crested Dog is heterozygous. The haired littermates with long fur are known as "powderpuffs"

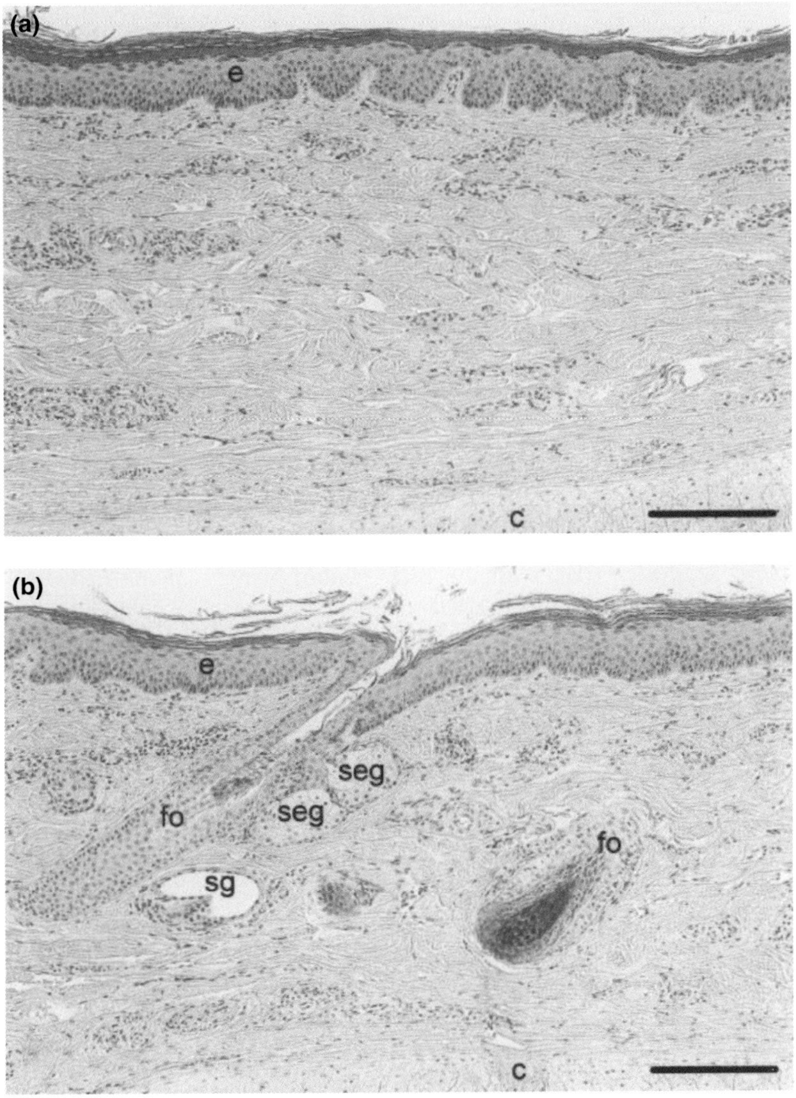

Fig. 3.1.5 X-linked ectodermal dysplasia (hypotrichosis and oligodontia) in a black and white German Holstein calf. Histology of the skin from the back of the ear pinna. (a) Hair follicles are completely absent; (b) a control animal of the same age and breed with normal skin and adnexa; scale bar = 75 μm; e, epidermis; fo, hair follicle; sg, apocrine sweat gland; seg, sebaceous gland; c, ear cartilage. (Reprinted with permission from Drögemüller et al. (2002a).)

(Robinson 1985) (Fig. 3.1.7). Hairless littermates are devoid of hair except for the crown of the head, lower parts of the extremities, and the tail. Adult Chinese Crested Dogs exhibit several hair follicle infundibula that are distorted and filled with abundant keratin squames (Fig. 2.2.10). Some hair follicles show a condensation of mesenchymal cells at the base of those comedones, suggesting remnants of an immature dermal papilla. Hairlessness is usually associated with defects in dentition, suggesting another variant of an ectodermal dysplasia in the dog. Although the phenotype has some similarities to X-linked anhidrotic ectodermal dysplasia, the distribution of alopecia is different as is the histopathological picture. Hence, it is unlikely that the ED1 gene is responsible for the hairless phenotype in the Chinese crested dog, as has recently been confirmed by linkage analysis (Sander et al. 2005).

3.1.2.1.2 Mexican Hairless Dog

The Mexican Hairless Dog (also known as "Xoloitzcuintli") is supposed to date back more than 5,700 years. The scientific literature on Mexican Hairless Dogs is sparse (Yankell et al. 1970a,b; Goto et al. 1987) and primarily focuses on their use in dermatological research, mostly describing descendants of Mexican Hairless Dogs crossbred with Beagles (Kimura et al. 1992, 1998; Kimura and Doi 1994a,b,

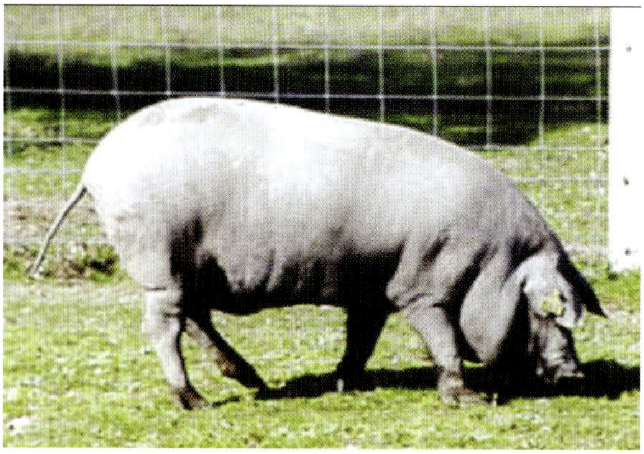

Fig. 3.1.6 Alopecic phenotype of the hairless Iberian pig. (Courtesy of M.A.T. Ibáñez.)

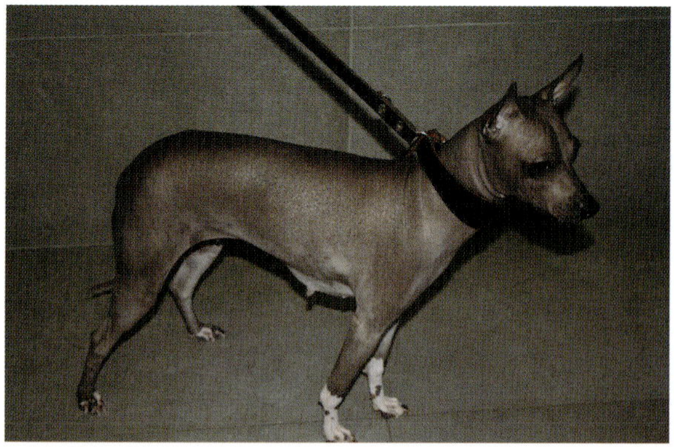

Fig. 3.1.8 Alopecic phenotype of the Mexican Hairless Dog. (Courtesy of J. Declercq.)

1998a,b, 1999). Hairlessness is inherited by an autosomal dominant trait, with the gene symbol being "Hm" (Kimura et al. 1992, 1993), and therefore litters reveal both hairless and coated individuals. The hairless siblings completely lack a hair coat except for some tufts of short, stiff hair on the head and on the tip of the tail (Fig. 3.1.8). Hairlessness is associated with dysplastic teeth and therefore represents another form of ectodermal dysplasia affecting more than one ectoderm-derived tissue. There are no immunological defects in hairless dogs (Hirota et al. 1990) and no significant abnormalities in hematological and serum biochemical parameters. Hairless dogs of less than

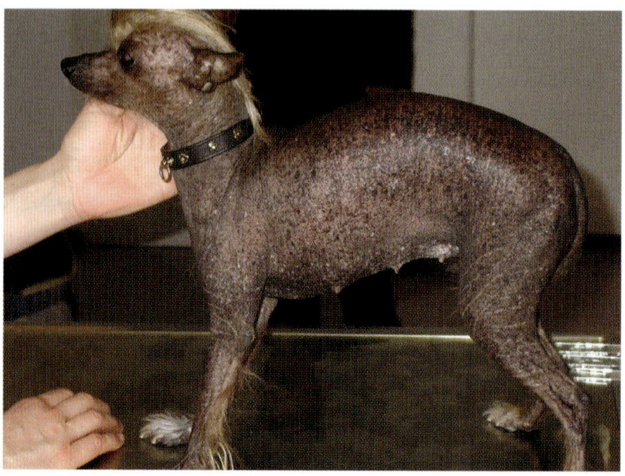

Fig. 3.1.7 Alopecic phenotype of the heterozygous Chinese Crested Dog. Note typical truncal alopecia with some tufts of hair at the crown of the head and the lower parts of the extremities.

2 weeks of age have a relatively thick epidermis with many melanocytes and prominent epidermal rete pegs (Fukuta et al. 1991; Kimura and Doi 1994a, b). There are several aborted hair follicle plugs that are unable to produce a hair shaft. Hair follicle plugs consist of an epidermal ingrowth with a mesenchymal condensation at its base, likely representing an immature dermal papilla. Those epidermal ingrowths do not develop into normal hair follicles and their number is finally reduced with age (Kimura and Doi 1996). Many of those aborted hair follicles form an infundibulum that accumulates masses of keratin squames and develops into a comedone. Comedones are most prominent on the dorsum, ventral neck, distal extremities, and prepuce. Most hair follicles likely undergo atrophy since biopsies from adult Mexican Hairless Dogs show a severely reduced number of cutaneous appendages. Whether a primary reduction of hair follicles is present in these dogs has not been clarified yet. Very few normal hair follicles with associated sebaceous and apocrine glands develop in the dorsal skin of hairless dogs (Kimura 1996). Interestingly, minoxidil, a potassium-channel agonist with hypotonic properties, has been reported to stimulate and improve postnatal hair follicle development in descendants of the Mexican Hairless Dog, but description of results and understanding of the underlying mechanism are poor (Kimura and Doi 1997).

3.1.2.1.3 Peruvian Hairless and Peruvian Inca Orchid Dog

The Peruvian Hairless Dog and the Peruvian Inca Orchid Dog (also known as Inca Hairless Dog) are distinct but very rare breeds. They resemble the Mexican hairless and Chinese Crested Dog in that hairlessness is caused by an autosomal dominant trait that produces normally haired and hairless littermates. Hairlessness is associated with dental abnormalities, suggesting an ectodermal dysplasia, most likely different from the anhidrotic form.

3.1.2.2 Hair follicle dysplasia with hair shaft formation

Once a hair follicle has undergone organogenesis, it starts producing a hair shaft (Fig. 3.1.1). This is the beginning of the differentiation phase of hair follicle morphogenesis (see Section 1.1.5) and it requires the anlage of a normal hair bulb. Many forms of congenital hair follicle dysplasia show histological evidence of hair shaft formation, ranging from severely dysplastic hair shafts to those that are almost normal (Fig. 3.1.9).

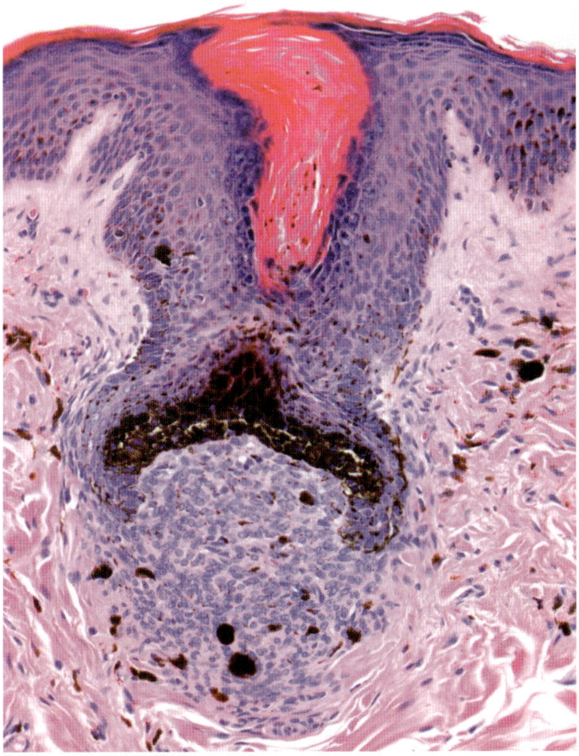

Fig. 3.1.9 Histology of congenital hair follicle dysplasia in a young Golden Retriever. Note formation of severely dysplastic dermal papilla and hair matrix cells.

If hair shafts are formed that penetrate the follicular ostium, alopecia usually results from frequent breaking of hair shafts. Hair follicle dysplasia with almost normal hair shaft formation may be difficult to detect morphologically, as the defects in hair shafts can be very subtle. It can be indistinguishable from mere trichomalacia (defects in hair shafts that are not associated with any abnormality in the hair follicle itself) (see Chapter 3.2).

Hair follicle dysplasia with some degree of hair shaft formation is common in laboratory animal models of alopecia. The prototypic hair follicle dysplasia with hair shaft formation is present in nude mice that have a defect in the Foxn1 transcription factor (see Chapter 1.1). In homozygous mice, hair shafts lack certain keratins and consequently they are soft and twist as they enter the follicular infundibulum. Most hair shafts are not able to penetrate the follicular ostium and instead coil within the infundibulum from which they are occasionally released during the still ongoing hair cycle. Although the nude phenotype has also been described in rats and humans, it has not been found in domestic animals so far.

3.1.2.2.1 Spiculosis in Kerry Blue Terriers

Hair shaft dysplasia with hair shaft formation has been described in Kerry Blue Terriers, where the disease is known as "spiculosis in Kerry Blue Terriers." Young male dogs are usually affected and will demonstrate thickened hair shafts that are known as thorns, spikes, or bristles. These symptoms are usually found around elbows, hocks, and on the feet. Hair follicles are dysplastic with premature keratinization (McKeever 1992).

3.1.2.2.2 Autosomal recessive congenital alopecia in cattle

There are various forms of autosomal recessive congenital alopecia in cattle. They are clinically distinct from X-linked anhidrotic ectodermal dysplasia (see Section 3.1.1.1.2). In many reports, however, histopathological descriptions are sparse (Eldridge and Atkeson 1953; Holmes and Young 1954; Ackerman 1983) and a more precise subclassification of these disease entities is currently impossible. An autosomal recessive hereditary form of progressive alopecia, occurring within the first weeks of life, is known in polled Hereford calves (Steffen et al. 1991, 1993). This "congenital progressive alopecia in polled Hereford cattle" might be the same condition that is known as "semihairlessness" (Craft and Blizzard 1934; Kidwell and Guilbert 1950; Young 1953; Hutt 1963). Calves have wiry and kinked or curled hair fibers at birth and present with alopecia over the bridge of the nose and the ears. Within weeks, alopecia progresses and affects head, lateral neck, shoulders, and dorsal lumbar areas (Fig. 3.1.10). Alopecia is associated with excessive scaling. Other consistent findings in affected animals are bone marrow erythroid hyperplasia with dyserythropoiesis and persistent macrocytic normochromic anaemia with mild reticulocytosis, subcapsular hepatic fibrosis, and subtle neurological findings (Steffen et al. 1992a,b). Histologically, the number of hair follicles is unaltered. Hair follicles are reported to show infundibular hyperkeratosis and degeneration of individual keratinocytes both within the infundibular epithelium and within the inner root sheath (Fig. 3.1.11). An increase in telogen hair follicles is described and there are atrophic sebaceous glands as well as dilated apocrine glands (Steffen et al. 1991).

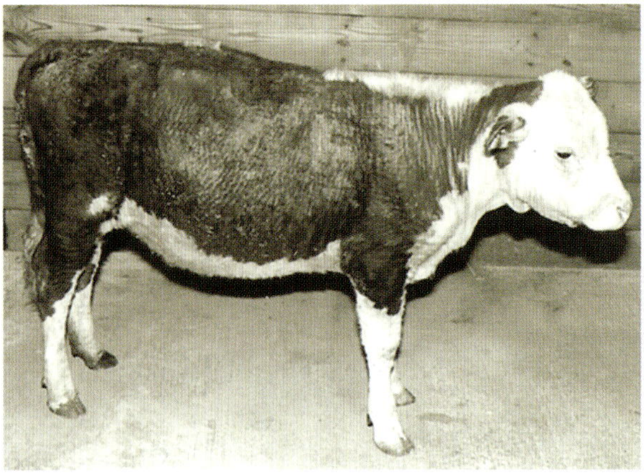

Fig. 3.1.10 Alopecic phenotype of polled Hereford cow. (Courtesy of D. Steffen.)

3.1.2.2.3 Autosomal dominant congenital alopecia in cattle

There is also an autosomal dominant congenital alopecia in cattle that has been described in the polled

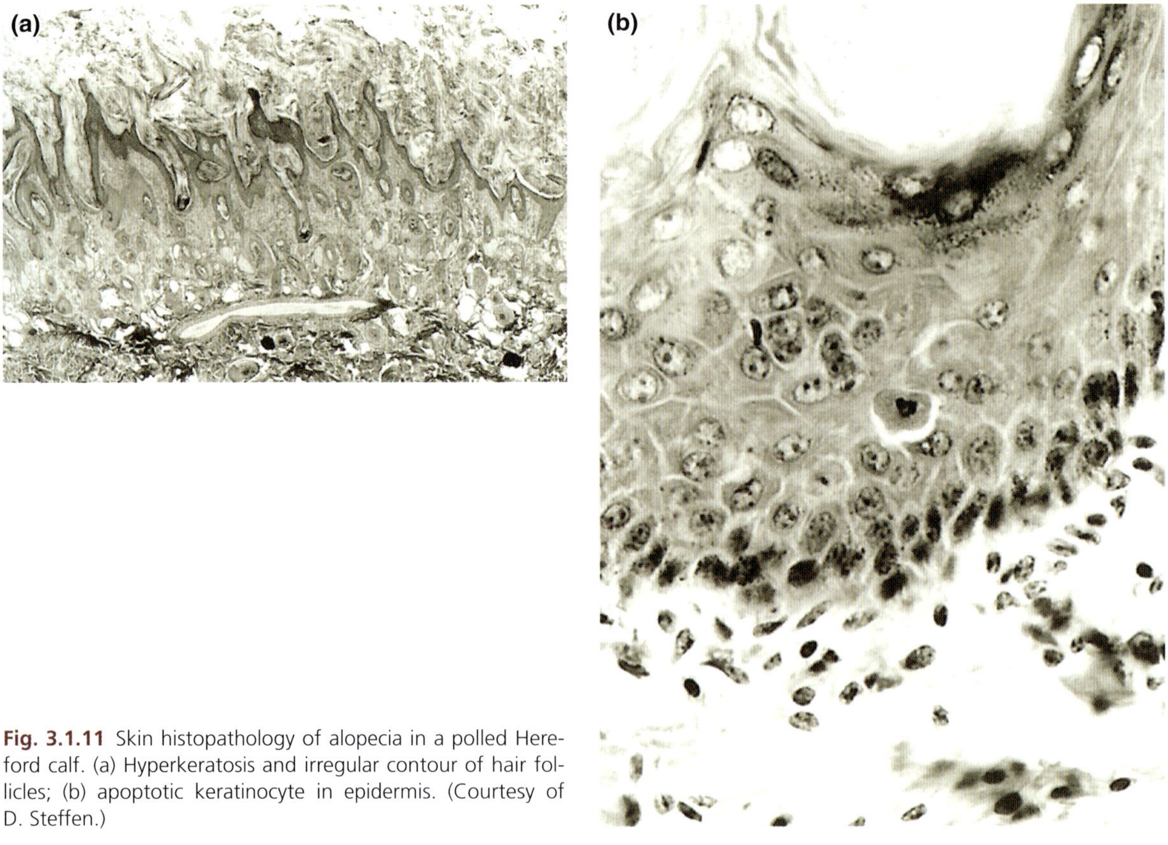

Fig. 3.1.11 Skin histopathology of alopecia in a polled Hereford calf. (a) Hyperkeratosis and irregular contour of hair follicles; (b) apoptotic keratinocyte in epidermis. (Courtesy of D. Steffen.)

Hereford breed. It is characterized by congenital alopecia with sparse curly hair, often associated with abnormalities of the hoofs. Hair follicles are hypoplastic and show vacuolization and enlarged trichohyalin granules in the inner root sheath (Jayasekera 1979; Rose et al. 1983; Bracho et al. 1984).

3.1.2.2.4 Hair follicle dysplasia in horses

Hair follicle dysplasia in horses is very rare and for most anecdotal cases detailed clinical and histopathological investigations are lacking. There is only one scientific report describing the clinical and histopathological features of hypotrichosis in a male blue roan Percheron draught horse (Valentine et al. 2001). The horse was born with patchy areas of alopecia over the trunk and extremities, whereas hair was present on mane, tail, and forelocks. With age, alopecia progressed and became generalized, with only sparse remaining vibrissae, mane, tail, and forelock hairs. Histopathology revealed a normal density of hair follicles, but hair shafts were mostly absent from follicles. Hair follicles had a severely reduced diameter (hypoplasia) and were often surrounded by a thickened connective tissue sheath, interpreted as an indication of "telogen." There was marked infundibular hyperkeratosis. Sebaceous glands as well as epitrichial apocrine glands were normal. Those features suggest a follicular dysplasia with dysplastic hair shafts.

3.1.2.2.5 Hair follicle dysplasia in cats

Hair follicle dysplasia in cats has appeared sporadically in various breeding programs throughout the world, but has rarely been reported in the scientific literature. First hairless individuals were reported from Mexico and France, but have not been bred systematically until hairlessness has occurred spontaneously in Canada in the 1960s and was finally maintained as the "Sphynx cat" breed. The hairless phenotype is symbolized by "hr" and is characterized by complete absence of fur except for tufts of short, soft hair on the ears, muzzle, tail, feet, and scrotum (Fig. 3.1.12). Whiskers are short and curled. Hairless cats with normal whiskers have been described as well, and the gene symbol "hi" has been suggested (Hendy-Ibbs 1984). Histopathological changes in Sphynx cats have not been sufficiently described. Biopsies from Sphynx cats that occasionally occur in diagnostic services show rather small and curved hair follicles that appear otherwise normal (Fig.

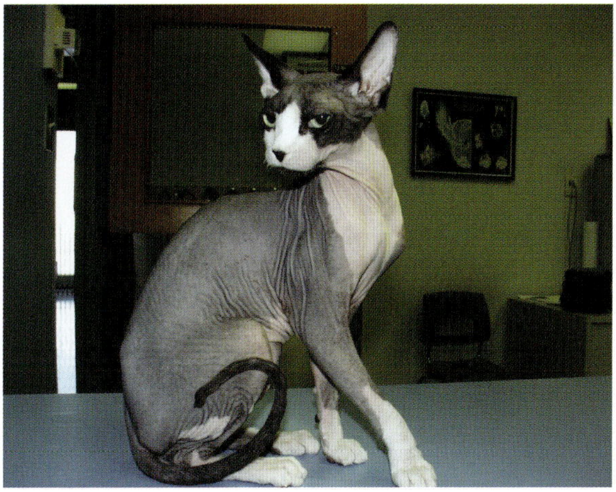

Fig. 3.1.12 Alopecic phenotype of a Sphynx cat.(Courtesy of M. Paradis.)

3.1.13). Most of those hair follicles are in anagen and they produce hair shafts. The latter, however, are very small in diameter, they bend within the dermis, and although some degree of hair shaft formation is evident, many hair follicle infundibula are empty.

3.1.2.3 Hair follicle dysplasia associated with congenital defects in hair follicle cycling

Hair follicle morphogenesis ends with initiation of the first hair growth cycle, which is initiation of hair follicle regression (catagen). A well-characterized phenotype of congenital alopecia in mice and humans is the "hairless" mutation. The hairless protein (that interacts with intranuclear histone deacetylases) functions as a transcription factor. Morphological studies suggest that hairless protein plays a crucial function in catagen development of hair follicles. Individuals with a nonfunctioning hairless protein develop a normal hair coat after birth but start loosing their hair shortly thereafter. In mice, alopecia progresses from the neck caudally, following initiation of the first postnatal hair growth cycle. In affected individuals the mesenchymal cells of the dermal papilla loose contact with the ectodermal cells of the hair germ. This results in formation of cystic hair follicle infundibula and a lack of anagen initiation. Instead cysts form in the deep dermis, possibly arising from an inductive potential of dermal papilla cells that lay in proximity to remnant epithelial cells. The morphological phenotype of the hairless mutation is rather characteristic and is almost

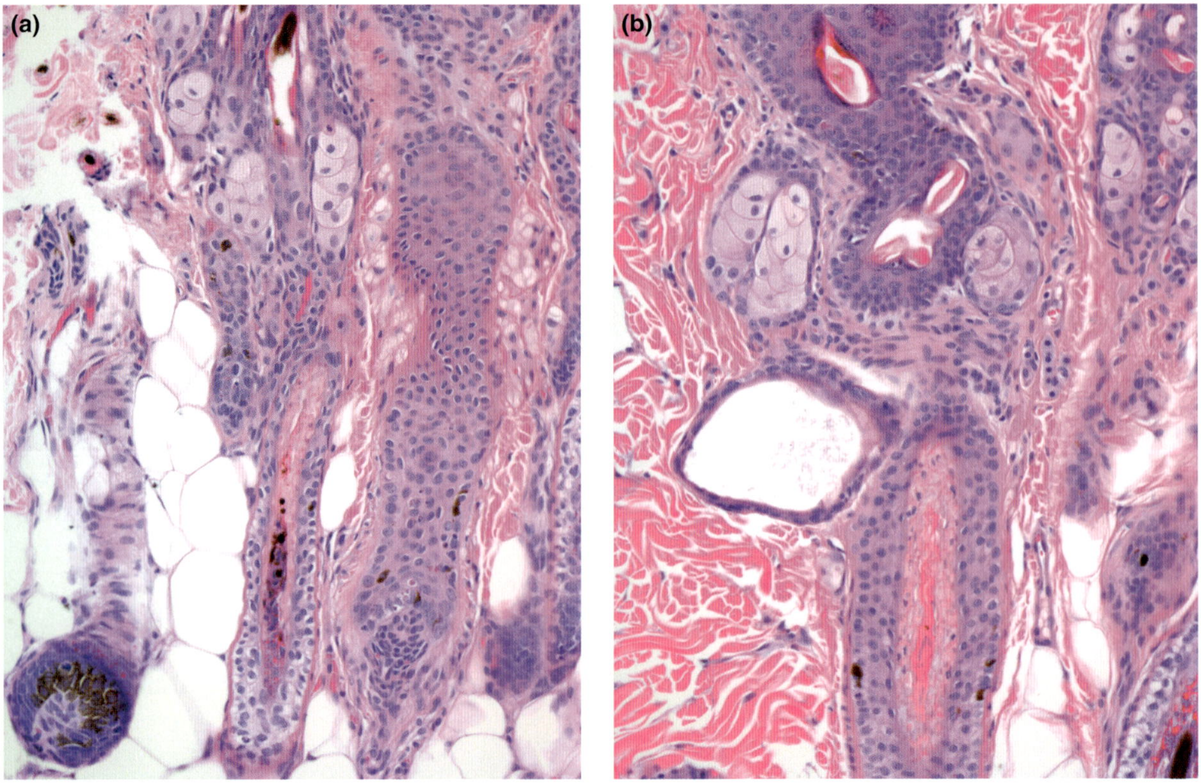

Fig. 3.1.13 Skin histology of a Sphynx cat. (a) Anagen and catagen hair follicles; (b) dysplastic hair shafts.

identical in mice and humans (where the disease is known as "papular atrichia").

3.1.2.3.1 Hairless cats

Recently, a hairless cat with congenital alopecia and a morpholgical phenotype that is somehow similar to hairless mice has been described (Figs 3.1.14 and 3.1.15). It is currently not known whether alopecia in this individual is linked to the analogous hairless gene, and more detailed investigations are warranted (Neuber et al. 2006).

3.1.2.3.2 Alopecia in Valle del Belice sheep

Mutations in the analogous hairless gene of sheep have been described in alopecic Valle del Belice sheep (Fig. 3.1.16). Exon 3 of the hairless gene shows a high frequency of recombination and conversion in alopecic individuals, suggesting a pathogenetic involvement of the sheep hairless gene (Finocchiaro et al. 2003).

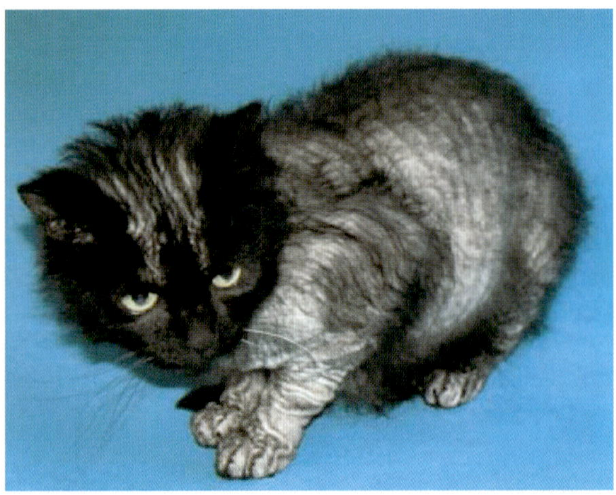

Fig. 3.1.14 Cat with congenital hairlessness. Extensive alopecia on head, trunk, and extremities. (Reprinted with permission from Neuber et al. (2006).)

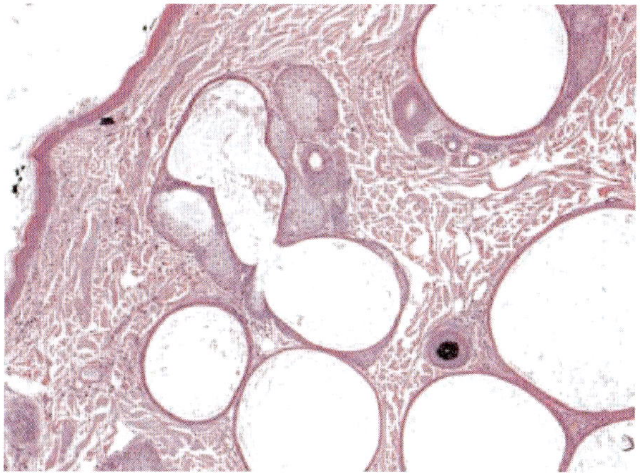

Fig. 3.1.15 Cat with congenital hairlessness. Skin histology with cystic dilation of hair follicles. (Reprinted with permission from Neuber et al. (2006).)

3.1.2.3.3 Lethal and viable hypotrichosis in cattle

Some cases of hypotrichosis in cattle show a strikingly similar morphology to hairless mice. Diseases described as "lethal hypotrichosis" and "viable hypotrichosis" in cattle are associated with dysplastic hair follicles that do not produce hair shafts (Fig. 3.1.17). However, morphology shows trichilemmal keratinization, suggesting that inner root sheath formation, which is always associated with hair shaft formation, has once been present. Hair shafts may have been lost during improper telogen formation. Alopecia is due to dysplastic hair follicles that do not form hair. The number of hair follicles, however, is reported to be normal, as are sebaceous glands. Apocrine glands undergo cystic degeneration. Lethal hypotrichosis occurs in Holstein–Friesians as an autosomal recessive trait and is clinically characterized by generalized alopecia with only sparse hair on muzzle, eyelids, ears, tail, and pastern (Mohr and Wreidt 1928). Affected calves die within a few hours after birth. Viable hypotrichosis has been described in the Guernsey, Jersey, Holstein, and Hereford breeds (Surrarrer 1943; Hutt and Saunders 1953; McGavin and Alexander 1961; Becker et al. 1963; Schleger 1967). It is inherited as an autosomal recessive trait and is characterized by generalized congenital alopecia, with sparse hair on legs, tail, eyelids, and ear pinnae.

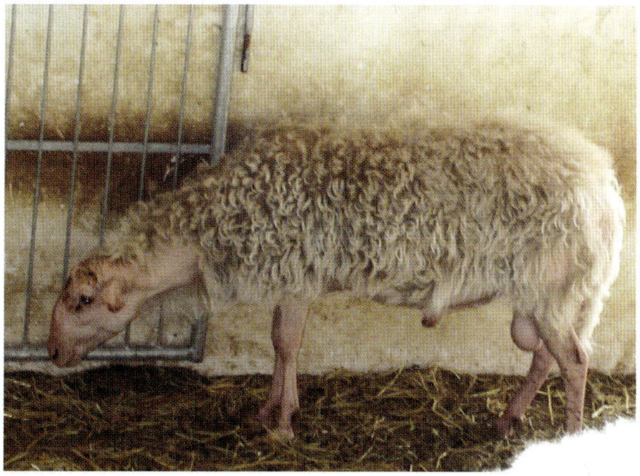

Fig. 3.1.16 Alopecic phenotype of hairless Valle del Belice sheep. (Courtesy of R. Finocchiaro.)

3.1.2.4 Dysplasia of hair follicle pigmentation

The forms of congenital alopecia that were discussed so far involve abnormalities in epithelial and mesenchymal cells of the hair follicle. However, the neuroectoderm-derived follicular melanocytes also contribute to the formation of a pigmented hair shaft, and abnormalities in melanocytes have been described that are associated with alopecia, primarily in the dog.

3.1.2.4.1 Canine black hair follicle dysplasia

Black hair follicle dysplasia (BHFD) in dogs was first described in 1972 as alopecia that is confined to black (or very dark brown) regions of the hair coat (Selmanowitz et al. 1972, 1977a). It has since been reported in a variety of breeds such as the Bearded Collie, Saluki, Border Collie, King Charles spaniel, Jack Russell Terrier, and Gordon Setter (Harper 1978; Gosselin et al. 1982; Hargis et al. 1991; Rest and Davies 1994; Delmage 1995; Dunn et al. 1995; Lewis 1995; Knottenbelt and Knottenbelt 1996; Bohnhorst et al. 2001). First clinical abnormalities are usually noted around 4 weeks of age and comprise fracture of hair shafts in black-coated regions, later resulting in partial alopecia and scaling (Fig. 3.1.18). Most severely affected regions are usually found on the head, ear pinnae, neck, and back, whereas other black-coated areas may exhibit almost normal hair. Trichograms will show pigment clumping in hair shafts (Fig. 2.1.7). Histopathology of affected skin reveals large clumps of melanin within melanocytes of the hair matrix, the

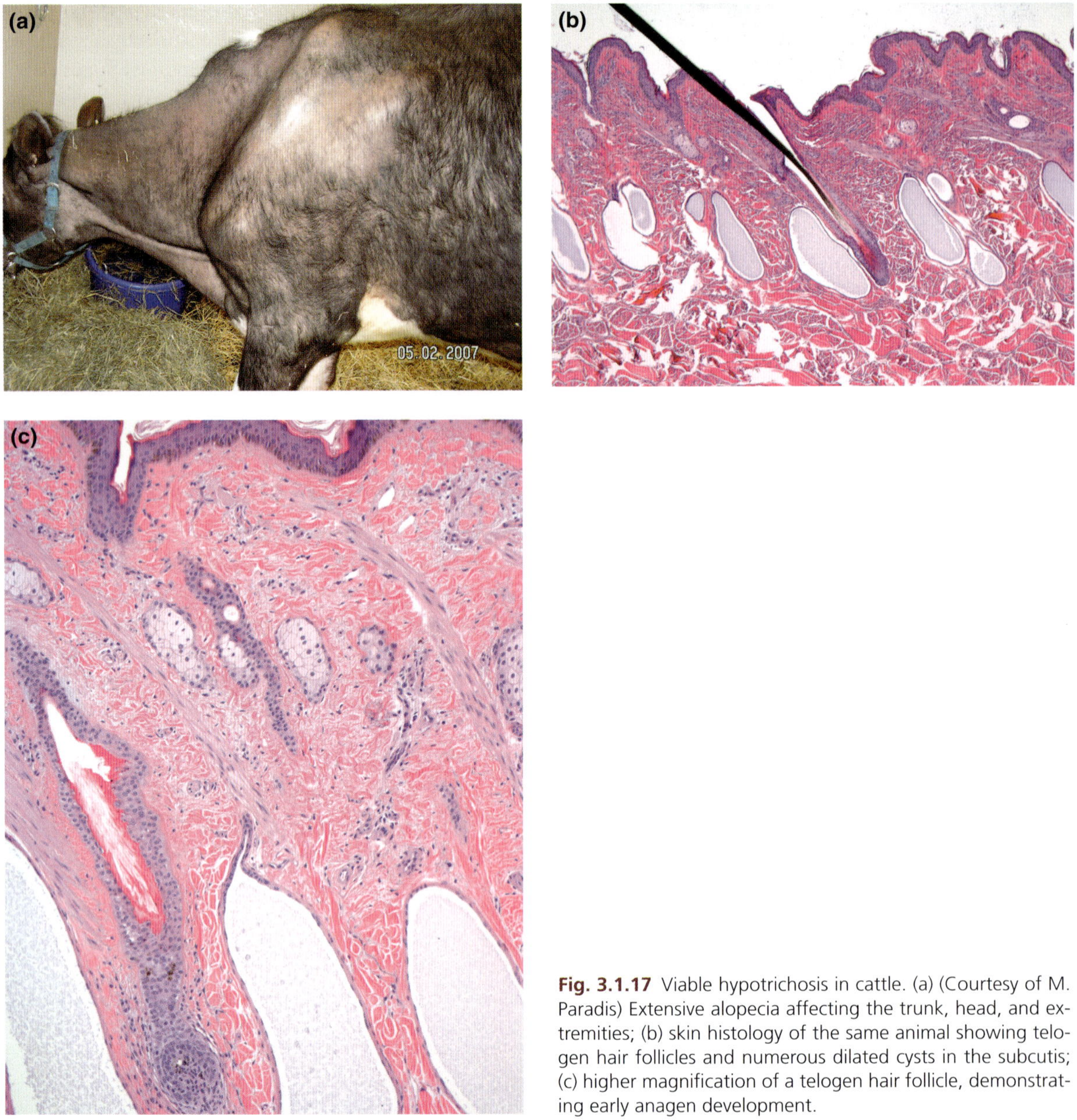

Fig. 3.1.17 Viable hypotrichosis in cattle. (a) (Courtesy of M. Paradis) Extensive alopecia affecting the trunk, head, and extremities; (b) skin histology of the same animal showing telogen hair follicles and numerous dilated cysts in the subcutis; (c) higher magnification of a telogen hair follicle, demonstrating early anagen development.

outer root sheath and, if pigmented, the epidermis. Irregularly distributed clumps of melanin are also found within the medulla and the cortex of hair shafts and the inner root sheath (Fig. 3.1.19). Those hair shafts frequently break within the hair canal resulting in a distorted follicular infundibulum that is filled with keratin squames, fragmented hairs, and large irregular clumps of melanin. These changes have been described as early as 20 days after birth but may develop much later. Chronic lesions may reveal atrophic hair follicles and large numbers of perifollicular melanophages (Selmanowitz et al. 1977a,b; Hargis et al. 1991) (Fig. 3.1.19). Scanning electron microscopy has shown that the cuticle is absent over large areas of the hair fiber, and the cortex may show multiple pits or be fragmented (Hargis et al. 1991). BHFD is inherited in

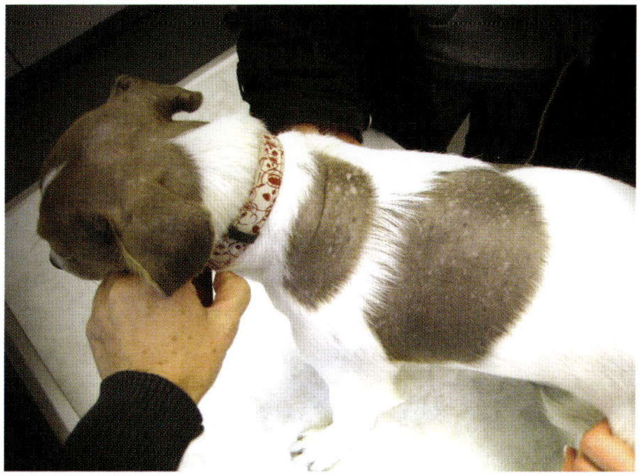

Fig. 3.1.18 Black hair follicle dysplasia in a Jack Russell Terrier. Note extensive alopecia restricted to dark-colored skin areas.

an autosomal recessive mode. Its etiology and pathogenesis are still obscure. It is known that the MSH receptor gene is not linked to BHFD (Schmutz et al. 1998). BHFD has been repeatedly compared to alopecia areata (Selmanowitz et al. 1977a,b; Bohnhorst et al. 2001), but until today there is no evidence that an inflammatory process causes this follicular disease. Association with symmetric lupoid onychitis has been made in a Gordon Setter affected with BHFD and positive antinuclear antibodies have been demonstrated in a few affected dogs (Bohnhorst et al. 2001), but further evidence of any causative link is lacking and seems unlikely. BHFD has been classified as an ectodermal dysplasia by some authors (Foil 1990; Knottenbelt and Knottenbelt 1996), but morphological and genetic evidence points to a neuroectodermal rather than an ectodermal defect.

3.1.2.4.2 Canine color dilution alopecia

With regard to histopathology, color dilution alopecia (CDA) in dogs is identical to BHFD. CDA, also known as color mutant alopecia, has been described in various breeds such as Chihuahua, Chow Chow, Dachshund, Doberman Pinscher, Great Dane, Irish Setter, Italian Greyhound, Poodle, Rhodesian Ridgeback, Saluki, Schnauzer, Shetland Sheepdog, Silky Terrier, whippet, Yorkshire Terrier, as well as some crossbreeds, and Mongrels (Conroy et al. 1975; Briggs and Botha 1986; Ferrer et al. 1988; Miller 1990a,1991; Malik and France 1991; Finnie and Tham 1993; Roperto et al. 1995; Kim et al. 2005). In those breeds, CDA is associated with certain coat colors, known as blue, gray, fawn, and red. Those colors are considered "dilute" since they are brighter shades of black or brown (Laukner 1998). Clinically, a variable degree of alopecia and scaling affects primarily the trunk, and rarely the head and extremities (Fig. 3.1.20). First clinical signs are usually noticed between 3 and 12 months of age, rarely later in life. Affected dogs are prone to secondary bacterial folliculitis, and lesions are usually slowly progressive with age. Scanning electron microscopy reveals cortical defects with large vacuoles that contain melanin granules in medullary, subcortical, and intracortical areas (Beco et al. 1996) (Fig. 3.1.21).

3.1.2.4.3 Etiology and pathogenesis of canine coat color dilution and black hair follicle dysplasia

The etiology of both BHFD and CDA is still not completely understood. Both diseases have been considered an ectodermal defect, although it is most likely that its origin is manifest in neuroectodermal melanocytes. Miller (1990a) was the first to compare the histopathological phenotype of CDA-affected dogs with certain strains of mice and cats (Maltese dilution). He considered a central role of the "*d*" locus that controls intensity of hair shaft pigmentation by influencing size, shape, and distribution of melanin granules within the hair shaft (Silvers 1979; Miller 1991). In mice, there are three spontaneous mutations at the "*d*" locus that cause coat color dilution and similar histomorphological changes as seen in CDA and BHFD. These are mutations in the leaden (*ln*), the dilute (*d*), and the ashen (*ash*) gene (Silvers 1979) corresponding to the human Griscelli syndrome, a rare autosomal recessive disorder that is characterized by diffuse skin pigmentation, silvery hair, and the occurrence of either a primary neurological impairment or a severe immune disorder (Westbroek et al. 2001). It has been shown that those three mutations are linked to defects in the intracellular transport mechanisms within cutaneous melanocytes. Melanocytes synthesize melanosomes in the cell center and transport them into long cytoplasmic dendrites that reach between multiple surrounding keratinocytes of the epidermis or the hair matrix. This transport of melanosomes involves both microtubules and actin filaments (Kelleher and Titus 1998; Rodionov et al. 1998; Rogers

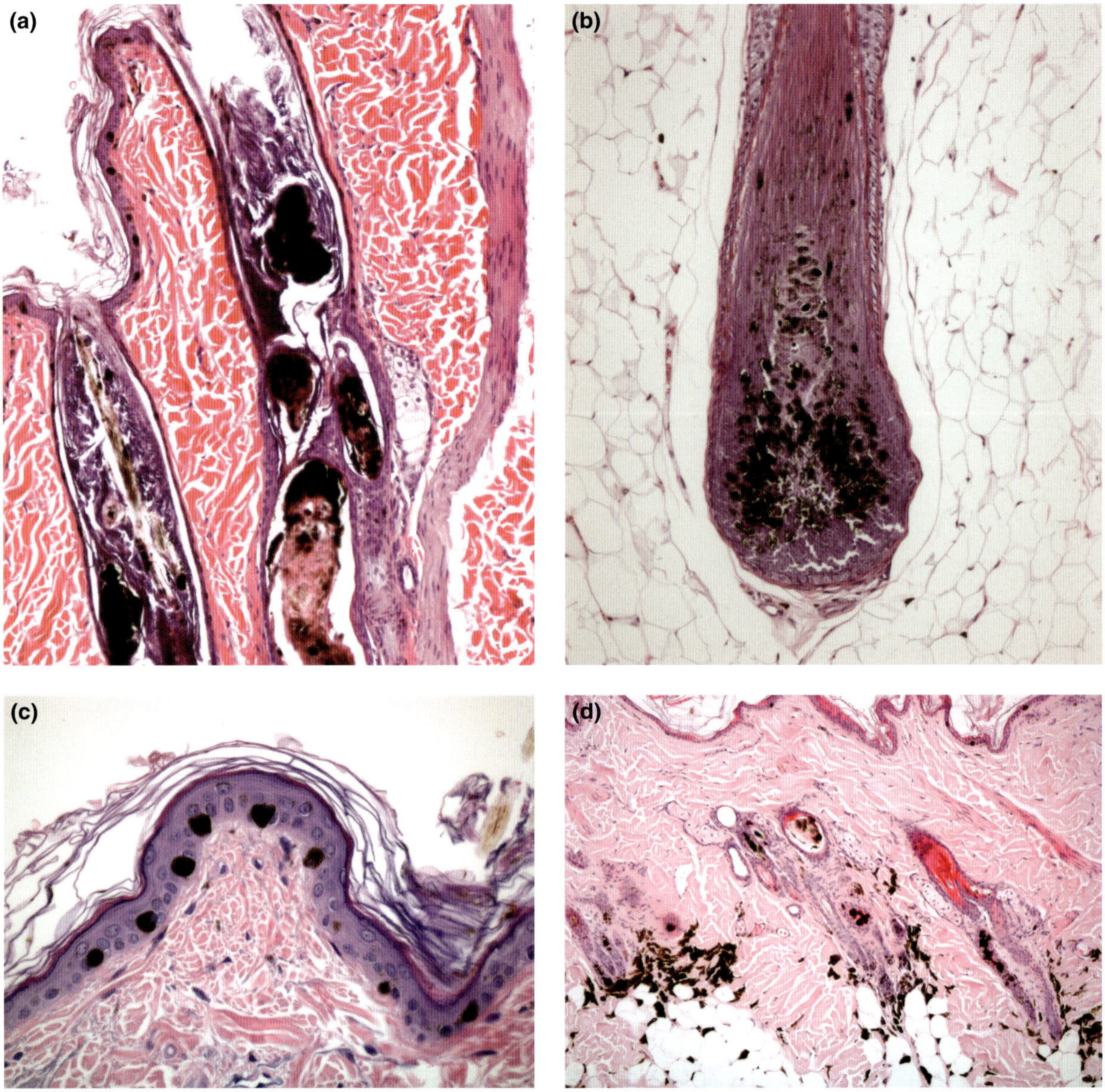

Fig. 3.1.19 Skin histology of black hair follicle dysplasia. (a) Dysplastic hair shafts with irregular pigmentation; (b) pigment clumping in the hair follicle matrix; (c) pigment clumping in epidermal melanocytes; (d) catagen hair follicles with dysplastic hair shafts and numerous pigmented cells in the dermis (melanophages).

and Gelfand 1998). Transport along actin filaments in the cell periphery requires the proteins myosin Va (product of the dilute locus), Rab27a (product of the ashen locus) (Wilson et al. 2000), and melanophilin (product of the leaden locus) (Hume et al. 2002) (Fig. 3.1.22). Myosin Va is part of a motor protein that facilitates direct movement along actin filaments in an ATP-dependent manner. Both Rab27a and melanophilin link melanosomes to myosin (Hume et al. 2002; Nagashima et al. 2002). Consequently, functional deficits in any of those three proteins will result in a lack of melanosome transport into cytoplasmic dendrites (Provance et al. 1996, 2002). This transport, however, is crucial to allow coordinated

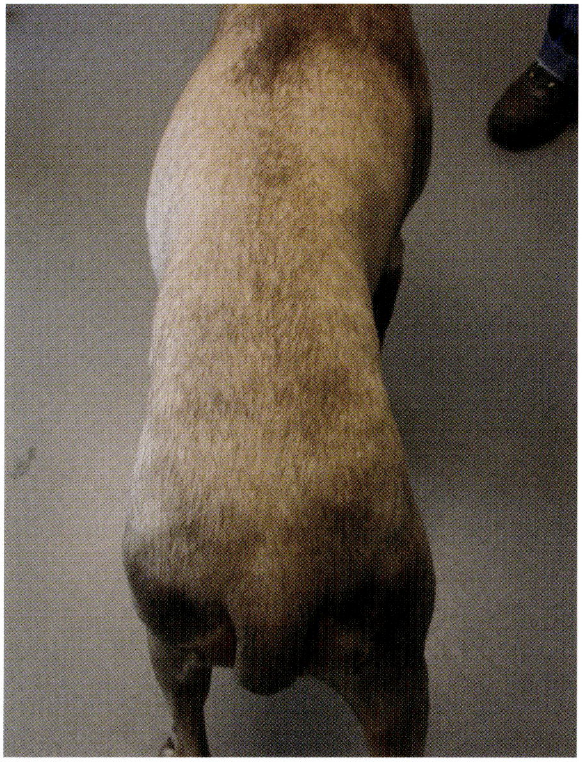

Fig. 3.1.20 Color dilution alopecia in a brown-colored Doberman Pinscher.

transfer of melanosomes from melanocytes into surrounding keratinocytes. Light microscopic evaluation of plucked hair shafts from CDA- and BHFD-affected dogs reveals large packets of clumped pigment within the hair shaft cortex and medulla. Those packets correlate to cortical and medullary vacuoles that are filled with abundant melanosomes, as demonstrated by transmission electron microscopy (Beco et al. 1996). As those melanosomes appear to be of normal size, the term "macromelanosomes" is rather inaccurate and should be replaced by "aggregated melanosomes." Whether the aggregation of melanosomes occurs in terminally differentiating keratinocytes or in melanocytes that originate from the hair bulb and have accidentally been integrated into the hair shaft is still unknown. Recently, evidence was provided that coat color dilution in several dog breeds is caused by one or more mutations within or near the melanophilin gene (Philipp et al. 2005), indicating the similarity to the leaden mutation in mice and the Griscelli syndrome type 3 in humans (Ménasché et al. 2003). A recent study has demonstrated a wide breed distribution of the melanophilin mutation, suggesting an old mutation event that most likely occurred before the foundation of our modern dog breeds (Drögemüller et al. 2008). Although the current data clearly indicate that the dilute mutation increases the risk for CDA and BHFD, there seem to be breed-specific modifying factors.

In summary, there are various dog breeds with characteristic aggregation of melanosomes within hair follicles and epidermis. These abnormalities are associated with black (or dark brown) hair or various shades of blue, silver, and red. The occurrence of pigment clumping in black hairs demonstrates that it is not necessarily associated with coat color dilution. It is likely that black hair fibers in BHFD are so heavily pigmented that even the irregular distribution of

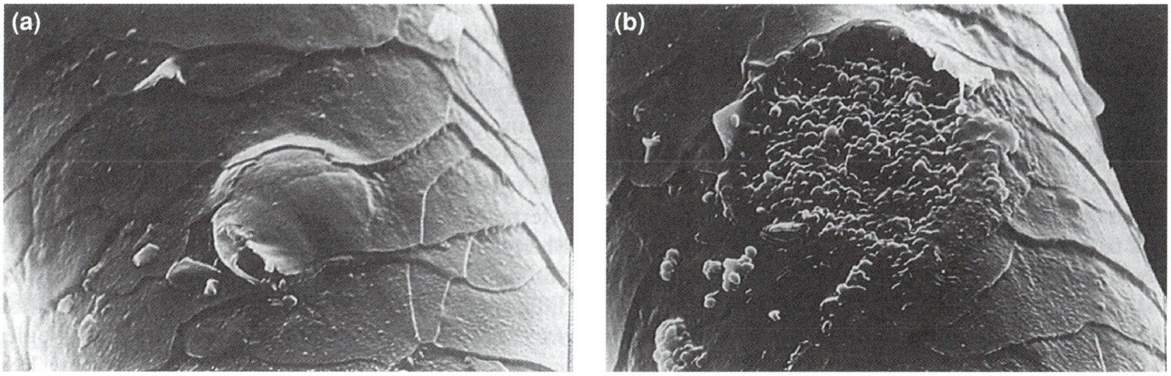

Fig. 3.1.21 Scanning electron microscopy of a hair shaft from a Dachshund with color dilution alopecia, 3,500×. (a) Swelling of the hair shaft cuticle; (b) rupture of cuticle with release of cortical material, assumed to be melanin granules. (Reprinted with permission from Beco et al. (1996).)

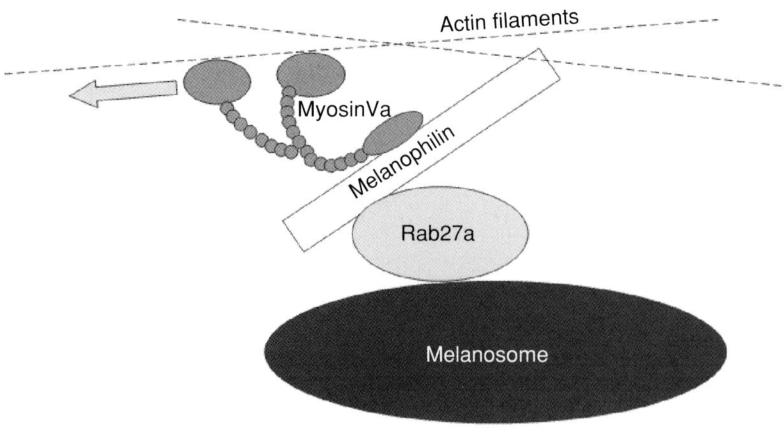

Fig. 3.1.22 Schematic demonstration of proteins involved in melanosome transport along actin filaments.

pigment does not affect its color. The abnormality manifests in cutaneous melanocytes that show impaired melanosome transport. Evidence exists that, at least in some dog breeds, this melanosome transport defect is linked to the melanophilin gene, one of three genes that occur at the "*d*" (dilute) locus. Some dogs with this phenotype (e.g., Weimaraner) are healthy, whereas others develop alopecia and scaling in the first months of life. The degree of melanosome aggregation is variable among breeds and individuals, and so is the expressivity of the clinical disease. It is most likely that BHFD and CDA are based on similar genetic defects and that they merely represent various forms of severity. This would be in line with previous observations, suggesting that BHFD has pigment clumps of larger size than CDA (Hargis et al. 1991). There is no doubt that hair fibers with very irregular pigmentation are prone to fracture. Therefore, alopecia in many cases of BHFD and CDA can be explained by the fracture of hair shafts within or outside of the hair canal. In addition, both BHFD and CDA are reported to show nongrowing hair follicles (i.e., telogen hair follicles or follicle atrophy). This is usually associated with marked hyperkeratosis within the follicular infundibulum. It is possible that hair cycle arrest is a consequence of melanin release. Alternatively, an independent secondary disease process could explain follicular inactivity, and further studies are needed to ultimately clarify the pathogenesis.

Some dogs with very mild coat color dilution may present alopecia later in life. This has particularly been described in black- and red-coated Doberman Pinschers (Miller 1990b), where alopecia clinically and histopathologically resembled CDA with the difference that dogs were between 1 and 4 years of age at the onset of clinical disease. Another difference was the severity of pigmentary clumping that was reported to be much milder compared to most dogs with typical early-onset CDA. Consequently, none of these dogs was described to have typical dilute coat color. It is still not known whether this CDA-like disease in adult dogs is simply a very mild and retarded form of CDA or whether it is caused by a secondary hair cycling abnormality that triggers expressivity of pigmentary changes that do not become clinically apparent otherwise.

3.1.2.4.4 Hair follicle dysplasia in the Weimaraner dog

A specific type of alopecia has been described in young adult Weimaraners (Laffort-Dassot et al. 2002). All Weimaraners have a diluted coat color. As in CDA (see Section 3.1.2.4.2), this coat color dilution is based on an irregular distribution of melanosomes within the hair shaft. Normal Weimaraners have few melanin aggregates (clumps) in both cortex and medulla of hair shafts. These melanin aggregates occur with a moderate density and are quite evenly distributed along the hair shaft. The cuticle is normal. Histologically, melanocytes with aggregated melanosomes are present in the epidermis and the hair bulb. However, melanosome aggregation has usually no clinical significance as only about 20% of hair follicles in normal Weimaraners are slightly distorted with mild infundibular hyperkeratosis.

There is a distinct form of alopecia in Weimaraners that has been named "Follicular dysplasia of the Weimaraner." A genetic defect is assumed but the

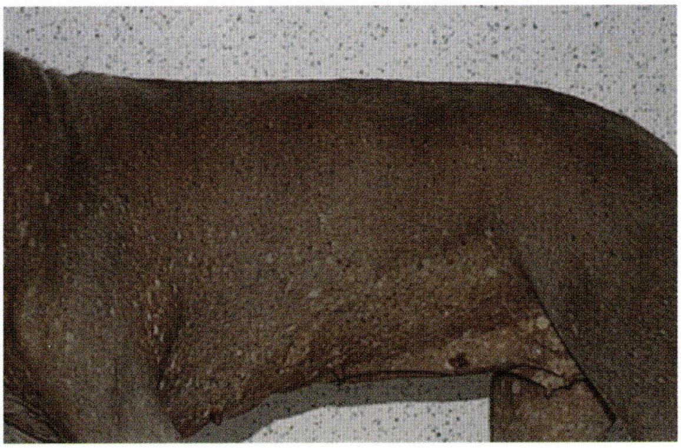

Fig. 3.1.23 Multifocal alopecia in a Weimaraner with follicular dysplasia. (Reprinted with permission from Laffort-Dassot et al. (2002).)

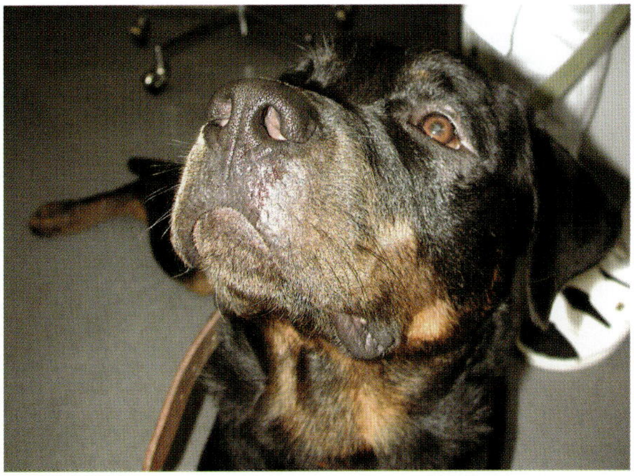

Fig. 3.1.24 Follicular lipidosis in a Rottweiler. Subtle alopecia of mahogany-colored skin areas. (Courtesy of C. Favrot.)

underlying pathogenesis has not been elucidated yet. Alopecia occurs in young adults of both gender, usually between 1 and 3 years of age. Alopecia involves the back, lateral and ventral thorax, flanks, and abdomen, but spares the head and limbs (Fig. 3.1.23). In the affected region, hair fibers break and follicles are prone to recurrent bacterial infection. No pruritus is seen with the disease. Plucked hair shafts from affected areas contain large aggregates of melanin. In contrast to normal Weimaraners, the aggregates are larger and more numerous. In addition, large circular cuticular defects (craters) are found (best demonstrated by scanning electron microscopy). Histology bears many similarities to CDA, but findings are less severe. Hair bulbs and hair shafts show melanocytes with large aggregates of melanosomes. Many hair follicles are distorted by large amounts of infundibular keratin. In summary, macroscopical and histological findings are almost identical to color dilution alpecia, except that their degree of severity is milder. This suggests that "follicular dysplasia in Weimaraners" is another variant of a neuroectodermal dysplasia of the follicular pigmentary unit. The quantitative differences may be explained by the overall smaller amount of melanin in Weimaraners (compared to the breeds classically affected by CDA). Because of the morphological similarities to CDA, it can be assumed that one of the proteins that are crucially involved in melanosome transport (melanophilin, Rab27a, myosin Va) is also involved in the pathogenesis of alopecia in Weimaraners. Whether the mutation in this protein is similar to or different from the one in CDA has to be investigated in more detail. The overall milder degree of pigmentation and pigmentary abnormalities may also explain why alopecia in Weimaraners occurs much later in life than CDA.

3.1.2.4.5 Hair matrix lipidosis in the Rottweiler dog

Another color-linked and presumably hereditary disease of hair follicles that develops within the first months after birth is canine follicular lipidosis (Gross et al. 1997). This disease has only been described in young Rottweilers so far, is rare, and is associated with early onset of alopecia, affecting mahagony-colored areas on the feet and face (Fig. 3.1.24). Follicular lipidosis is characterized by intracytoplasmic lipid-filled vacuoles within cells of the hair follicle matrix (Fig. 3.1.25). Whether lipid vacuoles occur in keratinocytes or melanocytes has not been clarified yet, and the underlying pathogenesis is not known. Alopecia is most likely a result of increased hair shaft fragility.

3.1.2.4.6 Follicular pigmentary abnormalities in other domestic animals species

Morphological features similar to BHDF and CDA have been reported in horses and cattle (Ayers et al. 1989; Miller and Scott 1990), but are extremely rare.

3.1.3 Unclassified forms of congenital alopecia

As suggested above, congenital alopecia can be classified as hair follicle aplasia, hair follicle dysplasia

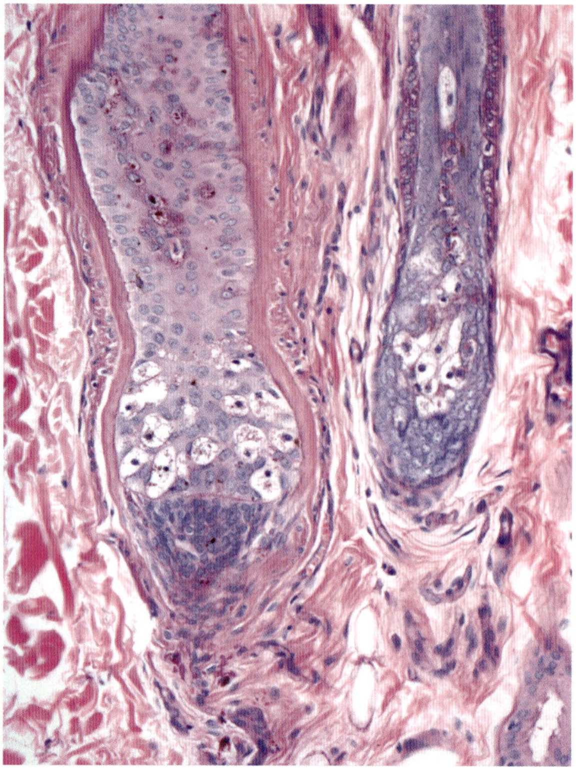

Fig. 3.1.25 Skin histology of follicular lipidosis in a Rottweiler. Large cytoplasmic vacuoles (presumed to be fat) within the hair bulb matrix.

(with or without hair shaft formation), and dysplasia of the hair follicle pigmentary unit (neuroectodermal dysplasia). This classification requires a detailed histopathological evaluation of the skin. There are some forms of congenital alopecia in domestic animals, where such investigations have not been performed or have been reported insufficiently, not allowing further classification. Among these is the "American hairless terrier," a dog breed that originated from the American Rat Terrier. Hairlessness spontaneously occurred in Rat Terriers in 1972 and was maintained as an individual breed with an autosomal recessive trait. The phenotype is symbolized as "Ha." Affected dogs are born with a sparse hair coat that is eventually shed and never replaced. Dogs are completely bald by 6 weeks of age with only whiskers and eyebrows remaining. Dentition of these dogs is normal, suggesting that they are not analogous to the Chinese Crested or Mexican Hairless Dog.

Furthermore, congenital alopecia has been described in Poll Dorset sheep (viable hypotrichosis) and in Karakul sheep, but information on its clinical and morphologic phenotype or its genetic background is too sparse for further subclassification (Nel 1964; Dolling and Brooker 1966; Mackie and Mcintyre 1992).

References

Ackerman L. 1983. Inheritance of baldy calf syndrome. *Modern Veterinary Practice* 64:807.

Ayers JR, Leipold HW, Schalles R, Cole D. 1989. Pathological studies of cross-related congenital hypotrichosis in cattle. *Zentralblatt für Veterinärmedizin A* 36:447–452.

Becker RB, Simpson CF, Wilcox CA. 1963. Hairless Guernsey cattle. Hypotrichosis – a nonlethal character. *Journal of Heredity* 54:1.

Beco L, Fontaine J, Gross TL, Charlier G. 1996. Color dilution alopecia in seven Dachshunds. A clinical study and the hereditary, microscopical and ultrastructural aspect of the disease. *Veterinary Dermatology* 7:91–97.

Bohnhorst JO, Hanssen I, Moen T. 2001. Antinuclear antibodies (ANA) in Gordon Setters with symmetrical lupoid onychodystrophy and black hair follicular dysplasia. *Acta Veterinaria Scandinavica* 42:323–329.

Bracho GA, Beeman K, Johnson JL, Leipold HW. 1984. Further studies of congenital hypotrichosis in Hereford calves. *Zentralblatt für Veterinärmedizin A* 31:72.

Braun U, Ansari HA, Hediger, R, Süss U, Ehrensperger F. 1988. Hypotrichosis and oligodontia associated with a chromosomal Xq-deletion in a Simmental/red Holstein crossbreed. *Tierärztliche Praxis* 16:39–44.

Briggs OM, Botha WS. 1986. Color mutant alopecia in a blue Italian greyhound. *Journal of the American Animal Hospital Association* 22:611–614.

Casal ML, Jezyk PF, Greek JM, Goldschmidt MH, Patterson DF. 1997. X-linked ectodermal dysplasia in the dog. *Journal of Heredity* 88:513–517.

Casal ML, Mauldin EA, Ryan S, Scheidt JL, Kennedy J, Moore PF, Felsburg PJ. 2005. Frequent respiratory tract infections in the canine model of X-linked ectodermal dysplasia are not caused by an immune deficiency. *Veterinary Immunology and Immunopathology* 107:95–104.

Chastain CB, Swayne DE. 1985. Congenital hypotrichosis in male Basset Hound littermates. *Journal of the American Veterinary Medical Association* 187:845–846.

Cole LJ. 1919. A defect of hair and teeth in cattle, probably hereditary. *Journal of Heredity* 10:303.

Conroy JD, Rasmusen BA, Small E. 1975. Hypotrichosis in miniature poodle siblings. *Journal of the American Veterinary Medical Association* 166:697–699.

Craft WA, Blizzard WL. 1934. The inheritance of semihairlessness in cattle. *Journal of Heredity* 25:385.

David LT. 1932. Histology of the skin of the mexican hairless swine (sus scrofa). *American Journal of Anatomy* 50:283–292.

Delmage DA. 1995. Black hair follicular dysplasia. *Veterinary Record* 136:79–80.

Distl O, Drögemüller C, Kuiper H, Kutschke L, Hermanns W, Kehler W, Scholz H. 2000. Genetische untersuchung von kongenitaler hypotrichose mit anodontie bei deutschen Holstein Kälbern. *Tierärztliche Umschau* 55:72–79.

Dolling CHS, Brooker MG. 1966. A viable hypotrichosis in Poll Dorset sheep. *Journal of Heredity* 57:87–90.

Drieux H, Priouzeau M, Thiery G, Priouzeau ML. 1950. Hypotrrichose congenitale avec anodontie, acerie et macroglossie chez le veau. *Recueility de Medicine Veterinaire* 126:385–399.

Drögemüller C, Distl O, Leeb T. 2001. Partial deletion of the bovine ED1 gene causes anhidrotic ectodermal dysplasia in cattle. *Genome Research* 11:1699–1705.

Drögemüller C, Distl O, Leeb T. 2003. X-linked anhidrotic ectodermal dysplasia (ED1) in men, mice, and cattle. *Genetics, Selection, Evolution* (1 Suppl):S137–S145.

Drögemüller C, Haase B, Philipp U, Günzel-Apel AR, Leeb T. 2008. The non-coding MLPH c.-22G>A SNP associated with dilute coat color is found in genetically diverse dogs with and without symptoms of color dilution alopecia. Abstract, International Congress on Transposable Elements, Saint Malo.

Drögemüller C, Karlsson EK, Hytönen MK, Perlaski M, Dolf G, Saimio K, Lohi H, Limdblad-Toh K, Leeb T. 2008. A mutation in hairless dogs implicates FOX13 in ectodermal development. *Science* 321:1462.

Drögemüller C, Kuiper H, Peters M, Guionaud S, Distl O, Leeb T. 2002a. Congenital hypotrichosis with anodontia in cattle: a genetic, clinical and histological analysis. *Veterinary Dermatology* 13:307–313.

Drögemüller C, Peters M, Pohlenz J, Distl O, Leeb T. 2002b. A single point mutation within the ED1 gene disrupts correct splicing at two different splice sites and leads to anhidrotic ectodermal dysplasia in cattle. *Journal of Molecular Medicine* 80:319–323.

Dunn KA, Russell M, Boness JM. 1995. Black hair follicular dysplasia. *Veterinary Record* 137:412.

Eldridge FE, Atkeson FW. 1953. Streaked hairlessness in Holstein Friesian cattle. *Journal of Heredity* 44:265.

Fernandez A, Silio L, Noguera JL, Sanchez A, Ovilo C. 2003. Linkage mapping of the porcine hairless gene (HR) to chromosome 14. *Animal Genetics* 34:317–318.

Ferrer L, Durall I, Closa J, Mascort J. 1988. Color mutant alopecia in Yorkshire terriers. *Veterinary Record* 122:360–361.

Finnie JW, Tham VL. 1993. Colour mutant alopecia in a kelpie × border collie dog. *Australian Veterinary Journal* 70:388–389.

Finocchiaro R, Portolano B, Damiani G, Caroli A, Budelli E, Bolla P, Pagnacco G. 2003. The hairless (hr) gene is involved in the congenital hypotrichosis of Valle del Belice sheep. *Genetics, Selection, Evolution* 35:S147–S156.

Foil CS. 1990. The skin. In: Hoskins JD (ed.), *Veterinary Pediatrics*, pp. 359–403. Philadelphia, PA: WB Saunders.

Freire-Maia N, Lisboa-Costa T, Pagnan NAB. 2001. Ectodermal dysplasias: how many? *American Journal of Medical Genetics* 104:84.

Fukuta K, Koizumi N, Imamura K, Goto N, Hamada H. 1991. Microscopic observation of skin and lymphoid organs in the hairless dog derived from the Mexican hairless. *Experimental Animals* 40:69–76.

Gosselin Y, Papageorges M, Teuscher E. 1982. Black hair follicular dysplasia in dogs. *Canine Practice* 9:8–15.

Goto N, Imamura K, Miura Y, Ogawa T, Hamada H. 1987. The Mexican hairless dog, its morphology and inheritance. *Experimental Animals* 40:69–76.

Grieshaber TL, Blakemore JC, Yaskulski S. 1986. Congenital alopecia in a Bichon frise. *Journal of the American Veterinary Medical Association* 188:1053–1054.

Gross TL, Pascal-Tenorio A, Munn RJ, Hargis AM, Kline A. 1997. Follicular lipidosis in three Rottweilers. *Veterinary Dermatology* 8:33–39.

Hargis AM, Brignac MM, Al-Bagdadi FAK, Muggli F, Mundel A. 1991. Black hair follicular dysplasia in black and white saluki dogs: differentiation from color mutant alopecia in the Doberman pinscher by microscopic examination of hairs. *Veterinary Dermatology* 2:69–83.

Harper RC. 1978. Congenital black hair follicular dysplasia in bearded collie puppies. *Veterinary Record* 102:87.

Hendy-Ibbs PM. 1984. Hairless cats in Great Britain. *Journal of Heredity* 75:506–507.

Hirota Y, Koizumi N, Matsubara Y, Imamura K, Fukuta K. 1990. Immunological features in hairless descendants derived from Mexican hairless dogs. *The Japanese Journal of Veterinary Science* 52:1117–1121.

Holmes JR, Young GB. 1954. Symmetrical alopecia in cattle. *Veterinary Record* 66:704.

Hume AN, Collinson LM, Hopkins CR, Strom M, Barral DC, Bossi G, Griffiths GM, Seabra MC. 2002. The leaden gene product is required with Rab27a to recruit myosin Va to melanosomes in melanocytes. *Traffic* 3:193–202.

Hutt FB. 1963. A note of six kinds of genetic hypotrichosis in cattle. *Journal of Heredity* 54:186.

Hutt FB, Saunders LZ. 1953. Viable genetic hypotrichosis in Guernsey cattle. *Journal of Heredity* 44:97.

Jayasekera MY. 1979. Pathological changes in congenital hypotrichosis in Hereford cattle. *Zentralblatt für Veterinärmedizin A* 26:744.

Kelleher JF, Titus MA. 1998. Intracellular motility: how can we all work together? *Current Biology* 8:R394–R397.

Kidwell JF, Guilbert HR. 1950. A recurrence of the semihairless gene in cattle. *Journal of Heredity* 41:190.

Kim JH, Kang KI, Sohn HJ, Woo GH, Jean YH, Hwang EK. 2005. Color-dilution alopecia in dogs. *Journal of Veterinary Science* 6:259–261.

Kimura T. 1996. Studies on development of hairless descendants of Mexican hairless dogs and their usefulness in dermatological science. *Experimental Animals* 45:1–13.

Kimura T, Doi K. 1994a. Age-related changes in skin color and histologic features of hairless descendants of Mexican hairless dogs. *American Journal of Veterinary Research* 55:480–486.

Kimura T, Doi K. 1994b. Response of the skin over the dorsum to sunlight in hairless descendants of Mexican hairless dogs. *American Journal of Veterinary Research* 55:199–203.

Kimura T, Doi K. 1996. Spontaneous comedones on the skin of hairless descendants of Mexican hairless dogs. *Experimental Animals* 45:377–384.

Kimura T, Doi K. 1997. The effect of topical minoxidil treatment on hair follicular growth of neonatal hairless descendants of Mexican hairless dogs. *Veterinary Dermatology* 8:107–113.

Kimura T, Doi K. 1998a. Effects of all-trans retinoic acid on the dorsal skin of hairless dogs. *Toxicologic Pathology* 26:595–601.

Kimura T, Doi K. 1998b. Efficacy of hydroquinone in the treatment of cutaneous hyperpigmentation in hairless descendants of Mexican hairless dogs. *Laboratory Animal Science* 48:469–475.

Kimura T, Doi K. 1999. Dorsal skin reactions of hairless dogs to topical treatment with corticosteroids. *Toxicologic Pathology* 27:528–535.

Kimura T, Kuroki K, Doi K. 1998. Dermatotoxicity of agricultural chemicals in the dorsal skin of hairless dogs. *Toxicologic Pathology* 26:442–447.

Kimura T, Ohshima S, Doi K. 1992. Haematological and serum biochemical values in hairless and haired descendants of Mexican hairless dogs. *Laboratory Animals* 26:214–218.

Kimura T, Ohshima S, Doi K. 1993. The inheritance and breeding results of hairless descendants of Mexican hairless dogs. *Laboratory Animals* 27:55–58.

Knottenbelt CM, Knottenbelt MK. 1996. Black hair follicular dysplasia in a tricolour Jack Russell terrier. *Veterinary Record* 138:475–476.

Kral F, Schwartzman RM (eds). 1964. *Veterinary and Comparative Dermatology*, pp. 183–184. Philadelphia, PA: Lippincott.
Kuiper H, Kutschke L, Drögemüller C, Leeb T, Distl O. 2001. Assignment of the bovine ectodysplasin A gene (ED1) to bovine Xq22-q24 by fluorescence in situ hybridization. *Cytogenetics and Cell Genetics* 92:356–357.
Kunkle GA. 1984. Congenital hypotrichosis in two dogs. *Journal of the American Veterinary Medical Association* 185:84–85.
Laffort-Dassot C, Beco L, Carlotti D. 2002. Follicular dysplasia in five Weimaraners. *Veterinary Dermatology* 13:253.
Laukner A. 1998. Coat color in dogs. 1: Basics of coat color genesis. *Tierärztliche Praxis Ausgabe Klientiere und Heimtiere* 26:49–54.
Lemus-Flores C, Ulloa-Arvizu R, Ramos-Kuri M, Estrada FJ, Alonso RA. 2001. Genetic analysis of Mexican hairless pig populations. *Journal of Animal Sciences* 79:3021–3026.
Lewis CJ. 1995. Black hair follicular dysplasia in UK bred salukis. *Veterinary Record* 137:294–295.
Mackie JT, Mcintyre B. 1992. Congenital hypotrichosis in Poll Dorset sheep. *Australian Veterinary Journal* 69:146–147.
Malik R, France MP. 1991. Hyperpigmentation and symmetrical alopecia in three silky terriers. *Australian Veterinary Practitioner* 21:135–138.
McGavin MD, Alexander GI. 1961. Viable hypotrichosis in a Jersey calf. *Queensland Journal of Agricultural Science* 18:105.
McKeever PJ. 1992. Spiculosis. *Journal of the American Animal Hospital Association* 28:257.
Ménasché G, Ho CH, Sanal O, Feldmann J, Tezcan I, Ersoy F, Houdusse A, Fischer A, de Saint Basile G. 2003. Griscelli syndrome restricted to hypopigmentation results from a melanophilin defect (GS3) or a MYO5A F-exon deletion (GS1). *Journal of Clinical Investigation* 112:450–456.
Mecklenburg L. 2006. An overview on congenital alopecia in domestic animals. *Veterinary Dermatology* 17(6):393–410.
Meyer VH, Drommer W. 1968. Erbliche hypotrichie beim Schwein. *Deutsche Tierärztliche Wochenschrift* 75:13.
Miller WH. 1990a. Color dilution alopecia in Doberman pinschers with blue or fawn coat colours: a study on the incidence and histopathology of this disorder. *Veterinary Dermatology* 1:113–122.
Miller WH. 1990b. Follicular dysplasia in adult black and red Doberman pinschers. *Veterinary Dermatology* 1:181–187.
Miller WH. 1991. Alopecia associated with coat color dilution in two Yorkshire terriers, one saluki, and one mix-breed dog. *Journal of the American Animal Hospital Association* 27:39–43.
Miller WH, Scott DW. 1990. Black-hair follicular dysplasia in a Holstein cow. *The Cornell Veterinarian* 80:273–277.
Mohr OL, Wreidt C. 1928. Hairless, a new recessive lethal in cattle. *Journal of Genetics* 19:315.
Moura E, Cirio SM. 2004. Clinical and genetic aspects of X-linked ectodermal dysplasia in the dog—a review including three new spontaneous cases. *Veterinary Dermatology* 15:269–277.
Muller GH, Kirk RW (eds). 1976. *Small Animal Dermatology*, 2nd edn, pp. 495–496. Philadelphia, PA: WB Saunders.
Nagashima K, Torii S, Yi Z, Igarashi M, Okamoto K, Takeuchi T, Izumi T. 2002. Melanophilin directly links Rab27a and myosin Va through its distinct coiled-coil regions. *FEBS Letters* 517:233–238.
Nel JA. 1964. Hypotrichosis congenita in Karakul sheep. *South African Journal of Agricultural Science* 7:875–877.
Neuber AE, Van Den Broek AH, Rhind SM, Hill PB, Thoday KL. 2006. Generalized alopecic and cystic dermatosis in a cat: a counterpart to the hairless mouse phenotype or a unique congenital dermatosis? *Veterinary Dermatology* 17(1):63–69.
Ojo SA. 1987. The characteristics of bovine congenital hypodontia. *Veterinary Medicine* 82:192.
Philipp U, Hamann H, Mecklenburg L, Nishino S, Mignot E, Günzel-Apel AR, Schmutz SM, Leeb T. 2005. Polymorphisms within the canine MLPH gene are associated with dilute coat color in dogs. *BMC Genetics* 16:34.
Provance DW, James TL, Mercer JA. 2002. Melanophilin, the product of the leaden locus, is required for targeting of myosin-Va to melanosomes. *Traffic* 3:124–132.
Provance DW, Wei M, Ipe V, Mercer JA. 1996. Cultured melanocytes from dilute mutant mice exhibit dendritic morphology and altered melanosome distribution. *Proceedings of the National Academy of Sciences of the United States of America* 93:14554–14558.
Rest JR, Davies JBA. 1994. Black hair follicular dysplasia. *Veterinary Record* 135:607.
Rieck GW. 1985. Hypotrichie-hypodontie syndrom beim Rind. *Deutsche Tierärztliche Wochenschrift* 92:328–329.
Roberts E, Carroll WE. 1931. The inheritance of hairlessness in swine. *Journal of Heredity* 22:125.
Robinson R. 1985. Chinese crested dog. *Journal of Heredity* 76:217–218.
Rodionov VI, Hope AJ, Svitkina TM, Borisy GG. 1998. Functional coordination of microtubule-based and actin-based motility in melanophores. *Current Biology* 8:165–168.
Rogers SL, Gelfand VI. 1998. Myosin cooperates with microtubule motors during organelle transport in melanophores. *Current Biology* 8:161–164.
Roperto F, Cerundolo R, Restucci B, Vincensi MR, de Caprariis D, De Vico G, Maiolino P. 1995. Colour dilution alopecia (CDA) in 10 Yorkshire terriers. *Veterinary Dermatology* 6:171–178.
Rose R, Smith JE, Leipold HW. 1983. Increased solubility of hair from hypotrichotic Herefords. *Zentralblatt für Veterinärmedizin A* 30:363.
Sander P, Drögemüller C, Cadieu E, André C, Leeb T. 2005. Analysis of the canine EDAR gene and exclusion as a candidate for the hairless phenotype in the Chinese crested dog. *Animal Genetics* 36:168–171.
Schleger AV. 1967. Histopathology of hypotrichosis in calves. *Australian Journal of Biology Science* 20:661.
Schmutz SM, Moker JS, Clark EG, Shewfelt R. 1998. Black hair follicular dysplasia, an autosomal recessive condition in dogs. *Canadian Veterinary Journal* 39:644–646.
Seeliger F, Drögemüller C, Tegtmeier P, Baumgärtner W, Distl O, Leeb T. 2005. Ectodysplasin-1 deficiency in a German Holstein bull associated with loss of respiratory mucous glands and chronic rhinotracheitis. *Journal of Comparative Pathology* 132:346–349.
Selmanowitz VJ, Kramer KM, Orentreich N. 1970b. Congenital ectodermal defect in miniature poodles. *Journal of Heredity* 61: 196–199.
Selmanowitz VJ, Kramer KM, Orentreich N. 1972. Canine hereditary black hair follicular dysplasia. *Journal of Heredity* 63:43–44.
Selmanowitz VJ, Markofsky J, Orentreich N. 1977a. Black-hair follicle dysplasia in dogs. *Journal of the American Veterinary Medical Association* 171:1079–1081.
Selmanowitz VJ, Markofsky J, Orentreich N. 1977b. Heritability of an ectodermal defect—a study of affected dogs. *Journal of Dermatologic Surgery and Oncology* 3:623–626.
Selmanowitz VJ, Kramer KM, Orentreich N, Hyman AB. 1970a. Congenital ectodermal dysplasia in male miniature poodle siblings. *Archives of Dermatology* 101:613–615.
Silvers WK (ed.). 1979. *The Coat Colors of Mice: A Model for Mammalian Gene Action and Interaction*, pp. 83–90. New York: Springer.
Steffen DJ, Elliott GS, Leipold HW, Smith JE. 1992a. Congenital dyserythropoiesis and progressive alopecia in polled Hereford calves: hematologic, biochemical, bone marrow cytologic, electrophoretic, and flow cytometric findings. *Journal of Veterinary Diagnostic Investigation* 4:31–37.

Steffen DJ, Leipold HW, Elliott GS, Smith JE. 1992b. Ultrastructural findings in congenital anemia, dyskeratosis, and progressive alopecia in polled Hereford calves. *Veterinary Pathology* 29:203–209.

Steffen DJ, Leipold HW, Gibb J, Smith JE. 1991. Congenital anemia, dyskeratosis, and progressive alopecia in polled Hereford calves. *Veterinary Pathology* 28:234–240.

Steffen DJ, Leipold HW, Schalles R, Kemp K, Smith JE. 1993. Epidemiologic findings in congenital anemia, dyserythropoiesis, and dyskeratosis in polled Hereford calves. *Journal of Heredity* 84: 263–265.

Surrarrer TC. 1943. Bulldog and hairless calves. *Journal of Heredity* 34:175.

Thomsett LR. 1961. Congenital hypotrichia in the dog. *Veterinary Record* 73:915–917.

Valentine BA, Hedstrom OR, Miller WH Jr, Scott DW, Mathies S. 2001. Congenital hypotrichosis in a Percheron draught horse. *Veterinary Dermatology* 12:215–217.

Westbroek W, Lambert J, Naeyaert JM. 2001. The dilute locus and Griscelli syndrome: gateways towards a better understanding of melanosome transport. *Pigment Cell Research* 14:320–327.

Wijeratne WVS, O'Toole D, Wood L, Harkness JW. 1988. A genetic, pathological and virological study of congenital hypotrichosis and incisor anodontia in cattle. *Veterinary Record* 122:149–152.

Wilson SM, Yip R, Swing DA, O'Sullivan TN, Zhang Y, Novak EK, Swank RT, Russell LB, Copeland NG, Jenkins NA. 2000. A mutation in Rab27a causes the vesicle transport defects observed in ashen mice. *Proceedings of the National Academy of Sciences of the United States of America* 97:7933–7938.

Yankell SL, Khemani L, Dolan MM. 1970a. Sunscreen recovery studies in the Mexican hairless dog. *Journal of Investigative Dermatology* 55:31–33.

Yankell SL, Schwartzman RM, Resnick B. 1970b. Care and breeding of the Mexican hairless dog. *Laboratory Animal Care* 20:940–945.

Young JB. 1953. A note on the occurrence of an epithelial defect in a grade Hereford herd. *Australian Veterinary Journal* 9:298.

3.2

Trichomalacia

Lars Mecklenburg

Trichomalacia describes a form of alopecia where hair follicles are normal but hair shafts show subtle abnormalities that lead to increased fragility and finally breaking of hair fibers. The value of histopathology to diagnose trichomalacia is limited, since no morphological abnormalities in hair follicles are found. These conditions are best diagnosed clinically and by the use of plucked hair shafts that are investigated under a light microscope (see Section 2.1.4.2).

Trichomalacia can occur very early in life and therefore may be confused with congenital alopecia. In fact, some forms of congenital alopecia may actually be restricted to subtle hair fiber malformations, and thus a clear distinction between these two conditions may not always be possible. Some forms of trichomalacia may occur with a familial predisposition, although they are not monogenetically inherited. Most trichomalacias, however, are likely acquired and occur spontaneously in single animals of any age. Defining the underlying etiology may be difficult, and often there is spontaneous remission without further treatment.

3.2.1 Trichomalacia due to nutritional deficiencies

Trichomalacia is rare in domestic animal species. It can be associated with nutritional deficiencies, particularly in young individuals suffering from infectious intestinal diseases or in old animals suffering from any kind of serious chronic disease. Malnutrition may be caused by insufficient dietary intake, malabsorption, poor utilization of nutrients, or increased catabolism. Chronic indigestion can result in alopecia, and the mechanism of alopecia is most likely due to the lack of minerals and vitamins (Stocker et al. 1999). Protein/calorie deficiency will impact the growth rate of hair follicle matrix cells and will thus result in structurally normal hair shafts of less quality and less durability. Hair fibers become brittle and break off easily. If malnutrition is severe, it is conceivable that anagen hair follicles may actually cease proliferation, which means that they will undergo catagen development and may remain in telogen until proper nutrition is restored. Therefore, both effects on hair shaft synthesis and hair follicle cycling are possible. Effects on hair shaft synthesis, however, will become clinically apparent much earlier.

On the basis of the clinical phenotype of alopecia, it is impossible to specifically determine the deficient nutrient. Several nutritional deficiencies have been described to cause alopecia: *Copper deficiency in ruminants* occurs either as a primary disease or is secondary to molybdenosis, as molybdenum impairs intestinal absorption of copper. Copper deficiency results in alopecia associated with anorexia, diarrhea, osteoporosis, and heart failure (Frank 1998). Nonalopecic areas often show a decrease in pigmentation of hair, due to a depression of tyrosinase activity (Whitelaw et al. 1979). Trichomalacia is known in humans with hereditary copper deficiency (due to defects in a copper transport protein), where the disease is called "kinky hair syndrome" or "Menkes syndrome." *Zinc deficiency in ruminants* results in alopecia and parakeratotic hyperkeratosis. In addition, hoofs grow abnormally and most animals show anorexia. Alopecia is due to malformed hair fibers that become distorted within the follicular infundibulum (Nelson et al. 1984; Masters et al. 1985). Hypovitaminosis can also be a cause of trichomalacia and alopecia. Such an example is *folic acid deficiency* that has been described in a 3-week-old male Charolais calf that had a history of progressive hair loss (Bouvet et al. 1988). Folic acid is required for cellular turnover, and its lack will likely impair proliferation of hair matrix cells. Daily oral administration of folic acid (1 mg/kg/day) resulted in a steady regrowth of hair within 2 months. *Vitamin A* and *biotin deficiencies* are other examples of trichomalacia and alopecia caused by hypovitaminosis (Colomb et al. 1970; Rubisz-Brzezinska 1974; Nyhan 1987; Mock 1991; Fujimoto et al. 2005).

3.2.2 Trichomalacia due to intoxications

Several toxicoses can be associated with trichomalacia and alopecia. *Selenium intoxication in ruminants* results in alopecia and cracking and enlargement of the hoof. Selenium induces oxidative stress and hampers hair shaft synthesis. In addition to alopecia, there is often gangrene at the tip of the tail of calves (Kaur et al. 2003). *Hypervitaminosis A, D, and E* have been described as causes of alopecia in calves, associated with cranial chondrodysplasia (Yamamoto et al. 2003). Sheep experimentally intoxicated with *thallium* will also develop alopecia (Spikermann 1981), eventually associated with hair follicle dystrophy (see Chapter 3.4). Similarly, alopecia has been described as a consequence of chronic thallium intoxication in dogs (Thomas and McKeever 1993; Gassner et al. 2000).

3.2.3 Familial feline and canine trichomalacias

Familial trichomalacias with increased hair shaft fragility are rare but well-characterized diseases in humans, classified as monilethrix, pili torti, or trichorrhexis nodosa. Most of these diseases have not been described in domestic animals so far. Familial *pili torti* have once been described in a cat litter. Kittens presented with generalized hair loss associated with periocular and pedal dermatitis. Hair fibers showed flattening and rotation. Only a subset of hairs (i.e., secondary hairs) was involved whereas others were normal. Biopsies showed normal hair follicles, except for some infundibular hyperkeratosis and dilation (Geary and Baker 1986). Familial *trichorrhexis nodosa* has been described in Abyssinian cats (Wilkinson and Kristensen 1989). Trichorrhexis nodosa is defined as one or multiple thickenings along the hair fiber (nodes). In affected Abyssinian cats, hair shafts exhibit an onion-shaped swelling at the tip. This swelling is due to a focally enlarged hair shaft medulla. The hair coat feels lusterless and rough. The disease is inherited in an autosomal recessive trait. *Trichoptilosis* is characterized by a splitting of hair fibers at the tip (the term derives from the Greek root "tricho" meaning hair and "ptilosis" meaning "falling out of the eyelashes"). A familial form of trichoptilosis has been described in Golden Retrievers (Miller 2004). *Familial trichomalacia in German Shepherds* has been described with multifocal alopecia affecting the dorsolateral trunk (Fig. 3.2.1a). Affected dogs are otherwise healthy. Microscopic examination of hair shafts revealed focal areas of medullary swelling, followed by longitudinal splitting and breakage of the hair shaft (Fig. 3.2.1b). The disease recovers spontaneously but relapses may occur (Tieghi et al. 2003).

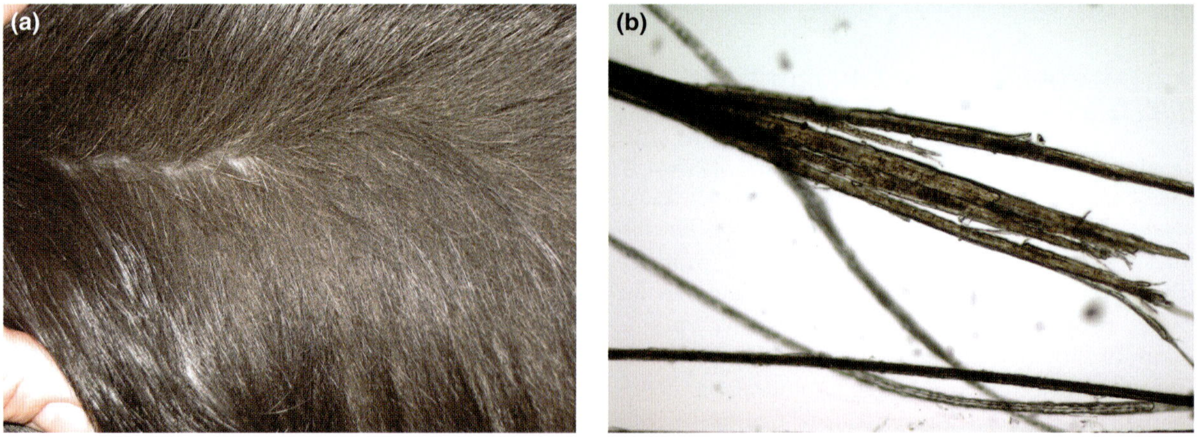

Fig. 3.2.1 Medullary trichomalacia in German Shepherd. (a) Broken hair shafts on the dorsum; (b) trichogram showing split hair shafts.

3.2.4 Trichomalacia caused by external damage to the hair fiber

Hair shaft abnormalities morphologically similar to those described above can occur spontaneously as a sequela of solar, chemical, or physical trauma to the hair shaft. Most cases will present with trichoptilosis, that is, splitting of the tip of hair fibers. Spontaneous trichorrhexis nodosa has been described in a cat (Alhaidari et al. 1996) and in dogs (Scott et al. 2001). Small regularly spaced nodular swellings occur along the hair shaft that are associated with cuticular defects.

References

Alhaidari Z, Olivry T, Ortonne JP. 1996. Acquired feline hair shaft abnormality resembling trichorrhexis nodosa in humans. *Veterinary Dermatology* 7:235–238.

Bouvet A, Baired JD, Basrur PK. 1988. Folic acid therapy for alopecia in a Charolais calf. *Veterinary Record* 123:533–536.

Colomb D, Cretin J, Vibert J, Steiner HG. 1970. Trichorrhexis nodosa in a hypothrepsic child with hypovitaminosis A. *Lyon Medical* 223:337.

Frank A. 1998. Mysterious moose disease in Sweden. Similarities to copper deficiency and/or molybdenosis in cattle and sheep. Biochemical background of clinical signs and organ lesions. *Science of the Total Environment* 208:17–26.

Fujimoto W, Inaoki M, Fukui T, Inoue Y, Kuhara T. 2005. Biotin deficiency in an infant fed with amino acid formula. *Journal of Dermatology* 32:256.

Gassner G, Tholen V, Ternes W. 2000. Chronic thallium intoxication in five German pointers of one litter. *Berliner und Munchener Tierarztliche Wochenschrift* 113:295–298.

Geary MR, Baker KP. 1986. The occurrence of pili torti in a litter of kittens in England. *Journal of Small Animal Practice* 27:85.

Kaur R, Sharma S, Rampal S. 2003. Effect of sub-chronic selenium toxicosis on lipid peroxidation, glutathione redoc cycle and antioxidant enzymes in calves. *Veterinary and Human Toxicology* 45:190–192.

Masters DG, Chapman RE, Vaughan JD. 1985. Effects of zinc-deficiency on the wool growth, skin and wool follicles of preruminant lambs. *Australian Journal of Biological Sciences* 38:355–364.

Miller WH. 2004. Structural follicular dysplasia. *Proceedings of 29th World Congress of the World Small Animal Veterinary Association.* Available at www.vin.com\proceedings.

Mock DM. 1991. Skin manifestations of biotin deficiency. *Seminars in Dermatology* 10:296–302.

Nelson DR, Wolff WA, Blodgett DJ, Luecke B, Ely RW, Zachary JF. 1984. Zinc deficiency in sheep and goats: three field cases. *Journal of the American Veterinary Medical Association* 184:1480–1485.

Nyhan WL. 1987. Inborn errors of biotin metabolism. *Archives of Dermatology* 123:1696.

Rubisz-Brzezinska J. 1974. Effect of vitamin A deficiency on hair growth in rats. *Przeglad Dermatologiczny* 61:19.

Scott DW, Miller WH, Griffin CE (eds). 2001. *Small Animal Dermatology*, 6th edn. Philadelphia, PA: WB Saunders.

Spikermann AR. 1981. Loss of wool in sheep following experimental thallium poisoning. *Deutsche Tierarztliche Wochenschrift* 88:252–253.

Stocker H, Lutz H, Ruesch P. 1999. Clinical, hematological and biochemical findings in milk-fed calves with chronic indigestion. *Veterinary Record* 145:307–311.

Thomas ML, McKeever PJ. 1993. Chronic thallium toxicosis in a dog. *Journal of the American Animal Hospital Association* 29:211.

Tieghi C, Miller WH, Scott DW, Pasquinelli G. 2003. Medullary trichomalacia in 6 German shepherd dogs. *Canadian Veterinary Journal* 44:132–136.

Whitelaw A, Armstrong RH, Evans CC, Fawcett AR. 1979. A study of the effects of copper deficiency in Scottish blackface lambs on improved hill pasture. *Veterinary Record* 104:455–460.

Wilkinson GT, Kristensen TS. 1989. A hair abnormality in Abyssinian cats. *Journal of Small Animal Practice* 30:27.

Yamamoto K, Sasahito K, Yoshikawa M, Nobuyuki O, Mikami O, Yamada M, Nakamura K, Yasuyuki N. 2003. Hyena disease (premature physeal closure) in calves due to overdose of vitamins A, D3, E. *Veterinary and Human Toxicology* 45:85–87.

3.3

Disorders of hair follicle cycling

3.3.1 Hypothyroidism

Monika Linek

The thyroid gland lies on the lateral aspect of the trachea, and physiologically it is often not palpable (Rijnberk 1996). The functional units of the gland are follicles composed of a single-layered epithelium surrounding a central lumen filled with colloid. The colloid consists of thyroglobulin (Tg), a large glycoprotein that binds to and stores the actual thyroid hormones. Thyroid hormone biosynthesis includes the active transport of iodide (the main element of thyroid hormones) from the blood into the thyroid epithelial cell, oxidation of iodine by the enzyme thyroid peroxydase, and transfer to tyrosine residues of the Tg molecule. These iodotyrosines can then combine with monoiodotyrosine (MIT) or diiodotyrosine (DIT), and thus can form the thyroid hormones thyroxin (T4, composed of two DIT) or triiodothyronine (T3, composed of one MIT and one DIT). For secretion of thyroid hormones into the circulatory system, Tg with its bound thyroid hormones reenters into the follicle epithelial cell where Tg is hydrolyzed in phagolysosomes and thyroid hormones secreted (Feldman and Nelson 2004).

Although most of the metabolic activity of thyroid hormones can be ascribed to T3, T4 secretion from the thyroid gland is four times higher than that of T3. In the blood, thyroid hormones are primarily bound to proteins (thyroid binding globulin and some low-affinity albumins like the thyroxin-binding prealbumin transthyretin). Less than 0.05% of T4 and less than 0.5% of T3 are not protein bound (Larsen and Berry 1995). Protein binding acts as a reservoir and maintains a steady thyroid hormone concentration, regulated by a feedback mechanism. The free form of T4 (fT4) can enter cells in the periphery. In the cell, 80% of fT4 is then deiodinated to free T3 (fT3), which then mediates its biological activity. During phases of fasting or nonthyroidal diseases, fT4 can also be deiodinated to reverse T3 (rT3), a metabolically inactive form (Mason and Wilkinson 1973; Kallfelz 1977; Feldman and Nelson 2004).

The thyroid function is mainly regulated by thyrotropin (also named thyroid-stimulating hormone, TSH), a glycoprotein that is secreted by the anterior lobe of the pituitary. TSH secretion from the pituitary is inhibited by fT3 (within the pituitary produced from fT4). A second modulation derives from the hypothalamus that secretes both thyreotropin-releasing hormone (TRH, stimulating TSH secretion from the pituitary), and somatostatin as well as other neuropeptides that inhibit TSH release. A third autoregulatory system enables the thyroid to adapt to insufficient or excessive concentrations of iodine. Iodine deficiency will cause increased thyroid function and goiter development, whereas long-term excessive iodine uptake will result in inhibition of peroxidase activity and hypothyroidism (Feldman and Nelson 2004).

As mentioned above, only free thyroid hormones (fT3/fT4) will diffuse across cell membranes and produce biological effects. fT3 enters cells more rapidly, has a more rapid onset of action, and is three to five times more potent than fT4. Both thyroid hormones bind to intranuclear receptors and activate the transcription of a variety of regulatory enzymes, resulting in increased oxygen consumption and an increased metabolic rate of mitochondria. Thyroid hormones are essential for skeletal and neurological development. They have a positive inotropic and chronotropic effect on the heart, increase the number and affinity of beta-adrenergic receptors, and enhance the response to catecholamines. They elicit catabolic effects on adipose tissue and muscle. Due to this wide variety of physiological effects, a deficiency in thyroid hormones will produce variable and profound clinical changes (Greenspan 2001).

With regard to hair follicles, thyroid hormones influence cell cycle kinetics of hair bulbs. Dissected human scalp hair follicle bulbs from hypothyroid patients show a significant decrease in proliferative activity compared to normal controls. In hyperthyroid patients a significant increase was found (Schell et al. 1991; Kiesewetter and Schell 1994). In hypothyroid dogs, hair regrows slower after clipping (Credille et al. 2001). Furthermore, there are more telogen hair follicles in hypothyroid dogs than in euthyroid controls. This suggests that both a slower elongation of hair shafts and a hair cycle arrest contribute to the development of alopecia in hypothyroid dogs.

3.3.1.1 Canine hypothyroidism

3.3.1.1.1 Etiology and pathogenesis

Hypothyroidism may result from a dysfunction of any part of the hypothalamic–pituitary–thyroid axis and may be acquired or congenital. In general, three pathogenetic groups can be differentiated: Primary hypothyroidism is defined as the absence or loss of thyroid function and is the most common cause of hypothyroidism in the dog. Secondary hypothyroidism or central hypothyroidism is the deprivation of stimulation by TSH followed by inactivity of the thyroid glands. Tertiary hypothyroidism is caused by a congenital malformation or acquired destruction of the hypothalamus, which so far has not been recognized in animals.

Canine hypothyroidism in most cases is acquired. Congenital hypothyroidism can occur in almost any mammalian species. Congenital primary hypothyroidism results from dysgenesis of the thyroid gland or from cellular defects in iodine uptake. Congenital secondary hypothyroidism has been described in the giant schnauzer, the Scottish Deerhound, and boxer with a TSH production defect and in German Shepherds associated with cyst formation and pituitary hypoplasia leading to proportional dwarfism (Kooistra et al. 2000; Graham et al. 2007). Independently of the underlying pathogenesis the clinical consequences are a sequela of the decreased production of thyroid hormones and therefore similar. In some forms, however, additional clinical signs such as goiter, growth retardation, or other signs of pituitary dysfunction are present.

3.3.1.1.1.1 Primary hypothyroidism

Adult onset primary hypothyroidism is the most common dysfunction of the thyroid gland in the dog. In 95% of cases, hypothyroidism in the dog is caused by a successive irreversible destruction of the thyroid gland. This destruction can be histologically divided into two main pathologic categories. First, an autoaggressive lymphocytic process, named autoimmune lymphocytic thyroiditis or, second, an idiopathic thyroid degeneration without an inflammatory infiltrate but with replacement of the thyroid parenchyma by adipose or fibrous tissue (Benjamin et al. 1996; Graham et al. 2001b). Distinction between these two processes, however, may be artificial, as some of the noninflammatory cases are considered as an end stage of the autoaggressive damage. Autoimmune thyroiditis is usually associated with the occurrence of autoantibodies against the Tg protein (TgAA). A large research database at the Michigan State University found an overall average of 50% TgAA-positive (suggestive of autoimmune thyroiditis) and 50% TgAA-negative (suggestive of noninflammatory thyroid atrophy) cases of hypothyroidism (Graham et al. 2007). However, the distribution of the two types differed between breeds. Whereas, for example, 80% of hypothyroid cases in the English Setter were TgAA positive, less than 30% of Doberman Pinschers showed TgAA (Nachreiner et al. 1998; Graham et al. 2007).

TgAA and less often other thyroid colloidal and microsomal antigens have been identified in dogs with lymphocytic thyroiditis with and without manifest hypothyroidism and irrespectively of the thyroid hormone status (Table 3.3.1). It is believed that these autoantibodies initiate an antibody-dependent, complement-mediated lymphocytic infiltration and may eventually destroy the thyroid gland. However, the mechanisms that lead to the formation of autoantibodies have not yet been characterized. The high prevalence of TgAA among certain breeds suggests some heritability. Several heritability studies in Beagles, Doberman Pinschers, English Setters, and Rhodesian Ridgebacks confirm an association with a particular major histocompatibility complex subtype (Kennedy et al. 2006, 2007). The causes for autoimmunity are most likely multifactorial. Antigenic

Table 3.3.1 Association of TgAA with different stages of hypothyroidism in the dog

Stage of thyroiditis	Clinical signs	tT4, fT4	TSH	TgAA
Subclinical thyroiditis	Negative	Normal	Normal	Positive
Subclinical hypothyroidism	Negative	Normal	Increased	Positive
Overt hypothyroidism	Present	Decreased	Increased	Positive or negative
Atrophic hypothyroidism	Present	Decreased	Increased	Negative

tT4, total thyroxine; fT4, free thyroxine; TSH, thyroid stimulating hormone; TgAA, thyroglobuline autoantibodies. Adapted from Graham et al. (2001b).

mimicry of thyroid antigens by viral or bacterial antigens has been suggested in human thyroiditis (Tomer and Davies 1993). An association between routine vaccinations and canine thyroiditis, however, has not been confirmed (Scott-Moncrieff et al. 2006). Some veterinarians report a geographical difference in the prevalence of thyroiditis; others report a seasonal influence (Graham et al. 2007).

The mere presence of TgAA antibodies is not predictive for thyroid dysfunction. In a 12-month prospective study in 234 TgAA-positive dogs, 1 out of 5 had progressive dysfunction within 1 year and only 1 out of 20 became hypothyroid (Graham et al. 2001a). The detection of TgAA is, therefore, not an appropriate tool to diagnose hypothyroidism. However, TgAA can interfere with the T3/T4 measurements (see Section 3.3.1.1.2.3).

Autoantibodies to T3 (T3AA) are recognized in less than 1% of all laboratory samples and even rarer are T4 autoantibodies (T4AA). The relative absence of T3AA/T4AA can be explained by the small molecular size of T3 and T4. Only when attached to Tg do they provide an antigenic stimulus (Nachreiner et al. 2002). If present, T3AA and T4AA can interfere with T3/T4 measurements in serum, falsely increasing or decreasing their levels.

Iodine deficiency as a cause of primary hypothyroidism is very rare in dogs because iodine requirements are low in this species. Even when dietary iodine is restricted, fT4 concentrations remain in the normal range (Feldman and Nelson 2004).

There are rare cases of hypothyroidism in the dog where follicular hyperplasia develops without iodine deficiency and without the presence of circulating autoantibodies. The etiology of the hypothyroidism in these cases could not be determined. Excessive dietary iodine uptake has been suggested in some cases, since it can significantly impair iodine uptake and thyroid hormone production with a subsequent increase in TSH secretion (Castillo et al. 2001).

3.3.1.1.1.2 Secondary hypothyroidism

Secondary hypothyroidism in young animals is mostly a congenital pituitary hypoplasia (see below). In the adult dog, acquired defects in the pituitary thyrotropic cells are very rare, and destruction by a pituitary neoplasm is uncommon. Most pituitary neoplasms are accompanied by additional endocrinopathies such as Addison's disease, diabetes insipidus, and reproductive dysfunctions. The most common pituitary tumor in the dog is an ACTH-producing adenoma of the pars distalis, resulting in hyperadrenocorticism. This tumor rarely destroys the thyrotropic cells, but rather suppresses TSH production by the excessive activity of glucocorticoids. Secondary hypothyroidism due to the suppression of pituitary thyrotrophic cells is most commonly caused by concurrent illness (i.e., euthyroid sick syndrome), drugs, or hormones (steroids). In secondary forms of hypothyroidism, TSH levels are low or even undetectable.

3.3.1.1.1.3 Congenital hypothyroidism

Congenital hypothyroidism due to agenesis of the thyroid gland is rare and most often results in early postnatal death. If affected animals survive, they will show mental retardation, hypoactivity, impaired skeletal maturation, and retarded growth. Congenital hypothyroidism due to pituitary malformations has been recognized in many dog breeds and has been studied most thoroughly in the German Shepherd Dog. Hypoplasia of the anterior pituitary in these dogs results in impaired TSH, growth hormone, follicle stimulating hormone, luteotropic hormone, and prolactin production. This leads to proportionate dwarfism, opposed to disproportionate dwarfism that is caused by a selective deficiency of growth hormone (Kooistra et al. 2000).

Inherited defects in thyroid hormone synthesis as known in the sheep, cattle, and goat (congenital dyshormonogenetic goiter) are very rare in dogs (Wilson 1975; Dolling and Good 1976). In most of theses cases hypothyroidism is associated with high TSH levels and goiter formation.

3.3.1.1.2 Diagnosis

Correctly diagnosing hypothyroidism is a very difficult task for the clinical veterinarian. Several assays exist that are more or less appropriate to assist in diagnosis, but regardless of the chosen combination of assays, all results have to be interpreted in context with the clinical presentation and general clinical findings. Best screening tests for hypothyroidism are assays with a high sensitivity. They allow exclusion of hypothyroidism, if the measured hormone is within the normal range (Table 3.3.2).

3.3.1.1.2.1 Clinical presentation

Clinical features of canine hypothyroidism are very important for the diagnosis, since no single endocrine assay can confirm the diagnosis on its own. The predictive values of thyroid function tests are greatly enhanced when combined with clinical signs and results of general medical diagnostic tests. The clinical picture reflects the multisystemic character of the disease, is unspecific, and can vary from mild to severe. Although, in general, hypothyroidism is more common in large breeds than in small breeds, reports of breed incidence must be interpreted with great caution because they can be biased by the tests that were used to confirm the diagnosis and by breed popularity. Age of onset is usually between 4 and 6 years of age, but may vary between 2 and 9 years. There is no apparent gender predisposition. As thyroid hormones are required to maintain cellular metabolism, a deficiency affects many organs. Clinical signs may vary depending on age at onset, stage of disease, and breed (Panciera 2001; Scott-Moncrieff 2007) (Table 3.3.3). The most common, although very unspecific, clinical observations in the dog are reduced activity, lethargy, mental dullness, and weight gain. Dermatological changes are reported in 60–80% of hypothyroid dogs (Panciera 1994b; Dixon et al. 1999). The initial abnormality is a dull, dry, and brittle hair coat with some degree of nonpruritic, noninflammatory, and symmetrical truncal alopecia (Fig. 3.3.1). Clipped hair fails to regrow properly, and telogen hairs are lost at friction areas where they are not replaced (Credille et al. 2001). Some dogs may show alopecia at the bridge of the nose. In some breeds such as the Irish setter, hair fails to shed normally, leading to temporary hypertrichosis. In boxers and Doberman Pinschers,

Table 3.3.2 Diagnostic value of screening tests for canine hypothyroidism

Test	Abnormality	Sensitivity	Specificity	Remarks
tT4	Decreased	89–100% (normal values exclude hypothyroidism)	75–82% (influenced by euthyroid sick syndrome and by many drugs)	Inexpensive
fT4*	Decreased	80–90%	~93% (more reliable than tT4)	Not readily available in all countries
TSH	Increased	63–87% (1/4 of all hypothyroid dogs have normal values)	82–100%	Inexpensive; can be used in combination with tT4 or fT4*
Combination of tT4 and TSH	tT4 decreased, TSH increased	63–91% (inconclusive results are possible)	92–100%	Inexpensive
Combination of fT4* and TSH	fT4* decreased, TSH increased	74–80% (inconclusive results are possible)	97–98%	
rhTSH-stimulation test	Insufficient stimulation	High	High	Expensive; needs 4–6 h

tT4, total thyroxine; fT4*, free thyroxine measured by equilibrium dialysis; rhTSH, recombinant human TSH. (Based on data from Ferguson (2005) and Daminet (2005).)

Table 3.3.3 Clinical signs of hypothyroidism in the adult dog

Affected organ system	Clinical sign
General condition	Lethargy* Weight gain* Mental dullness*
Cardiovascular	Bradycardia Arrhythmia
Hematology	Anemia (normochromic, normocytic)*
Skin	Alopecia, symmetric* Loss of hair regrowth after clipping* "Rat" tail (alopecia of the tail)* Thin, dry, brittle hair coat* Hyperpigmentation Pyoderma* Otitis externa Seborrhea Facial myxedema
Clinical chemistry	Hyperlipidemia Slightly elevated liver enzymes (ALT, ALP) Coagulopathy
Eye	Corneal lipidosis Uveitis
Reproductive system	Persistent anestrus Prolonged estrus Gynecomastia
Behavior	Aggressiveness
Neuromuscular system	Exercise intolerance* Ataxia Peripheral and central vestibular dysfunction† Facial nerve paralysis (N. facialis, N. trigeminus) Seizures

*Common.
†Peripheral vestibular dysfunction—ataxia, loss of balance, nystagmus; central vestibular dysfunction—ataxia, loss of balance, nystagmus, and loss of proprioception.

focal hair retention rather than hair loss may predominate (Feldman and Nelson 2004), giving the coat a very dense, brush-like appearance with different color shades (Fig. 3.3.2). In addition to alopecia (or hypertrichosis), the skin may show seborrhea and hyperpigmentation. Many dogs with hypothyroidism have an increased susceptibility to develop recurrent skin infections (pyoderma) after a reasonable course of antimicrobial therapy. Facial myxedema (i.e., cutaneous mucinosis), often referred to as the "tragic face," is rare.

Clinical workup for dogs with suspected hypothyroidism should include a complete blood count, a biochemical screen, and urinalysis. Most consistent findings with hypothyroidism are mild nonregenerative anemia and elevated cholesterol levels. Fructosamine levels have been reported to be increased (Reusch et al. 2002).

3.3.1.1.2.2 Histopathology

Skin biopsies are often performed in animals with hair coat changes or with suspected endocrine alopecias. However, histopathological findings in skin biopsies from hypothyroid dogs reveal nondiagnostic unspecific changes such as orthokeratotic hyperkeratosis, follicular inactivity, and telogenization. Dermal mucinosis or hypertrophic and vacuolated arrector pili muscles, if present, may support the diagnosis of hypothyroidism, but again are not conclusive to allow a final diagnosis to be made. Many biopsy specimens from hypothyroid dogs will show some degree of pyoderma.

3.3.1.1.2.3 Laboratory tests

Endocrine laboratory tests are indispensable to diagnose hypothyroidism, but need to be interpreted with great caution. Thyroid hormone levels are not only decreased in hypothyroidism but also in numerous other diseases and with several drugs. In addition, measurements of thyroid hormone levels and of TSH need to be performed with sufficient skills, since assays that were developed for humans cannot be used in veterinary medicine without proper adaptations.

Hypothyroidism should be associated with low levels of circulating thyroid hormone and high levels of TSH. In humans, the diagnostic accuracy of concurrent measurements of fT4 and endogenous TSH is almost 100% (Wiesli and Schmid 2001). In dogs, however, only about 50% of hypothyroid dogs will show a classical test result that will allow a straightforward diagnosis of hypothyroidism. Unfortunately, the diagnostic accuracy of thyroid hormone measurements in dogs, particularly that for fT4 levels, is not comparable to that in humans. This is mostly due to differences in the protein-binding capacity between canine and human thyroid hormone. Dogs have less thyroxine-binding globuline (TBG) and a lower affinity of thyroid hormone to bind to TBG. This results in higher concentrations of fT4 in animals. However, most commercial radioimmunoassay (RIA) fT4 assays that are employed in veterinary laboratories very much depend on TBG concentrations. Therefore, they

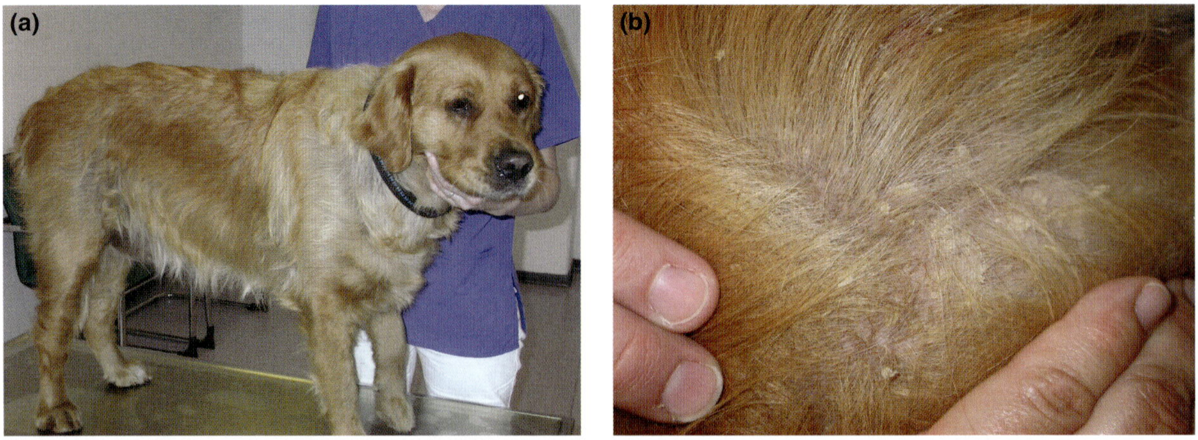

Fig. 3.3.1 Hypothyroidism in a golden retriever. (a) "Tragic" face and the dull appearance of the hair coat; (b) closer inspection of the hair coat reveals extensive scaling.

frequently produce inappropriately low fT4 results in animals, and are less useful for assisting in the diagnosis of canine hypothyroidism (Witherspoon et al. 1988; Ferguson 1995; Nelson et al. 2004).

Total T4

Most veterinary laboratories measure total T4 (tT4), the sum of protein-bound and free T4. Either a RIA or an enzyme-linked immunoassay (ELISA) can be used. Although the RIA is considered the gold standard, its sensitivity has to be evaluated by each laboratory, particularly for detecting low T4 levels, and it can be influenced by autoantibodies to Tg (TgAA). The ELISA is reported to be less sensitive to TgAA interference. Snap T4 test kits are available but their accuracy and usefulness in the diagnosis of hypothyroidism has not been elucidated sufficiently yet (Lurye et al. 2002; Peterson et al. 2003).

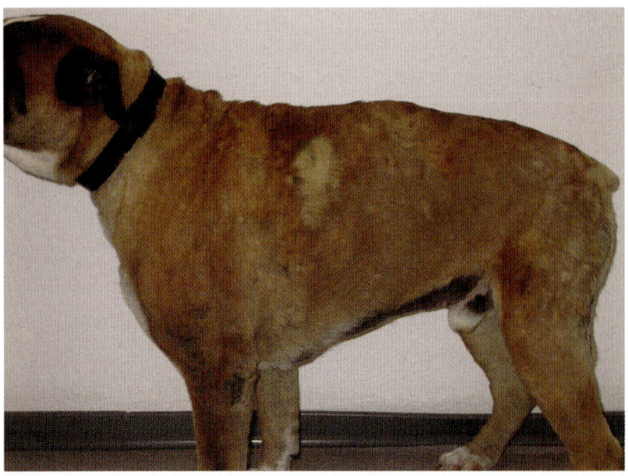

Fig. 3.3.2 Boxer with hypothyroidism and extensive patchy hypertrichosis. Note variety in hair length and color.

The main diagnostic value of measuring tT4 is the fact that hypothyroidism can be ruled out, if tT4 values are within the normal limits. Less than 10% of hypothyroid dogs may show normal tT4 levels due to the interference with TgAA (Peterson et al. 1997). These patients represent a particular diagnostic challenge and require further workup such as determination of TgAA (see below). Once again, this emphasizes the importance of clinical findings being considered for the diagnosis of hypothyroidism. Low tT4 levels are by no means sufficient to accurately diagnose hypothyroidism. Although most hypothyroid dogs will have low tT4 levels, other diseases or drug interference can cause low tT4 levels that are not due to impaired thyroid function.

Free T4

The measurement of free T4 would allow a more precise evaluation of the thyroid hormone fraction that is actually available to the cells. However, as it has been mentioned before, the commercial fT4 radioimmuneassay is severely influenced by the TBG concentration, producing falsely low measurements and overestimating hypothyroidism. Therefore, there is no advantage to measuring free T4 in lieu of total T4. A new assay technique, that is, equilibrium dialysis, uses a dialysis step to separate free T4 from protein-bound T4. This measurement is not affected by circulating autoantibodies and seems to be less influenced by nonthyroidal illnes than tT4. Some studies found a high specificity (93%), high sensitivity (98%), and a high diagnostic accuracy (90%) (Peterson et al. 1997; Dixon and Mooney 1999; Ferguson 2007). Others, however, conclude that fT4 (measured by equilibrium dialysis) adds only minimal supplementary information compared to total T4 determination (Schachter et al. 2004). The equilibrium dialysis assay is far more laborious and expensive than the conventional RIA. Whereas many U.S. laboratories perform fT4 measurements with equilibrium dialysis, this technique is only offered by a few European veterinary diagnostic laboratories.

Effects of nonthyroidal illness or drugs on T4

A low tT4 (or a low fT4 measured by equilibrium dialysis) is not diagnostic for hypothyroidism. Many other causes may provoke low tT4 and fT4 levels. First of all, there are normal random fluctuations as T4 is secreted pulsatile and not constantly. Nelson et al. (1991) reported, that the range of fT4 concentration in healthy dogs is 1.0–3.3 μg/dL, overlapping with 0–1.5 μg/dL in hypothyroid dogs. Breed, age, body weight, and reproductive stage of females may influence the hormone level. Sighthounds such as Salukis, Whippet and Greyhounds have lower tT4 and fT4 levels than other breeds (Hill et al. 2001; van Geffen et al. 2006). Therefore, breed-specific reference ranges are urgently needed. Serum analysis of healthy sled dogs revealed a significant decrease in tT4 and fT4 concentrations and a significant increase in TSH concentration in dogs that were in the peak training state (Evason et al. 2004).

In any severe illness, the body physiologically adapts with reduced cellular metabolism by decreasing T4 synthesis, reducing conversion of T4 to T3, and subsequently decreasing T4 and T3 levels. This is referred to as the "euthyroid sick syndrome" (Kantrowitz et al. 2001; Mooney et al. 2008). The severity of the illness is reflected by the suppression of serum thyroid hormones. Furthermore, nonthyroidal diseases with hypoproteinemia, or production of hormone-binding inhibitors, or administration of drugs that are highly protein bound, may inhibit protein binding of thyroxin and thus can increase fT4. This temporary increase in fT4 will subsequently lead to a decreased TSH secretion and reduced thyroid hormone production with decreased tT4 and fT4 levels. Additionally, TSH- and TRH-stimulation tests will be influenced by the euthyroid sick syndrome, further complicating the accurate diagnosis of hypothyroidism.

In dogs with endocrine alopecia, a diagnostic dilemma may exist in the differentiation of hyperadrenocorticism and hypothyroidism, particularly if clinical signs and results of routine blood and urine tests are not diagnostic for the one or the other disease. Glucocorticoids reduce baseline serum tT4 and fT4 concentrations in 60% of cases (Peterson et al. 1984; Ferguson and Peterson 1992). This is most likely mediated by suppression of TSH secretion, since 75% of hypercortisolemic dogs have low TSH levels. Therefore, dogs with naturally acquired hyperadrenocorticism can develop secondary hypothyroidism due to TSH deficiency. On the other hand, about 25% of dogs with hyperadrenocorticism have low tT4 levels and high TSH levels over 0.6 ng/mL. Although these dogs mimic primary hypothyroidism, they actually do not need any therapy. To accurately diagnose hypothyroidism, it is therefore very important to rule out hyperadrenocorticism, firstly by a thorough history and physical examination, and secondly by additional tests such as ultrasound, urine cortisol/creatinine ratio, low-dose dexamethasone suppression test, or ACTH stimulation test (see 3.3.2.1.2). It cannot be overemphasized that high dosages and even short-term administration of exogenous glucocorticoids have the same effect on thyroid testing as spontaneous hyperadrenocorticism, resulting in falsely low tT4 levels and a frequent misdiagnosis of hypothyroidism (Daminet et al. 1999). Ideally, glucocorticoids should be discontinued for 4–8 weeks before thyroid hormones are measured.

Except for exogenous glucocorticoids, other drugs can affect serum thyroid hormone levels as well (Daminet and Ferguson 2003). Of particular importance are phenobarbital and sulfonamides (Gookin et al. 1999; Kantrowitz et al. 1999; Gieger et al. 2000; Muller et al. 2000; Williamson et al. 2002; Frank et al. 2005). It may take up to 8 weeks or even longer after cessation of treatment, until normal thyroid hormone levels are reestablished. Some NSAIDs influence thyroid function tests, too. For example, treatment with caprofen for 5 weeks causes a significant decrease in tT4 levels. The knowledge about the interferences between drugs and thyroid hormones is still sparse (Table 3.3.4). Therefore, until proven otherwise, any

Table 3.3.4 Drug influences on tT4, fT4, and TSH

Drugs	tT4	fT4	TSH
Glucocorticoids	↓	↓	↓/–
Sulfonamides	↓	↓	↑
Phenobarbital	↓	↓	↑/–
Propranolol	–	nd	–
Potassium bromide	–	nd	–
Clomipramin	↓	↓	–
Ketoprofen	↓/–	–	–
Carprofen	↓/–	↓/–	↓/–
Etodolac	–	–	–
Furosemid	↓	nd	nd
Cephalexine	–	–	–
Iodine	↓	↓	↑
Propythiouracil	↓	↓	↑
Methimazol	↓	↓	↑

↓, decreased; ↑, increased; –, no effect; nd, no data available.

drug should be suspected to have an influence on thyroid hormone test results.

Total T3 and free T3

T3 is secreted in very low amounts by the thyroid gland. Most T3 is produced within the target cells by deiodination from fT4. Either fT3 or rT3 is formed. The latter is a metabolically inactive form that is used to counteract thyroid hormone activity in certain metabolic states such as illness or starvation. The accuracy of tT3 or fT3 measurements for the diagnosis of hypothyroidism is low and thus both are generally considered as poor screening tests for hypothyroidism (Ferguson 2007).

TSH

In humans, serum TSH levels have a high sensitivity for hypothyroidism, correlate well with the disease status, and can be used as a screening test. In the dog, serum TSH levels also have a high specificity, but their sensitivity is only 63–82%. One-fourth of all hypothyroid dogs have normal TSH levels (Boretti and Reusch 2004). Possible reasons for this may be a pulsatile release of TSH, a concurrent drug administration that interferes with thyroid hormone metabolism, a concurrent illness that suppresses pituitary TSH release, an exhaustion of pituitary TSH release, or inability of the assays to detect all isoforms of circulating TSH (Peterson et al. 1997; Ramsey et al. 1997; Kemppainen and Behrend 2001). Most laboratories use immunoradiometric or chemiluminescence assays to measure TSH. Normal values for serum TSH concentrations are up to 0.6 ng/mL. Levels below 0.03 ng/mL cannot be detected by most assays. Since abnormally low TSH levels cannot be detected in dogs, there is no use of TSH measurements for the diagnosis of secondary hypothyroidism or thyrotoxicosis under levothyroxine treatment.

Serum TSH concentrations should always be interpreted in conjunction with tT4 levels (or fT4 measured in equilibrium dialysis). A low tT4 level together with a high TSH concentration, and compatible clinical signs and history support the diagnosis of primary hypothyroidism. Normal tT4 levels combined with a normal TSH concentration rule out hypothyroidism (Scott-Moncrieff et al. 1998; Dixon and Mooney 1999). Any other combination, however, is difficult to interpret and represents a diagnostic dilemma. High TSH concentrations and normal T4 levels may suggest an early stage of hypothyroidism, but should not be associated with clinical signs of hypothyroidism. High TSH concentrations can also be found in dogs with euthyroid sick syndrome (see above).

For differentiating between hypothyroidism and euthyroid sick syndrome and other nonthyroidal low T4 level, endocrine function tests are required.

TRH stimulation test

The TSH-releasing hormone (TRH) stimulation test evaluates the responsiveness of the pituitary gland to TRH and the responsiveness of the thyroid gland to TSH. Different protocols have been described (Scott-Moncrieff and Nelson 1998; Feldman and Nelson 2004). After blood is obtained for baseline tT4 and TSH levels, TRH is administered intravenously. Blood samples for measuring TSH are taken after 20 min and those for measuring T4 are taken after 2 and/or 3 h. The TSH and T4 increase is often low, and the interpretation of the results can be difficult. In an euthyroid dog, the post-TRH serum tT4 levels should be greater than 2.0 ng/mL and should increase at least 0.5 ng/mL over the baseline level. Levels between 1.0 and 2.0 ng/mL are not diagnostic for hypothyroidism (Frank 1996). Serum TSH levels should increase by 100%. But even then, the diagnostic accuracy to diagnose euthyroidism is only about 90%. Furthermore, the plasma TSH concentration at 30 min after TRH administration does not differ significantly between primary hypothyroidism and nonthyroidal illness (Diaz Espineira et al. 2007). Thus, the TRH stimulation test does not offer any additional diagnostic benefit over the TSH stimulation test.

TSH stimulation test

The TSH stimulation test evaluates the responsiveness of the thyroid gland to exogenous TSH administration, and is regarded as the gold standard for differentiating hypothyroidism from euthyroid sick syndrome or nonthyroidal illness. Bovine TSH, which has been used for decades, has been removed from the market. Therefore, recombinant human TSH (rhTSH) has to be used (Sauve and Paradis 2000; Boretti et al. 2006a). The recommended dose of rhTSH for testing is 50–75 μg/dog administered intravenously. A peak increase in T4 levels is expected at 6 h after TSH administration. rhTSH is quite expensive and one vial contains 1.1 mg of lyophilized rhTSH that can be used for 12 tests. To lower costs, aliquots can be frozen at −20°C for 8 weeks without loosing its biological activity (De Roover et al. 2006). Interpretation of the test needs to be based on a comparison of T4 levels before and after TSH stimulation. In general, any increase larger than 1.5 times is considered euthyroid and excludes hypothyroidism. Two recent studies, however, revealed substantial overlap in hypothyroid and nonhypothyroid dogs (Boretti et al. 2006b; Diaz-Espineira et al. 2007).

Autoantibodies

As discussed before, detection of TgAA supports a diagnosis of lymphocytic thyroiditis, but it is by no means a diagnostic criterion for hypothyroidism. Dogs with hypothyroidism can be TgAA negative and euthyroid dogs can be TgAA positive. One study in 234 dogs confirmed that only 20% of TgAA-positive dogs develop hypothyroidism (Graham et al. 2001a).

Recently, autoantibodies against thyroid peroxidase have been identified in hypothyroid dogs with TgAA, but the value of antithyroid peroxidase autoantibodies as a diagnostic tool for hypothyroidism has yet to be evaluated in further studies (Skopek et al. 2006).

Autoantibodies to T3 (T3AA) and T4 (T4AA) are very rare. In a large survey, autoantibodies against T4 or T3 were only found in 6.3% (Nachreiner et al. 2002). T4AA and T3AA are always associated with TgAA, thus indicating autoimmune thyroiditis (Ferguson 2007). Some breeds show a higher prevalence of thyroid hormone autoantibodies, such as Pointer, English Setter, English Pointer, Skye Terrier, German Wirehaired Pointer, Old English Sheepdog, Boxer, Maltese, Kuvasz, and Petit Basset Griffon Vendeen. Measuring T4AA or T3AA does not add information on the severity or the progression of thyroiditis, nor is it an indicator of thyroid gland function. Measurement of T3AA and T4AA is therefore only indicated, if unexpectedly high or low serum T4 levels have to be explained.

Thyroid ultrasonography

Ultrasonography with high resolution can effectively evaluate the size, shape, capsule delineation, volume, echogenicity, and homogenicity of the thyroid gland. Recent studies have shown that determination of thyroid volume and mean cross-sectional surface area by ultrasonography can accurately differentiate between euthyroid and hypothyroid dogs (Reese et al. 2005; Bromel et al. 2006). When all five parameters (size, shape, volume, echogenicity, and homogenicity) are combined, ultrasonography has an overall diagnostic sensitivity of 94.1% (Taeymans et al. 2007). Thus, ultrasonography is helpful to differentiate hypothyroidism from euthyroid sick syndrome. However, breed-specific reference ranges for thyroid size and volume have not been elaborated yet.

3.3.1.1.3 Therapy and monitoring

The initial treatment of choice is synthetic levothyroxine at a dosage of 0.02 mg/kg body weight every 12 h. The twice-daily dosage leads to a more constant level of thyroxin concentration closer to the physiological range. As intestinal absorption is influenced by dietary factors and proteins that bind levothyroxine, it is best administered without food. The high dosage in dogs compared with humans can be explained by the overall low absorption. Some authors recommend the dosing of levothyroxine be based on body surface area (0.5 mg/m^2), as the body surface area is more closely related to the metabolic rate than the body weight (Feldman and Nelson 2004). Lowering the initial dose of levothyroxine is indicated in dogs with concurrent cardiomyopathy, since a sudden increase of metabolism and oxygen demand may result in heart failure (Panciera 1994a).

An increase in mental alertness and activity usually occurs within the first weeks after levothyroxine supplementation, whereas complete resolution of dermatological and neurological changes may take several months (Dixon et al. 2002; Feldman and Nelson 2004).

Response to treatment should be evaluated 6–8 weeks after initiating therapy. Total T4 and TSH are measured 4–6 h after administration of levothyroxine. Serum T4 levels should be in the high normal range or above the reference range, and TSH levels should have returned to the normal range. In principle, tT4 levels should be higher than 1.5 ng/mL at any time point after levothyroxine administration. A 6-h postpill level above the reference range does not require a dose reduction as long as there are no signs of thyrotoxicosis, such as panting, nervousness, polyphagia, weight loss, and diarrhea. Thyrotoxicosis is rare in the dog and most commonly occurs in euthyroid patients that have been misdiagnosed as being hypothyroid due to nonthyroidal illness. Discontinuation for a few days should resolve the clinical signs of thyrotoxicosis.

A response to levothyroxine administration is by no means specific for hypothyroidism. Other conditions with poor coat quality, such as canine recurrent flank alopecia may appear to be levothyroxine responsive, even in euthyroid patients. Therefore, trial levothyroxine therapy without confirmed diagnosis of hypothyroidism should not be conducted.

Short-term treatment of healthy dogs with levothyroxine will decrease T4 and T3 responses to TSH-stimulation for more than 4 weeks (Panciera et al. 1990). Therefore, levothyroxine should be discontinued for at least 6 weeks if thyroid function is to be evaluated by TRH or TSH stimulation tests.

Failures to respond to levothyroxin therapy can have several possible reasons. The most common cause is an inappropriate diagnosis of hypothyroidism, especially if hyperadrenocorticism has not been sufficiently ruled out. Concurrent illnesses such as allergic dermatitis or medications may interfere with the efficacy of levothyroxine therapy. Insufficient owner compliance and improper tablet administration should also be considered. Impaired absorption of levothyroxine is extremely rare. In confirmed cases, treatment with liothyronine sodium (T3) is indicated.

3.3.1.2 Feline hypothyroidism

In the cat, spontaneous hypothyroidism is very rare, whereas the iatrogenic form occurring due to radioiodine therapy of hyperthyroidism, thyroidectomy, or overdosing of antithyroid drugs is seen frequently in this species. The risk to develop hypothyroidism after treatment with iodine 131 is about 30.3% and is twice as likely with a bilateral scintigraphic pattern than a unilateral scintigraphic pattern (Meric and Rubin 1990; Nykamp et al. 2005).

Causes of spontaneous feline hypothyroidism include congenital hypothyroidism that has been recognized in domestic shorthair cats and in Abyssinian cats (Arnold et al. 1984; Sjollema et al. 1991; Jones et al. 1992). In the latter, it is autosomal recessive. Long-term prognosis for cats with congenital hypothyroidism is poorly documented. Clinical signs may resolve without treatment, but frequently patients show continued musculoskeletal abnormalities, mental dullness, and gastrointestinal motility problems (Tobias and Lobato 2001).

Spontaneous lymphocytic thyroiditis was recorded in one cat only (Rand et al. 1993). Thyroid gland atrophy, cystic follicles, amyloidosis, and goiter have been demonstrated by histopathology (Feldman and Nelson 2004).

The clinical signs of feline hypothyroidism are similar to those reported for dogs, with lethargy and obesity being most prominent. In contrast to dogs, cats can develop a severe inappetence. Bradycardia and hypothermia can additionally occur. Hypercholesterolemia and normocytic, normochromic, nonregenerative anemia have been found in iatrogenic hypothyroid cats (Scott-Moncrieff 2007). Dermatological signs are variable and often represent a sequela to decreased grooming. Easily epilated hairs and poor regrowth of hair may be seen at pressure points and at the dorsal and lateral tail base. An asymmetric or symmetric alopecia may involve the neck, thorax, and abdomen.

Initial screening tests and their limitations are similar to those in the dog. A low serum concentration of tT4 in an adult cat is almost always caused by euthyroid sick syndrome (Mooney et al. 1996; Peterson et al. 2001). fT4 in dialysis is presumably more sensitive and specific for assessing thyroid function, but most research is done on hyperthyroid cats. Assays for endogenous TSH in cats have been hampered by the lack of feline-specific TSH and standards (Graham et al. 2000). Tests for autoantibodies have not been established in cats.

The TRH stimulation test is limited due to common adverse reactions to TRH administration in cats. Furthermore, interpretation of results is difficult (Tomsa et al. 2001). Since bovine TSH is no longer available, rhTSH must be used for stimulation tests. The TSH stimulation test has been evaluated in euthyroid cats and can be performed by intravenous administration of 0.025–0.2 mg of rhTSH. The serum tT4 concentration is measured at the time of TSH administration and 6 h later (Stegeman et al. 2003). However, data on results of hypothyroid cats are not available at the time of writing. The treatment is similar as for dogs.

3.3.1.3 Equine hypothyroidism

Equine hypothyroidism remains a controversial endocrine disorder, because extrathyroidal factors, including the administration of drugs and systemic diseases, affect serum thyroid hormone concentrations in horses (Sojka et al. 1993; Frank et al. 2002; Reed et al. 2003). Major cause of hypothyroidism in the foal is inadequate or excessive iodine uptake with goiter formation (Allen et al. 1996). There is only one report on idiopathic primary hypothyroidism and alopecia in the horse (Stanley and Hillidge 1982). Diagnosis of equine hypothyroidism is currently limited to clinical signs, low thyroxine hormone levels, and the TRH response test (Breuhaus 2002; Breuhaus et al. 2006).

References

Allen AL, Townsend HG, Doige CE, Fretz PB. 1996. A case-control study of the congenital hypothyroidism and dysmaturity syndrome of foals. *Canadian Veterinary Journal* 37:349–351.

Arnold U, Opitz M, Grossier I, Bader R, Eigenmann JE. 1984. Goitrous hypothyroidism and dwarfism in a kitten. *Journal of the American Animal Hospital Association* 20:753–758.

Benjamin SA, Stephens LC, Hamilton BF, Saunders WJ, Lee AC, Angleton GM, Mallinckrodt CH. 1996. Associations between lymphocytic thyroiditis, hypothyroidism, and thyroid neoplasia in beagles. *Veterinary Pathology* 33(5):486–494.

Boretti FS, Reusch CE. 2004. Endogenous TSH in the diagnosis of hypothyroidism in dogs. *Schweizer Archiv Fur Tierheilkunde* 146(4):183–188.

Boretti FS, Sieber-Ruckstuhl NS, Favrot C, Lutz H, Hofmann-Lehmann R, Reusch CE. 2006a. Evaluation of recombinant human thyroid-stimulating hormone to test thyroid function in dogs suspected of having hypothyroidism. *American Journal of Veterinary Research* 67(12):2012–2016.

Boretti FS, Sieber-Ruckstuhl NS, Willi B, Lutz H, Hofmann-Lehmann R, Reusch CE. 2006b. Comparison of the biological activity of recombinant human thyroid-stimulating hormone with bovine thyroid-stimulating hormone and evaluation of recombinant human thyroid-stimulating hormone in healthy dogs of different breeds. *American Journal of Veterinary Research* 67(7):1169–1172.

Breuhaus BA. 2002. Thyroid-stimulating hormone in adult euthyroid and hypothyroid horses. *Journal of Veterinary Internal Medicine* 16:109–115.

Breuhaus BA, Refsal KR, Beyerlein SL. 2006. Measurement of free thyroxine concentration in horses by equilibrium dialysis. *Journal of Veterinary Internal Medicine* 20:371–376.

Bromel C, Pollard RE, Kass PH, Samii VF, Davidson AP, Nelson RW. 2006. Comparison of ultrasonographic characteristics of the thyroid gland in healthy small-, medium-, and large-breed dogs. *American Journal of Veterinary Research* 67(1):70–77.

Castillo VA, Pisarev MA, Lalia JC, Rodriguez MS, Cabrini RL, Marquez G. 2001. Commercial diet induced hypothyroidism due to high iodine. A histological and radiological analysis. *Veterinary Quarterly* 23(4):218–223.

Credille KM, Slater MR, Moriello KA, Nachreiner RF, Tucker KA, Dunstan RW. 2001. The effects of thyroid hormones on the skin of beagle dogs. *Journal of Veterinary Internal Medicine* 15(6):539–546.

Daminet S. 2005. *Proceedings of the ESVD Workshop on Endocrinology*, Spa, Belgium, pp. 24–45.

Daminet S, Ferguson DC. 2003. Influence of drugs on thyroid function in dogs. *Journal of Veterinary Internal Medicine* 17(4):463–472.

Daminet S, Paradis M, Refsal KR, Price C. 1999. Short-term influence of prednisone and phenobarbital on thyroid function in euthyroid dogs. *Canadian Veterinary Journal* 40(6):411–415.

De Roover K, Duchateau L, Carmichael N, van Geffen C, Daminet S. 2006. Effect of storage of reconstituted recombinant human thyroid-stimulating hormone (rhTSH) on thyroid-stimulating hormone (TSH) response testing in euthyroid dogs. *Journal of Veterinary Internal Medicine* 20(4):812–817.

Diaz Espineira MM, Mol JA, Peeters ME, Pollak YW, Iversen L, van Dijk JE, Rijnberk A, Kooistra HS. 2007. Assessment of thyroid function in dogs with low plasma thyroxine concentration. *Journal of Veterinary Internal Medicine* 21(1):25–32.

Dixon RM, Mooney CT. 1999. Evaluation of serum free thyroxine and thyrotropin concentrations in the diagnosis of canine hypothyroidism. *Journal of Small Animal Practice* 40(2):72–78.

Dixon RM, Reid SW, Mooney CT. 1999. Epidemiological, clinical, haematological and biochemical characteristics of canine hypothyroidism. *Veterinary Record* 145:481–487.

Dixon RM, Reid SW, Mooney CT. 2002. Treatment and therapeutic monitoring of canine hypothyroidism. *Journal of Small Animal Practice* 43(8):334–340.

Dolling CE, Good BF. 1976. Congenital goitre in sheep: isolation of the iodoproteins which replace thyroglobulin. *Journal of Endocrinology* 71:179–192.

Evason MD, Carr AP, Taylor SM, Waldner CL. 2004. Alterations in thyroid hormone concentrations in healthy sled dogs before and after athletic conditioning. *American Journal of Veterinary Research* 65(3):333–337.

Feldman EC, Nelson RW. 2004. Hypothyroidism. In: Feldman EC, Nelson RW (eds), *Canine and Feline Endocrinology and Reproduction*, 3rd edn, pp. 88–155. Philadelphia: WB Saunders.

Ferguson DC. 1995. Free Thyroid hormone measurements in the diagnosis of thyroid disease. In: Bonagura J, Kirk RW (eds), *Current Veterinary Therapy XII*, pp. 360–364. Philadelphia: WB Saunders.

Ferguson DC. 2005. *Proceedings of the 20th Annual Congress of the ESVD/ECVD*, Chalkidiki, Greece, pp. 48–51.

Ferguson DC. 2007. Testing for hypothyroidism in dogs. *Veterinary Clinics of North America Small Animal Practice* 37(4):647–669.

Ferguson DC, Peterson ME. 1992. Serum free and total iodothyronine concentrations in dogs with hyperadrenocorticism. *American Journal of Veterinary Research* 53(9):1636–1640.

Frank LA. 1996. Comparison of thyrotropin-releasing hormone (TRH) to thyrotropin (TSH) stimulation for evaluating thyroid function in dogs. *Journal of the American Animal Hospital Association* 32(6):481–487.

Frank LA, Hnilica KA, May ER, Sargent SJ, Davis JA. 2005. Effects of sulfamethoxazole-trimethoprim on thyroid function in dogs. *American Journal of Veterinary Research* 66(2):256–259.

Frank N, Sojka J, Messer NT. 2002. Equine thyroid dysfunction. *Veterinary Clinics of North America Equine Practice* 18(2):305–319, vii.

Gieger TL, Hosgood G, Taboada J, Wolfsheimer KJ, Mueller PB. 2000. Thyroid function and serum hepatic enzyme activity in dogs after phenobarbital administration. *Journal of Veterinary Internal Medicine* 14(3):277–281.

Gookin JL, Trepanier LA, Bunch SE. 1999. Clinical hypothyroidism associated with trimethoprim-sulfadiazine administration in a dog. *Journal of the American Veterinary Medical Association* 214(7):1028–1031, 1021.

Graham P, Refsal K, Nachreiner R, Provencher AL. 2000. The measurement of feline thyrotropin using a commercial canine-specific immunoradiometric assay (abstract). *Journal of Veterinary Internal Medicine* 14:342.

Graham PA, Lundquist RB, Refsal KR. 2001a. 12-Month prospective study of 234 thyroglobulin antibody positive dogs which had no laboratory evidence of thyroid dysfunction. *Journal of Veterinary Internal Medicine* 14:298.

Graham PA, Nachreiner RF, Refsal KR, Provencher-Bolliger AL. 2001b. Lymphocytic thyroiditis. *Veterinary Clinics of North America Small Animal Practice* 31(5):915.

Graham PA, Refsal KR, Nachreiner RF. 2007. Etiopathologic findings of canine hypothyroidism. *Veterinary Clinics of North America Small Animal Practice* 37(4):17–31, v.

Greenspan FS. 2001. The thyroid gland. In: Greenspan FS, Gardner (eds), *Basic and Clinical Endocrinology*, 6th edn, pp. 201–205. New York: Lange Medical Books/McGraw Hill.

Hill RC, Fox LE, Lewis DD, Beale KM, Nachreiner RF, Scott KC, Sundstrom DA, Jones GL, Butterwick RF. 2001. Effects of racing and training on serum thyroid hormone concentrations in racing Greyhounds. *American Journal of Veterinary Research* 62(12):1969–1972.

Jones, BR, Gruffydd-Jones TJ, Sparkes AH, Lucke VM. 1992. Preliminary studies on congenital hypothyroidism in a family of Abyssinian cats. *Veterinary Record* 131(7):145–148.

Kallfelz FA.1977. Thyroid function in the dog. *Veterinary Clinics of North America* 7(3):497–512.

Kantrowitz LB, Peterson ME, Melian C, Nichols R. 2001. Serum total thyroxine, total triiodothyronine, free thyroxine, and thyrotropin concentrations in dogs with nonthyroidal disease. *Journal of the American Veterinary Medical Association* 219(6):765–769.

Kantrowitz LB, Peterson ME, Trepanier LA, Melian C, Nichols R. 1999. Serum total thyroxine, total triiodothyronine, free thyroxine, and thyrotropin concentrations in epileptic dogs treated with anticonvulsants. *Journal of the American Veterinary Medical Association* 214(12):1804–1808.

Kemppainen RJ, Behrend EN. 2001. Diagnosis of canine hypothyroidism. Perspectives from a testing laboratory. *Veterinary Clinics of North America Small Animal Practice* 31(5):951–962, vii.

Kennedy LJ, Barnes A, Short A, Brown JJ, Seddon J, Fleeman L, Brkljacic M, Happ GM, Catchpole B, Ollier WE. 2007. Canine DLA diversity: 3. Disease studies. *Tissue Antigens* 69(1 Suppl):292–296.

Kennedy LJ, Quarmby S, Happ GM, Barnes A, Ramsey IK, Dixon RM, Catchpole B, Rusbridge C, Graham PA, Hillbertz NS, Roethel C, Dodds WJ, Carmichael NG, Ollier WE. 2006. Association of canine hypothyroidism with a common major histocompatibility complex DLA class II allele. *Tissue Antigens* 68(1):82–86.

Kiesewetter H, Schell H. 1994. Cell kinetics of anagen scalp hairs under physiological and pathological conditions. *Skin Pharmacology* 7:55–60.

Kooistra HS, Voorhout G, Mol JA, Rijnberk A. 2000. Combined pituitary hormone deficiency in German shepherd dogs with dwarfism. *Domestic Animal Endocrinology* 19(3):177–190.

Larsen PR, MJ Berry. 1995. Nutritional and hormonal regulation of thyroid hormone deiodinases. *Annual Review of Nutrition* 15:323–352.

Lurye JC, Behrend EN, Kemppainen RJ. 2002. Evaluation of an in-house enzyme-linked immunosorbent assay for quantitative measurement of serum total thyroxine concentration in dogs and cats. *Journal of the American Veterinary Medical Association* 221(2):243–249.

Mason R, Wilkinson JS. 1973. The thyroid gland—a review. *Australian Veterinary Journal* 49(1):44–49

Meric SM, Rubin SI. 1990. Serum thyroxine concentrations following fixed-dose radioactive iodine treatment in hyperthyroid cats: 62 cases (1986–1989). *Journal of the American Veterinary Medical Association* 197(5):621–623.

Mooney CT, Little CJ, Macrae AW. 1996. Effect of illness not associated with the thyroid gland on serum total and free thyroxine concentrations in cats. *Journal of the American Veterinary Medical Association* 208(12):2004–2008.

Mooney CT, Shiel RE, Dixon RM. 2008. Thyroid hormone abnormalities and outcome in dogs with non-thyroidal illness. *Journal of Small Animal Practice* 49(1):11–16.

Muller PB, Wolfsheimer KJ, Taboada J, Hosgood G, Partington BP, Gaschen FP. 2000. Effects of long-term phenobarbital treatment on the thyroid and adrenal axis and adrenal function tests in dogs. *Journal of Veterinary Internal Medicine* 14(2):157–164.

Nachreiner RF, Refsal KR, Graham PA, Bowman MM. 2002. Prevalence of serum thyroid hormone autoantibodies in dogs with clinical signs of hypothyroidism. *Journal of the American Veterinary Medical Association* 220(4):466–471.

Nachreiner RF, Refsal KR, Graham PA, Hauptman J, Watson GL. 1998. Prevalence of autoantibodies to thyroglobulin in dogs with nonthyroidal illness. *American Journal of Veterinary Research* 59(8):951–955.

Nelson JC, Wang R, Asher DT, Wilcox RB. 2004. The nature of analogue-based free thyroxine estimates. *Thyroid* 14(12):1030–1036.

Nelson RW, Ihle SL, Feldman EC, Bottoms GD. 1991. Serum free thyroxine concentration in healthy dogs, dogs with hypothyroidism, and euthyroid dogs with concurrent illness. *Journal of the American Veterinary Medical Association* 198(8):1401–1407.

Nykamp SG, Dykes NL, Zarfoss MK, Scarlett JM. 2005. Association of the risk of development of hypothyroidism after iodine 131 treatment with the pretreatment pattern of sodium pertechnetate Tc 99m uptake in the thyroid gland in cats with hyperthyroidism: 165 cases (1990–2002). *Journal of the American Veterinary Medical Association* 226(10):1671–1675.

Panciera DL. 1994a. An echocardiographic and electrocardiographic study of cardiovascular function in hypothyroid dogs. *Journal of the American Veterinary Medical Association* 205(7):996–1000.

Panciera DL. 1994b. Hypothyroidism in dogs: 66 cases (1987–1992). *Journal of the American Veterinary Medical Association* 204:761–767.

Panciera DL. 2001. Conditions associated with canine hypothyroidism. *Veterinary Clinics of North America Small Animal Practice* 31(5):935–950.

Panciera DL, MacEwen EG, Atkins CE, Bosu WT, Refsal KR, Nachreiner RF. 1990. Thyroid function tests in euthyroid dogs treated with L-thyroxine. *American Journal of Veterinary Research* 51(1):22–26.

Peterson, ME, Ferguson DC, Kintzer PP, Drucker WD. 1984. Effects of spontaneous hyperadrenocorticism on serum thyroid hormone concentrations in the dog. *American Journal of Veterinary Research* 45(10):2034–2038.

Peterson, ME, Melian C, Nichols R. 1997. Measurement of serum total thyroxine, triiodothyronine, free thyroxine, and thyrotropin concentrations for diagnosis of hypothyroidism in dogs. *Journal of the American Veterinary Medical Association* 211(11):1396–1402.

Peterson ME, Melian C, Nichols R. 2001. Measurement of serum concentrations of free thyroxine, total thyroxine, and total triiodothyronine in cats with hyperthyroidism and cats with nonthyroidal disease. *Journal of the American Veterinary Medical Association* 218(4):529–536.

Peterson ME, Melian C, Nichols R. 2003. Total thyroxine testing: comparison of an in-house test kid with radioimmuno- and chemiluminescent assay (abstract). *Veterinary Internal Medicine* 17:396.

Ramsey IK, Evans H, Herrtage ME. 1997. Thyroid-stimulating hormone and total thyroxine concentrations in euthyroid, sick euthyroid and hypothyroid dogs. *Journal of Small Animal Practice* 38(12):540–545.

Rand JS, Levine J, Best SJ, Parker W. 1993. Spontaneous adult-onset hypothyroidism in a cat. *Journal of Veterinary Internal Medicine* 7(5):272–276.

Reed MS, Bayly WM, Sella DC. 2003. Hypothyroidism. In: Reed MS, Bayly WM, Sella DC (eds), *Equine Internal Medicine*, 2nd edn, pp. 1349–1351. New York: WB Saunders.

Reese S, Breyer U, Deeg C, Kraft W, Kaspers B. 2005. Thyroid sonography as an effective tool to discriminate between euthyroid sick and hypothyroid dogs. *Journal of Veterinary Internal Medicine* 19(4):491–498.

Reusch CE, Gerber B, Boretti FS. 2002. Serum fructosamine concentrations in dogs with hypothyroidism. *Veterinary Research Communications* 26(7):531–536.

Rijnberk A. 1996. Thyroids. In: Rijnberk A (ed.), *Clinical Endocrinology of Dogs and Cats*, pp. 35–55. Netherlands: Kluwer Academic Publishers.

Sauve F, Paradis M. 2000. Use of recombinant human thyroid-stimulating hormone for thyrotropin stimulation test in euthyroid dogs. *Canadian Veterinary Journal* 41(3):215–219.

Schachter S, Nelson RW, Scott-Moncrieff C, Ferguson DC, Montgomery T, Feldman EC, Neal L, Kass PH. 2004. Comparison of serum-free thyroxine concentrations determined by standard equilibrium dialysis, modified equilibrium dialysis, and 5 radioimmunoassays in dogs. *Journal of Veterinary Internal Medicine* 18(3):259–264.

Schell H, Kiesewetter F, Seidel C, von Hintzenstern J. 1991. Cell cycle kinetics of human anagen scalp hair bulbs in thyroid disorders determined by DANN flow cytometry. *Dermatologica* 182:23–26.

Scott-Moncrieff JC. 2007. Clinical signs and concurrent diseases of hypothyroidism in dogs and cats. *Veterinary Clinics of North America Small Animal Practice* 37(4):709–722, vi.

Scott-Moncrieff JC, Glickman NW, Glickman LT, HogenEsch H. 2006. Lack of association between repeated vaccination and thyroiditis in laboratory Beagles. *Journal of Veterinary Internal Medicine* 20(4):818–821.

Scott-Moncrieff JC, Nelson RW. 1998. Change in serum thyroid-stimulating hormone concentration in response to administration of thyrotropin-releasing hormone to healthy dogs, hypothyroid dogs, and euthyroid dogs with concurrent disease. *Journal of the American Veterinary Medical Association* 213(10): 1435–1438.

Scott-Moncrieff JC, Nelson RW, Bruner JM, Williams DA. 1998. Comparison of serum concentrations of thyroid-stimulating hormone in healthy dogs, hypothyroid dogs, and euthyroid dogs with concurrent disease. *Journal of the American Veterinary Medical Association* 212(3):387–391.

Sjollema BE, den Hartog MT, de Vijlder JJ, van Dijk JE, Rijnberk A. 1991. Congenital hypothyroidism in two cats due to defective organification: data suggesting loosely anchored thyroperoxidase. *Acta Endocrinologica* 125(4):435-440.

Skopek E, Patzl M, Nachreiner RF. 2006. Detection of autoantibodies against thyroid peroxidase in serum samples of hypothyroid dogs. *American Journal of Veterinary Research* 67(5):809–814.

Sojka JE, Johnson MA, Bottoms GD. 1993. Serum triiodothyronine, total thyroxine, and free thyroxine concentrations in horses. *American Journal of Veterinary Research* 54(1):52–55.

Stanley O, Hillidge CJ. 1982. Alopecia associated with hypothyroidism in a horse. *Equine Veterinary Journal* 14(2):165–167.

Stegeman JR, Graham PA, Hauptman JG. 2003. Use of recombinant human thyroid-stimulating hormone for thyrotropin-stimulation testing of euthyroid cats. *American Journal of Veterinary Research* 64(2):149–152.

Taeymans O, Daminet S, Duchateau L, Saunders JH. 2007. Pre- and post-treatment ultrasonography in hypothyroid dogs. *Veterinary Radiology and Ultrasound* 48(3):262–269.

Tobias S, Labato MA. 2001. Identifying and managing feline congenital hypothyroidism. *Veterinary Medicine* 96:719–726.

Tomer Y, Davies TF. 1993. Infection, thyroid disease, and autoimmunity. *Endocrine Reviews* 14(1):107–120.

Tomsa K, Glaus TM, Kacl GM, Pospischil A, Reusch CE. 2001. Thyrotropin-releasing hormone stimulation test to assess thyroid function in severely sick cats. *Journal of Veterinary Internal Medicine* 15(2):89–93.

van Geffen C, Bavegems V, Duchateau L, De Roover K, Daminet S. 2006. Serum thyroid hormone concentrations and thyroglobulin autoantibodies in trained and non-trained healthy whippets. *Veterinary Journal* 172(1):135–140.

Wiesli P, Schmid C. 2001. Hyper- and hypothyroidism: which tests are reliable in general practice? *Schweizerische Rundschau Fur Medizin Praxis* 90:877–881.

Williamson NL, Frank LA, Hnilica KA. 2002. Effects of short-term trimethoprim-sulfamethoxazole administration on thyroid function in dogs. *Journal of the American Veterinary Medical Association* 221(6):802–806.

Wilson JG. 1975. Hypothyroidism in ruminants with special reference to foetal goitre. *Veterinary Record* 97:161–164.

Witherspoon LR, el Shami AS, Shuler SE, Neely H, Sonnemaker R, Gilbert SS, Alyea K. 1988. Chemically blocked analog assays for free thyronines. I. The effect of chemical blockers on T4 analog and T4 binding by albumin and by thyroxin-binding globulin. *Clinical Chemistry* 34(1):9–16.

3.3.2 Hyperadrenocorticism

Rosario Cerundolo

The pilosebaceous unit is a major independent, peripheral endocrine organ (an equivalent of the hypothalamic–pituitary axis). Hair follicles respond to stimulation with corticotrophin-releasing hormone by changes in hair growth, pigmentation, cortisol production, and regulatory feedback (Ito et al. 2005). Even local application of steroids may induce suppression of the local intrafollicular endocrine axis. The cellular response to glucocorticoids is mediated via specific intracellular receptors that are present in the interfollicular epidermis, hair follicle bulge keratinocytes, and hair follicle matrix cells both of rodents and humans (Beato et al. 1995). Glucocorticoids affect the expression of estrogen receptors (ER) by increasing ER-β and decreasing ER-α (Thornton et al. 2006). Glucocorticoids have been reported to be potent suppressors of murine hair growth (Paus et al. 1994). However, the molecular mechanisms leading to hair loss in hyperadrenocorticism, particularly in dogs, have not been studied yet. Certain growth factors may play an important role as is suggested from in vitro and in vivo experiments (Stenn et al. 1993; Okada et al. 2006).

3.3.2.1 Canine hyperadrenocorticism

3.3.2.1.1 Etiology and pathogenesis

Spontaneous hyperadrenocorticism is a common clinical syndrome in dogs, resulting from an excessive circulating cortisol concentration. This is caused by an ACTH-secreting pituitary tumor (pituitary-dependent hyperadrenocorticism, PDH, or "Cushing's disease") in 85% of cases, but occasionally results from an adrenal gland tumor (adrenal-dependent hyperadrenocorticism, ADH). The two types of hyperadrenocorticism are indistinguishable clinically (Feldman and Nelson 2004). Hyperadrenocorticism occurs in middle-aged to older dogs. PDH is seen most frequently in smaller breeds and there is no sex predisposition. ADH is more common in larger breeds and two-thirds of cases are female. Very rarely hyperadrenocorticism is caused by an ectopic secretion of ACTH (Galac et al. 2005, 2007).

3.3.2.1.2 Diagnosis

Several laboratory tests have been described for confirming a diagnosis of canine hyperadrenocorticism. However, it is crucial to understand that all of these diagnostic tests have limitations and all can give both false-negative and false-positive results. The diagnosis should therefore not just rely upon the results of hormonal or diagnostic imaging tests, but also needs to be based on the clinical history, physical examination, and routine laboratory tests including hematology, biochemical profile, and urinalysis.

3.3.2.1.2.1 Clinical presentation

All clinical features of hyperadrenocorticism are caused by excessive circulating glucocorticoids. Clinical signs can vary considerably between individual animals. The most common clinical signs include polyuria, polydipsia, polyphagia, lethargy, muscle weakness, pot belly, excessive panting, and, in some cases, neurological signs secondary to a pituitary tumor (Feldman and Nelson 2004; Wood et al. 2007). Less common are stiff hindlimb gait (resulting from pseudomyotonia) and dyspnea (caused by pulmonary thromboembolism). The reader should refer to textbooks of internal veterinary medicine for more information about the systemic changes occurring in hyperadrenocorticism.

The most common dermatological signs are generalized alopecia, thin skin, bruising, and comedones. Less common are hair color change, phlebectasia, cutaneous hyperpigmentation, calcinosis cutis, chronic infections, or nonhealing wounds (Fig. 3.3.3).

Differential diagnoses include other endocrinopathies such as hyperestrogenism (see Section 3.3.3), hypothyroidism (see Section 3.3.1), and other hair cycle abnormalities such as alopecia X (see Section 3.3.4).

Hematology frequently shows a stress leukogram that is characterized by neutrophilia, monocytosis, lymphopenia, and eosinopenia. Neutrophilia and monocytosis occur due to demargination of these cells within capillaries and the prevention of egress of these cells from the vascular system. Lymphopenia occurs due to lympholysis, and eosinopenia occurs due to bone marrow sequestration of eosinophils. Thrombocytosis may be common and together with other coagulation abnormalities may predispose to the development of pulmonary thromboembolism.

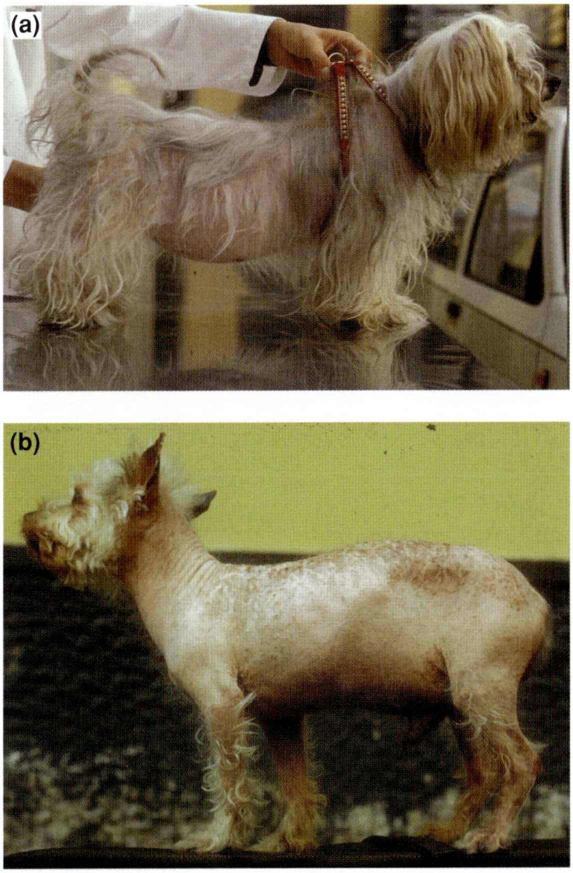

Fig. 3.3.3 Hyperadrenocorticism in a Yorkshire Terrier. (a) Alopecia of the trunk and tail with pendulous abdomen; (b) generalized alopecia.

Common abnormalities in the biochemical profile that are found in dogs with hyperadrenocorticism are elevated liver enzymes (aspartate aminotransferase (AST), alanine aminotransferase (ALT), alkaline phosphatase), hypercholesterolemia (resulting from increased fat catabolism), and mild hyperglycemia (due to an increase in gluconeogenesis and antagonism of insulin activity). Some cases may have a concurrent diabetes mellitus. Low blood urea nitrogen occurs due to polyuria. Hypophosphatemia may develop as glucocorticoids promote phosphorus excretion in the urine, and electrolyte abnormalities such as mild hypernatremia, hyperchloremia, and hypokalemia may be seen as well.

Urinalysis will reveal a low urine specific gravity (caused by polyuria) in most cases of canine hyperadrenocorticism. Some dogs may have proteinuria caused by hypertension. Glucosuria and urinary tract infections are further common findings in urinalysis. Therefore, urine samples in dogs with hyperadrenocorticism should routinely be cultured for bacteria.

3.3.2.1.2.2 Histopathology

Skin biopsies are frequently used to determine the cause of alopecia. Skin biopsy should be taken from the center of alopecia rather than the junctional zone of normal and alopecic skin. If there are plaques suggestive of calcinosis cutis, these should be biopsied as well. In canine hyperadrenocorticism, epidermis and the epithelium of the follicular infundibulum are frequently atrophic. Hair follicles are mostly in the telogen stage. Hair follicles in late stages of catagen are also frequently found. Sebaceous glands are often atrophic. Follicular hyperkeratosis is moderate to severe (Fig. 3.3.4). Comedones are frequently seen, but they are more common in dogs with iatrogenic hyperglucocorticoidism that often also present with marked calcinosis cutis. Phlebectasia (i.e., dilated and congested vessels in the superficial dermis) is a common finding in dogs that received topical corticosteroids (Gross 2005).

3.3.2.1.2.3 Laboratory tests

Dogs with hyperadrenocorticism have consistently higher levels of serum cortisol than normal patients. However, as the blood cortisol level fluctuates during the day, a single measurement of the serum cortisol level is inappropriate for diagnosing hyperadrenocorticism. Several endocrine tests have been developed that are discussed in more detail below. The urinary cortisol/creatinine ratio (UCCR), the low-dose dexamethasone suppression test (LDDST), and the ACTH stimulation test are the most commonly used screening tests for diagnosing canine hyperadrenocorticism. However, chronic stress from any disease process may result in adrenal hyperplasia and subsequent false-positive results in those screening assays. For this reason, hyperadrenocorticism should never be diagnosed on the basis of laboratory tests alone. The patient must also be exhibiting hallmark clinical signs of hyperadrenocorticism (see above). In dogs with nonadrenal illness, false-positive results are highest with the UCCR and lowest with the ACTH stimulation test. The most useful screening test for diagnosing canine hyperadrenocorticism is the LDDST. More detailed

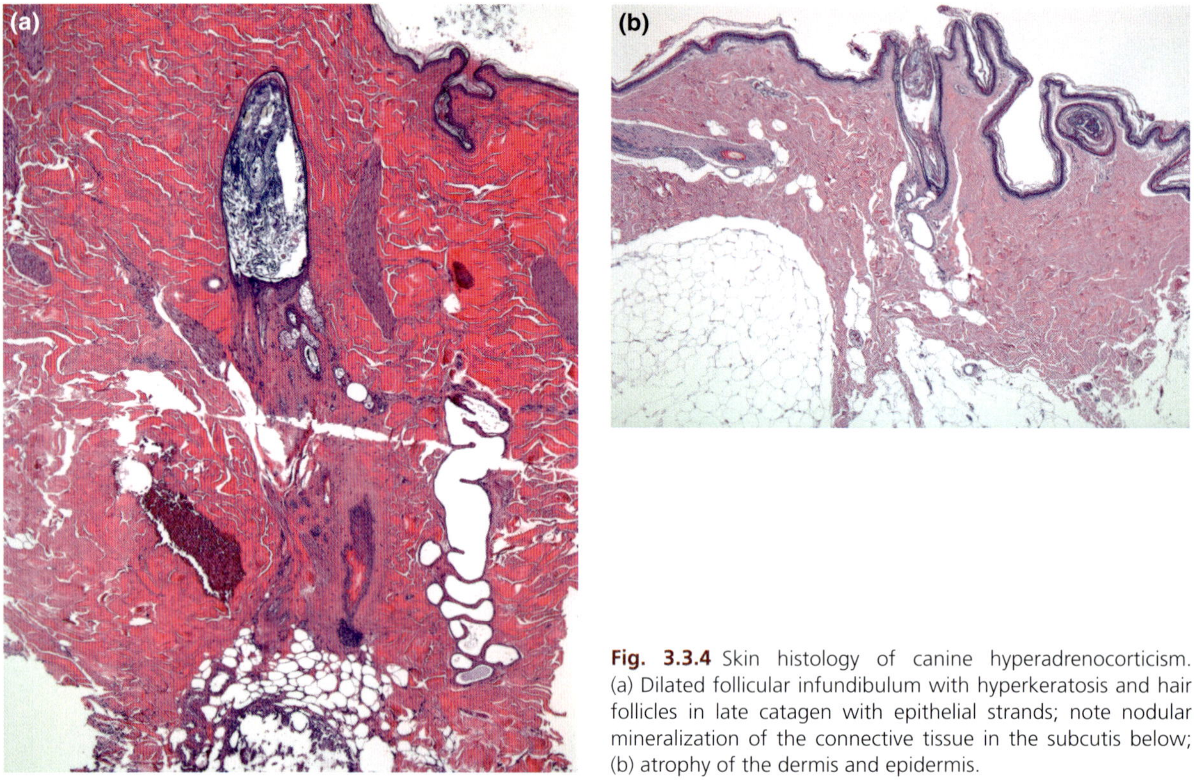

Fig. 3.3.4 Skin histology of canine hyperadrenocorticism. (a) Dilated follicular infundibulum with hyperkeratosis and hair follicles in late catagen with epithelial strands; note nodular mineralization of the connective tissue in the subcutis below; (b) atrophy of the dermis and epidermis.

information can be obtained from endocrinology textbooks (Rijnberk 1996; Feldman and Nelson 2004).

Differentiating between PDH and ADH can be difficult. The high-dose dexamethasone suppression test (HDDST) is more often used for differentiation. In addition, ultrasonography or other imaging techniques can be used by an experienced investigator.

Urinary cortisol/creatinine ratio

The consistently high serum cortisol concentration in dogs with hyperadrenocorticism results in a proportionately higher amount of cortisol in the urine. Therefore, the cortisol concentration in the urine can be used as a screening test for canine hyperadrenocorticism (Galac et al. 1997; Jensen et al. 1997). For exact quantification, cortisol levels are compared with creatinine levels in the urine. To minimize the impact of stress-induced endogenous cortisol production, a single urine sample should be collected in the morning by the dog owner at home. The UCCR test is very sensitive. Although original reports claim a 100% sensitivity, it is known that some patients with hyperadrenocorticism may show false-negative results with this test. Its specificity, however, is very poor, since many other chronic diseases or stress will cause abnormal results.

Urinary cortisol/creatinine ratio with dexamethasone suppression (oral LDDST)

A variant of the LDDST can be performed using oral dexamethasone administration (Vaessen et al. 2004). The oral LDDST requires a urine sample being taken for UCCR measurement. After the urine sample is collected, 0.01 mg/kg dexamethasone sodium phosphate is administered per os. Thereafter, two more urine samples are collected at 4 and 8 h after dexamethasone administration. The test is not used for the "routine" diagnosis of hyperadrenocorticism. It can be used to investigate the sensitivity to glucocorticoid feedback in cases in which the UCCR is not elevated, but the physical and biochemical changes still point to hyperadrenocorticism.

Low-dose dexamethasone suppression test

In normal dogs, administration of exogenous dexamethasone will cause a feedback inhibition of corticotropin-releasing hormone (CRH) and ACTH secretion, resulting in a suppression of endogenous levels of cortisol for 24 to 48 h. In dogs with hyperadrenocorticism, low levels of exogenous dexamethasone will not suppress cortisol levels, or will suppress them for a short time only. A blood sample for basal cortisol measurement is collected in the morning. Thereafter 0.01 mg/kg dexamethasone sodium phosphate is administered intravenously, and another blood sample for determination of cortisol levels is collected 4 and 8 h after dexamethasone administration. Normal dogs will exhibit suppressed post-dexamethasone cortisol levels. Animals with hyperadrenocorticism will not exhibit suppressed post-dexamethasone cortisol levels at the 8 h time point. Some dogs may have unusual test results (Mueller et al. 2006). The LDDST is more sensitive than the ACTH stimulation test, and will identify about 95% of dogs with hyperadrenocorticism. It is the most reliable screening test for this disease. Animals with chronic stress or severe nonadrenal disease, however, may have test results suggestive of hyperadrenocorticism and need diagnostic imaging techniques (see below) for further workup.

The LDDST can also be used to differentiate between PDH and ADH. PDH is likely, if cortisol levels are suppressed to less than 50% of the baseline level 4 h after dexamethasone administration, followed by high (equal to pre-suppression) cortisol levels 8 h after dexamethasone administration. If there is no suppression of cortisol levels at both 4 and 8 h, ADH can be suspected.

ACTH stimulation test

The ACTH stimulation test is very useful to confirm iatrogenic hyperadrenocorticism (see Section 3.3.2.2), but it is not the best test to detect and confirm spontaneous hyperadrenocorticism in dogs. The ACTH stimulation test determines the capacity of the adrenal cortex to secrete cortisol in response to ACTH. Dogs with both PDH and with ADH will show an exaggerated secretion of cortisol. Overnight fastening of the patient is recommended in order to avoid lipidemia. In the morning, a blood sample for measuring the baseline serum cortisol level is taken. Thereafter, synthetic ACTH is administered intravenously at a dose of 5 μg/kg (with a maximum dose of 250 μg). A poststimulation sample is collected 1 h later and cortisol levels are measured. About 85% of dogs with PDH and about 60% of dogs with ADH will show an increased cortisol level upon ACTH stimulation. Thus, a normal ACTH test does not rule out hyperadrenocorticism. Animals with chronic nonadrenal disease or severe stress may have falsely positive test results suggestive of hyperadrenocorticism.

17-Hydroxyprogesterone

Determination of serum 17-hydroxyprogesterone (17-OHP) levels (a precursor of cortisol) has newly been introduced into the diagnosis of canine hyperadrenocorticism (Norman et al. 1999; Chapman et al. 2003; Behrend et al. 2005). It is used in patients that have clinical signs of hyperadrenocorticism, but negative results with the LDDST and the ACTH stimulation test. In rare cases, 17-OHP is produced excessively and results in clinical signs of hyperadrenocorticism (also termed "atypical hyperadrenocorticism"). 17-OHP is measured in serum samples that are taken while performing an ACTH stimulation test (see above). Exaggerated levels of 17-OHP following ACTH administration are diagnostic for hyperadrenocorticism.

High-dose dexamethasone suppression test

As discussed above, dogs with PDH will show a temporary suppression of cortisol in the LDDST 4 h after dexamethasone administration, but cortisol levels will rise again at 8 h. Administering a higher dose of dexamethasone will overcome this resistance to the negative feedback mechanism. Therefore, a HDDST can be used to differentiate between PDH and ADH. As in the LDDST, 0.1 mg/kg dexamethasone sodium phosphate is used instead of 0.01 mg/kg, otherwise the test protocol is identical. Dogs with ADH will not show a suppression of cortisol levels, whereas most dogs with PDH (approximately 75%) will exhibit a greater than 50% suppression of post-dexamethasone cortisol levels at both 4 and 8 h.

ACTH

About 25% of dogs with PDH will still not show a marked suppression of cortisol levels after HDDST (see above). In these dogs, determination of the endogenous ACTH concentration can differentiate between PDH and ADH. Therefore, only the endogenous ACTH levels are measured, once a diagnosis of hyperadrenocorticism has been made. Dogs with PDH will have abnormally high levels of ACTH, whereas dogs with ADH will have abnormally low ACTH levels.

Samples for measuring ACTH levels should be taken in the morning (ideally after the dog has been hospitalized overnight to minimize stress). Sample handling requires special care, and instructions from the diagnostic laboratory should be followed carefully.

Imaging techniques

Abdominal radiographs may reveal hepatomegaly, dystrophic calcification (in kidneys, large vessels, and 50% of adrenal tumors), or an adrenal tumor (if large enough). Thoracic radiographs may reveal ectopic calcification and evidence of metastatic neoplasia.

Abdominal sonography is a reliable method to diagnose ADH, if performed by an experienced operator. Chronic stress, however, may result in findings similar to that of PDH hyperadrenocorticism. Adrenal glands should be symmetric and enlarged. Differentiation between focal nodular hyperplasia and a neoplasm can be challenging.

Computed tomography (CT) is helpful in the diagnosis of adrenal and pituitary tumors (Kooistra et al. 1997). However, it requires general anesthesia and an experienced interpreter. CT is not as sensitive as magnetic resonance imaging (MRI, see below), but is adequate for detection of pituitary masses that are larger than 8 mm in diameter.

MRI provides a superior soft-tissue contrast compared to CT. It is therefore more accurate for visualization of small pituitary tumors.

Similar to measuring endogenous ACTH levels, abdominal imaging techniques are not used to diagnose hyperadrenocorticism but rather to differentiate between PDH and ADH, once a screening test has confirmed hyperadrenocorticism.

3.3.2.1.3 Therapy

Before treating any dog with hyperadrenocorticism, it is worthwhile having a detailed discussion with the owner about the costs, benefits, and potential complications of the available therapies.

Routine ACTH stimulation tests should be carried out to evaluate the adrenal reserve and adjusting the therapy. CBC and biochemistry screenings including electrolytes should also be done to evaluate the response to the therapy, and to check for changes that may suggest the occurrence of hypoadrenocorticism. Survival time may vary from patient to patient depending on the type of tumor and the drug used (Barker et al. 2005).

Medical options for canine hyperadrenocorticism include mitotane, trilostane, and retinoic acid; other drugs (ketoconazole, L-deprenyl, aminoglutethimide) have also been suggested but are less effective (Reusch et al. 1999). Homeopathy has also been reported to be useful in 67% of the treated cases (Elliott 2001). Among the above-mentioned drugs, mitotane has most extensively been used in the treatment of canine hyperadrenocorticism. Trilostane has gained increased popularity among veterinarians during the last few years (Reine 2007), and the use of retinoic acid (isotretinoin) is a rather new but interesting option.

In dogs well controlled with medical therapy, the clinical signs resolve within a few weeks. Hair regrowth will occur within 4–8 weeks. Calcinosis cutis may take a few months to resolve. ACTH stimulation tests should be carried out repeatedly to monitor adrenal function. Biochemistry screens including electrolytes should also be performed to check for any evidence of hypoadrenocorticism.

3.3.2.1.3.1 Mitotane

Mitotane (*o,p*′-dichlorodiphenyldichloroethane) causes severe progressive necrosis of the adrenocortical zona fasciculata and reticularis, but usually spares the zona glomerulosa (Kintzer and Peterson 1991). The treatment needs to be monitored carefully, as prolonged treatment will cause Addison's disease. Appetite and water intake are excellent parameters to monitor therapeutic efficacy of mitotane. Thus, before initiating therapy, appetite and water intake should be carefully evaluated by the owner. Most of the dogs with hyperadrenocorticism are ravenous. Any appetite change during the loading dose period is important. As dogs reach the end of the loading dose phase, their appetite changes from ravenous to normal. If the loading dose goes beyond this point, the appetite changes from normal to poor or absent. Mitotane should be administered with a meal (preferably fatty), because this assures better absorption. The daily mitotane dose can be split to twice a day. Similar to the appetite, the patient's water intake will normalize under mitotane treatment.

Mitotane treatment should be split into a loading phase and a maintenance phase. Every dog is different, and it will depend on several factors (reduced appetite and water consumption, lethargy, duration, and dose of mitotane given) to determine when the end of the loading dose phase is reached. It is recommended to begin the dosage of mitotane on a Sunday so that the owner can maintain contact with the veterinarian during the entire week. Mitotane can be started at 25–50 mg/kg twice daily. Prednisone (5 mg/kg) should be available to mitigate any adverse effects that may occur during treatment. The owner should stop mitotane and call the veterinarian immediately, if any of the following signs are noted: lethargy, reduction in appetite, reduction in water intake (tell the owner what the average normal water intake should be), vomiting, or diarrhea. If one of the above signs is present, an ACTH stimulation test should be conducted, otherwise it will be performed on the 8th day of treatment. The test should show adequate suppression of the adrenal function. Most dogs will respond during the first 9 days of mitotane therapy, but some will not. If the ACTH stimulation test reveals high basal and/or post-ACTH cortisol concentrations, the loading dose phase is continued. In this case, another ACTH stimulation test is performed after 7 days. All dogs should have responded by then, and the maintenance dose phase is started.

The dosage of mitotane during maintenance depends on the response to the loading dose phase and the cortisol levels measured in the ACTH stimulation test. The maintenance dose of mitotane (25–50 mg/kg) will be given once or twice a week, divided into a morning and evening dose. Prednisone should be always available for any emergencies. ACTH stimulation tests will be performed after 1 month and after 3 months of maintenance treatment. Whenever the mitotane dose is adapted, an ACTH stimulation test should be performed after 1 month. Every dog's maintenance dose requirement will change over time. Therefore, regular clinical rechecks and ACTH stimulation tests need to be performed every 3–6 months.

In PDH patients that are poorly controlled with mitotane, therapy can be switched to trilostane. It is recommended to follow the guidelines for monitoring trilostane therapy as mentioned below. However, since mitotane destroys most of the adrenal cortex, it is recommended to perform an ACTH stimulation test before switching therapy.

3.3.2.1.3.2 Trilostane

Trilostane is a synthetic, orally administered, active steroid analogue that competitively inhibits 3β-hydroxysteroid dehydrogenase and hence reduces synthesis of several steroids, including cortisol and aldosterone (Fig. 3.3.11). This competitive inhibition is reversible and seems to be dose related. In many European countries, trilostane is the only drug that is approved for the treatment of canine hyperadrenocorticism.

It is recommended that trilostane be administered with food to enhance absorption. The currently suggested starting dose for dogs with hyperadrenocorticism is 3–5 mg/kg twice daily. The dose is adjusted according to clinical signs and serum cortisol values (Neiger et al. 2002; Ruckstuhl et al. 2002; Braddock et al. 2003; Alenza et al. 2006). Side effects are uncommon. A few days after starting therapy, some patients may show mild lethargy, decreased appetite (potentially due to corticosteroid withdrawal), and mild electrolyte changes. In one study of 78 dogs with confirmed PDH, 2 dogs developed signs and biochemical evidence of hypoadrenocorticism (Addison's disease); with appropriate treatment, one dog recovered and the other died. In a single case report, a dog receiving trilostane developed signs of hypoadrenocorticism, and histopathological evaluation of adrenal glands showed adrenal cortical necrosis with reactive inflammation and fibrosis (Chapman et al. 2004). Trilostane should not be used in pregnant animals, since it terminates pregnancy in monkeys. Trilostane appears to be safe with long-term (up to 3 years) daily administration.

Most dogs show resolution of polydipsia, polyuria, and polyphagia within 4 weeks of starting therapy. The skin problems resolve within 3 months of treatment in 62% of the dogs. Many biochemical changes, including elevated ALP and ALT activities, may resolve with treatment. The adrenal glands of dogs with PDH on this therapy may increase in size due to the continuous production of ACTH by the pituitary neoplasm (Mantis et al. 2003; Reusch et al. 2007).

It is currently recommended to perform an ACTH stimulation test after 10, 30, and 90 days of treatment and every 4–6 months thereafter. The ACTH stimulation test needs to be conducted between 4 and 6 h after trilostane administration. If the post-ACTH cortisol concentration is less than 20 nmol/L (0.7 μg/dL), trilostane is stopped for 48 h and then re-introduced at a lower dose. If the post-ACTH cortisol concentration is larger than 120 nmol/L (4.3 μg/dL), the trilostane dose is increased. If the post-ACTH cortisol concentration is between 20 and 120 nmol/L, and if the patients clinical signs have resolved, the trilostane dose is not altered. However, if clinical signs persist despite post-ACTH cortisol concentration in the range of 20 and 120 nmol/L, the trilostane dose should be adjusted.

Some patients may not respond adequately to trilostane therapy or the drug may cause side effects. In these cases, therapy can be switched from trilostane to mitotane. Experience with switching therapies is limited. Cortisol values are expected to rise within less than 24 h if trilostane treatment is stopped, and the patient may start to show signs of hyperadrenocorticism within a few days. An ACTH stimulation test is recommended before mitotane is started. Mitotane should only be started if post-ACTH cortisol concentrations are compatible with hyperadrenocorticism.

3.3.2.1.3.3 Retinoic acid

Retinoic acid has been shown to decrease corticotropin secretion in rodent models. Thus, it has recently been introduced into the therapy of canine hyperadrenocorticism. One study investigated the efficacy of isotretinoin (2 mg/kg) in PDH. Isotretinoin was administered daily per os. Clinical signs, plasma ACTH levels, and UCCR improved upon treatment, while the size of pituitary adenomas decreased. No adverse events or signs of hepatotoxicity were observed, but further studies are needed to elucidate the use of isotretinoin in the therapy of canine hyperadrenocorticism (Castillo et al. 2006).

3.3.2.1.3.4 Surgical therapy

Transsphenoidal hypophysectomy has been described for the treatment of pituitary tumors in dogs with PDH. However, this surgical technique requires an experienced surgeon and suitable facilities. The success rate is acceptable, but serious complications may occur (Hanson et al. 2007).

Unilateral adrenalectomy is indicated in canine ADH, but owner counseling is important, since this form of hyperadrenocorticism could be managed medically. The extent of any local invasion or metastatic spread should be investigated before surgery is performed. Animals with untreated ADH represent difficult surgical candidates because of the increased anesthetic risk (due to poor respiratory and hepatic function), hypercoagulability (leading to an increased risk of pulmonary thromboembolism), and poor vascular tone (leading to poor hemostasis). Furthermore, many adrenal tumors are quite friable and hemorrhagic. Primary wound healing is delayed, but wound breakdown is very rare. Acute postoperative hypoadrenocorticism due to preexisting contralateral adrenal atrophy is common. Therefore, postoperative intensive care facilities are mandatory. Even with experienced surgeons and appropriately equipped facilities, perioperative mortality rates can be as high as 30%. Medical treatment (trilostane) before sending dogs to surgery is mandatory to reduce such risks, although this has not been studied thoroughly yet. Previous mitotane therapy may be disadvantageous as tumors may become more friable. Adrenalectomy is best performed via a ventral midline laparotomy. The contralateral adrenal gland should be assessed for bilateral disease, and other abdominal organs should be checked for metastases. The renal vessels and caudal vena cava should be carefully examined for the presence of neoplasms. If there is local invasion, debulking surgery is still worthwhile, providing this can be accomplished safely. If not, a small biopsy should be taken for histopathological examination.

3.3.2.2 Canine iatrogenic corticosteroid-induced alopecia

Glucocorticoid hormones are potent inhibitors of keratinocyte proliferation and effective anti-inflammatory drugs, which have been widely used for the treatment of inflammatory skin disorders such as atopic dermatitis. However, their chronic use is accompanied by adverse effects. The most prominent side effects of glucocorticoid therapy are alopecia and skin atrophy that affects different skin components and compromises the barrier function of the skin. The skin atrophy is characterized by a reduction in epidermal thickness, a decreased number of keratinocytes, diminished intercellular lipids in the stratum corneum, loss of extracellular matrix, altered orientation and packing of collagen and elastic fibers combined with a decreased cellularity in the dermis, atrophy of the subcutaneous fat, and a decreased number of dermal mast cells.

The frequency of iatrogenic alopecia may be more common among colleagues who use and abuse corticosteroids than among veterinary specialists. Alopecia may be multifocal to generalized after corticosteroids have been given systemically, or focally at the administration site if given topically. Some dogs may be more sensitive than others.

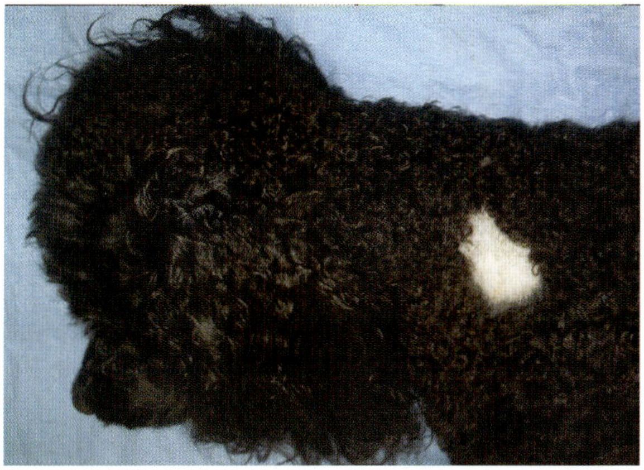

Fig. 3.3.5 Corticosteroid-induced alopecia in a Miniature Poodle following injection of a long-acting corticosteroid. (Courtesy of L. Beco.)

The changes at the skin level after topical application of corticosteroids or following a subcutaneous injection are similar to those seen with naturally occurring hyperglucocorticoidism. They occur 2–4 months after the application. There may be fragile and thin skin with alopecia and presence of comedones (Fig. 3.3.5).

The ACTH stimulation test is the only assay that identifies this condition reliably. The histological changes occurring in affected dogs are similar to those with the spontaneous disease.

Treatment other than discontinuation of steroid administration is not required. Hairs may take months to a year to regrow, and hairs may be lighter or darker than normal when regrown. Surgical excision is an option for dogs with permanent focal alopecia. If calcinosis cutis has developed, it will resolve within a few months depending on the severity of this condition. Treatment with DMSO gel may hasten the resolution of the lesions.

3.3.2.3 Feline hyperadrenocorticism

Feline hyperadrenocorticism or "feline Cushing's syndrome" is a disorder most often caused by a pituitary adenoma with excess adrenal cortisol secretion (Nelson et al. 1988; Watson and Herrtage 1998; Boord and Griffin 1999; Rossmeisl et al. 2000). Functioning benign adenomas or malignant adrenal carcinomas have also been reported in cats (Watson and Herrtage 1998). Iatrogenic hyperadrenocorticism is common in cats following prolonged glucocorticoid administration to control the clinical signs of allergy (Schaer and Ginn 1999; Ferasin 2001).

3.3.2.3.1 Diagnosis

3.3.2.3.1.1 Clinical presentation

Pituitary-dependent hyperadrenocorticism (PDH) is usually a disease of the middle-aged to older cat in the range of 5–16 years (with a median age of 10 years). No breed predilection has been found. There is a slight difference in sex distribution in feline hyperadrenocorticism; female cats are slightly more (60%) likely to develop the disease than males (Nelson et al. 1988).

In 80% of cases, feline hyperadrenocorticism is accompanied by diabetes mellitus (Nichols 1997). The most common clinical signs associated with hyperadrenocorticism in cats are insulin-resistance, polydypsia, polyuria, polyphagia, lethargy, abdominal enlargement, panting, obesity, muscle weakness, and recurrent upper respiratory and urinary tract infections. Lethargy (dullness) has been reported due to muscle weakness or due to a pituitary mass. Dermatological clinical signs are cutaneous atrophy and alopecia (Fig. 3.3.6).

Differential diagnoses include diabetes mellitus, acromegaly, liver or renal diseases, sex hormone-secreting adrenal tumors, pancreatic paraneoplastic alopecia, and hyperthyroidism.

Serum alkaline phosphatase is usually elevated, not because of the hypercortisolemia but rather as a result of the poorly regulated concomitant diabetes mellitus. This occurs because cats lack the glucocorticoid-induced isoenzyme for alkaline phosphatase.

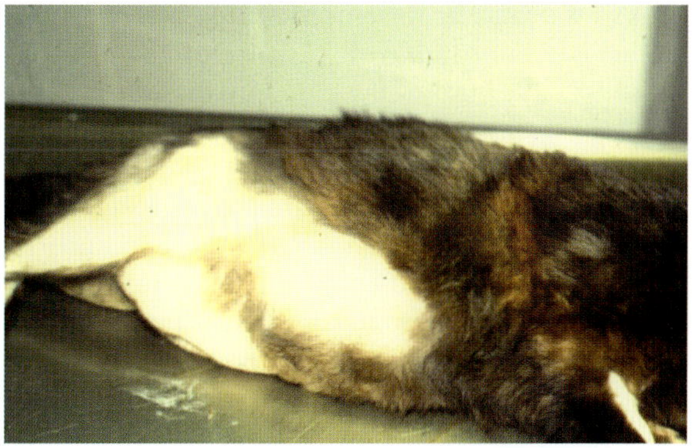

Fig. 3.3.6 Feline hyperadrenocorticism. Note extensive alopecia on the abdomen and proximal hindlegs. (Courtesy of M. Linek.)

High serum alanine amino, transferase activity, hypercholesterolemia, hyperglycemia, and low blood urea nitrogen are also common findings. The hemogram may reveal a mild erythrocytosis as well as a classical stress leukogram.

Cats often show increased urine specific gravity (>1,030) despite profound polydipsia and polyuria resulting from the concurrent diabetes mellitus. Many cats with hyperadrenocorticism have evidence of urinary tract infection.

3.3.2.3.1.2 Laboratory tests

Adequate screening tests for feline hyperadrenocorticism are UCCR, LDDT test, and ACTH stimulation test. The HDDT test, the plasma ACTH concentration, and imaging techniques can be used to differentiate between PDH and ADH.

Urinary cortisol/creatinine ratio

The UCCR is a simple and valuable screening test for hyperadrenocorticism in cats (Goossens et al. 1995). To perform this test, the owner is instructed to collect urine at home. To reduce stress, morning urine samples are collected from an empty litter box at the same time of day on two to three consecutive days. A mean value should be calculated from the two to three samples. A high mean UCCR is found in most cats with hyperadrenocorticism. To rule out a false-positive result in cats with nonadrenal illness, LDDST should be performed.

Low-dose dexamethasone suppression test

The LDDST is considered to be the test of choice for the diagnosis of hyperadrenocorticism in cats. It requires 10 times the dose used in dogs (0.1 mg/kg). Plasma is obtained for cortisol concentrations before, 4 and 8 h after intravenous dexamethasone administration. If this dose of dexamethasone (0.1 mg/kg) fails to adequately suppress circulating cortisol concentrations in a cat with compatible clinical signs, this is consistent with a diagnosis of hyperadrenocorticism. Normal cats and cats with nonadrenal illness will show adequate suppression of serum or plasma cortisol at 4 and 8 h post dexamethasone administration. However, in contrast to dogs with PDH, many cats with PDH will not suppress at 4 h and a few cats will suppress at 8 h after dexamethasone administration.

ACTH stimulation test

Similar to dogs, the ACTH stimulation test is mainly a test to evaluate the adrenal reserve capacity to produce cortisol. It can be used to verify iatrogenic hyperadrenocorticism. Only 50–60% of cats with hyperadrenocorticism will show an exaggerated response to ACTH administration. The preferred method for ACTH stimulation testing in cats is to determine serum cortisol concentrations 30 min before and 1 h after the intravenous or intramuscular injection of synthetic ACTH (0.125 mg/cat). Excess progesterone levels after ACTH stimulation have also been reported in cats with hyperadrenocorticism (Watson and Herrtage 1998; Boord and Griffin 1999).

High-dose dexamethasone suppression test

The HDDST is performed by administering a high dose of dexamethasone (1 mg/kg) in a protocol identical to the LDDST.

Plasma ACTH

Endogenous ACTH concentrations are normal to high in cats with PDH, whereas ACTH concentrations are usually low or undetectable in cats with adrenal tumors or with iatrogenic hyperadrenocorticism. As with dogs, samples must be collected in EDTA tubes and centrifuged immediately. The plasma is then stored in a plastic container (ACTH will stick to glass) and is immediately frozen until the assay is performed.

Imaging techniques

Ultrasonography can be used to detect PDH and ADH hyperadrenocorticism (Widmer and Guptill 1995). Symmetric adrenal glands of normal or enlarged size are suggestive of PDH, whereas unilateral enlargement supports ADH. With abdominal ultrasonography, small or noncalcified unilateral adrenal tumors can usually be detected, whereas bilateral adrenal enlargement can be visualized in cats with PDH. The contralateral adrenal gland would be expected to be small in cats with a unilateral cortisol-secreting tumor due to the fact that pituitary ACTH secretion has been chronically suppressed.

CT and MRI are reliable methods to image either the adrenals or the pituitary glands (Mauldin and Burk 1990). Similar to dogs, bilateral adrenal enlargement can be differentiated from a unilateral adrenal tumor in most cats. CT or MRI are the most helpful in the diagnosis of pituitary tumors. MRI provides superior soft-tissue contrast compared to CT, and is also more accurate for visualization of small pituitary tumors.

3.3.2.3.2 Therapy

Medical therapy has been successful in some cats with hyperadrenocorticism. Mitotane has been extensively used in the past (Schwedes 1997), but trilostane seems to be an effective adrenal steroid inhibitor in cats that is associated with minimal side effects (Skelly et al. 2003; Boag et al. 2004; Neiger et al. 2004). Trilostane is administered at a dose of 30–60 mg/cat/day. Trilostane therapy is monitored with routine ACTH stimulation tests to obtain adequate adrenal suppression.

Surgical treatment of feline hyperadrenocorticism consists of unilateral or, more commonly, bilateral adrenalectomy (Duesberg et al. 1995). The reader is referred to surgical texts for an explanation of the surgical procedure; however, medical management of the cat during the operative and postoperative period is essential for a good outcome. Before adrenalectomy, the cat should be treated with trilostane until the skin lesions of hyperadrenocorticism have resolved and diabetes mellitus, if present, is reasonably well controlled. Supplementation with glucocorticoid (10–20 mg methylprednisolone acetate) and mineralocorticoid (deoxycorticosterone acetate, 12.5 mg given intramuscularly) should be initiated immediately before bilateral adrenalectomy and monthly thereafter for the rest of the cat's life. Transsphenoidal hypophysectomy for the treatment of feline PDH is a viable alternative to adrenalectomy; however, this procedure is only performed by a few surgeons (Meij et al. 2001).

References

Alenza DP, Arenas C, Lopez ML, Melian C. 2006. Long-term efficacy of trilostane administered twice daily in dogs with pituitary-dependent hyperadrenocorticism. *Journal of American Animal Hospital Association* 42(4):269–276.

Barker EN, Campbell S, Tebb AJ, Neiger R, Herrtage ME, Reid SW, Ramsey IK. 2005. A comparison of the survival times of dogs treated with mitotane or trilostane for pituitary-dependent hyperadrenocorticism. *Journal of Veterinary Internal Medicine* 19(6):810–815.

Beato M, Herrlich P, Schultz G. 1995. Steroid hormone receptors: many actors in search of a plot. *Cell* 83:851–857.

Behrend EN, Kemppainen RJ, Boozer AL, Whitley EM, Smith AN, Busch KA. 2005. Serum 17-alpha-hydroxyprogesterone and corticosterone concentrations in dogs with nonadrenal neoplasia and dogs with suspected hyperadrenocorticism. *Journal of the American Veterinary Medical Association* 227(11):1762–1767.

Boag AK, Neiger R, Church DB. 2004. Trilostane treatment of bilateral adrenal enlargement and excessive sex steroid hormone production in a cat. *Journal of Small Animal Practice* 45(5):263–266.

Boord M, Griffin C. 1999. Progesterone secreting adrenal mass in a cat with clinical signs of hyperadrenocorticism. *Journal of American Veterinary Medical Association* 214(5):666–669.

Braddock JA, Church DB, Robertson ID, Watson AD. 2003. Trilostane treatment in dogs with pituitary-dependent hyperadrenocorticism. *Australian Veterinary Journal* 81:600–607.

Castillo V, Giacomini D, Páez-Pereda M, Stalla J, Labeur M, Theodoropoulou M, Holsboer F, Grossman AB, Stalla GK, Arzt E. 2006. Retinoic acid as a novel medical therapy for Cushing's disease in dogs. *Endocrinology* 147(9):4438–4444.

Chapman PS, Kelly DF, Archer J, Brockman DJ, Neiger R. 2004. Adrenal necrosis in a dog receiving trilostane for the treatment of hyperadrenocorticism. *Journal of Small Animal Practice* 45:307–310.

Chapman PS, Mooney CT, Ede J, Evans H, O'Connor J, Pfeiffer DU, Neiger R. 2003. Evaluation of the basal and post-adrenocorticotrophic hormone serum concentrations of 17-hydroxyprogesterone for the diagnosis of hyperadrenocorticism in dogs. *Veterinary Record* 153(25):771–775.

Duesberg CA, Nelson RW, Feldman EC, Vaden SL, Scott-Moncrieff CR. 1995. Adrenalectomy for treatment of hyperadrenocorticism in cats: 10 cases (1988–1992). *Journal of American Veterinary Medical Association* 207(8):1066–1070.

Elliott M. 2001. Cushing's disease: a new approach to therapy in equine and canine patients. *British Homeopathic Journal* 90:33–36.

Feldman EC, Nelson RW. 2004. *Canine and Feline Endocrinology and Reproduction*, 3rd edn. St. Louis: WB Saunders.

Ferasin L. 2001. Iatrogenic hyperadrenocorticism in a cat following a short therapeutic course of methylprednisolone acetate. *Journal of Feline Medicine and Surgery* 3(2):87–93.

Galac S, Kars VJ, Voorhout G, Mol JA, Kooistra HS. 2007. ACTH-independent hyperadrenocorticism due to food-dependent hypercortisolemia in a dog: a case report. *Veterinary Journal* 177: 141–143.

Galac S, Kooistra HS, Teske E, Rijnberk A. 1997. Urinary corticoid/creatinine ratios in the differentiation between pituitary-dependent hyperadrenocorticism and hyperadrenocorticism due to adrenocortical tumour in the dog. *Veterinary Quarterly* 19(1):17–20.

Galac S, Kooistra HS, Voorhout G, van den Ingh TS, Mol JA, van den Berg G, Meij BP. 2005. Hyperadrenocorticism in a dog due to ectopic secretion of adrenocorticotropic hormone. *Domestic Animal Endocrinology* 28:338–348.

Goossens MM, Meyer HP, Voorhout G, Sprang EP. 1995. Urinary excretion of glucocorticoids in the diagnosis of hyperadrenocorticism in cats. *Domestic Animal Endocrinology* 12(4):355–362.

Gross TL. 2005. Atrophic diseases of the adnexa. In: Gross TL, Ihrke PJ, Walder EJ, Affolter VK (eds), *Skin Diseases of the Dog and Cat: Clinical and Histopathologic Diagnosis*, 2nd edn, pp. 480–517. Oxford: Blackwell Science.

Hanson JM, Teske E, Voorhout G, Galac S, Kooistra HS, Meij BP. 2007. Prognostic factors for outcome after transsphenoidal hypophysectomy in dogs with pituitary-dependent hyperadrenocorticism. *Journal Neurosurgery* 107(4):830–840.

Ito N, Ito T, Kromminga A, Bettermann A, Takigawa M, Kees F, Straub RH, Paus R. 2005. Human hair follicles display a functional equivalent of the hypothalamic–pituitary–adrenal axis and synthesize cortisol. *FASEB Journal* 19(10):1332–1334.

Jensen AL, Iversen L, Koch J, Hoier R, Petersen TK. 1997. Evaluation of the urinary cortisol: creatinine ratio in the diagnosis of

hyperadrenocorticism in dogs. *Journal of Small Animal Practice* 38(3):99–102.
Kintzer PP, Peterson ME. 1991. Mitotane (o,p′-DDD) treatment of 200 dogs with pituitary-dependent hyperadrenocorticism. *Journal of Veterinary Internal Medicine* 5:182–190.
Kooistra HS, Voorhout G, Mol JA, Rijnberk A. 1997. Correlation between impairment of glucocorticoid feedback and the size of the pituitary gland in dogs with pituitary-dependent hyperadrenocorticism. *Journal of Endocrinology* 152(3):387–394.
Mantis P, Lamb CR, Witt AL, Neiger R. 2003. Changes in ultrasonographic appearance of adrenal glands in dogs with pituitary-dependent hyperadrenocorticism treated with trilostane. *Veterinary Radiology and Ultrasound* 44:682–685.
Mauldin GN, Burk RL. 1990. The use of diagnostic computerized tomography and radiation therapy in canine and feline hyperadrenocorticism. *Problems in Veterinary Medicine* 2(4):557–564.
Meij BP, Voorhout G, Van Den Ingh TS, Rijnberk A. 2001. Transsphenoidal hypophysectomy for treatment of pituitary-dependent hyperadrenocorticism in 7 cats. *Veterinary Surgery* 30(1):72–86.
Mueller C, Sieber-Ruckstuhl N, Wenger M, Kaser-Hotz B, Reusch CE. 2006. Low-dose dexamethasone test with "inverse" results: a possible new pattern of cortisol response. *Veterinary Record* 159(15):489–491.
Neiger R, Ramsey I, O'Connor J, Hurley KJ, Mooney CT. 2002. Trilostane treatment of 78 dogs with pituitary dependent hyperadrenocorticism. *Veterinary Record* 150:799–804.
Neiger R, Witt AL, Noble A, German AJ. 2004. Trilostane therapy for treatment of pituitary-dependent hyperadrenocorticism in 5 cats. *Journal of Veterinary Internal Medicine* 18(2):160–164.
Nelson RW, Feldman EC, Smith MC. 1988. Hyperadrenocorticism in cats: seven cases (1978–1987). *Journal of American Veterinary Medical Association* 193(2):245–250.
Nichols R. 1997. Complications and concurrent disease associated with diabetes mellitus. *Seminar in Veterinary Medicine and Surgery (Small Animals)* 12(4):263–267.
Norman EJ, Thompson H, Mooney CT. 1999. Dynamic adrenal function testing in eight dogs with hyperadrenocorticism associated with adrenocortical neoplasia. *Veterinary Record* 144:551–554.
Okada T, Ishii Y, Masujin K, Yasoshima A, Matsuda J, Ogura A, Nakayama H, Kunieda T, Doi K. 2006. The critical roles of serum/glucocorticoid-regulated kinase 3 (SGK3) in the hair follicle morphogenesis and homeostasis: the allelic difference provides novel insights into hair follicle biology. *American Journal of Pathology* 168(4):1119–1133.
Paus R, Handjiski B, Czarnetzki BM, Eichmüller S. 1994. A murine model for inducing and manipulating hair follicle regression (catagen): effects of dexamethasone and cyclosporin A. *Journal of Investigative Dermatology* 103(2):143–147.
Reine NJ. 2007. Medical management of pituitary-dependent hyperadrenocorticism: mitotane versus trilostane. *Clinical Technique in Small Animal Practice* 22(1):18–25.
Reusch CE, Sieber-Ruckstuhl N, Wenger M, Lutz H, Perren A, Pospischil A. 2007. Histological evaluation of the adrenal glands of seven dogs with hyperadrenocorticism treated with trilostane. *Veterinary Record* 160(7):219–224.
Reusch CE, Steffen T, Hoerauf A. 1999. The efficacy of L-Deprenyl in dogs with pituitary-dependent hyperadrenocorticism. *Journal of Veterinary Internal Medicine* 13:291–301.
Rijnberk A. 1996. Adrenals. In: Rijnberk A (ed.), *Clinical Endocrinology of Dogs and Cats*, pp. 61–88. Netherlands: Kluwer Academic Publishers.
Rossmeisl JH Jr, Scott-Moncrieff JC, Siems J, Snyder PW, Wells A, Anothayanontha L, Oliver JW. 2000. Hyperadrenocorticism and hyperprogesteronemia in a cat with an adrenocortical adenocarcinoma. *Journal of the American Animal Hospital Association* 36(6):512–517.
Ruckstuhl NS, Nett CS, Reusch CE. 2002. Results of clinical examinations, laboratory tests, and ultrasonography in dogs with pituitary-dependent hyperadrenocorticism treated with trilostane. *American Journal of Veterinary Research* 63:506–512.
Schaer M, Ginn PE. 1999. Iatrogenic Cushing's syndrome and steroid hepatopathy in a cat. *Journal of the American Animal Hospital Association* 35(1):48–51.
Schwedes CS. 1997. Mitotane (o,p′-DDD) treatment in a cat with hyperadrenocorticism. *Journal of Small Animal Practice* 38(11):520–524.
Skelly BJ, Petrus D, Nicholls PK. 2003. Use of trilostane for the treatment of pituitary-dependent hyperadrenocorticism in a cat. *Journal of Small Animal Practice* 44(6):269–272.
Stenn KS, Paus R, Dutton T, Sarba B. 1993. Glucocorticoid effect on hair growth initiation: a reconsideration. *Skin Pharmacology* 6:125–134.
Thornton MJ, Nelson LD, Taylor AH, Birch MP, Laing I, Messenger AG. 2006. The modulation of aromatase and estrogen receptor alpha in cultured human dermal papilla cells by dexamethasone: a novel mechanism for selective action of estrogen via estrogen receptor beta? *Journal of Investigative Dermatology* 126(9):2010–2018.
Vaessen MM, Kooistra HS, Mol JA, Rijnberk A. 2004. Urinary corticoid: creatinine ratios in healthy pet dogs after oral low-dose dexamethasone suppression tests. *Veterinary Record* 55:518–521.
Watson PJ, Herrtage ME. 1998. Hyperadrenocorticism in six cats. *Journal of Small Animal Practice* 39(4):175–184.
Widmer WR, Guptill L. 1995. Imaging techniques for facilitating diagnosis of hyperadrenocorticism in dogs and cats. *Journal of American Veterinary Medical Association* 206(12):1857–1864.
Wood FD, Pollard RE, Uerling MR, Feldman EC. 2007. Diagnostic imaging findings and endocrine test results in dogs with pituitary-dependent hyperadrenocorticism that did or did not have neurologic abnormalities: 157 cases (1989–2005). *Journal of the American Veterinary Medical Association* 231(7):1081–1085.

3.3.3 Canine hyperestrogenism

Lars Mecklenburg

Estrogens are potent modulators of hair growth. It is long known that injections of large doses of estradiol reduce hair growth in mice, rats, guinea pigs, and dogs (Hooker and Pfeiffer 1943; Trentin et al. 1952; Johnson 1958; Jackson and Ebling 1972). Independent of the gender, estrogens can delay initiation of anagen and thus are able to arrest hair follicles in the telogen phase (Oh and Smart 1996; Smart et al. 1999). Furthermore, estrogens can reduce the growth rate of anagen hair fibers, thus reducing the actual lengths of hair fibers (reviewed in Ohnemus et al. 2006). There is also evidence from experiments in mice that estrogens are able to terminate anagen and thus induce hair follicle regression (Ohnemus et al. 2004, 2005). This is supported by morphologic evidence from dogs experimentally treated with high doses of estradiol that also suggest a catagen-inductive (anagen terminating) activity of estrogens (Dow 1960; Jabara 1962).

Experimental studies in dogs that were treated with synthetic estrogens have clearly elucidated the estrogenic effects on the canine hair coat. Daily intramuscular injections of 1 mg stilbestrol dipropionate to young adult male and female Collies resulted in a dry hair coat, with thinning of the hair coat over the abdomen, at the inner thighs, and in the perianal region (Dow 1960). Alopecia was evident after 100 days of treatment and further progressed to involve the entire ventral trunk after 200 days of treatment. If continued, alopecia further progresses and will only spare head and distal extremities. Similar changes were found in male and female dogs receiving subcutaneous depot injections of diethylstilbestrol at intervals of 4–6 weeks (Jabara 1962). They developed alopecia after 11 months of treatment, affecting all areas of the trunk, sparing the head and distal parts of extremities. Hair regrew 3–7 months after discontinuation of estrogen application.

Interestingly, hyperestrogenism as a cause of alopecia is only known in the dog. Although ovarian follicular cysts and hyperestrogenism are frequently observed in the cat, alopecia has not been described in association with this condition. Hyperestrogenism is rare in other species including those that may ingest phytoestrogens, and alopecia is not a consistent phenomenon in these cases. This demonstrates once more the different susceptibility among various species of domestic animals.

3.3.3.1 Etiology and pathogenesis

The biologic effect that estrogens have on the hair follicle is very complex in as far as it shows great differences between species, genders, and skin sites (Hart 1990). In addition, metabolic activity of hair follicles varies between species, particularly with regard to androgen metabolism, clearly separating human scalp hair follicles from hair follicles of most other mammals (Bamberg et al. 2004). In humans, scalp hair follicles are androgen sensitive, and testosterone-mediated effects can be modulated by administration of estrogens. This is the reason why estrogens can prolong the anagen phase in male human scalp hair follicles, whereas they inhibit hair growth in female human scalp hair follicles and in pelage follicles of most other mammals. Gender differences are also based on different metabolic capacities of hair follicle subunits (Smart et al. 1999; Conrad et al. 2005). Site-dependent differences may be either caused by variations in the metabolic capacity and/or by variations in estrogen receptor (ER) expression patterns (Eigenmann et al. 1984; Bratka-Robia et al. 2002; Robia et al. 2003).

In the female, estrogens are primarily produced in the ovary. Cells of the theca interna of developing follicles produce androstenedione from cholesterol. Androstenedione is a substance of moderate androgenic activity. This compound crosses the basal membrane into the surrounding granulosa cells, where it is converted to estrone or estradiol, either immediately or through testosterone. The conversion of testosterone to estradiol, and of androstenedione to estrone, is catalyzed by the enzyme aromatase. Estrogen synthesis in the ovary is controlled by hypothalamic hormones, that is, follicle-stimulating hormone and luteinizing hormone. Besides the ovary there are several other tissues that can synthesize estrogens, particularly the adrenal cortex, the liver, and the mammary gland. These secondary sources of estrogens are of particular importance in males and in spayed females. The hair follicle itself also possesses aromatase enzyme activity and thus is able to convert androgens to estrogens. The biological significance of this finding, however, is yet unknown.

Estrogens act via the ER, a member of the nuclear hormone family of intracellular receptors, which mainly acts as a DNA-binding transcription factor that regulates gene expression. There are two different forms of the ER, usually referred to as α and β, each encoded by a separate gene. Hormone-activated ERs form dimers, and since the two forms are coexpressed in many cell types, the receptors may form ER-α ($\alpha\alpha$) or ER-β ($\beta\beta$) homodimers or ER-$\alpha\beta$ ($\alpha\beta$) heterodimers. The different forms of estrogen differ in their affinity to the alpha and beta isoforms of the ER. ERs have been demonstrated in the dermal papilla of hair follicles from various mammalian species (mouse, dog, man) (Oh and Smart 1996; Bratka-Robia et al. 2002; Frank et al. 2006). Both ER-α and ER-β are expressed in the hair follicle dermal papilla, but their quantities differ throughout the hair growth cycle.

Their expression is highest in catagen and telogen and lowest in anagen. It is now known from experiments in mice that catagen promotion is mediated via ER-α, whereas ER-β likely functions as a silencer of ER-α action during anagen (Chanda et al. 2000; Moverare et al. 2002; Ohnemus et al. 2005).

Despite the unequivocal effect that estrogens have on hair follicles, they are not essential for normal hair growth. In most cases, ovariectomy and thus significant reduction of circulatory estrogen levels does not have any influence on the hair coat. In rare cases (but more frequently in certain breeds such as Setters, long-haired Dachshunds, Small Munsterlander, and long- and smooth-haired Retrievers) coat quality may change after ovariectomy, but the pathogenesis of this effect is yet unknown and gonadotropins rather than estrogens may represent the major mediators of this effect (Welle et al. 2006). Furthermore, estrogenic effects on hair follicles must be counteracted physiologically, since all intact females exhibit an increase in plasma estrogen levels preceding estrus, while only few ever develop alopecia.

3.3.3.2 Diagnosis and therapy

Hair coat effects of hyperestrogenism comprise a dry hair coat and thinning of the hair coat over the abdomen, at the inner thighs, and in the perianal region. The head and distal parts of extremities are spared.

Clinical differential diagnoses of canine hyperestrogenism are limited as clinical signs are usually not restricted to the skin. With regard to alopecia, differential diagnoses include hyperadrenocorticism (see Section 3.3.2), canine recurrent flank alopecia (see Section 3.3.5), hypothyroidism (see Section 3.3.1), Alopecia X (see Section 3.3.4), or other breed-specific hair cycle abnormalities (see Section 3.3.9).

Skin histology in canine hyperestrogenism is similar in male and female dogs and is independent of its cause. Hair follicles show infundibular orthokeratotic hyperkeratosis. There are many hair follicles in late catagen stages and some in telogen, whereas the number of anagen hair follicles is reduced (Fig. 3.3.7). Depending on the duration of hyperestrogenism, the epidermis and sebaceous glands may eventually

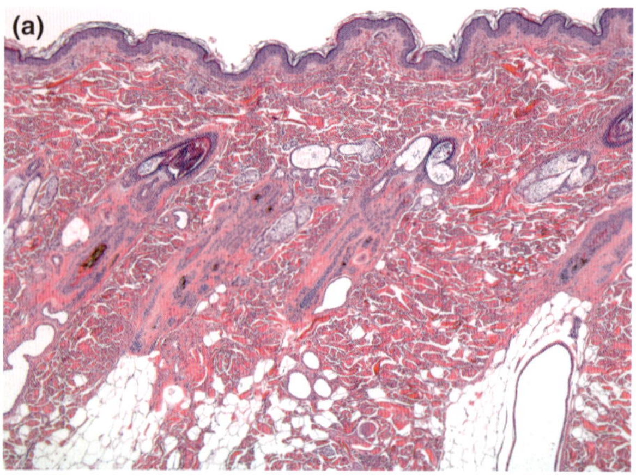

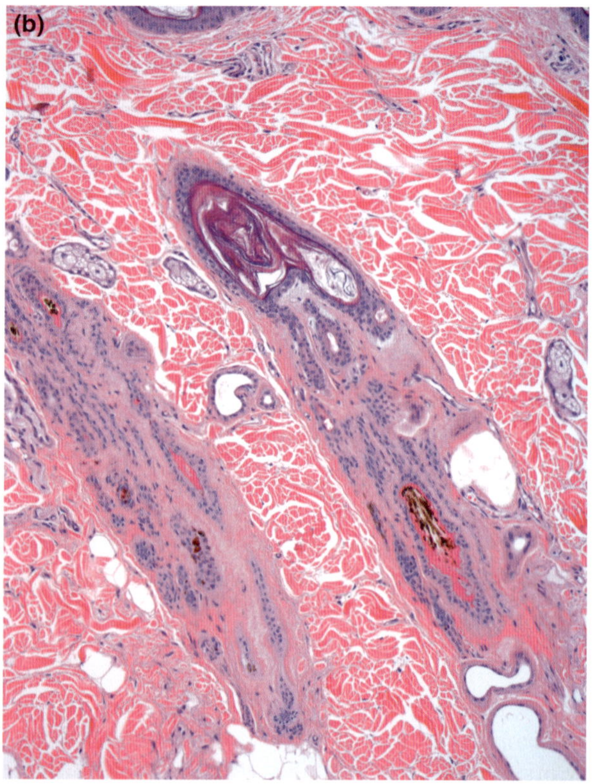

Fig. 3.3.7 Skin histology of canine hyperestrogenism. (a) All hair follicles are in late catagen/telogen; mild hyperkeratosis of follicular infundibula; (b) higher magnification showing catagen hair follicles with epithelial strand and thickened connective tissue sheath.

become atrophic. Apocrine glands may show dilatation. The dermis appears denser than normal with thicker, closely packed collagen bundles and fewer fibrocyte nuclei. As pyoderma is a frequent sequela of hyperestrogenism, biopsies may show variable degrees of purulent inflammation, eventually involving hair follicles (folliculitis and furunculosis). In general, histopathology is not sufficiently diagnostic for hyperestrogenism but merely suggests an endocrine disease.

3.3.3.2.1 Hyperestrogenism in intact bitches

Hyperestrogenism can occur in intact bitches in conjunction with ovarian cysts or tumors that derive from sex-cord stromal tissue of the ovary (mostly granulosa cell tumors, rarely thecomas or other sex-cord stromal neoplasms) (Fiorito 1992). Estrogen production by these cysts or tumors is autonomous and is no longer controlled by hypothalamic gonadotropins. Plasma estrogen levels may exceed the normal range, but it is not always possible to demonstrate consistent elevation of estrogen levels.

Besides alopecia, hyperestrogenism in bitches may result in gynecomastia (eventually with formation of mammary tumors), cystic endometrial hyperplasia, uterine leiomyomas, irregular estrus cycles, or persistent estrus, characterized by vulval enlargement, persistence of sanguinous discharge, vaginal cornification, and estrus behavior. Another serious side effect of very high levels of estrogens is myelosuppression with subsequent nonregenerative anemia, leukopenia, and thrombocytopenia. In contrast to hyperadrenocorticism (see Section 3.3.2), no polydypsia and polyuria develops and liver enzyme activity in serum is within normal limits.

Alopecia caused by hyperestrogenism begins in the genital and perianal region and progresses to the abdomen, ventral thorax, medial thighs, flanks, and proximal extremities (Fig. 3.3.8). The color of remaining hair may lighten. Over time, alopecic areas become hyperpigmented with dry seborrhea. Miliary sebaceous cysts may be present. In later stages the skin becomes thin. Secondary pyoderma is not uncommon and may change the clinical picture of the alopecic skin to erythema, crusting, and epidermal collarettes.

Ovarian cysts can be treated with GnRH (10 μg/kg), once or repeatedly, but this does not always resolve the problem. If the problem persists, estrus can be stopped by oral administration of low doses of megestrol acetate (once daily, first week: 0.1 mg/kg; second week: 0.05 mg/kg) with the risk of inducing pyometra. If therapy fails, ovariectomy is warranted. Neoplasms need to be surgically removed. Removal of the estrogen source will result in regrowth of hair within 2–4 months.

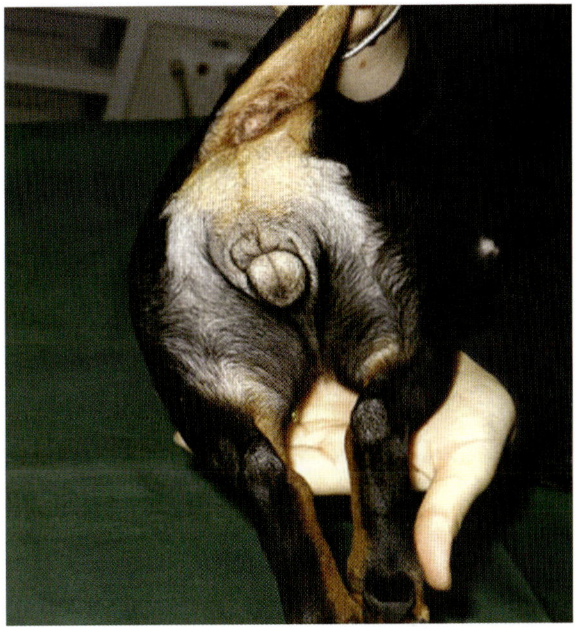

Fig. 3.3.8 Hyperestrogenism in an intact bitch with extensive alopecia of the caudal thighs. Note enlarged vulva.

3.3.3.2.2 Hyperestrogenism in neutered females

Hyperestrogenism with alopecia in neutered female dogs can occur after treatment with diethylstilbestrol for urinary incontinence (Barsanti et al. 1983). Hyperestrogenism may also be found in bitches that have undergone incomplete ovariectomy with subsequent development of ovarian cysts or neoplasms (Pluhar et al. 1995). Remnants of ovarian tissue can be detected by the human choriogonadotropin (hCG) stimulation test. Upon stimulation with hCG a successfully ovariectomized dog should not demonstrate an increase in estrogen and progesterone concentrations, whereas a significant increase is found in dogs that have been incompletely ovariectomized. Superficial to intermediate and nucleated as well as enucleated superficial cells in vaginal cytology verify estrogenic activity.

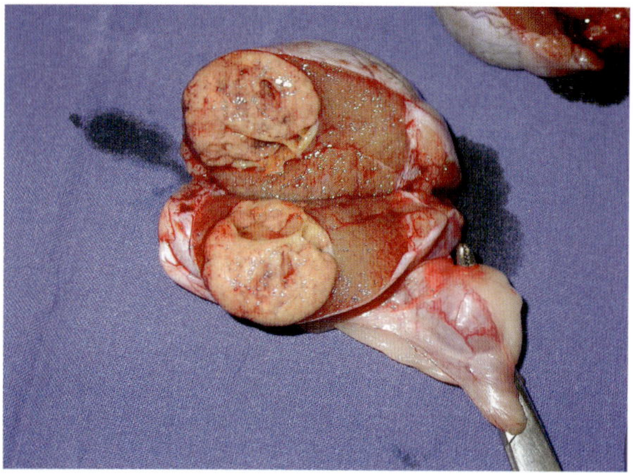

Fig. 3.3.9 Gross pathology of Sertoli cell tumor in the testis of a dog.

3.3.3.2.3 Hyperestrogenism in males

Hyperestrogenism in intact male dogs is mostly caused by estrogen-secreting sex-cord stromal tumors of the testis (mostly Sertoli cell tumor) (Medleau 1989; Schmeitzel 1990; Kim and Kim 2005). Sertoli cell neoplasms in the dog occur frequently in cryptorchids (the incidence of Sertoli cell tumors is reported to be 23 times higher in cryptorchid compared to normal dogs). They are firm, multinodular, and well demarcated from the surrounding testicular tissue (Fig. 3.3.9). Most Sertoli cell tumors are benign, particularly when they are less than 2 cm in diameter. A high incidence of Sertoli cell tumors is reported in Boxers, Cairn Terriers, Collies, Pekingese, Shetland Sheepdogs, and Weimaraners. There are rare reports on other testicular neoplasms associated with hyperestrogenism in the male dog, but their significance and pathogenesis is yet unknown. Other rare cases of reported hyperestrogenism in phenotypically male dogs were cases of

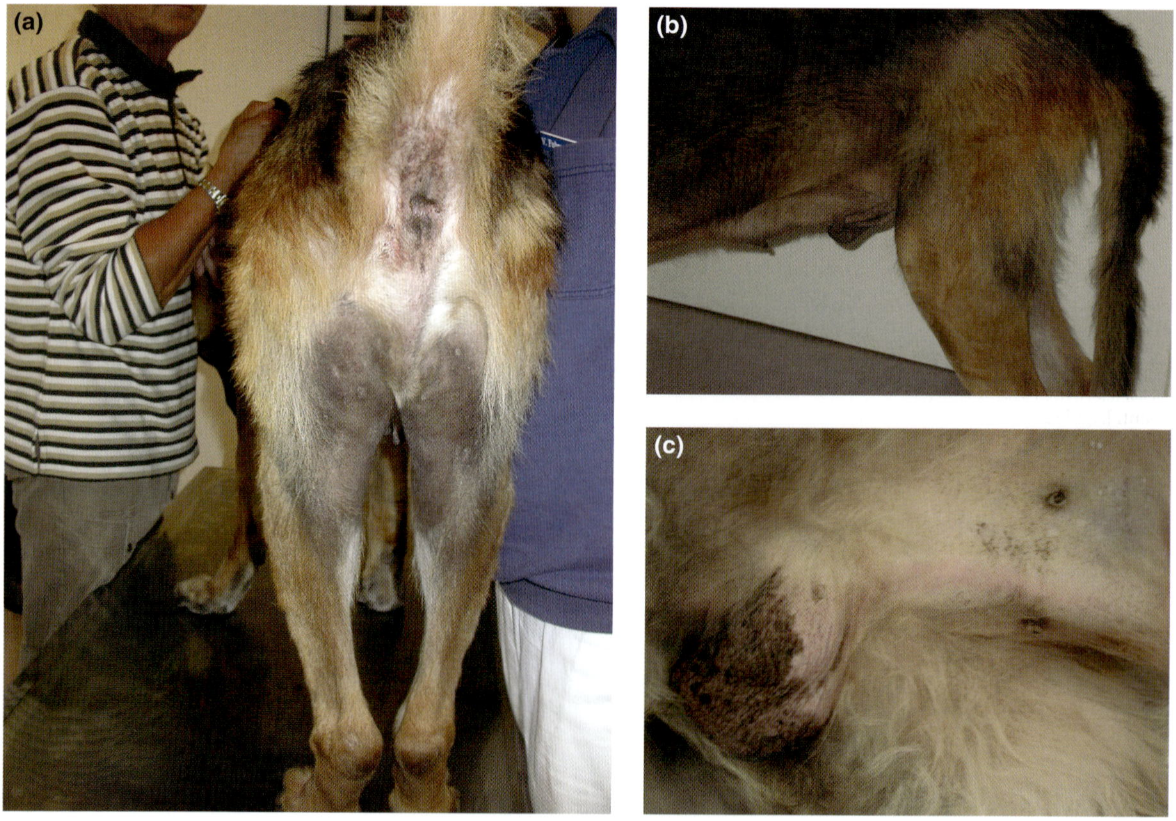

Fig. 3.3.10 Hyperestrogenism in a male dog with Sertoli cell tumor. (a) Extensive alopecia of caudal thighs; (b) gynecomastia; (c) linear erythema of the prepuce.

female pseudohermaphroditism, where ovarian tissue caused high levels of estrogen. In castrated male dogs, the adrenal cortex produces significant amounts of estrogens. Spontaneous hyperestrogenism with alopecia in castrated male dogs, however, has not been reported so far.

Alopecia in male dogs with Sertoli cell tumors follows the same pattern as with hyperestrogenism in intact bitches. Alopecia begins in the perineum and extends to the abdomen, ventral chest, neck, thighs, and flanks (Fig. 3.3.10). Beside alopecia, clinical signs of hyperestrogenism in male dogs are feminization (i.e., gynecomastia and attractiveness to male dogs), a pendulous prepuce, atrophy of the penile sheath, aspermatogenesis, and myelosuppression, resulting in anemia, leukopenia, and thrombocytopenia. A linear erythema along the prepuce is a specific, pathognomonic, clinical finding in male dogs with hyperestrogenism (Fig. 3.3.10). Unilateral testicular neoplasia is mostly associated with enlargement of one testicle and atrophy of the other. Elevated plasma levels of estradiol cannot always be demonstrated in dogs with Sertoli cell tumors. A diminished testosterone/estradiol ratio is more frequently found than a mere increase in the estradiol concentration (Mischke et al. 2002).

Testicular neoplasms are treated by orchiectomy. Clinical signs, including alopecia, usually resolve within a few months.

References

Bamberg E, Aichinger A, Mitteregger G. 2004. In vitro metabolism of dehydroepiandrosterone and testosterone by canine hair follicle cells. *Veterinary Dermatology* 15:19–24.

Barsanti JA, Medleau L, Latimer K. 1983. Diethylstilbestrol-induced alopecia in a dog. *Journal of the American Veterinary Medical Association* 182:63.

Bratka-Robia CB, Egerbacher M, Helmreich M, Mitteregger G, Benesch M, Bamberg E. 2002. Immunohistochemical localization of androgen and oestrogen receptors in canine hair follicles. *Veterinary Dermatology* 13:113–118.

Chanda S, Robinette CL, Couse JF, Smart RC. 2000. 17beta-estradiol and ICI182780 regulate the hair follicle cycle in mice through an estrogen receptor-alpha pathway. *American Journal of Physiology. Endocrinology and Metabolism* 278:E202–E210.

Conrad F, Ohnemus U, Bodo E, Biro T, Tychsen B, Gerstmayer B, Bosio A, Schmidt-Rose T, Altgilbers S, Bettermann A, Saathoff M, Meyer W, Paus R. 2005. Substantial sex-dependent differences in the response of human scalp hair follicles to estrogen stimulation in vitro advocate gender-tailored management of female versus male pattern balding. *Journal of Investigative Dermatology. Symposium Proceedings* 10:243–246.

Dow C. 1960. Oestrogen and skin atrophy. *Journal of Pathology and Bacteriology* 80:434.

Eigenmann JE, Poortman J, Koeman JP. 1984. Estrogen-induced flank alopecia in the female dog: evidence for local rather than systemic hyperestrogenism. *Journal of the American Animal Hospital Association* 20:621.

Fiorito DA. 1992. Hyperestrogenism in bitches. *Compendium on Continuing Education for the Practicing Veterinarian* 14:727.

Frank LA, Donnell RL, Kania SA. 2006. Oestrogen receptor evaluation in Pomeranian dogs with hair cycle arrest (alopecia X) on melatonin supplementation. *Veterinary Dermatology* 17:252–258.

Hart JE. 1990. Endocrine pathology of estrogens: species differences. *Pharmacology and Therapeutics* 47:203–218.

Hooker CW, Pfeiffer CA. 1943. Effects of sex hormones on spontaneous hair growth, skin, hair and sebaceous glands in the rat. *Endocrinology* 32:69.

Jabara AG. 1962. Some tissue changes in the dog following stilboestrol administration. *Australian Journal of Experimental Biology* 40:293.

Jackson D, Ebling FJ. 1972. The activity of hair follicles and their response to oestradiol in the guinea-pig *Cavia porcellus* L. *Journal of Anatomy* 111:303.

Johnson E. 1958. Quantitative studies of hair growth in the albino rat. II. The effect of sex hormones. *Journal of Endocrinology* 16:351.

Kim O, Kim KS. 2005. Seminoma with hyperesterogenemia in a Yorkshire terrier. *Journal of Veterinary Medical Science* 67:121–123.

Medleau L. 1989. Sex hormone-associated endocrine alopecias in dogs. *Journal of the American Animal Hospital Association* 25:689–694.

Mischke R, Meurer D, Hoppen HO, Ueberschar S, Hewicker-Trautwein M. 2002. Blood plasma concentrations of oestradiol-17beta, testosterone and testosterone/oestradiol ratio in dogs with neoplastic and degenerative testicular diseases. *Research in Veterinary Science* 73(3):267–272.

Moverare S, Lindberg MK, Faergemann J, Gustafsson JA, Ohlsson C. 2002. Estrogen receptor alpha, but not estrogen receptor beta, is involved in the regulation of the hair follicle cycling as well as the thickness of epidermis in male mice. *Journal of Investigative Dermatology* 119:1053–1059.

Oh HS, Smart RC. 1996. An estrogen receptor pathway regulates the telogen–anagen hair follicle transition and influences epidermal cell proliferation. *Proceedings of the National Academy of Sciences of the United States of America* 93:12525.

Ohnemus U, Uenalan M, Conrad F, Handjiski B, Mecklenburg L, Nakamura M, Inzunza J, Gustafsson JA, Paus R. 2005. Hair cycle control by estrogens: catagen induction via estrogen receptor (ER)-α is checked by ERβ signaling. *Endocrinology* 146:1214–1225.

Ohnemus U, Uenalan M, Handjiski B, Paus R. 2004. Topical estrogen accelerates hair regrowth in mice after chemotherapy-induced alopecia by favoring the dystrophic catagen response pathway to damage. *Journal of Investigative Dermatology* 122:7.

Ohnemus U, Uenalan M, Inzunza J, Gustafsson JA, Paus R. 2006. The hair follicle as an estrogen target and source. *Endocrine Reviews* 27:677–706.

Pluhar GE, Memon MA, Wheaton LG. 1995. Granulosa cell tumor in an ovariohysterectomized dog. *Journal of the American Veterinary Medical Association* 207:1063.

Robia CB, Mitteregger G, Aichinger A, Benesch M, Bamberg E. 2003. Effect of testosterone and oestradiol-17beta on canine hair follicle culture. *Journal of Veterinary Medicine. A, Physiology, Pathology, and Clinical Medicine* 50:225–229.

Schmeitzel LP. 1990. Sex hormone-related and growth hormone-related alopecias. *Veterinary Clinics of North America. Small Animal Practice* 20:1579.

Smart RC, Oh HS, Chanda S, Robinette CL. 1999. Effects of 17-beta-estradiol and ICI182780 on hair growth in various strains of mice. *Journal of Investigative Dermatology. Symposium Proceedings* 4:285–289.
Trentin JJ, Devita J, Gardner WU. 1952. Effect of moderate doses of estrogen and progesterone on mammary growth and hair growth in dogs. *Anatomical Record* 113:163–177.
Welle M, Reichler I, Barth A, Forster U, Sattler U, Arnold S. 2006. Immunohistochemical localization and quantitative assessment of GnRH-, FSH-, and LH-receptor mRNA Expression in canine skin: a powerful tool to study the pathogenesis of side effects after spaying. *Histochemistry and Cell Biology* 126(5):527–535.

3.3.4 Canine alopecia X

Linda Frank

Breeders of dogs with a double coat and dense undercoat, such as *Pomeranians*, *Alaskan Malamutes*, *Chow Chows*, and *Keeshonds*, have long recognized an alopecic condition in their breeds consisting of bilaterally symmetrical alopecia with hyperpigmentation of the skin that is not caused by hypothyroidism, hyperadrenocorticism, or hyperestrogenism. This condition has also been described in *Miniature* and *Toy Poodles*. In the veterinary literature it has been called pseudo-Cushing's syndrome, adult-onset growth hormone deficiency (hyposomatotropism), growth hormone-responsive alopecia, castration-responsive alopecia, biopsy-responsive alopecia, congenital adrenal hyperplasia-like syndrome, and, most recently, "alopecia X." This term reflects the mystery behind the cause of the alopecia, but it fails to reflect what we do know about the condition, that is, that all cases of "alopecia X" show a disturbance in the hair growth cycle. For the ease of classification, the alopecic conditions known under the term "alopecia X" are all mentioned in this chapter, but the reader should keep in mind that it is not yet proven that "alopecia X" in the above-mentioned breeds is actually a single disease entity with similar etiology and pathogenesis.

3.3.4.1 Etiology and pathogenesis

Hair cycle arrest in plush-coated dogs was first described by Siegel in 1977. He referred to the condition as pseudo-Cushing syndrome because the clinical appearance resembled dogs with Cushing syndrome but lacked the biochemical abnormalities. Adult-onset growth hormone deficiency was one of the first theories for the alopecia (Eigenmann and Patterson 1984a; Scott and Walton 1986). This theory was disproved when various studies showed many dogs with this condition, including 14/19 Chow Chows and 3/4 Keeshonds, to have normal growth hormone responses to stimulatory factors and normal insulin-like growth factor-1 (IGF-1) concentrations (Eigenmann et al. 1984b; Lothrop 1988). In addition, castration resulted in hair regrowth in six intact dogs with hair cycle arrest in spite of continued low growth hormone concentrations in the four dogs evaluated (Rosser 1990). Even without true growth hormone deficiency, growth hormone supplementation did result in hair growth in many dogs with this condition (Lothrop 1988). Growth hormone may induce anagen initiation of the hair follicle, although the exact mechanism is not known.

In 1990, Schmeitzel and Lothrop suggested that the alopecia may be attributed to an overproduction of adrenal cortical steroid hormone intermediates. Adrenal steroid hormones were evaluated before and after ACTH stimulation in 7 intact Pomeranians with bilateral alopecia and hyperpigmentation and in 12 normal-coated intact Pomeranians. Both groups demonstrated abnormal serum concentrations of adrenal steroid intermediates and sex hormones (most notably high 17-hydroxyprogesterone), compared to 19 mixed-breed control dogs. The authors hypothesized that the dogs had a partial deficiency of the 21-hydroxylase enzyme (as described in people with congenital adrenal hyperplasia) that may account for the laboratory and clinical findings. This enzyme is important for cortisol formation and its deficiency results in an increase in serum 17-hydroxyprogesterone, which provides substrate for making additional androstenedione and estradiol (Fig. 3.3.11). In humans with late-onset congenital adrenal hyperplasia, clinical signs are attributed to hyperandrogenism and may include premature development of testosterone-dependent hairs in children, hirsutism in women, early fusion of epiphyseal growth plates, and severe acne (Speiser et al. 1992). In addition, male pattern baldness may be the only clinical presentation in young women. It is, however, unlikely that hyperandrogenism is the cause of the hair cycle arrest in dogs with alopecia X. The reason for this is multifactorial. The most obvious is that dogs do not have androgen-dependent hair follicles. Dogs do not have substantial changes in hair coat upon maturation, nor do they have abrupt

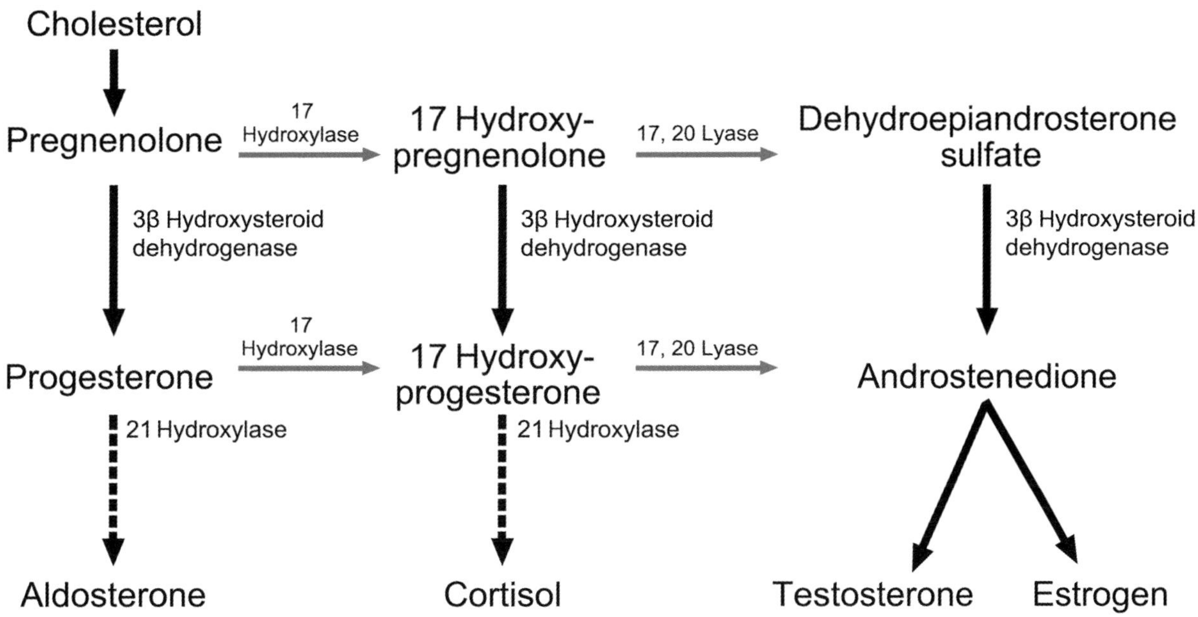

Fig. 3.3.11 Schematic demonstration of enzymes involved in steroid hormone production.

hair coat changes associated with castration or ovariohysterectomy. In addition, administration of methyltestosterone has resulted in hair regrowth in some dogs with this condition (Lothrop 1988; Rosser 1990). Another reason that congenital adrenal hyperplasia is an unlikely explanation for the hair cycle arrest is that dogs do not have clinical signs other than the coat abnormality associated with this condition.

To further investigate the role of adrenal steroid intermediates and sex hormones in the pathogenesis of hair cycle arrest, a retrospective evaluation of hormone concentrations in dogs with this condition was undertaken (Frank et al. 2003). From this study it was concluded that not all dogs with alopecia X had detectable abnormalities in serum concentrations of sex hormones and adrenal steroid hormone intermediates, and seldom were values substantially greater than the upper limits of the reference ranges. In a prospective study (Frank et al. 2004), sex hormones and adrenal steroid hormone intermediate concentrations were measured from dogs with alopecia X before and during treatment with melatonin or mitotane. Results from this study showed hair regrowth not to be associated with decrease in serum concentrations of sex or adrenal steroid hormones, and many dogs with hair regrowth still had hormonal abnormalities. More recently, the canine 21-hydroxylase gene has been cloned and sequenced in Pomeranians with hair cycle arrest and no mutations in the gene were identified (Takada et al. 2002). Lastly, the adrenal and pituitary glands of 14 Pomeranian dogs with hair cycle arrest were evaluated using MRI scanning and found to be no different than controls (Shibata et al. 2005).

Hypercortisolemia has been reexamined as a cause of hair loss in dogs with alopecia X (Cerundolo et al. 2007). Miniature Poodles and Pomeranians with hair cycle arrest had increased urinary cortisol to creatinine ratios; however, substantial overlap of the ranges occurred among alopecic Pomeranians and Poodles, non-alopecic Pomeranians, and healthy control dogs. In addition, not all alopecic Pomeranians and Poodles had abnormal low-dose dexamethasone suppression (Cerundolo et al. 2007). Since hypercortisolemia is associated with many clinical signs including dilute urine, polyuria, polydipsia, polyphagia, and urinary tract infections in addition to coat abnormalities, this explanation seems unlikely. In addition, one of the unique features associated with alopecia X is hair regrowth at a site of trauma such as a biopsy or surgical site. Trauma-induced anagen is a known phenomenon of the hair follicle (Argyris 1967) and is inhibited by corticosteroids (Stenn and Paus 2001).

Hair regrowth at a site of trauma in dogs with hair cycle arrest implies a local inhibition of anagen at the level of the follicle that can be overridden rather than a systemic hormonal inhibition. New theories on the pathogenesis of hair cycle arrest in plush-coated dogs are focusing on genetics and hair follicle receptors. Both extrinsic (hormones) and intrinsic (cytokines, growth factors, and receptors) factors influence the hair cycle (Stenn and Paus 2001; Botchkarev and Kishimoto 2003) (see Section 1.2.1.5). Anagen initiation involves complex interactions between estrogen receptors, bone morphogenic protein 4, sonic hedgehog signaling, and noggin, among others (Botchkarev and Kishimoto 2003). A recent study investigated the use of a pure estrogen receptor antagonist, fulvestrant, in treating Pomeranian dogs with hair cycle arrest (Frank 2007). Both a 10 mg/kg dose (Frank 2007) and a 20 mg/kg dose (unpublished observations) were found to be ineffective in causing hair regrowth in the majority of dogs. It is, therefore, likely that hair follicles in dogs with alopecia X require stimulation from multiple molecules, such as noggin or even IGF, in conjunction with blocking of the estrogen receptor.

Recently, the cathepsin L2 (CTSL2) gene was investigated as a potential candidate gene for canine alopecia X. However, none of the found polymorphisms affected the coding sequence, and haplotype analysis did not reveal an association of one particular CTSL2 haplotype with the disease phenotype. It was therefore concluded that the CTSL2 gene is not the causative gene for alopecia X (Mausberg et al. 2007).

3.3.4.2 Diagnosis

Alopecia X has been recognized in many plush-coated breeds, especially Pomeranians, Chow Chows, Keeshonds, Alaskan Malamutes, Siberian Huskies, and Samoyeds, with Pomeranians by the far most common breed affected (Frank et al. 2003). In addition, this condition occurs in Toy and Miniature Poodles that have a more curly rather than a plush hair coat. While originally reported to occur in dogs between the ages of 1 and 3 years, coat changes may occur anytime between 1 and 10 years of age (Frank et al. 2004). Both male and female dogs may be affected regardless of neuter status. If the hair loss occurs in an intact dog, hair regrowth may occur following neutering, but a relapse within 1 to 2 years is likely.

3.3.4.2.1 Clinical presentation

The dermatologic changes in these dogs mimic those of endocrine alopecias such as hyperadrenocorticism, with alopecia and other coat changes, sparing the head and distal extremities. Initially, there may be preferential loss of guard hairs resulting in a dull, dry coat. Increased matting of the coat may be an early clinical complaint. Sometimes a more generalized loss of guard hairs gives the coat a "puppy" appearance (Fig. 3.3.12). The hair coat may also appear lighter or a different color with the loss of guard hairs (Fig. 3.3.13).

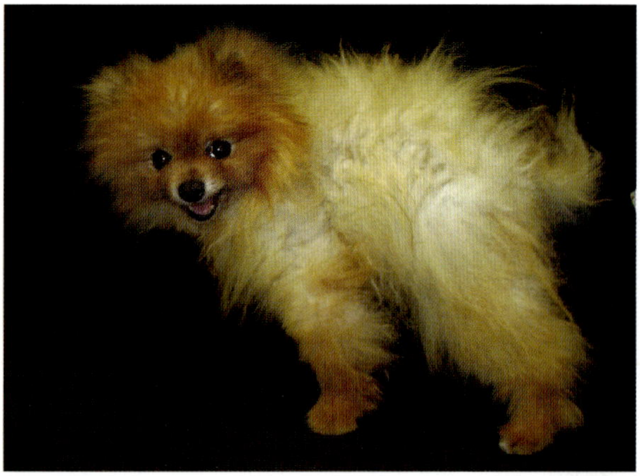

Fig. 3.3.12 Alopecia X in a 5-year-old intact male Pomeranian with loss of guard hairs giving the appearance of a puppy coat.

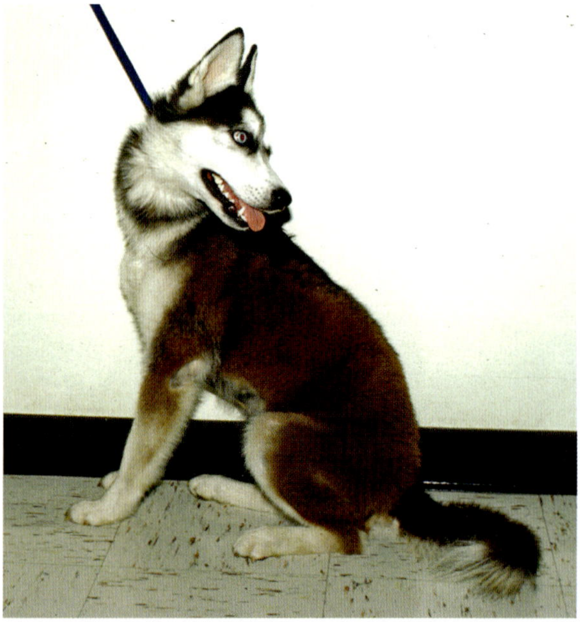

Fig. 3.3.13 Alopecia X in a young adult spayed, female Siberian Husky with loss of guard hairs resulting in a change in coat color. (Courtesy of University of Florida.)

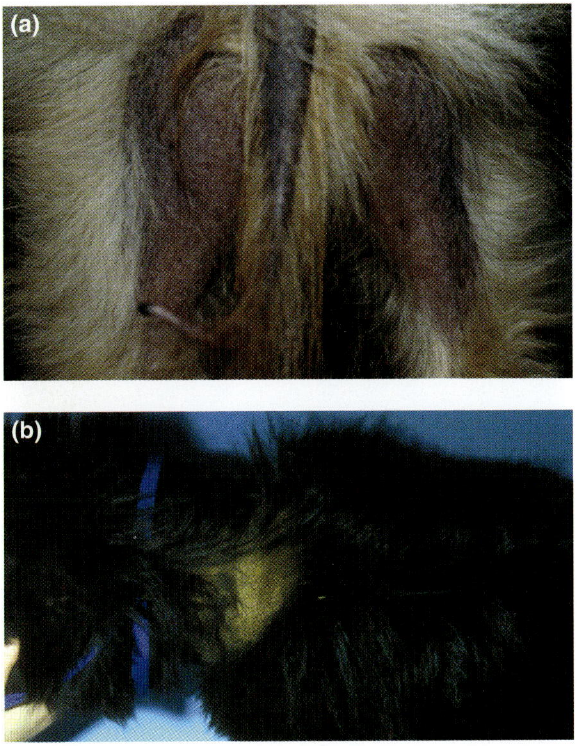

Fig. 3.3.14 Alopecia X. (a) 3-year-old male castrated Pomeranian with alopecia of the caudal thighs and tail; (b) 2-year-old intact male Chow Chow with alopecia of the neck. (Courtesy of University of Tennessee.)

Hair loss may first be noted on frictional areas such as the collar, tail head region, and caudal thighs and these areas will become more severely involved with time (Fig. 3.3.14). These early coat changes may be subtle, making it difficult to determine the time frame to hair loss. From early changes to complete hair loss may take several years in some dogs (Fig. 3.3.15). The retained secondary hairs are also lost with time, resulting in complete alopecia of the affected areas (Fig. 3.3.16). The exposed skin often becomes intensely hyperpigmented (Fig. 3.3.17); however, not all dogs develop hyperpigmentation. Likely, the increased pigmentation is a function of sun exposure and can be minimized with sun restriction or clothing. These dogs tend to regrow tufts of hair at sites of surgical trauma such as a skin biopsy or surgery site (Fig. 3.3.18).

Owners may first become aware of a problem when their dog's hair coat fails to regrow after clipping. This can be seen with endocrine diseases but can also be a normal feature of these plush-coated breeds. Nordic breeds have been shown to have a longer haired telogen phase naturally that may last for years (Credille 2000). Conversely, the dog could have hair cycle arrest before guard hair loss or overt alopecia has occurred.

The coat changes seen in dogs with alopecia X are not accompanied by any systemic signs. These dogs are otherwise healthy. If signs of systemic disease are present, then other endocrine diseases such as hyperadrenocorticism, hypothyroidism, hyperestrogenism, or diabetes mellitus should be investigated.

Diagnosis of alopecia X is by exclusion. The primary differential diagnoses include hyperadrenocorticism (see Section 3.3.2), hypothyroidism (see Section 3.3.1), hyperestrogenism (see Section 3.3.3), canine recurrent flank alopecia (see Section 3.3.5.), and other breed-specific hair cycle abnormalities (see Section 3.3.9). In addition, sebaceous adenitis (see Section 4.8) can present with a similar clinical presentation, especially in breeds such as Samoyeds, known to develop this condition. Sebaceous adenitis can be readily excluded by skin biopsy.

3.3.4.2.2 Laboratory tests

Because diagnosis of hair cycle arrest is by exclusion of other diseases, dogs need to be screened with routine laboratory tests (hematology, chemistry panel, urinalysis) that should be unremarkable. In addition, thyroid and adrenal function should be assessed with appropriate tests. Sometimes dogs will have thyroid results suggestive of hypothyroidism but hair fails to regrow on appropriate supplementation. Once systemic disease has been ruled out, a skin biopsy is helpful to support the diagnosis of hair cycle arrest and eliminate inflammatory disease such as sebaceous adenitis or folliculitis.

3.3.4.2.3 Histopathology

Skin biopsies will not allow final differentiation of alopecia X from most other forms of hair cycle arrest such as underlying endocrine disease. Histopathologic changes noted are those typical of an endocrinopathy and include orthokeratotic hyperkeratosis, follicular keratosis, follicular dilatation, epidermal melanosis, and telogenization of hair follicles (Fig. 3.3.19). In addition, many hair follicles show excessive trichilemmal keratinization ("flame follicles") that is a sign of late catagen, suggesting that catagen development is actually delayed. This feature is prominent in

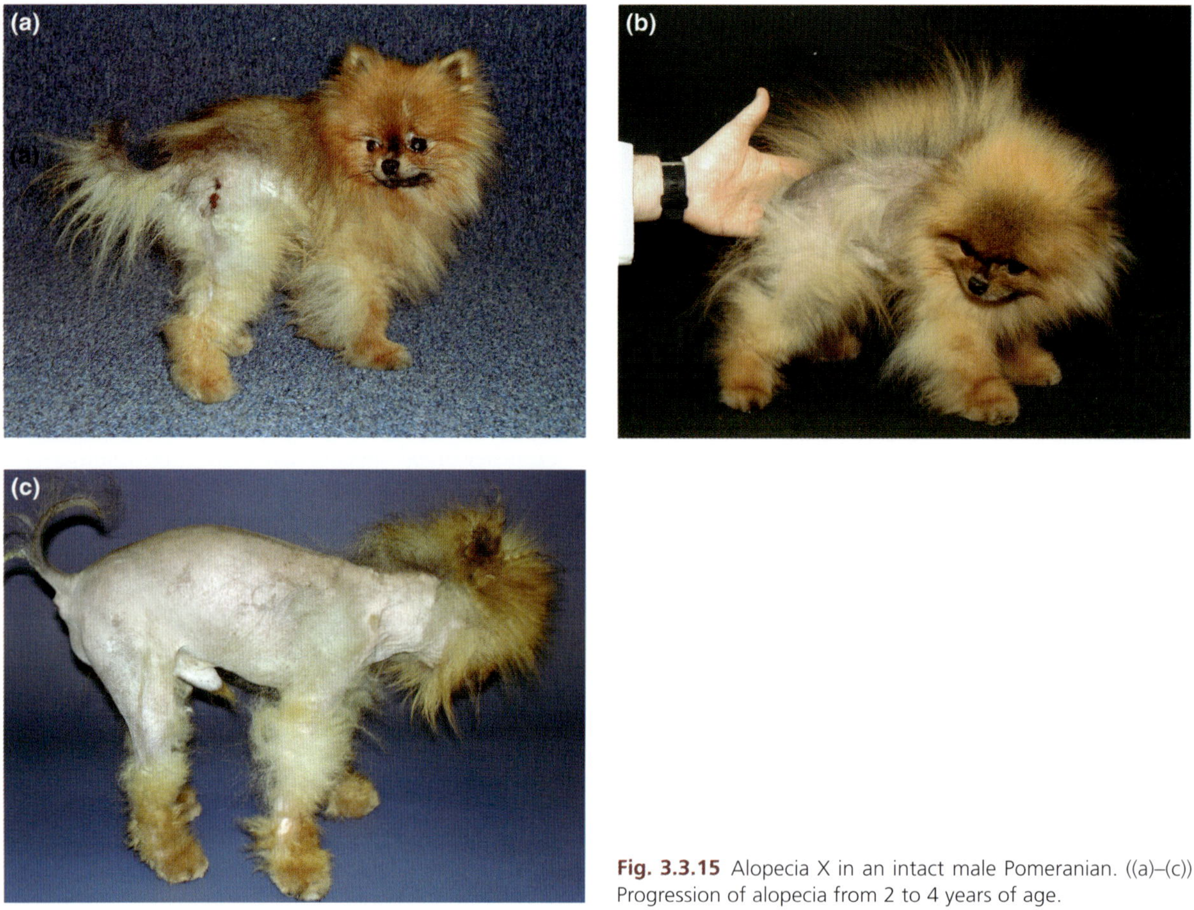

Fig. 3.3.15 Alopecia X in an intact male Pomeranian. ((a)–(c)) Progression of alopecia from 2 to 4 years of age.

alopecia X but is also observed in other hair cycle abnormalities, and is therefore not exclusively diagnostic for this condition. The presence of "flame follicles" may simply reflect the specific nature of plush-coated dogs. Histopathology can also show misshapen telogen follicles with abnormal accumulations of melanin in hair shafts, follicular epithelium, and sebaceous glands (Frank et al. 2006) (Fig. 3.3.20).

3.3.4.3 Therapy

In intact dogs neutering is the initial treatment of choice. Many dogs experience hair regrowth for some period of time after surgery, from months to years. If the hair loss initially occurred after neutering, recurred after neutering, or failed to respond to neutering, treatment options include melatonin, methyltestosterone, growth hormone supplementation, mitotane, trilostane, or doing nothing. Recently, treatment with an oral antiandrogen was reported to result in partial (9 dogs) to complete hair regrowth (1 dog) in 13 alopecic Pomeranians (Paradis and Cerundolo 2005). Unfortunately, the various treatments are not always effective. In addition, the new hair is rarely permanent and will often fall out in months to years despite continued treatment.

3.3.4.3.1 Melatonin

First line treatment for dogs with alopecia X following neutering is melatonin. Melatonin treatment results in partial to complete hair regrowth in approximately 40% of cases and is very safe. It is contraindicated in dogs with diabetes because it can cause insulin resistance at high doses. Melatonin's mechanism of action is not known. Melatonin may influence

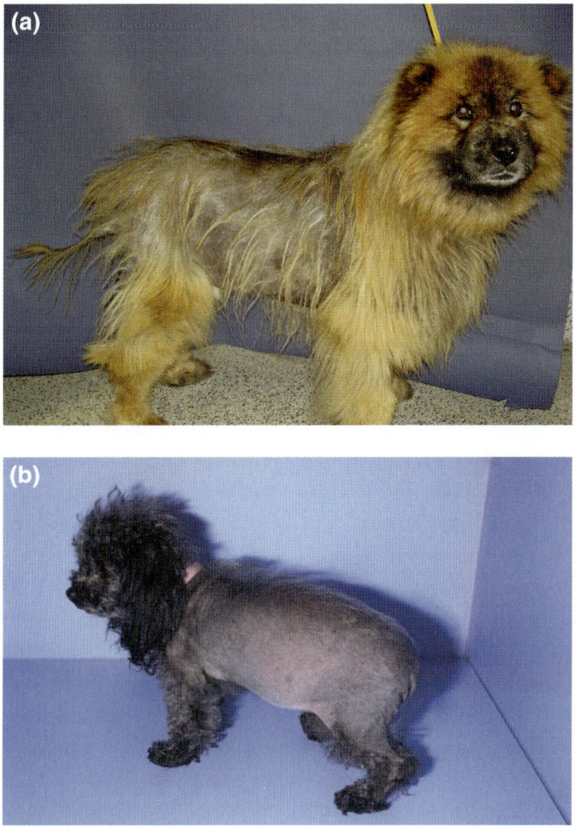

Fig. 3.3.16 Alopecia X. (a) 7-year-old male castrated Chow Chow with alopecia and hyperpigmentation of his trunk; (b) 11-year-old female spayed Miniature Poodle with alopecia and hyperpigmentation of her trunk. (Courtesy of University of Tennessee.)

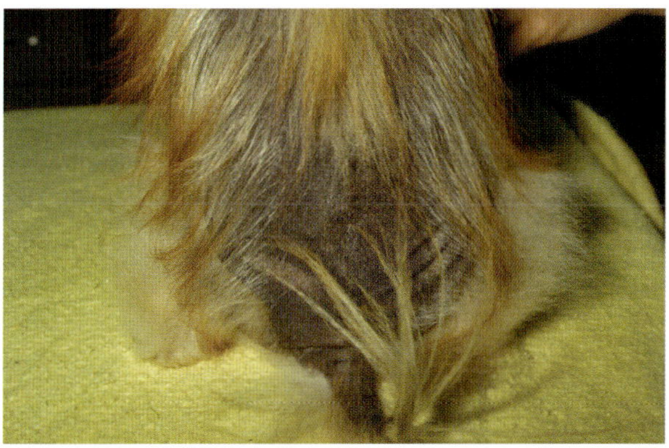

Fig. 3.3.17 Alopecia X in an adult male Pomeranian with hyperpigmentation and alopecia of the caudodorsum. (Courtesy of University of Florida.)

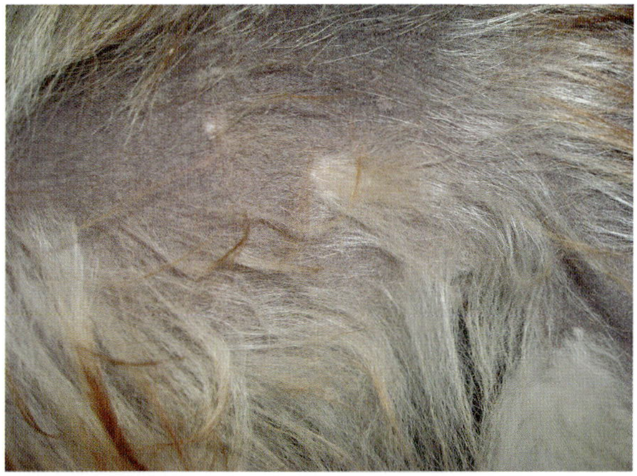

Fig. 3.3.18 Alopecia X. Note hair regrowth at site of previous biopsy.

hair growth by altering serum sex hormones in sexually intact dogs (Ashley et al. 1999); however, this mechanism is unlikely in neutered dogs (Frank et al. 2004). Hair follicles do not have melatonin receptors (Dicks et al. 1996); therefore, melatonin may influence hair growth through its activity on estrogen receptors. Estrogen receptors may have a regulatory role in the hair cycle by stimulating the expression of bone morphogenic protein (BMP-4) that is associated with downregulation of certain molecules resulting in inhibition of hair growth (Oh and Smart 1996; Smart et al. 1999; Botchkarev and Kishimoto 2003), and melatonin has been shown

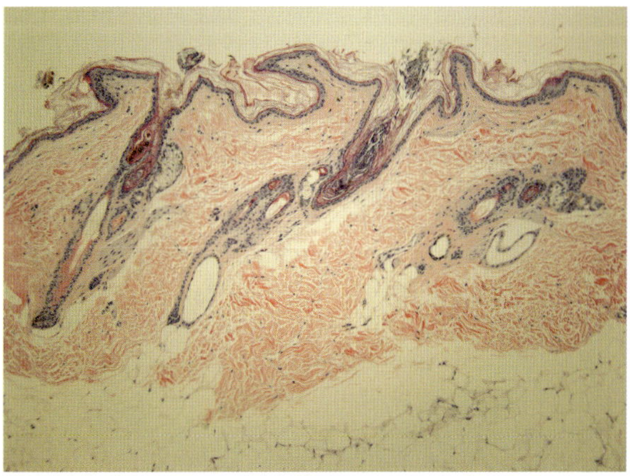

Fig. 3.3.19 Skin histology of alopecia X. Characteristic features include orthokeratotic hyperkeratosis and presence of flame follicles.

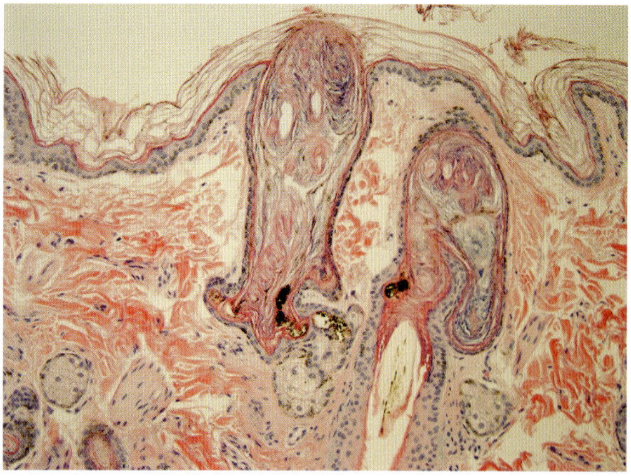

Fig. 3.3.20 Skin histology of alopecia X. Note large deformed follicles with pigment accumulation in the sebaceous glands and ducts.

to block estrogen receptors in human breast cancer cells (Rato 1999; Kiefer et al. 2002). Estrogen receptors are prominent in the canine telogen hair and dermal papilla of dogs with hair cycle arrest (Frank et al. 2006). The recommended dose of melatonin is 3 mg BID for small breeds and 6–12 mg BID for large breeds (Frank et al. 2004). There seems to be an increased efficacy noted in the small breeds. This may be associated with a discrepancy in dosing of small versus large breed dogs with the average dosage for Pomeranians and Poodles being 1.4 mg/kg every 12 h as compared to 0.3 mg/kg every 12 h for Siberian Huskies and Keeshonds (Frank et al. 2004). Many dogs will subsequently lose hair even if current treatment is maintained; therefore, it is recommended to stop treatment once hair regrowth is established. This may preserve the usefulness of this treatment again in the future.

While growth hormone administration has been effective in causing hair regrowth in a number of dogs (Eigenmann and Patterson 1984a; Lothrop 1988; Bell et al. 1993), growth hormone may induce diabetes mellitus and is not readily available. Treatment with methyltestosterone may result in hair regrowth (Lothrop 1988; Rosser 1990) but may also be associated with unwanted side effects including increased aggression and cholangiohepatitis.

Two drugs used to treat hyperadrenocorticism, mitotane and trilostane, have been used to manage some dogs with hair cycle arrest. The exact mechanisms by which *o,p'*-DDD or trilostane cause hair regrowth in dogs with hair cycle arrest are unknown. These drugs may work through hormone manipulation since hormones are known to have both stimulatory and inhibitory effects on the hair follicle cycle (Stenn and Paus 2001). In addition, trilostane has been shown to inhibit estrogen receptors (Puddefoot et al. 2002).

3.3.4.3.2 Mitotane

Mitotane (*o,p'*-DDD), a chlorinated hydrocarbon derivative that causes selective necrosis and atrophy of the zona fasciculata and zona reticularis of the adrenal cortex, has been used successfully to treat dogs with hair cycle arrest at daily induction doses of 15–25 mg/kg followed by twice weekly maintenance (Rosenkrantz and Griffin 1992; Frank et al. 2004). Twelve Chow Chows treated with mitotane had partial (2 dogs) to complete (10 dogs) hair regrowth (Rosenkrantz and Griffin 1992). That degree of success is not always reported. Of six Pomeranians treated with mitotane, three had complete hair regrowth, one had partial hair regrowth, and two failed to regrow their hair (Frank et al. 2004). Response to treatment was not related to cortisol or adrenal steroid hormone concentrations. However, ACTH stimulation tests should be performed to monitor cortisol concentrations and prevent hypocortisolemia. Dogs may subsequently lose hair in spite of good hormonal control and continued treatment with mitotane. Therefore, it is recommended that dogs be removed from treatment once a full hair coat is established.

3.3.4.3.3 Trilostane

Trilostane, an inhibitor of 3-beta hydroxysteroid dehydrogenase, has also been used with success to treat some dogs with hair cycle arrest (Cerundolo et al. 2004; Leone et al. 2005). Dosages used in these studies ranged from 3.0 to 3.6 mg/kg twice a day in 3 Alaskan Malamutes (Leone et al. 2005) to 10.8 mg/kg per day in 16 Pomeranians and 8 Miniature Poodles (Cerundolo et al. 2004). Complete hair regrowth was seen in all 3 Alaskan Malamutes, all 8 Miniature Poodles, and 14/16 Pomeranians within 6 months. No adverse effects were observed in those studies; however, two dogs died in the study although the cause of death was not believed to be related to treatment (Cerundolo et al. 2004). In addition, trilostane has been reported to cause adrenal necrosis in a dog (Chapman et al. 2004) and, therefore, should be used with caution.

References

Argyris TS. 1967. Hair growth induced by damage. *Advances in Biology of the Skin* 9:339–356.

Ashley PF, Frank LA, Schmeitzel LP, Bailey EM, Oliver JW. 1999. Effect of oral melatonin administration on sex hormone, prolactin, and thyroid hormone concentrations in adult dogs. *Journal of the American Veterinary Medical Association* 215(8):1111–1115.

Bell AG, Jones BR, Scott MF. 1993. Growth hormone responsive dermatosis in three dogs. *New Zealand Veterinary Journal* 41:195–199.

Botchkarev VA, Kishimoto J. 2003. Molecular control of epithelial–mesenchymal interactions during hair follicle cycling. *Journal of Investigative Dermatology Symposium Proceedings* 8:46–55.

Cerundolo R, Lloyd DH, Persechino A, Evans H, Cauvin A. 2004. Treatment of canine alopecia X with trilostane. *Veterinary Dermatology* 15:285–293.

Cerundolo R, Lloyd DH, Vaessen MM, Mol JA, Kooistra HS, Rijnberk A. 2007 March 24. Alopecia in Pomeranians and miniature poodles in association with high urinary corticoid:creatinine ratios and resistance to glucocorticoid feedback. *Veterinary Record* 160(12):393–397. Erratum in: *Veterinary Record* 2007;160(16):547.

Chapman PS, Kelly DF, Archer J, Brockman DJ, Neiger R. 2004. Adrenal necrosis in a dog receiving trilostane for the treatment of hyperadrenocorticism. *Journal of Small Animal Practice* 45:307–310.

Credille KM. 2000. The role of nutrition on the canine hair follicle: a preliminary report. In: Reinhart GA, Carey DP (eds), *Recent Advances in Canine and Feline Nutrition*, Vol. 3, pp. 37–53. Wilmington: Orange Frazer Press.

Dicks P, Morgan CJ, Morgan PJ, Kelly D, Williams LM. 1996. The localization and characterization of insulin-like growth factor-1 receptors and the investigation of melatonin receptors on the hair follicles of seasonal and nonseasonal fibre-producing goats. *Journal of Endocrinology* 151:55–63.

Eigenmann JE, Patterson DF. 1984a. Growth hormone deficiency in the mature dog. *Journal of the American Animal Hospital Association* 20:741–746.

Eigenmann JE, Patterson DF, Froesch ER. 1984b. Body size parallels insulin-like growth factor 1 levels but not growth hormone secretory capacity. *Acta Endocrinologica* 106:448–453.

Frank LA. 2007. Oestrogen receptor antagonist and hair regrowth in dogs with hair cycle arrest (alopecia X). *Veterinary Dermatology* 18:63–66.

Frank LA, Donnell RL, Kania SA. 2006. Oestrogen receptor evaluation in Pomeranian dogs with hair cycle arrest (alopecia X) on melatonin supplementation. *Veterinary Dermatology* 17:252–258.

Frank LA, Hnilica KA, Bohrbach BW, Oliver JW. 2003. Retrospective evaluation of sex hormones and steroid hormone intermediates in dogs with alopecia. *Veterinary Dermatology* 14:91–97.

Frank LA, Hnilica KA, Oliver JW. 2004. Adrenal steroid hormone concentrations in dogs with hair cycle arrest (alopecia X) before and during treatment with melatonin and mitotane. *Veterinary Dermatology* 15:278–284.

Kiefer T, Ram PT, Yuan L, Hill SM. 2002. Melatonin inhibits estrogen receptor transactivation and cAMP levels in breast cancer cells. *Breast Cancer Research and Treatment* 71:37–45.

Leone F, Cerundolo R, Vercelli A, Lloyd DH. 2005. The use of trilostane for the treatment of alopecia X in Alaskan malamutes. *Journal of the American Animal Hospital Association* 41:336–342.

Lothrop CD. 1988. Pathophysiology of canine growth hormone-responsive alopecia. *Compendium of Small Animal Practice* 10:1346–1349.

Mausberg EM, Drogemuller C, Leeb T, Dolf G, Rufenacht S, Welle M. 2007. Evaluation of the CTSL2 gene as a candidate gene for alopecia X in Pomeranians and Keeshonden. *Animal Biotechnology* 18(4):291–296.

Oh H-S, Smart RC. 1996. An estrogen receptor pathway regulates the telogen–anagen hair follicle transition and influences epidermal cell proliferation. *Proceedings of the National Academy of Sciences of the United States of America* 93:12525–12530.

Paradis M, Cerundolo R. 2005. Genodermatosis: alopecia and hypotrichoses. *Advances in Veterinary Dermatology* 5:360–364.

Puddefoot JR, Barker S, Glover HR, Malouitre SDM, Vinson GP. 2002. Non-competitive steroid inhibition of oestrogen receptor functions. *International Journal of Cancer* 101:17–22.

Rato AG. 1999. Melatonin blocks the activation of estrogen receptor for DNA binding. *FASEB Journal* 13:857–868.

Rosenkrantz WS, Griffin C. 1992. Lysodren therapy in suspect adrenal sex hormone dermatosis. *Proceedings of the Second World Congress of Veterinary Dermatology*, 13–16 May, Montréal, Québec, Canada, p. 121.

Rosser EJ. 1990. Castration responsive dermatosis in the dog. In: von Tscharner C, Halliwell REW (eds), *Advances in Veterinary Dermatology*, Vol. 1, pp. 34–42. Philadelphia: Baillière Tindall.

Schmeitzel LP, Lothrop CD. 1990. Hormonal abnormalities in Pomeranians with normal coat and in Pomeranians with growth hormone-responsive dermatosis. *Journal of the American Veterinary Medical Association* 197:1333–1341.

Scott DW, Walton DK. 1986. Hyposomatotropism in the mature dog: a discussion of 22 cases. *Journal of the American Animal Hospital Association* 22:467–473.

Shibata K, Koie H, Nagata M. 2005. Clinicopathologic and morphologic analysis of the adrenal gland in Pomeranians with non-illness alopecia. *Japanese Journal of Veterinary Dermatology* 11:115–120.

Siegel ET (ed). 1977. Hypofunction of the anterior pituitary gland. In: *Endocrine Diseases of the Dog*, pp. 23–32. Philadelphia: Lea & Febiger.

Smart RC, Oh H-S, Chanda S, Robinette CL. 1999. Effects of 17-β-estradiol and ICI 182 780 on hair growth in various strains of mice. *Journal of Investigative Dermatology Symposium Proceedings* 4:285–289.

Speiser PW, White PC, New MI. 1992. Congenital adrenal hyperplasia. In: Vivian HT James (ed.), *The Adrenal Gland*, 2nd edn, pp. 327–371. New York: Raven Press.

Stenn KS, Paus R. 2001. Controls of hair follicle cycling. *Physiological Reviews* 81:449–494.

Takada K, Kitamura H, Takiguchi M, Saito M, Hashimoto A. 2002. Cloning of canine 21-hydroxylase gene and its polymorphic analysis as a candidate gene for congenital adrenal hyperplasia-like syndrome in Pomeranians. *Research in Veterinary Science* 73:159–163.

3.3.5 Canine recurrent flank alopecia

Manon Paradis

Canine recurrent flank alopecia (CRFA) is a skin disorder of unknown etiopathogenesis that is characterized by episodes of truncal hair loss that often reoccurs on an annual basis. This fascinating problem was first reported in the literature in ovariohysterectomized dogs (Scott 1990), although earlier reports of adult onset hyposomatotropism (Scott and Walton 1986; Shanley and Miller 1987) most likely included some true cases of CRFA. Several names for this disorder (e.g., seasonal flank alopecia, idiopathic cyclic flank alopecia, cyclic follicular dysplasia, recurrent flank alopecia) were proposed in subsequent reports (Cieslowski and Paradis 1993; Miller and Dunstan 1993; Waldman 1995; Curtis et al. 1996; Fontaine et al. 1998). It soon became evident that the disease was not limited to ovariohysterectomized dogs and that none of the proposed names fit perfectly (e.g., hair loss not always confined the flank area, recurrence not a constant feature).

3.3.5.1 Etiology and pathogenesis

The etiology of CRFA remains obscure. To date, underlying causes, such as usual endocrinopathies, have not been identified (Miller and Dunstan 1993; Curtis et al. 1996; Daminet and Paradis 2000). The high incidence in some breeds and the familial character of CRFA observed in Boxers, Airedales, Affenpinschers, Griffon Korthals, and Bearded Collies suggest a genetic predisposition (Waldman 1995; Fontaine et al. 1998; Scott et al. 2001).

The seasonal nature and annual recurrence suggest that photoperiod may be involved. The higher incidence of CRFA at higher latitude (around or north of the 45° parallel) supports the importance of light exposure to this disorder. Moreover, in Australia and New Zealand, the onset of CRFA appears to be the reverse of what we see in the Northern Hemisphere (also during their short photoperiod season) (Paradis 1998).

Melatonin is involved in the neuroendocrine control of photoperiod-dependent molting in several mammalian species such as mink and foxes. Called the hormone of darkness, melatonin is primarily synthesized by the pineal gland and secreted mainly at night, with its production directly proportional to the length of the dark period. As the length of photoperiod decreases in late summer, melatonin concentration increases, initiating autumn molt and growth of winter pelage. Melatonin has been used to manipulate seasonal coat changes in a variety of species including mink and foxes (Rose et al. 1987; Valtonen et al. 1995). Mink treated with implants of melatonin in June, when natural melatonin production is very low, exhibit an early onset of autumn molt, and produced precocious prime winter pelage by mid October, 6–8 weeks earlier than normal (Rose et al. 1987).

In view of the role of melatonin in molting and hair growth, it was proposed that photoperiod might be implicated in the pathological process of CRFA and that a genetically influenced dysregulation in this hormone could be responsible for the clinical signs (Paradis 1995). At high latitude we expect high melatonin secretion in early autumn. However, it is possible that exposure to abnormally long photoperiods associated with indoor housing, characteristic to dogs living in colder climate, may contribute to the pathogenesis of CRFA. Increased daily retinal exposure to artificial light may result in a decrease in endogenous melatonin secretion, resulting in alopecia in genetically predisposed animals.

3.3.5.2 Diagnosis

CRFA is most commonly seen in Boxers, which may account for approximately half of all cases, but Airedale Terriers and English Bulldogs are also commonly affected. Other predisposed breeds include Schnauzers (miniature, standard and giant), French Bulldog, Doberman, Bouvier des Flandres, Bearded Collie, Griffon Korthals, shorthair and wirehair German Pointers, Briard, Bullmastiff, Mastiff, Rhodesian Ridgeback, Affenpinscher, Scottish Terrier, Staffordshire Terrier, Rottweiler, Labrador Retriever, Golden Retriever, and Dalmatian (Cieslowski and Paradis 1993; Miller and Dunstan 1993; Waldman 1995; Curtis et al. 1996; Fontaine et al. 1998). Although CRFA appears to affect virtually any breed, this condition is rare to absent in the plush-coated Nordic breeds, German Shepherd Dogs, and Cocker Spaniels.

3.3.5.2.1 Clinical presentation

Mean age at the onset of the first episode is 4 years, but can be quite variable (range: 8 months to 11 years). The alopecia usually develops during periods of short daylength with an onset, for the majority of dogs, between November and March in the Northern Hemisphere. Dogs of either sex and of any reproductive status can be affected. In addition, the actual month of onset does not appear to be affected by breed, age,

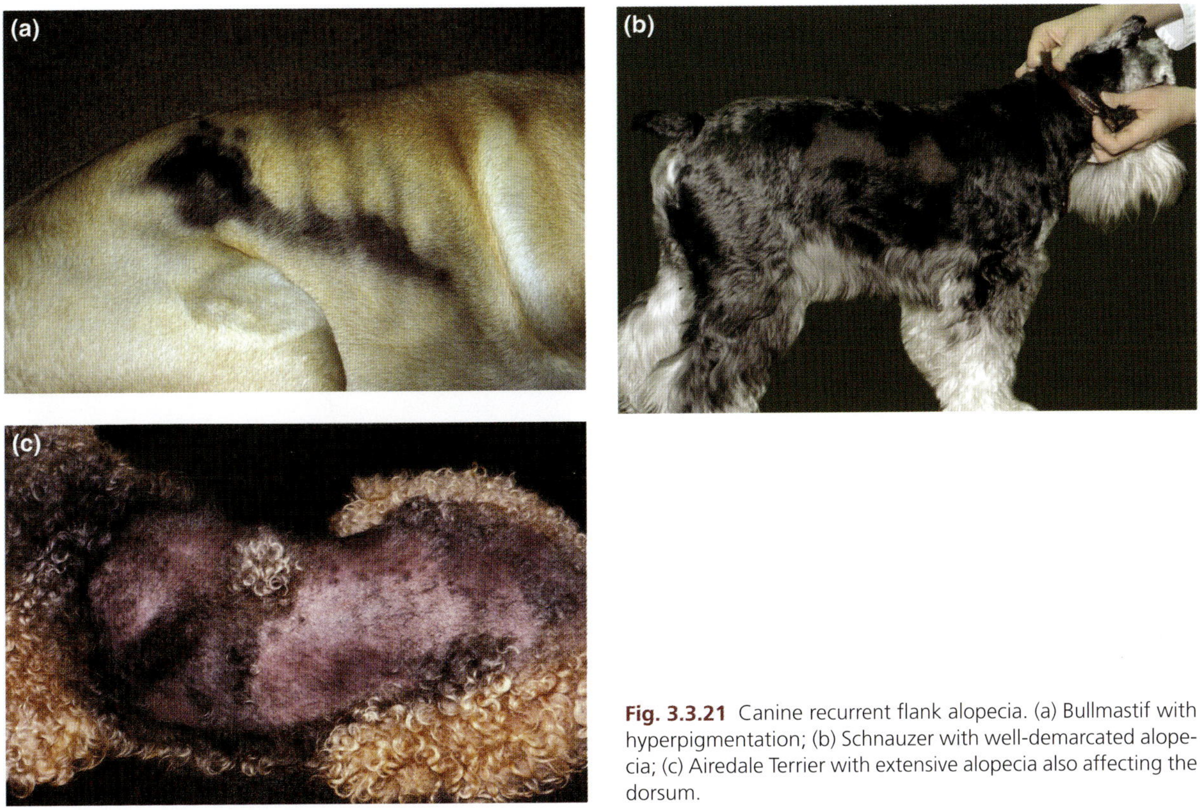

Fig. 3.3.21 Canine recurrent flank alopecia. (a) Bullmastif with hyperpigmentation; (b) Schnauzer with well-demarcated alopecia; (c) Airedale Terrier with extensive alopecia also affecting the dorsum.

sex, or sexual status (Paradis 1998; Scott et al. 2001; Paradis and Cerundolo 2003).

CRFA is characterized by a usually rapidly developing alopecia most often confined to the thoracolumbar region. Lesions are nonpruritic, nonscarring, and typically bilaterally symmetric, but on occasion only one side of the body is affected or one side is more affected than the other. The visually striking alopecic lesions have well-demarcated borders conferring a geographic image (Fig. 3.3.21). Alopecic areas are often markedly hyperpigmented and range in size from 2 cm in diameter to extensive lesions involving the whole thoracolumbar area with patch of normal coat occasionally remaining in the alopecic area (Fig. 3.3.21). Whereas hyperpigmentation is usually prominent in Boxers, it is usually absent in Wirehaired Pointers (Linek, unpublished observation).

Spontaneous regrowth of hair usually occurs within 3–8 months, but it can take much longer in some cases (range: 1–14 months). New hair growth usually consists of normal pelage quality and density. Some individuals (particularly boxers) may grow darker hair in the previously affected areas and some Miniature Schnauzers may regrow hair of a golden color (aurotrichia) (Fig. 3.3.22). Uncommonly, hair regrowth may become less complete following several episodes of affliction. Rarely, some cases eventually progress

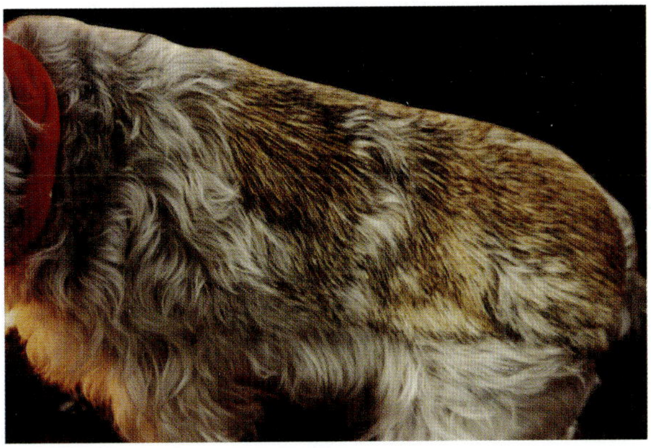

Fig. 3.3.22 Aurotrichia in CRFA. Miniature Schnauzer with regrowth of darker and golden hair.

to a permanent flank alopecia and marked skin hyperpigmentation (Paradis and Cerundolo 2003; Gross et al. 2005).

The majority of the CRFA cases develop recurrent alopecic episodes year after year; however, up to 20% of cases may only have one isolated episode of flank alopecia during their whole life. Some dogs have an occasional year when the alopecia does not recur. The extent of alopecia is variable, with some dogs developing a virtually identical area and duration of hair loss year after year, and other dogs developing more extensive areas and/or longer episodes of hair loss as years go by (Paradis and Cerundolo 2003).

Rarely, alopecias at the bridge of the nose, the base of the ears, the base of the tail, and/or the perineum, which also manifest a spontaneous regrowth and recurrence, have been observed in conjunction with thoracolumbar alopecia in some Airedales, Golden Retrievers, Griffon Korthals, Dobermans, Wirehaired Pointers, and Giant Schnauzers (Paradis and Cerundolo 2003).

The diagnosis of CRFA is based on history, clinical signs, exclusion of endocrinopathies such as hypothyroidism, and skin biopsies.

3.3.5.2.2 Histopathology

The histopathologic findings are greatly influenced by the stage of the disease when biopsy specimens are obtained. The fairly distinctive findings in active lesions are characterized by follicles with marked infundibular orthokeratotic hyperkeratosis extending to secondary follicles ("witch's feet" or "octopus-like hair follicles"). Most hair follicles are in various stages of catagen; some may be in telogen (Fig. 3.3.23). Most hair follicles will be in early or late stages of anagen, if biopsies are taken during the regression phase, shortly before new hair shafts appear on the skin (Fig. 3.3.24). The described follicular findings are suggestive of, but not pathognomonic of, CRFA (Miller and Dunstan 1993; Yager and Wilcock 1994; Scott et al. 2001; Gross et al. 2005). These changes are not always present and may be found occasionally in other alopecic diseases. In lesions with profound follicular inactivity and hyperpigmentation, one might also observe sebaceous gland hyperpigmentation and melanin aggregates in the follicular lumen (Bagladi et al. 1996; Scott et al. 2001), suggesting a rapid and premature catagen induction similar to hair follicle dystrophy.

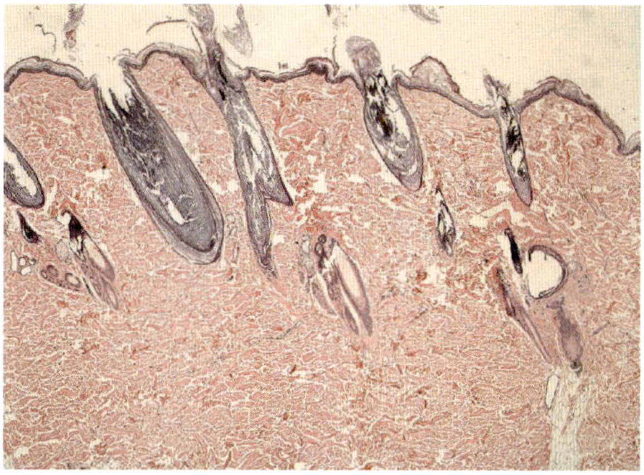

Fig. 3.3.23 Skin histology of CRFA. Dilation and hyperkeratosis of the follicular infundibulum. All hair follicles are in late catagen/telogen with club hairs.

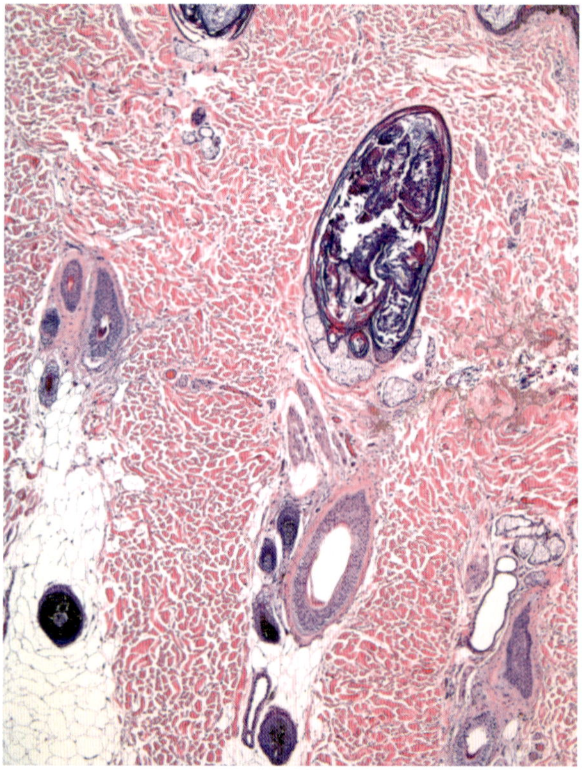

Fig. 3.3.24 Skin histology of CRFA in remission. Note presence of dilated follicular infundibula and anagen hair bulbs.

3.3.5.2.3 Differential diagnoses of CRFA

In dogs presented for a first episode, endocrinopathies, such as hypothyroidism (see Section 3.3.1), hyperadrenocorticism (see Section 3.3.2), hyperestrogenism (see Section 3.3.3), or breed-specific hair cycle abnormalities (see Section 3.3.9), need to be ruled out. Hypothyroidism, considering its high incidence in dogs, is an important differential diagnosis. Some canine breeds predisposed to lymphocytic thyroiditis and hypothyroidism (e.g., Airedales, Boxers, and German Pointers) are also at high risk for developing CRFA. Age of onset is also similar for these two disorders. Of note, some cases of CRFA can occur in dogs as young as 10 months; however, clinical hypothyroidism is virtually nonexistent in dogs less than 2 years of age. Not unexpected, however, hypothyroidism and CRFA can both occur in the same animal (Daminet and Paradis 2000). This can occasionally represent a real diagnostic and therapeutic challenge. On the other hand, hypothyroidism is not commonly associated with the rapid onset, bilaterally symmetrical, noninflammatory alopecia. Instead, cutaneous changes are typically insidious, slowly progressive, and usually begin with a dull brittle hair coat and seborrhea. Hypotrichosis and eventually alopecia often develop along the bridge of the nose, tail, and other frictional areas, much before the development of flank alopecia. When the latter occurs, metabolic signs (e.g., lethargy, weight gain) are generally obvious. Fortunately, results of thyroid function in cases of CRFA will often be within normal reference values and hypothyroidism ruled out in most cases. However, results may occasionally suggest a diagnosis of hypothyroidism and hair regrowth may coincide with levothyroxine administration. It is only several months later, when the hair loss occurs again in spite of the levothyroxine administration, that the puzzled clinician will then realize that the initial hair growth was coincidental and not related to thyroid hormone supplementation. In any case, due to lack of sensitivity and specificity of the various diagnostic tests currently available to evaluate canine thyroid function, one must always be vigilant when interpreting test results.

The hair cycle abnormality described in Portuguese Water Dogs (see Section 3.3.9.2) appears to be a distinct clinical disorder from CRFA, even if the hair loss can spontaneously regress and recur (Miller and Scott 1995). Distinctive histopathologic findings have been reported. These include abnormal melanization of the pilosebaceous units, prominent apoptosis of keratinocytes in the inner and outer root sheaths, and dissolution of the hair matrix of anagen hair follicles. The Irish Water Spaniel is also inflicted by a similar follicular disease that is often cyclical initially (Cerundolo et al. 2000). Histopathology reveals features similar to CRFA and abnormal melanization (as in color dilution alopecia and black hair follicular dysplasia) as well as, occasionally, excessive trichilemmal keratinization ("flame follicles") as seen in alopecia X.

Recently, a puzzling recurrent or persistent flank alopecia and interface dermatitis were reported in nine Boxers (Rachid et al. 2003). The interface dermatitis was characterized by multifocal annular, crusted lesions confined to the areas of follicular disease. The inflammatory lesions were neither pruritic nor painful, and affected dogs were otherwise healthy. Histopathologically, the inflammatory lesions were characterized by an interface dermatitis. Immunohistochemical studies failed to demonstrate immunoglobulins or complement at the basement membrane zone or within blood vessel walls. In dogs with recurrent or persistent disease, the follicular disease and interface dermatitis ran parallel courses of spontaneous remission and recurrence, or persistence, respectively. The relationship between the two histological reaction patterns is not known. It is possible that mild lesions of erythema ab igne (radiant heat dermatitis) are superimposed on CRFA lesions in some of those cases.

At last, spontaneous hair regrowth can be observed in telogen effluvium (see Section 3.3.6), post-clipping alopecia (see Section 3.3.7), erythema ab igne (radiant heat dermatitis), and some cases of demodicosis (see Section 4.1.3) and dermatophytosis (see Section 4.1.2) (Scott et al. 2001; Paradis and Cerundolo 2003). However, the distinctive history and clinical features of CRFA generally allows easy differentiation from these conditions.

3.3.5.3 Therapy

Aside for the cosmetic aspect of the disease, dogs with CRFA are healthy otherwise. Nonetheless, the apparent familial implication of CRFA requires caution when selecting breeding animals, as it may be preferable not to reproduce dogs affected by this disorder.

3.3.5.3.1 *Melatonin*

The efficacy of melatonin in preventing CRFA was evaluated in a pilot study of nine dogs who had previously suffered at least three consecutive episodes of CRFA (Paradis 1995). They received subcutaneous melatonin implants around the autumnal equinox, approximately 2 months before the next anticipated episode of alopecia. None of them developed alopecia in the winter following the melatonin treatment. The unpredictable course of CRFA and the spontaneous regrowth of hair render the evaluation of any therapeutic agent difficult, whether used to prevent an anticipated episode of alopecia or to shorten an existing episode, and all attempts at conducting randomized placebo-controlled trials have failed. Nevertheless, several veterinary dermatologists have since used melatonin in CRFA either to prevent recurrence or, more frequently, to shorten the duration of an existing alopecic episode. On the basis of the anecdotal information, apparent successes are obtained in approximately 50–75% of cases, with melatonin administered either orally or subcutaneously (Paradis 1999, 2002). Randomized placebo-controlled trials are needed to corroborate the anecdotal claims of efficacy.

Although implants commercially available in the fox fur industry were used in the initial study, oral administration of melatonin is currently recommended (Paradis 1999, 2002). Melatonin tablets are sold in either drug stores or health food stores in several countries. Treatment regimen for CRFA consists typically of 3–6 mg/dog administered orally every 8–12 h for 1–2 months, although it is becoming apparent that this relatively high dose and/or frequency of administration is not always essential. Treatment should be initiated shortly after the onset of alopecia or 1–2 months before an anticipated episode. It is unlikely that treatment duration beyond 2 months will result in an increased success rate because it was shown in mink that activation of hair follicles by melatonin occurs during a 4–6 week period and this photoperiodic signal does not seem necessary for later pelage growth and maturation (Valtonen et al. 1995). Therefore, this treatment regimen would seem appropriate if melatonin is used as a nonspecific anagen hair cycle inducer. On the other hand, a longer duration of treatment and possibly a much higher dose of melatonin might be needed, if modulation of sex-hormone secretion is required.

Melatonin is apparently safe but owners should be informed on the off-label use of this drug. In addition, due to its interaction with reproductive hormone it is preferable to avoid its use in breeding animals (Ashley et al. 1999), although it is not recommended to reproduce dogs affected with CRFA.

3.3.5.3.2 *Minoxidil*

Minoxidil, a vasodilator used topically in humans with androgenic alopecia, was used orally in dogs with what appears to be CRFA (Scott et al. 2001). Some dogs regrew hair; however, this might have been due to the spontaneous regrowth normally seen in CRFA. In any case, side effects (e.g., weakness, lethargy, collapses) were seen in 50% of the dogs treated; oral minoxidil treatment is therefore not recommended.

References

Ashley P, Frank LA, Schmietzel LP, Bailey EM, Olivier JW. 1999. Effect of oral melatonin administration on sex hormone, prolactin, and thyroid hormone concentrations in adult dogs. *Journal of American Veterinary Medical Association* 215:1111–1115.

Bagladi MS, Scott DW, Miller WH. 1996. Sebaceous gland melanosis in dogs with endocrine skin disease or follicular dysplasia. A retrospective study. *Veterinary Dermatology Journal* 7:85–90.

Cerundolo R, Lloyd DH, McNeil PE, Evans H. 2000. An analysis of factors underlying hypotrichosis and alopecia in Irish water Spaniels in the United Kingdom. *Veterinary Dermatology Journal* 11:107–122.

Cieslowski D, Paradis M. 1993. Alopécie saisonnière canine. *Médecin Vétérinaire du Québec* 23:98.

Curtis CF, Evans H, Lloyd DH. 1996. Investigation of reproductive and growth hormone status of dogs affected by idiopathic recurrent flank alopecia. *Journal of Small Animal Practice* 37:417–422.

Daminet S, Paradis M. 2000. Evaluation of thyroid function in dogs suffering from recurrent flank alopecia. *Canadian Veterinary Journal* 41:699–703.

Fontaine J, Beco L, Paradis M. 1998. Alopécie récidivante des flancs: à propos de 12 cas chez le griffon Korthals. *Point Vétérinaire* 29:445–449.

Gross TL, Ihrke PJ, Walder EJ, Affolter VK. 2005. *Skin Diseases of the Dog and Cat: Clinical and Histopathologic Diagnosis*, 2nd edn. Oxford: Blackwell Publishing.

Miller MA, Dunstan RW. 1993. Seasonal flank alopecia in boxers and Airedale terriers: 24 cases (1985–1992). *Journal of the American Veterinary Medical Association* 203:1567–1572.

Miller WH, Scott DW. 1995. Follicular dysplasia of the Portuguese water dogs. *Veterinary Dermatology Journal* 6:67–74.

Paradis M. 1995. Canine recurrent flank alopecia: treatment with melatonin. *Proceedings of the 11th AAVD/ACVD Meeting*, Santa Fe, NM, p. 49.

Paradis M. 1998. Canine flank alopecia. Derm Dialogue. *Bulletin of the American Academy of Veterinary Dermatology* Summer:10–13.

Paradis M. 1999. Melatonin therapy in canine alopecia. In: Bonadura ED (ed.), *Kirk's Current Veterinary Therapy XIII*, pp. 546–549. Philadelphia: WB Saunders.

Paradis M. 2002. Melatonin. Roundtable summaries. *Derm Dialogue* Winter:12–13.
Paradis M, Cerundolo R. 2003. An approach to symmetrical alopecia in the dog. In: Foster A, Foil C (eds), *BSAVA Manual of Small Animal Dermatology*, 2nd edn. Ames, Iowa: Wiley-Blackwell. pp. 83–93.
Rachid MA, Demaula CD, Scott DW, Miller WH, Senter DA, Myers S. 2003. Concurrent follicular dysplasia and interface dermatitis in Boxer dogs. *Veterinary Dermatology Journal* 14:159–166.
Rose J, Oldfield J, Stromshak F. 1987. Apparent role of melatonin and prolactin in initiating winter fur growth in mink. *General and Comparative Endocrinology* 65:212–215.
Scott DW. 1990. Seasonal flank alopecia in ovariohysterectomized dogs. *Cornell Veterinarian* 80:187–195.
Scott DW, Miller WH, Griffin CE (eds). 2001. *Muller and Kirk's Small Animal Dermatology*, 6th edn. Philadelphia: WB Saunders.
Scott DW, Walton DK. 1986. Hyposomatotropism in the mature dog: a discussion of 22 cases. *Journal of American Animal Hospital Association* 22:467–473.
Shanley KJ, Miller WH. 1987. Adult onset growth hormone deficiency in siblings Airedale terriers. *Compendium of Continuing Education for the Practicing Veterinarian* 9:1076–1082.
Valtonen M, Vakkuri P, Blomsted L. 1995. Autumnal timing of photoperiodic manipulation critical via melatonin to winter pelage development in mink. *Journal of Animal Sciences* 61:589–596.
Waldman L. 1995. Seasonal flank alopecia in affenpinschers. *Journal of Small Animal Practice* 36:272–273.
Yager JA, Wilcock BP. 1994. *Color Atlas and Text of Surgical Pathology of the Dog and Cat.* London, England: Mosby Year Book.

3.3.6 Telogen effluvium

Rosario Cerundolo

3.3.6.1 Canine telogen effluvium

Telogen effluvium (syn. defluxion) is an abnormality of hair follicle cycling, characterized by excessive loss of telogen hairs. It is the result of synchronization of the hair follicle cycle that leads all the hair follicles to undergo simultaneous anagen development. This results clinically in simultaneous shedding of the old club hair and hence may cause temporary alopecia, known as "telogen effluvium." This condition is commonly associated with stressful events such as pregnancy, parturition, lactation, severe systemic illness, marked febrile episodes, shock, surgery, and various drugs (Harrison and Sinclair 2002).

3.3.6.1.1 Etiology and pathogenesis

In human dermatology, hair follicle effluvium is subdivided into five different clinical types (Headington 1993). These are (i) immediate anagen release, (ii) delayed anagen release, (iii) short anagen syndrome, (iv) immediate telogen release, and (v) delayed telogen release. The first two are conditions where the hair growth cycle of many follicles becomes synchronized. Immediate anagen release is a short onset effluvium where follicles are stimulated to leave anagen and enter telogen prematurely, resulting in an increased hair shedding at the end of telogen approximately 2–3 months later. It is common after a physiologic stress such as severe illness, and with drug-induced hair loss. Reversal is associated with resumption of the normal cycle. Delayed anagen release is the cause of postpartum hair loss. During pregnancy, hairs remain in prolonged anagen rather than cycling into telogen. If a large number of follicles are involved, postpartum telogen conversion will be accompanied by increased shedding some months later. Short anagen syndrome is due to an idiopathic shortening of the duration of anagen and can cause a persistent telogen hair shedding in some individuals. Immediate telogen release results from a shortening of normal telogen with release of club hairs as the follicles are stimulated to reenter anagen. This is common in patients starting therapy with minoxidil. Discontinuation of minoxidil, which prolongs the duration of anagen, will precipitate telogen release. Delayed telogen release occurs after a prolonged telogen followed by transition to anagen. It occurs in animals with synchronous hair cycles during shedding of their winter coats. It may occur in some humans seasonally.

A similar subdivision has not been elaborated for domestic animals yet, and it is unlikely that it would contribute to a better understanding or management of this condition in veterinary medicine. No scientific studies have been published on telogen effluvium in domestic animals. There are only anecdotal reports or book citations that describe telogen effluvium in dogs and cats (Scott et al. 2000).

3.3.6.1.2 Diagnosis

Patchy to diffuse alopecia occurs within a few weeks or months and usually affects the trunk. Hairs are easily epilated (Fig. 3.3.25). Differential diagnoses of telogen effluvium are chemotherapy-induced alopecia and endocrine alopecia such as hypothyroidism, hyperadrenocorticism, and hyperestrogenism. The history should help to identify chemotherapy-induced alopecia, since histologically, during its late stage, it is

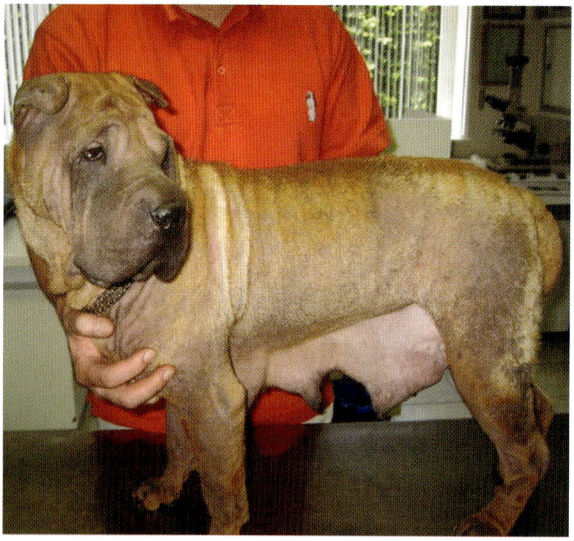

Fig. 3.3.25 Telogen effluvium in a Shar-Pei that developed 4 weeks postpartum. Note extensive alopecia of the face and trunk. (Courtesy of J. Declercq.)

similar to telogen effluvium caused by other mechanisms. Endocrine alopecia can be ruled out by other clinical signs and laboratory tests.

Diagnosis of telogen effluvium should be based on a trichogram that shows telogen hairs, characterized by minimal or absent pigmentation. Skin biopsies should be collected from the most severely affected areas in the early phase of hair loss, because samples collected late will only show normal anagen hair follicles indicative of the recovery phase. In early lesions, hair follicles are in telogen, but in the remission phase they are predominantly in anagen. There is no evidence of follicular atrophy and there may be diminution of follicular size compatible with the hair cycle (Gross 2005).

3.3.6.1.3 Therapy

Specific therapy is not required as hair regrowth occurs completely a few months after the cause of the underlying stress has been resolved.

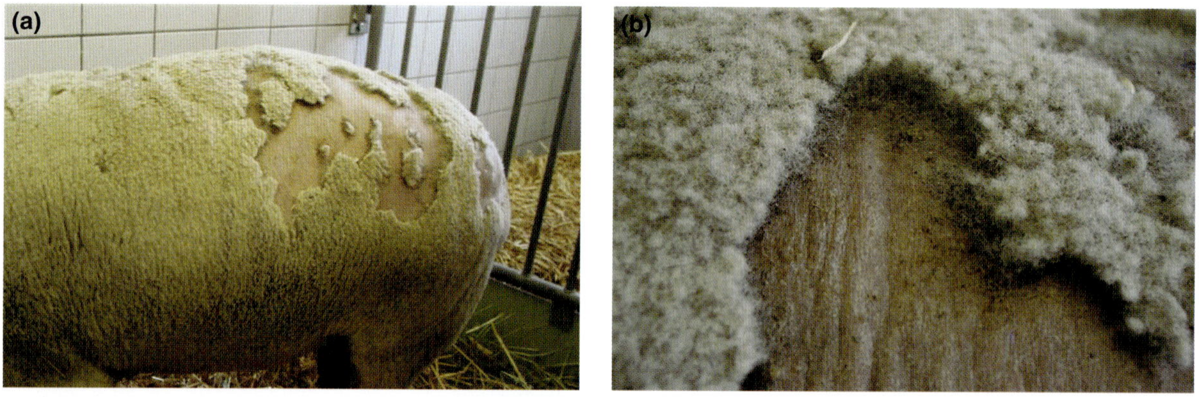

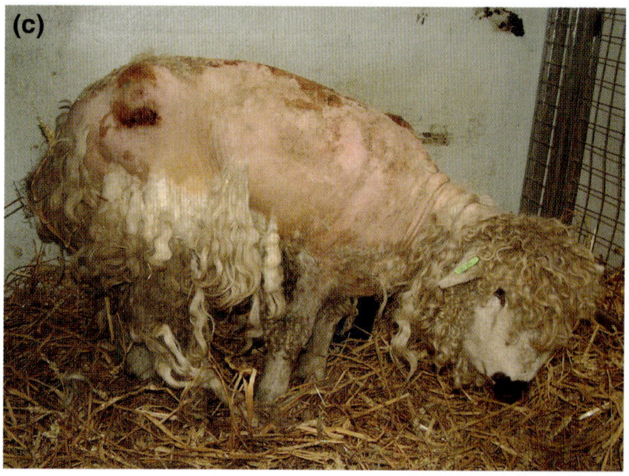

Fig. 3.3.26 Telogen arrest in sheep known as "wool slip." Well-demarcated alopecia on the trunk. ((a,b) Courtesy of S. Rüfenacht; (c) Courtesy of N. Sargison.)

3.3.6.2 Ovine telogen effluvium (wool slip)

"Wool slip" in sheep is a form of patchy alopecia developing in housed ewes that are shorn in winter (Morgan et al. 1986). It may, however, also occur in the summer months (French et al. 1990). The pathogenesis of this condition is still unknown. It has been suggested that wool slip is due to stressful events such as housing and shearing. It is likely that stressful shearing may induce release of high levels of corticosteroids as the hair loss is similar to the one induced by the use of corticosteroids in sheep. Wool slip does not occur when sheep are sheared during the summer months. The reason for this discrepancy is unclear. It is possible that other factors such as the low environmental temperature combined with shearing may play a role in hair loss. Wool slip occurring during the summer months may be triggered by post-lambing early lactation (French et al. 1990).

No breed or sex predisposition has been described. Affected sheep show multifocal areas of alopecia occurring on the back (Fig. 3.3.26). Skin biopsies from affected areas show early anagen hair follicles. Unaffected sheep at the same time of the year would normally show telogen hair follicles, thus suggesting that wool slip is a premature, synchronous shedding of hair (i.e., telogen effluvium), most likely due to high levels of corticosteroids that occur as a result of the combination of housing and shearing (Morgan et al. 1986).

No specific therapy has been reported. Changes in housing and husbandry management may avoid the occurrence of this condition.

References

French NP, Morgan KL, Fell C. 1990. Wool slip in Wiltshire horns. *Veterinary Record* 127(10):267.

Gross TL. 2005. Atrophic diseases of the adnexa. In: Gross TL, Ihrke PJ, Walder EJ, Affolter VK (eds), *Skin Diseases of the Dog and Cat: Clinical and Histopathologic Diagnosis*, 2nd edn, pp. 480–517. Oxford: Blackwell Science.

Harrison S, Sinclair R. 2002. Telogen effluvium. *Clinical and Experimental Dermatology* 27(5):389–385.

Headington JT. 1993. Telogen effluvium. New concepts and review. *Archives in Dermatology* 129(3):356–363.

Morgan KL, Brown PJ, Wright AI, Steele FC, Baker AS. 1986. An investigation into the aetiology of 'wool slip': alopecia in ewes which are housed and shorn in winter. *Veterinary Record* 119(25–26):621–625.

Scott DW, Miller WH, Griffin CE. 2000. *Muller & Kirk's Small Animal Dermatology*, 6th edn. Philadelphia: WB Saunders.

3.3.7 Canine postclipping alopecia

Rosario Cerundolo

3.3.7.1 Etiology and pathogenesis

Postclipping alopecia (PCA) is a very confusing disease for many veterinarians. It is characterized by a lack of hair regrowth after close clipping. It usually affects Northern breeds that have guard hairs and thick undercoats, such as the Siberian Husky, Alaskan Malamute, Samoyed, and the American Eskimo Dog. True plush-coated dogs such as Pomeranians and Chow Chows, which lack guard hairs, are also reported to be predisposed to true PCA. It has been proposed that these breeds normally have a hair follicle cycle with a prolonged telogen phase, which possibly developed as an energy-saving device in extremely cold climates, so they do not have to shed and regrow their coat (Credille et al. 2001). Possible pathogenetic factors are a yet unexplained pathological hair cycle arrest or thermal factors such as decreased temperature caused by shaving, since the undercoat would normally be expected to keep a high temperature at the skin level.

The geographic region where dogs live might also play an important role in this condition. If they are genetically meant to live in an environment with prolonged darkness and low temperature, it may be that they become abnormal when they are moved to a different environment.

Although there have been studies on hair regrowth after clipping in various canine breeds, no scientific studies or case reports have been published on this topic in Nordic breeds, but there are only anecdotal reports or book citations (Scott et al. 2000; Diaz et al. 2004, 2006).

3.3.7.2 Diagnosis

There is a lack of hair regrowth at the site of the previous clipping that may have occurred months before. Common sites are the one clipped for venipuncture, surgery, mat removal, or procedures such as myelography or epidural anesthesia (Fig. 3.3.27). Mild scaling may be occasionally seen. Differential diagnoses are endocrinopathies such as hypothyroidism (see Section 3.3.1) or hyperadrenocorticism (see Section 3.3.2) that

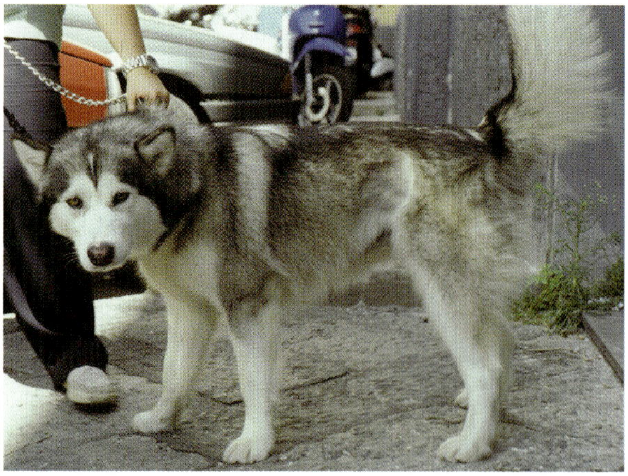

Fig. 3.3.27 Postclipping alopecia in an Alaskan Malamute following clipping for sonography. Note the well-circumscribed area of alopecia in the flank region; the hair coat regrew after 10 months.

also often cause lack of hair regrowth after clipping, and alopecia X (see Section 3.3.4).

Postclipping alopecia is diagnosed by the signalment, the history, and the clinical presentation. Routine blood/urine and hormonal tests should be carried out to rule out an underlying endocrinopathy. Skin biopsies should be collected from areas of complete alopecia. They will reveal mostly telogen hair follicles and eventually mild epidermal hyperkeratosis. Telogen hair shafts are retained. Very few hair follicles in late catagen may be seen (Gross 2005; Walder 2005).

3.3.7.3 Therapy

If there is no underlying endocrinopathy, the hair regrows in 6–12 months, which is a longer period of time than the 3-month average recently documented in Labrador Retrievers (Diaz et al. 2004). Newly regrown hairs may be initially dark in color, especially in breeds with "pointed" hairs such as the Siberian Husky and the Alaskan Malamute (Gross 2005). It is recommended to never shave sled dogs, unless it is absolutely necessary.

References

Credille KM, Slater MR, Moriello KA, Nachreiner RF, Tucker KA, Dunstan RW. 2001. The effects of thyroid hormones on the skin of Beagle dogs. *Journal of Veterinary Internal Medicine* 15:539–546.

Diaz SF, Torres SM, Dunstan RW, Lekcharoensuk C. 2004. An analysis of canine hair re-growth after clipping for a surgical procedure. *Veterinary Dermatology* 15(1):25–30.

Diaz SF, Torres SM, Nogueira SA, Gilbert S, Jessen CR. 2006. The impact of body site, topical melatonin and brushing on hair regrowth after clipping normal Siberian husky dogs. *Veterinary Dermatology* 17(1):45–50.

Gross TL. 2005. Atrophic diseases of the adnexa. In: Gross TL, Ihrke PJ, Walder EJ, Affolter VK (eds), *Skin Diseases of the Dog and Cat: Clinical and Histopathologic Diagnosis*, 2nd edn, pp. 480–517. Oxford: Blackwell Science.

Scott DW, Miller WH, Griffin CE. 2000. *Muller and Kirk's Small Animal Dermatology*, 6th edn. Philadelphia: WB Saunders.

Walder EJ. 2005. Genodermatosis: alopecia and hypotrichosis. In: Hillier A, Foster AP, Kwochka KW (eds), *Advances in Veterinary Dermatology*, Vol. 5, pp. 360–364. Oxford: Blackwell Science.

3.3.8 Canine pattern alopecia

Manon Paradis

Canine pattern alopecia (CPA, syn. canine pattern baldness) is a relatively common but poorly studied skin disorder characterized by an acquired bilaterally symmetric hair loss. Different syndromes have been described depending on the body areas involved.

3.3.8.1 Etiology and pathogenesis

CPA is a breed-specific folliculopathy, somehow similar to but clearly not identical to "human pattern baldness," that is, human androgenetic alopecia (Kaufman et al. 1998; Whiting 2001). The term "canine pattern baldness," initially used by analogy to the human disease, should be abandoned and replaced by "canine pattern alopecia," because an androgen receptor dysfunction, as seen in man with androgenic alopecia, has not been proven. The pathogenesis of CPA is currently not known. A central endocrine disorder has been ruled out, but the involvement of an abnormality in a hormone receptor on the hair follicle is still debatable.

CPA may be an overshoot reaction to artificial selection pressure favoring the fine, delicate coat sought by breeders who often attempt to manipulate the appearance of a dog without considering possible genetic damage (Paradis and Cerundolo 2005). Over the last decades, smooth hair Dachshund breeders have been able to significantly decrease the incidence of "ventral type" CPA by selective breeding but with the result of dogs generally having a coat not as fine.

3.3.8.2 Diagnosis

The diagnosis of CPA is based on history, dermatological examination, and exclusion of endocrinopathies such as hypothyroidism (see Section 3.3.1) and hyperadrenocorticism (see Section 3.3.2) and of inflammatory diseases such as alopecia areata (see Chapter 4.7). However, the early onset of CPA and breed predisposition make it quite distinctive from most of these disorders. Congenital alopecia (see Chapter 3.1) may need to be excluded in some cases.

3.3.8.2.1 Clinical presentation

3.3.8.2.1.1 Ventral-type pattern alopecia

The most common syndrome "CPA ventral type" is characterized by a progressive alopecia developing along the ventral neck, chest and abdomen, the caudomedial aspect of thighs, perineum, and the postauricular regions (base of the ear pinnae). These dogs are born with normal coats, but after 6 months of age a gradually progressing hair loss develops in these body regions (Fig. 3.3.28). This will progress for one year or so, leaving the affected areas partially to completely alopecic. The remaining hairs appear finer than normal. It has been reported that this syndrome is seen almost exclusively in females (Scott et al. 2001); however, the disease is also seen quite frequently in male dogs. The actual prevalence in males and females is unknown.

"CPA ventral type" is seen in several breeds of dogs with a "short/fine" type of hair coat such as Dachshund, Chihuahuas, Miniature Pinschers, Whippets, Greyhound, Italian Greyhound, Boston Terrier, Manchester Terrier, and Boxer. (Scott et al. 2001; Gross et al. 2005; Paradis and Cerundolo 2005). Due to awareness of Dachshund breeders and careful breeding program, the frequency of occurrence of this syndrome has apparently decreased in this breed.

"Bald thigh syndrome of Greyhound dogs" is a poorly defined disorder generally described as hair loss at the caudolateral and/or lateral aspect of the thighs of racing Greyhounds (Schoning and Cowan 2000). It may represent "CPA ventral type," but could also be caused by a yet unknown hair cycle abnormality (see Section 3.3.9.5).

3.3.8.2.1.2 Pinnal-type pattern alopecia

"CPA pinnal type" (syn. "canine pinnal alopecia") is another syndrome of CPA, seen much less commonly than "CPA ventral type." It is observed mainly in Smooth-haired and Wirehaired Dachshunds. The dogs are born with a normal hair coat but develop a characteristic progressive alopecia restricted to the entire convex aspect of pinna (Fig. 3.3.29). It is reported that the alopecia starts around 6–9 months of age and may progress over several years to a completely bald and hyperpigmented pinna (Scott et al. 2001). However, in some cases, the alopecia may be apparent only after 2 years of age and may spontaneously regress with possible recurrences over the years. Some dogs may also develop alopecia on the bridge of the nose.

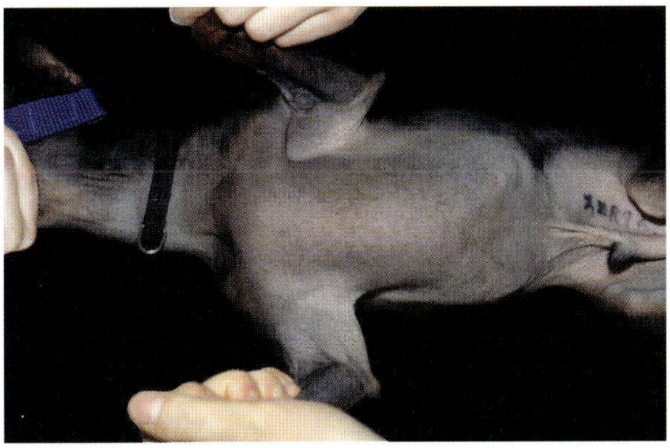

Fig. 3.3.28 Canine pattern alopecia, ventral type, in a Miniature Pinscher. Note alopecia of neck, axilla, and abdomen.

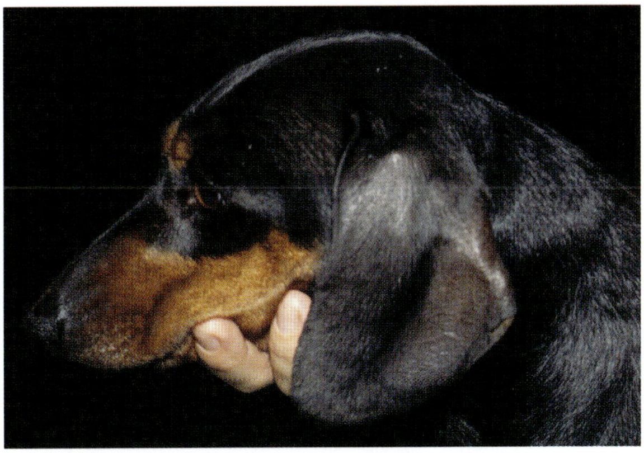

Fig. 3.3.29 Canine pattern alopecia, pinnal type, in a dachshund. Multifocal alopecia on ear pinna and nose.

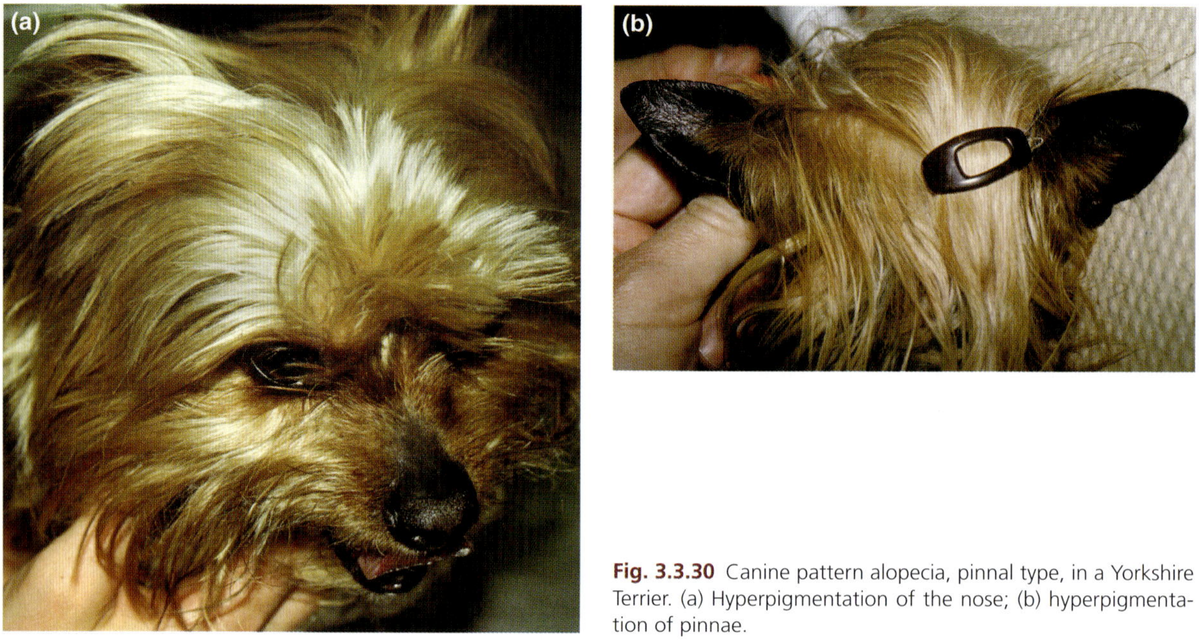

Fig. 3.3.30 Canine pattern alopecia, pinnal type, in a Yorkshire Terrier. (a) Hyperpigmentation of the nose; (b) hyperpigmentation of pinnae.

Although it is reported in the literature that males are most commonly affected (Scott et al. 2001), it is also seen in females. The actual prevalence in males and females is not known.

"Alopecia and melanoderma of Yorkshire Terrier" is clinically very similar to "CPA pinnal type" and may in fact be a different appellation for the same disorder. It is characterized by an acquired alopecia and progressive hyperpigmentation restricted to the convex aspect of pinnae and bridge of the nose (Scott et al. 2001) (Fig. 3.3.30). Although most dogs remain affected throughout their lifetime, some may recover spontaneously.

Pinnal alopecia can also be seen in Dachshunds with canine ear margin seborrhea. However, scaling and crusting is the predominant feature and alopecia is mostly marginal (Scott et al. 2001; Gross et al. 2005).

3.3.8.2.2 Histopathology

Skin biopsies are rarely required to confirm a diagnosis of CPA, but might be useful in some cases, at least to rule out other disorders. Skin biopsies are not frequently performed in CPA, in part due to the biopsy sites often requiring general anesthesia and the possible permanent visible scarring at biopsy sites. If hair loss is present on regions besides the pinnae, other sites should be selected as pinnal biopsies may lead to damaged cartilage, prominent scarring, and distortion (Gross et al. 2005).

The dermatohistopathologic findings in CPA are not well defined, and in early cases abnormal features can only be appreciated if a section from an affected skin is compared with a normal one. The changes observed can be subtle and at low power CPA might look like an endocrinopathy, so clinicopathologic correlation is critical.

The findings are characterized by miniaturization of anagen hair follicles (Yager and Wilcock 1994; Scott et al. 2001; Gross et al. 2005). Since many biopsies are taken in a late stage of the disease, it might be difficult to confirm the presence of anagen follicles (Paradis and Cerundolo 2005). Proliferation markers such as Ki67 could be used to prove that the cells of the follicular bulb are cycling, confirming that attenuated anagen follicles are present. Hair follicles are characterized by moderate to severe decrease in size and length with fine residual hair shaft, but overall hair follicle units are present in normal numbers and most are in anagen (Yager and Wilcock 1994; Gross et al. 2005) (Fig. 3.3.31).

Secondary features of CPA are keratin accumulation in the small follicles and infundibular melanin clumping caused by shrinkage following apoptosis that

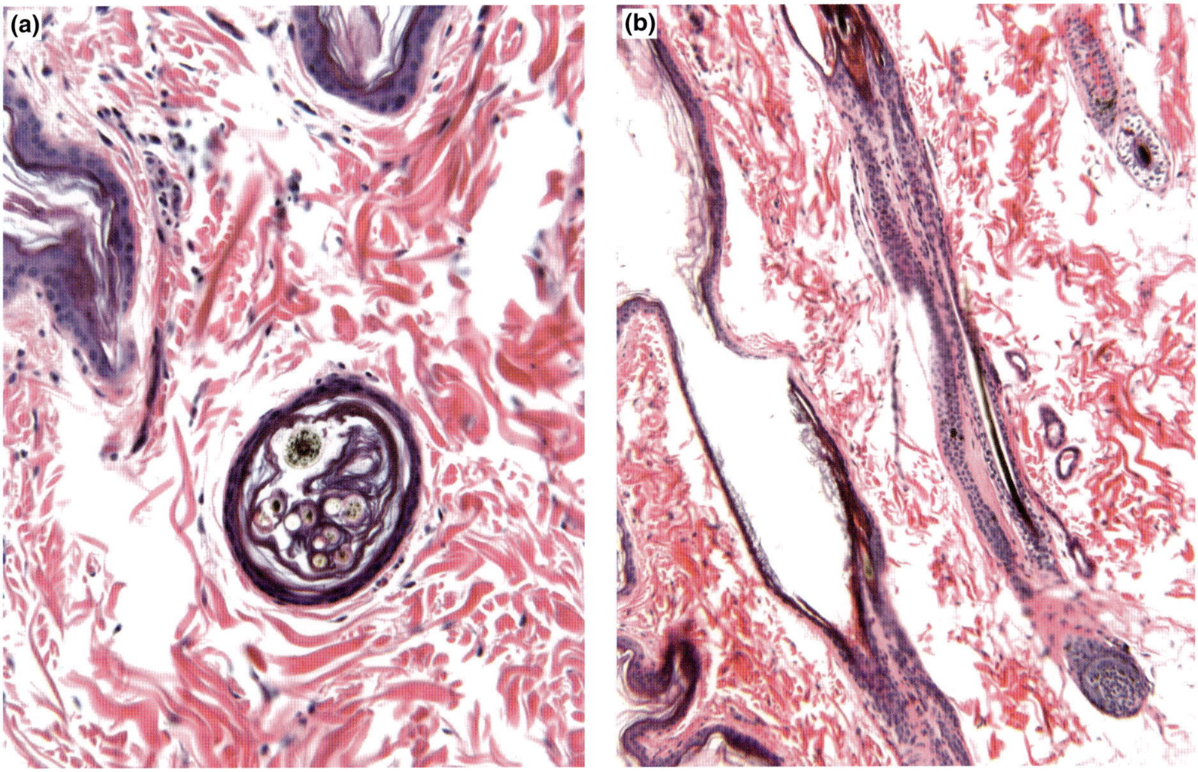

Fig. 3.3.31 Skin histology of canine pattern baldness. (a) Small diameter hair shafts in the follicular infundibulum; (b) both anagen and catagen hair follicles occur; hair shafts are small.

then drops out and accumulates in macrophages. The epidermis is generally unremarkable except for some degree of hyperpigmentation in chronic alopecic cases (Paradis and Cerundolo 2005).

3.3.8.3 Therapy

Spontaneous hair regrowth in CPA is uncommon, but it has been observed, at least in occasional cases of "CPA pinnal type." Most dogs with CPA are not treated, because it is a cosmetic problem only and also because there is no known effective treatment, aside for the possible beneficial effect of melatonin, estrogen, and finasteride.

3.3.8.3.1 Estrogen

Estrogen is indeed potentially effective if the so-called estrogen-responsive alopecia and "CPA ventral type" are the same entity (Scott et al. 2001). Indeed, the existence of this distinct disorder is doubtful since most cases described in the literature were most likely the cases of "CPA ventral type," or less commonly cases of canine recurrent flank alopecia and canine alopecia X. Nevertheless, because of serious adverse reactions seen with exogenous administration of estrogens, therapeutic trial with this hormone is not recommended for such a benign and purely aesthetic disorder.

3.3.8.3.2 Melatonin

In a study evaluating the efficacy of melatonin in canine recurrent flank alopecia, two Boxers with concurrent CPA ventral type experienced an impressive hair growth in the chest and ventral neck areas where hair coat was previously sparse to absent (Paradis 1995). On the basis of these unexpected findings, a pilot study was then conducted to evaluate the efficacy of melatonin in the treatment of canine CPA (Paradis 1996). Eleven purebred dogs affected with "CPA ventral type"

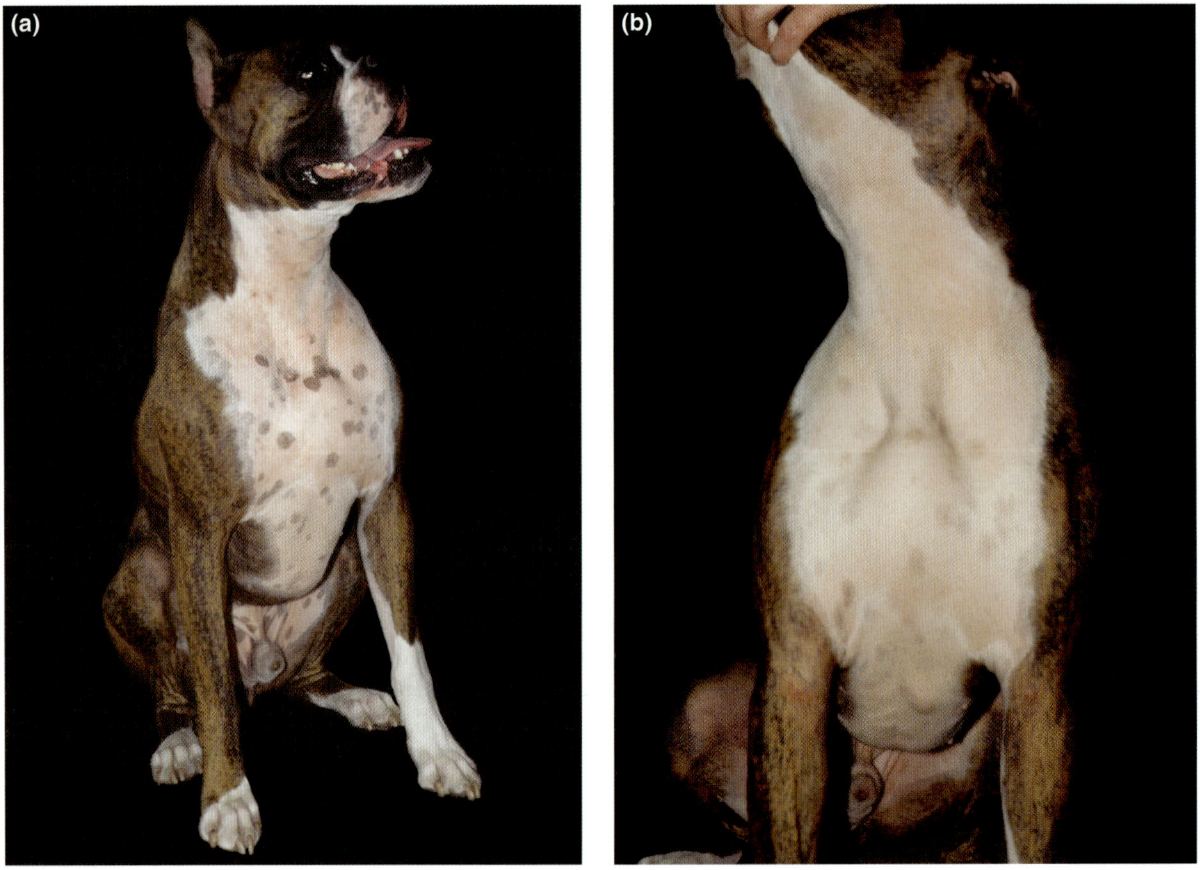

Fig. 3.3.32 Canine pattern alopecia, ventral type, in a Boxer. (a) Before melatonin therapy; (b) after melatonin therapy.

treated with melatonin (subcutaneous implants or oral tablets) experienced mild to moderate hair growth in the affected areas (Fig. 3.3.32). Hair growth was noticed as early as 6 weeks following initiation of treatment and maximal growth was achieved 3–4 months later.

No controlled studies investigating the efficacy of melatonin in CPA are yet available. However, in this pilot study, many cases of "CPA ventral type" and a few cases of "CPA pinnal type" have been treated with melatonin by several veterinary dermatologists and good to excellent results have been observed in approximately 50–70% of dogs (Paradis 2000).

3.3.8.3.3 Finasteride

Finasteride, a 5α-reductase inhibitor preventing the conversion of testosterone to dihydrotestosterone, has been used with success in some cases of CPA ventral type, but again controlled clinical trials are lacking (Paradis and Cerundolo 2005).

References

Gross TL, Ihrke PJ, Walder EJ, Affolter VK. 2005. *Skin Diseases of the Dog and Cat: Clinical and Histopathologic Diagnosis*, 2nd edn. Oxford: Blackwell Publishing.

Kaufman KD, Olsen EA, Whiting D, Savin R, DeVillez R, Bergfeld W, Price VH, Van Neste D, Roberts JL, Hordinsky M, Shapiro J, Binkowitz B, Gormley GJ. 1998. Finasteride in the treatment of men with androgenic alopecia. *Journal of the American Academy of Dermatology* 39:578–589.

Paradis M. 1995. Canine recurrent flank alopecia: treatment with melatonin. *Proceedings of the 11th AAVD/ACVD Meeting*, Santa Fe, NM, p. 49.

Paradis M. 1996. Melatonin therapy in canine pattern baldness. *Proceedings of the Third World Congress of Veterinary Dermatology, Edinburgh, Scotland*, p. 53.

Paradis M. 2000. Melatonin therapy in canine alopecia. In: Bonagura JD (ed.), *Kirk's Current Veterinary Therapy XIII*, pp. 546–549. Philadelphia: WB Saunders.

Paradis M, Cerundolo R. 2005. Genodermatis: alopecia and hypotrichoses. In: Hillier A, Foster AP, Kwochka KW (eds), *Advance in Veterinary Dermatology*, Vol. 5, pp. 360–364. Oxford: Blackwell Publishing.
Schoning PR, Cowan LA. 2000. Bald thigh syndrome of Greyhound dogs: Gross and microscopic findings. *Veterinary Dermatology* 11:49–51.
Scott DW, Miller WH, Griffin CE (eds). 2001. *Muller and Kirk's Small Animal Dermatology*, 6th edn. Philadelphia: WB Saunders.
Whiting DA. 2001. Possible mechanisms of miniaturization during androgenetic alopecia or pattern hair loss. *Journal of the American Academy of Dermatology* 45:S81–S86.
Yager JA, Wilcock BP. 1994. *Color Atlas and Text of Surgical Pathology of the Dog and Cat*. London, England: Mosby Year Book.

3.3.9 Breed-specific canine hair cycle abnormalities

Rosario Cerundolo, Manon Paradis, and Lars Mecklenburg

Hair cycle disorders that have been discussed so far are those that can be clearly distinguished on the basis of clinical, morphological, and other parameters. Still, there are a variety of alopecic diseases in dogs that are frequently referred to as "follicular dysplasia" that have not been reviewed so far. Most of these diseases are actually hair cycle abnormalities. The term "dysplasia," however, is inaccurate to classify these diseases as, first, they do not represent a developmental abnormality (such as in congenital alopecia) and, second, they do not represent a specific disease. In fact, the diseases are very different between the breeds. Therefore, it is more accurate to talk about a hair cycle abnormality that occurs in a specific breed where it has characteristic features. Although the etiology is not understood so far, a marked breed and family predisposition suggests hereditary factors being involved in the pathogenesis.

3.3.9.1 Alopecia in the Irish Water Spaniel

The Irish Water Spaniel is an old Irish dog breed that is characterized by lack of hair on the throat and the tail (Fig. 3.3.33). Beside these "desired" patches of alopecia, unwanted or "pathologic" hair loss has been described in the Irish Water Spaniel (Cerundolo et al. 2000).

3.3.9.1.1 Clinical presentation

Alopecia in the Irish Water Spaniel is most likely inherited in a dominant autosomal trait (Cerundolo et al. 1999). In a recent survey, 28% Irish Water Spaniels were affected by abnormal hair loss that was distributed on the laterodorsal neck, flanks, dorsum, rump, or caudal parts of the thighs, or any combination thereof. The rump was most consistently affected, followed by the thighs, neck, and trunk (Fig. 3.3.34). Remaining hair in affected skin areas shows a brighter color and is easily epilated. The coat may have a frizzy, wooly, or puppy-like appearance due to loss of primary hairs. Pruritus is rare, unless secondary infection is present.

In females, alopecia develops 6–8 weeks after the first or second estrus cycle with subsequent hair regrowth 3–4 weeks later. Alopecia may reoccur during subsequent estrus cycles and may become permanent. In some dogs, alopecia did not occur when estrus cycles were suppressed by progestagens, but reoccured when estrus cycle suppression was discontinued.

In males, alopecia starts later in life, mostly between 5 and 6 years of age. There is usually no variation of alopecia with season. Hair loss progresses continuously and finally becomes permanent. Both intact and neutered male dogs can be affected.

No consistent endocrine abnormalities have been demonstrated in Irish Water Spaniels with alopecia. Although some patients will show decreased T4 serum concentrations, most dogs had a normal response to TSH stimulation, excluding hypothyroidism as the primary cause of alopecia. Hyperadrenocorticism had been excluded in all cases, on the basis of a lack of appropriate clinical and biochemical signs and a normal ACTH stimulation test. Although an estrogenic influence on hair follicles is quite likely in this disease, estrogen concentrations are usually not significantly elevated. Increased 17-OHP concentrations have been found after ACTH stimulation, but their significance has not been elucidated so far (Cerundolo et al. 2000).

Clinical differential diagnoses of Irish Water Spaniel alopecia include endocrinopathies such as hypothyroidism, hyperadrenocorticism, and hyperestrogenism. Canine recurrent flank alopecia has not been described in the Irish Water Dog, but, if present, may overlap with the breed-specific alopecia described herein. Canine recurrent flank alopecia, however, does not progress to the caudal thighs or the neck.

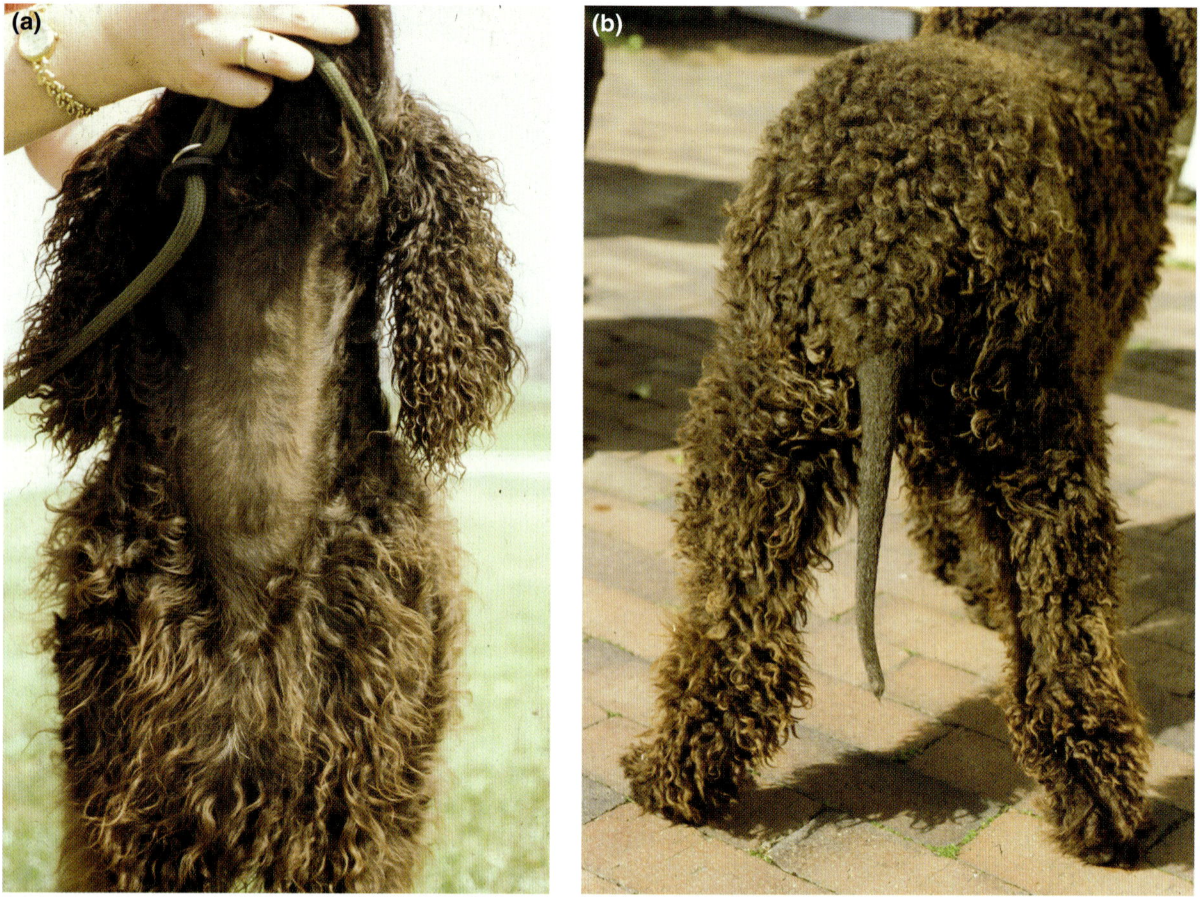

Fig. 3.3.33 Normal alopecia in the Irish Water Spaniel. (a) Lack of hairs on the ventral surface of the neck; (b) alopecia on the tail. (Reprinted with permission from Cerundolo et al. (2000).)

3.3.9.1.2 Histopathology

Histopathology will show most hair follicles in late catagen or telogen, with a markedly dilated follicular infundibulum, filled with orthokeratotic hyperkeratosis (Fig. 3.3.35). Thus, hair follicle morphology resembles that of canine recurrent flank alopecia. In addition, slight aggregation of pigment may be observed either within the hair shaft or within the hair follicle outer root sheath, associated with few perifollicular melanophages. Pigmentary clumping is most likely a sequela of premature catagen induction rather than a sign of an inherited pigmentary dysplasia. Inflammatory changes suggestive of a secondary superficial pyoderma do frequently occur in alopecic skin from Irish Water Spaniels. Trichomalacia, characteristic of trichorrhexis nodosa, has been noted in rare cases of Irish Water Spaniel alopecia. However, trichorrhexis nodosa always resolved within weeks and may have been a sequela of weathering or external trauma to the hair shaft rather than a sign of follicular dysplasia.

3.3.9.1.3 Therapy

Since etiology and pathogenesis of alopecia in Irish Water Dogs are unknown, no specific treatment can be initiated. Some cases have well responded to a fish and corn diet. However, even if this treatment improves the skin condition and may stimulate temporary growth of fine hair, in most cases alopecia is progressive and usually permanent. Affected dogs are healthy as this

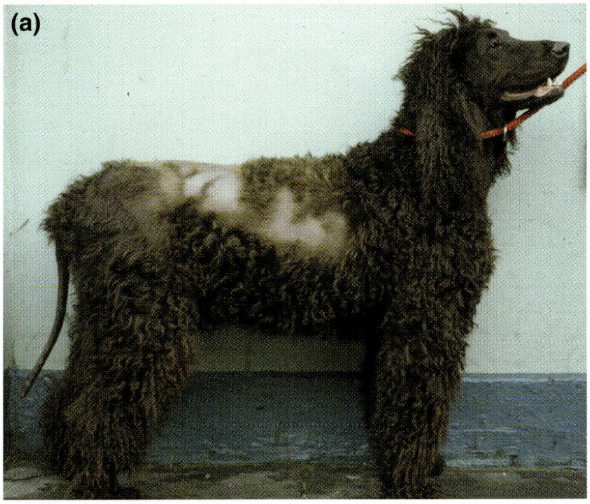

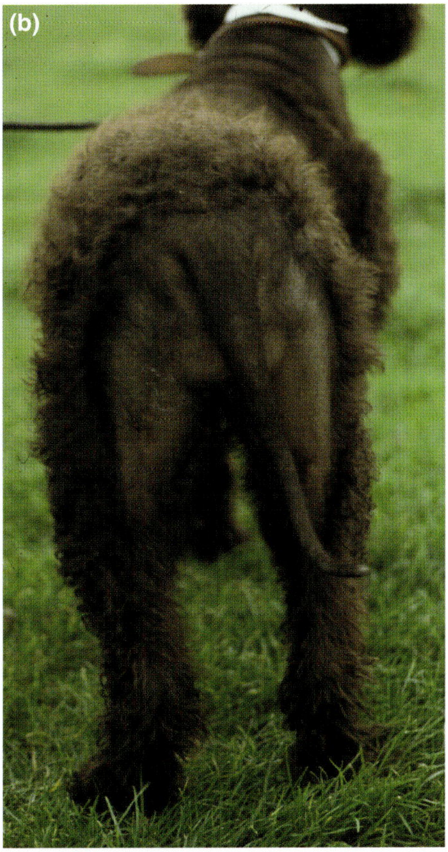

Fig. 3.3.34 Hereditary alopecia in an Irish Water Spaniel. (a) Alopecia of the dorsal and lateral trunk; (b) alopecia of the thighs. (Reprinted with permission from Cerundolo et al. (2000).)

is just an aesthetic condition, but they should not be bred. Levothyroxine administration does not improve the condition. Pyoderma, if present, needs to be treated with systemic antibiotics and mild antiseborrheic or antibacterial shampoos (see 4.1.1.3.).

3.3.9.2 Alopecia in the Portuguese Water Dog

Portuguese Water Dogs are thought to derive from the Standard Poodle. Like Poodles they have a curly

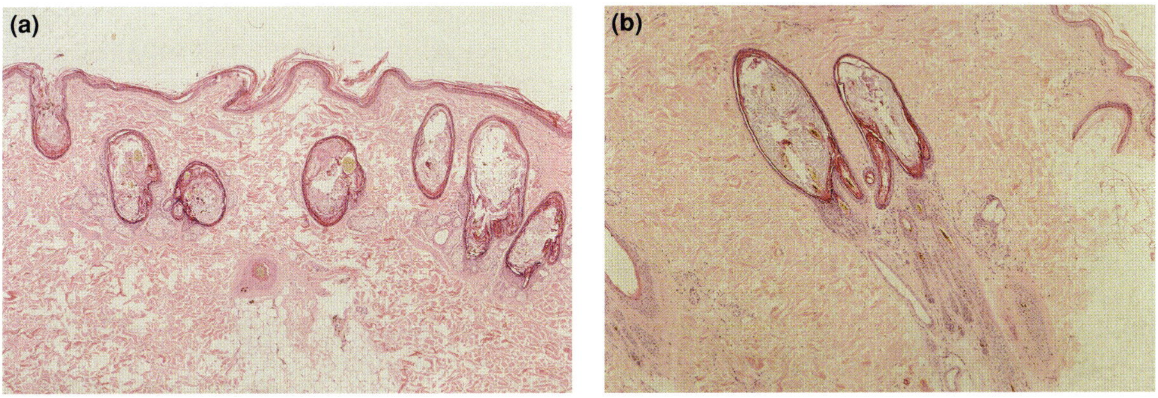

Fig. 3.3.35 Skin histology of Irish Water Spaniel with hereditary alopecia. (a) Severely dilated and hyperkeratotic follicular infundibula with lack of anagen hair follicles; (b) hair follicles in catagen. (Reprinted with permission from Cerundolo et al. (2000).)

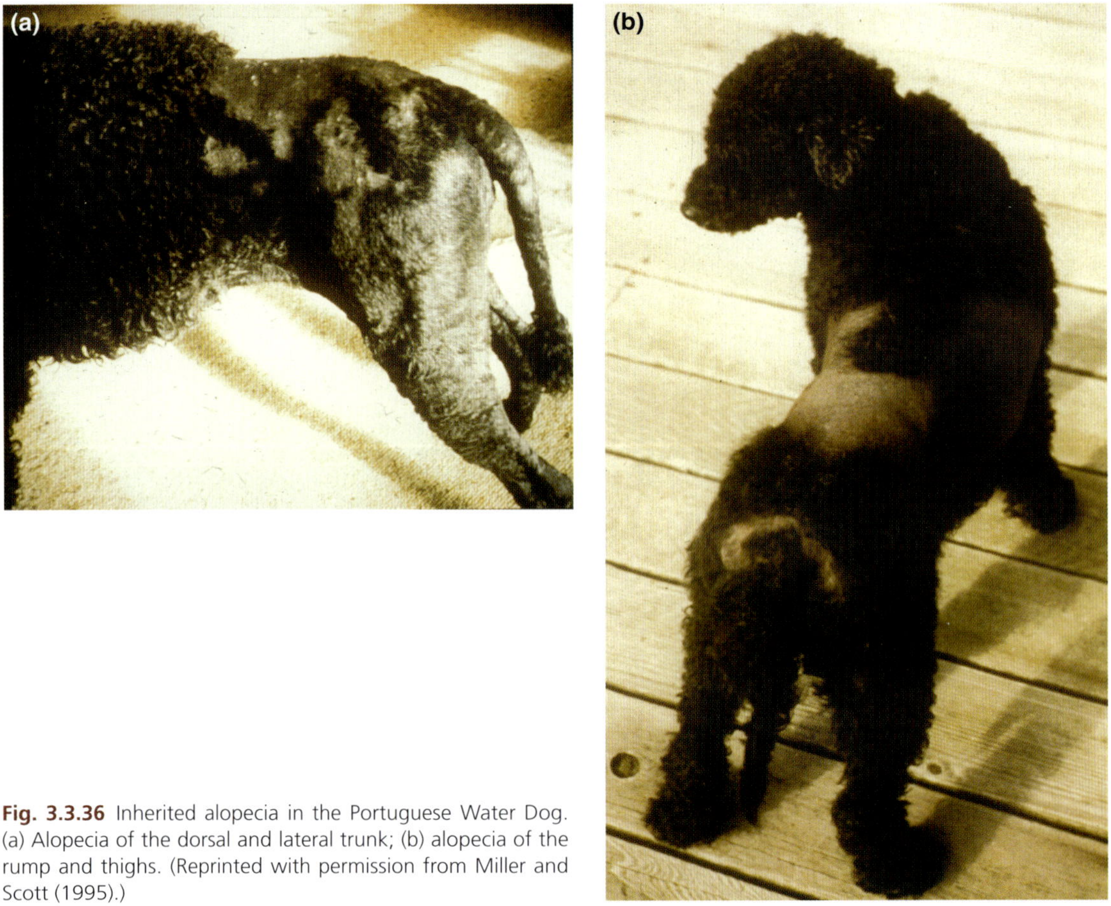

Fig. 3.3.36 Inherited alopecia in the Portuguese Water Dog. (a) Alopecia of the dorsal and lateral trunk; (b) alopecia of the rump and thighs. (Reprinted with permission from Miller and Scott (1995).)

coat. A particular form of alopecia has been described in the Portuguese Water Dogs that is clinically and morphologically similar to the alopecia found in Irish Water Spaniels (Miller and Scott 1995).

Hair loss occurs in the saddle and flank region at a median age of 2 years. Both males and females are affected. Periocular skin or caudal thighs may show alopecia as well. Hair may spontaneously regrow after several months, but in most cases falls out again during subsequent episodes. Regrown hair is reported abnormal, being dull, dry, and fragile (Fig. 3.3.36).

Histopathology will reveal a marked infundibular orthokeratotic hyperkeratosis with hair follicles mostly being in the catagen and telogen phase. Similar to Irish Water Spaniels, pigmentary clumping is usually found in hair shafts in the hair follicle outer root sheath. Misshapen small anagen hair bulbs and vacuolar alteration in the hair matrix and the inner root sheath have been described, but their significance is yet unknown (Miller and Scott 1995).

3.3.9.3 Alopecia in the Chesapeake Bay retriever

The Chesapeake Bay Retriever is a hunting dog that originates from North America by breeding Curly-coated and Flat-coated Retrievers with Irish Water Spaniels and some other breeds. The Chesapeake Bay Retriever has a dense and short hair coat. Recently, an alopecic condition has been described in the Chesapeake Bay Retriever (Cerundolo et al. 2005) that clinically and morphologically resembles alopecia in the Irish Water Spaniel (see above).

Hair loss can start as early as 5 months of age but usually affects dogs between 1.5 and 4 years of age.

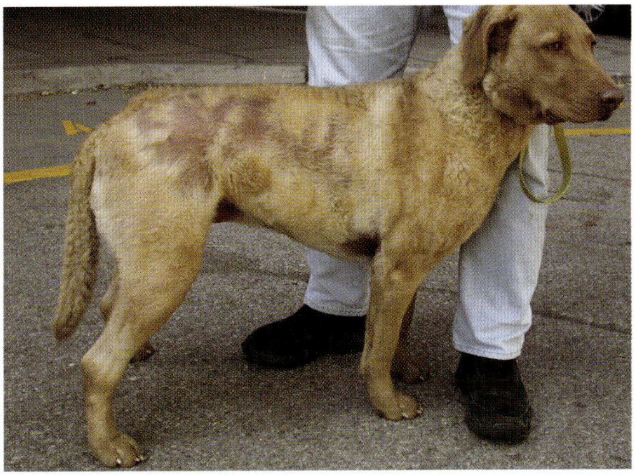

Fig. 3.3.37 Hereditary alopecia in the Chesapeake Bay Retriever. Hair loss affects the lateral side of the body and the thighs.

Alopecia can occur in intact and neutered male and female individuals, and ranges from sparse hair to complete baldness. Axillae, ventrum, flanks, rump, latero-ventral thorax, or caudal thighs or any combination thereof are affected (Fig. 3.3.37). Secondary pyoderma may occur. Routine hematological and biochemical investigations are within normal limits, and no consistent endocrine abnormalities have been detected in alopecic Chesapeake Bay Retrievers. Hypothyroidism, hyperadrenocorticism, and hyperestrogenism have been ruled out in all described cases.

Histopathology is identical to the alopecia described in Irish Water Spaniels and resembles canine recurrent flank alopecia, although the disease is distinct clinically, since alopecia is not confined to the flank area and alopecia does not show cyclic regression (Fig. 3.3.38). Miniaturized hair follicles have been described, but their significance is yet unknown. As with the alopecia in Irish Water Spaniels, the alopecia in Chesapeake Bay Retrievers does not respond to treatment with levothyroxine or melatonin.

3.3.9.4 Alopecia in the curly-coated retriever

The authors are aware of a form of alopecia in curly-coated retrievers that is clinically and histologically similar to the alopecia described in Irish Water Spaniels, Portuguese Water Dogs, and the Chesapeake Bay Retrievers. However, no scientific studies have yet been published on this topic.

3.3.9.5 Alopecia in the greyhound

Some Greyhounds, particularly male racing dogs, develop a form of alopecia on the lateral and caudal thighs, eventually spreading to the abdomen and ventral thorax (Fig. 3.3.39) (Schoning and Cowan 2000; Scott et al. 2001; Paradis and Cerundolo 2005).

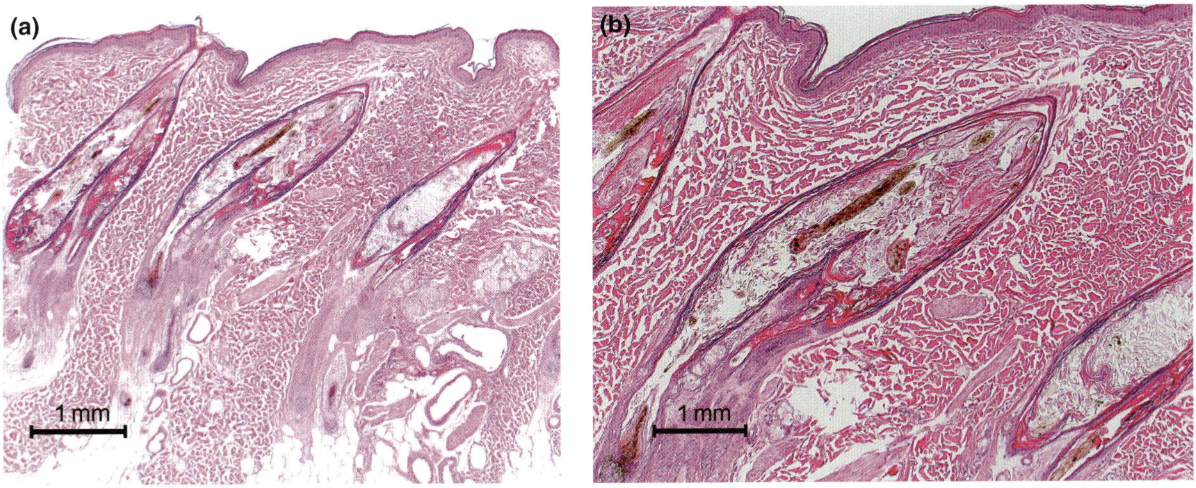

Fig. 3.3.38 Skin histology of hereditary alopecia in the Chesapeake Bay Retriever. (a) Pronounced distension of follicular infundibula by marked orthokeratotic hyperkeratosis; (b) dysplastic hair shafts with abnormal pigmentation. (Reprinted with permission from Cerundolo et al. (2005).)

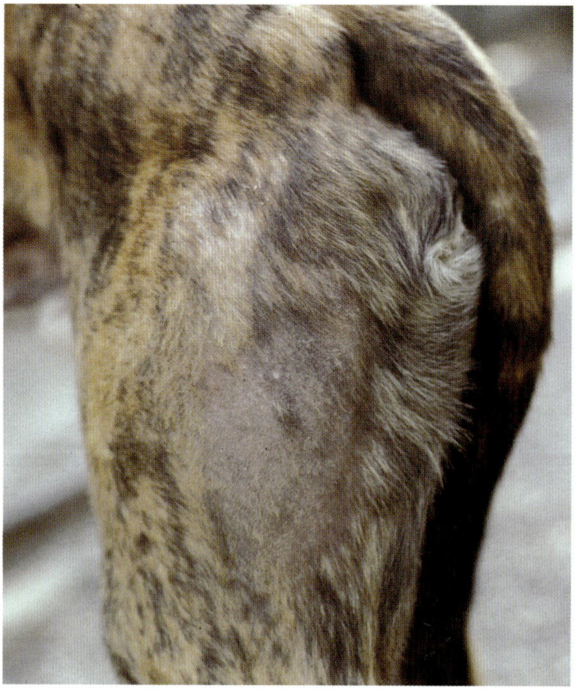

Fig. 3.3.39 Alopecia of the thighs in a Greyhound (bald thigh syndrome).

The disease is known as "bald thigh syndrome" in greyhounds and it occurs in young adults with an age of approximately 2–3 years. Histology shows infundibular hyperkeratosis and a lack of anagen hair follicles. Most hair follicles are in late catagen or telogen stages. Bald thigh syndrome shares some aspects with "CPA ventral type," but it is yet unclear whether it is pathogenetically related to CPA ventral type as seen in dogs with a "short/fine" type of hair coat (see Section 3.3.8).

The pathogenesis of this hair cycle abnormality in greyhounds has not been sufficiently investigated yet. It is possible that a few cases may be due to, or may at least be aggravated by, endogenous testosterone (Paradis and Cerundolo 2005). Low thyroid hormone concentrations during the racing period could also trigger the disease (Hill et al. 2001). To make a final diagnosis, hypothyroidism, hyperadrenocorticism, and hyperestrogenism have to be ruled out. No treatment has been suggested in the literature. Hair generally regrows (at least at the lateral aspect of thighs) when racing activity is stopped (Paradis and Cerundolo 2005).

3.3.9.6 Alopecia in the Pont Audemer Spaniel

The Pont Audemer spaniel originates from France and derives from the Irish Water Spaniel. It has a brown hair coat. Recently, a specific form of alopecia has been described in the Pont Audemer spaniel (Guaguere et al. 2000). Alopecia affected the trunk and ears and firstly appeared at the age of 7–18 months. Biopsies from affected skin regions showed infundibular hyperkeratosis, pigment clumping in hair shafts and outer root sheath, and some degree of vacuolar degeneration and apoptosis of keratinocytes from the outer and inner root sheath. No information on hair cycle stages was provided in the original report of this disease. Endocrine tests were all normal, ruling out hypothyroidism, hyperadrenocorticism, or hyperestrogenism. Melatonin treatment has not been effective.

3.3.9.7 Alopecia in the Siberian Husky and the Alaskan Malamute

Nordic dog breeds such as the Siberian Husky and the Alaskan Malamute normally have a dense hair coat. These breeds may be affected with alopecia X, that is, a rather unspecific hair cycle arrest that occurs in many plush-coated dogs and the Miniature and Toy Poodle (see Section 3.3.4.). The "follicular dysplasia" that has been described in the Siberian Husky and the Alaskan Malamute (Post et al. 1988) is most likely identical to the disease "alopecia X."

References

Cerundolo R, Lloyd DH, Pidduck HG. 1999. Studies on the inheritance of hair loss in the Irish Water spaniel. *Veterinary Record* 145:542.

Cerundolo R, Mauldin EA, Goldschmidt MH, Beyerlein SL, Refsal KR, Oliver JW. 2005. Adult-onset hair loss in Chesapeake Bay retrievers: as clinical and histological study. *Veterinary Dermatology* 16:39.

Cerundolo R, McEvoy F, MacNeil PE, Evans H. 2000. An analysis of factors underlying hypotrichosis and alopecia in Irish Water Spaniel in the United Kingdom. *Veterinary Dermatology* 11:107.

Guaguere E, Degorce-Rubiales F, Poujade A, Lecanu J, Petriowski M, Prelaud P. 2000. Genetic follicular dysplasia in Pont Audemer Spaniel dog: A report of eight cases. *Veterinary Dermatology* 11(1 Suppl):53.

Hill RC, Fox LE, Lewis DD, Beale KM, Nachreiner RF, Scott KC, Sundstrom DA, Jones GL, Butterwick RF. 2001. Effects of racing and training on serum thyroid hormone concentrations in racing Greyhounds. *American Journal of Veterinary Research* 62(12):1969–1972.

Miller WH, Scott DW. 1995. Follicular dysplasia of the Portuguese water dog. *Veterinary Dermatology* 6:67.
Paradis M, Cerundolo R. 2005. Genodermatis: Alopecia and hypotrichoses. In: Hillier A, Foster AP, Kwochka KW (eds), *Advance in Veterinary Dermatology*, Vol. 5, pp. 360–364. Blackwell Publishing.
Post K, Dignean MA, Clark EG. 1988. Hair follicle dysplasia in a Siberian husky. *Journal of the American Animal Hospital Association* 24:659–662.
Schoning PR, Cowan LA. 2000. Bald thigh syndrome of Greyhound dogs: Gross and microscopic findings. *Veterinary Dermatology* 11:49.
Scott DW, Miller WH, Griffin CE. 2001. *Muller & Kirk's Small Animal Dermatology*, 6th edn. Philadelphia: Ed Saunders.

3.4 Hair follicle dystrophy and atrophy

Rosario Cerundolo and Lars Mecklenburg

Hair follicles, as it has been mentioned and extensively described in other chapters, lose cells (i.e., keratinocytes) when they undergo cyclic regression (catagen) and rest (telogen). These physiological stages of hair growth cycling should not be termed "atrophy," since they do not necessarily represent a pathological change (Dunstan et al. 2001). True atrophy is represented by a loss of hair follicle cells beyond the physiological telogen phase. Such atrophy of hair follicles indeed exists in domestic animals, although it is comparatively rare. Atrophic hair follicles have also been named "fading follicles," emphasizing their small size compared to the overall size of dermis and other cutaneous adnexa. Atrophic hair follicles are histopathologically characterized by small remnants of keratinocyte strands that are surrounded by a markedly thickened connective tissue sheath (see Section 2.2.3.5).

Dystrophy by definition is a degenerative process that is due to "malnutrition" of an organ. Morphological hallmarks of hair follicle dystrophy are uncoordinated vacuolar degeneration or apoptosis of keratinocytes that is distinct from apoptosis occurring during catagen (see Section 2.2.3.4). Further characteristics of hair follicle dystrophy are uneven distribution of melanin within the hair shafts, perifollicular melanophages, a wide-open hair canal, distortion of the entire follicle, and an irregular diameter of hair follicles (Hendrix et al. 2005). The most typical form of hair follicle dystrophy occurs with cytotoxic drugs, that is, drugs that interfere with mitosis. Although hair follicles of domestic animals are much less sensitive to such a treatment than are human hair follicles, hair follicle dystrophy may still appear in domestic animals. Since dogs are increasingly treated with cytotoxic drugs against malignancies, dystrophic alopecia is being seen more frequently in this species nowadays. Hair follicle dystrophy has also been named "anagen effluvium" emphasizing that affected anagen hair follicles lose their hair shafts. However, it has been demonstrated that both a dystrophic anagen and a dystrophic catagen can exist (Hendrix et al. 2005). Therefore, the term "dystrophy" is more appropriate. Hair follicle dystrophy may precede atrophy of hair follicles and both conditions may blend into one another.

3.4.1 Chemotherapy-induced hair follicle dystrophy in dogs and cats

Chemotherapy-induced alopecia is a very well-known and widely dreaded adverse event in human cancer patients. The human hair follicle appears to be particularly vulnerable for cytotoxic drugs. Chemotherapeutic agents that cause alopecia are alkylating agents (e.g., melphalan, chlorambucil, cyclophosphamide, and cisplatin), antimetabolites (e.g., methotrexate and 5-fluorouracil), vinca alkaloids (e.g., vincristine and vinblastine), topoisomerase inhibitors (e.g., doxorubicin), and antitumoral antibiotics (e.g., actinomycin D and bleomycin) (Herzberg 1966; Fitzpatrick 2003). Toxic substances (e.g., selenium, molybdenum, thallium, and arsenic) have also been reported to cause alopecia (Yun and Kim 2007).

Cancer chemotherapy is nowadays more popular in veterinary medicine. Dogs and cats are increasingly treated for internal malignancies with drugs such as doxorubicin. Therefore, hair loss is being seen in dogs and cats as well, although its clinical and morphological characteristics are by far less striking than in humans (Chun et al. 2001; Kisseberth and MacEwen 2001).

Doxorubicin and other cytotoxic cancer drugs interfere with cell division and thus target rapidly proliferating cell populations such as bone marrow stem cells, gastrointestinal epithelium, and finally hair follicle matrix cells. Impaired mitotic and metabolic processes in actively growing hair follicles will lead to thinning of the hair shaft that becomes fragile and susceptible to fracture with minimal trauma. Hair loss in chemotherapy-induced alopecia can be mainly due to hair breakage rather than hair loss (Crounse and Van Scott 1960). Disruption of proliferation of matrix cells will also result in uncoordinated cessation of hair shaft elongation. Melanin pigment will eventually spill out of the hair follicle, which is then taken up by perifollicular macrophages (melanophages). This results in the typical morphology of dystrophic hair follicles.

Studies in mice have demonstrated that the morphology of hair follicle dystrophy after chemotherapy is variable and depends on simultaneous stimulation or inhibition of hair growth (Ohnemus et al. 2004; Hendrix et al. 2005). Dystrophic hair follicles can remain in anagen, most likely when the toxic insult still allows some proliferation of matrix cells. On the other hand, dystrophic hair follicles can undergo premature catagen development. This will lead to telogen hair follicles that can recover from the chemotherapy-induced insult and can grow normally once treatment has been discontinued. In humans, dystrophic anagen is a common feature with chemotherapy-induced alopecia, whereas this has rarely been observed in dogs. Most dogs with doxorubicin-induced alopecia reveal telogen hair follicles, suggesting that they have undergone the dystrophic catagen pathway and await stimulation of a new anagen phase. Therefore, many dogs show biopsies that are compatible with telogen effluvium rather than hair follicle dystrophy (Gross et al. 2005). However, the description of morphological lesions in biopsies from dogs and cats treated with chemotherapeutic agents is still very sparse.

3.4.1.1 Clinical presentation

Clinically, chemotherapy-induced hair loss can be very variable. The severity of hair loss after chemotherapy depends on the route of administration, the dose, and the treatment schedule. Hair loss usually begins 7–10 days following the initiation of chemotherapy and becomes most clinically apparent within 1–2 months.

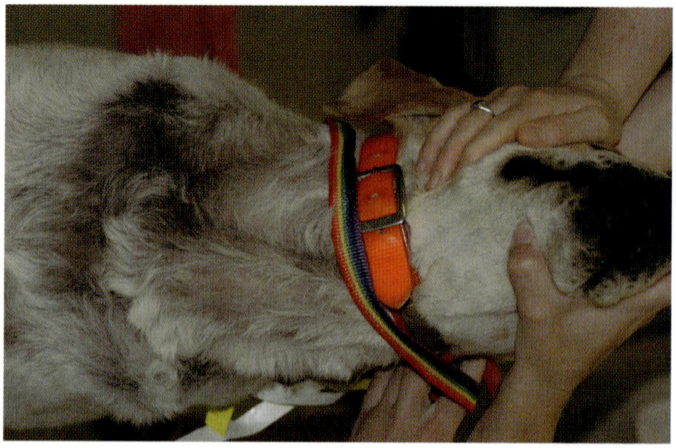

Fig. 3.4.1 Chemotherapy-induced alopecia in a Labrador following treatment with doxorubicin. Hair loss of the ventral neck.

Alopecia may begin on the head (Fig. 3.4.1) to become multifocal and then diffuse affecting the trunk, and occasionally the extremities. Hairs are easily epilated. The severity of alopecia may depend on the drug as well as the individual predisposition. Dry skin may be present in animals receiving doxorubicin due to sebaceous glands degeneration (Van Vleet and Ferrans 1980; Selleri et al. 2006). Clipped areas may show delayed hair regrowth. Beagles receiving weekly standard doses of intravenous doxorubicin develop alopecia within 4–6, weeks, affecting the head (lips, muzzle, and eyes) and then the thorax, abdomen, and the proximal inner areas of the limbs. They may also develop erythema and pruritus in alopecic areas, occasionally resulting in dry and scaly skin and ulceration (Van Vleet and Ferrans 1980). Cats can lose their guard hairs and whiskers. Hair regrowth may vary in color and texture (Van Vleet and Ferrans 1980; Chun et al. 2007).

Diagnosis of chemotherapy-induced alopecia should be straightforward. The history of previous treatments or possible contact with toxic substances is suggestive of the disease. A trichogram will show both telogen hairs and fractured hair shafts, often characterized by irregular pigmentation and structural defects. In localized forms of alopecia, causes of folliculitis should be ruled out.

3.4.1.2 Histopathology

Skin biopsies may reveal changes in the anagen hair bulbs with the presence of pyknotic and karyorrhectic

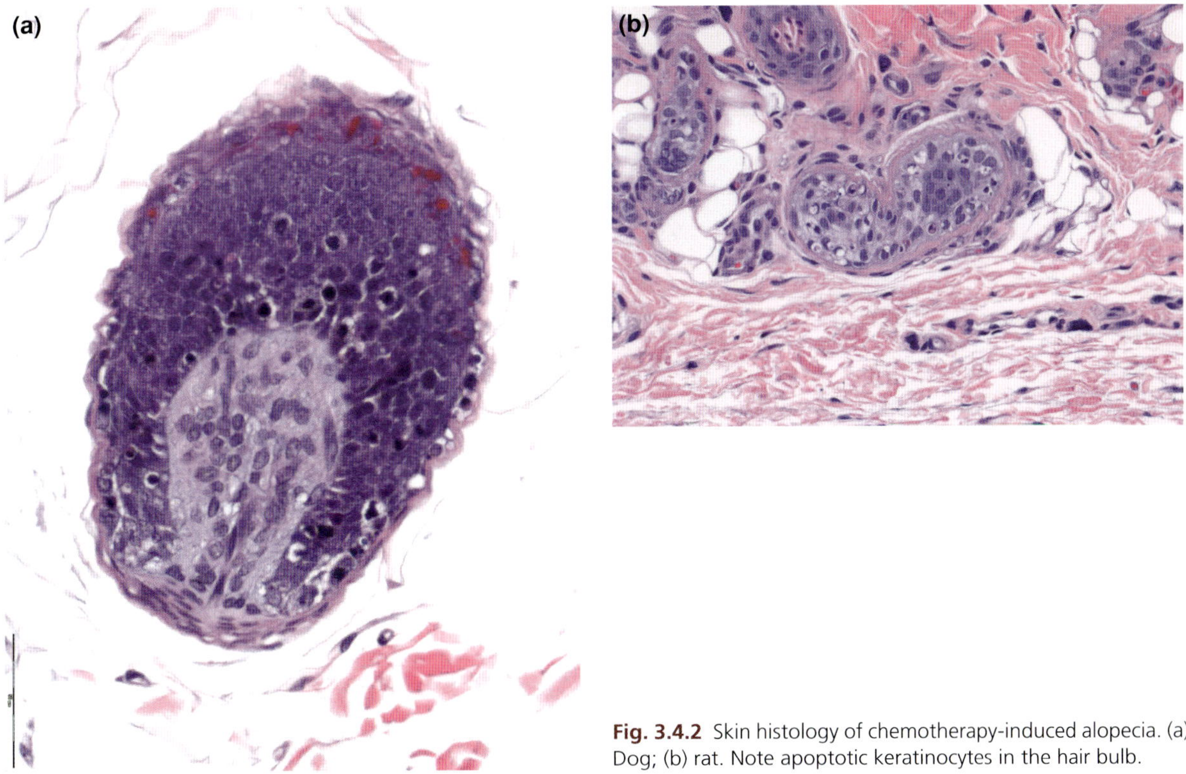

Fig. 3.4.2 Skin histology of chemotherapy-induced alopecia. (a) Dog; (b) rat. Note apoptotic keratinocytes in the hair bulb.

nuclei in the hair matrix (Fig. 3.4.2). Keratinization within the inner and outer root sheath will be disturbed and dysplastic hair shafts may be seen within the hair canal. No inflammation should target the hair bulb. Epidermis and dermis can be normal or may show signs of atrophy (Van Vleet and Ferrans 1980; Yager 1994).

Poodles, Old English Sheepdogs, and Terriers are reported to be at increased risk (Chun et al. 2007). It is quite likely that dog breeds with many anagen hair follicles are more susceptible to chemotherapy-induced alopecia than are dogs with a predominance of telogen hair follicles, as a lack of cell proliferation will protect from the influence of the chemotherapeutic agent. As in humans, chemotherapy-induced alopecia is an acceptable side effect that is outweighed by the benefit of the treatment. No treatment is available other than cessation of the chemotherapeutic agent. Alopecia is reversible, since hair follicle stem cells are usually not affected (Amoh et al. 2007). Hair regrowth begins several weeks after the cessation of chemotherapy. In humans, approximately 65% of patients experience a change in the color, texture, and type of hair (Yun and Kim 2007).

3.4.2 Canine dermatomyositis

Dermatomyositis is a well-characterized disease in Collies and Shetland Sheepdogs (Hargis et al. 1984; Ferguson et al. 2000). It occurs in young dogs less than 6 months of age that show a familial predisposition (*familial dermatomyositis*). A similar disease that is indistinguishable from familial dermatomyositis occurs spontaneously in other breeds. Again, very young individuals are affected, but no familial predisposition is known (*spontaneous dermatomyositis*). Dermatomyositis starts on the head where crusting and alopecia occur in the periorbital and perioral skin (Fig. 3.4.3). Similar lesions may develop on the tips of the ear pinnae, at the claw fold (eponychium), at the tip of the tail, or at any bony prominence. Ulceration may develop in severely affected patients. In addition to skin lesions, claws may become dystrophic. Most dogs show some degree of skeletal muscle involvement that

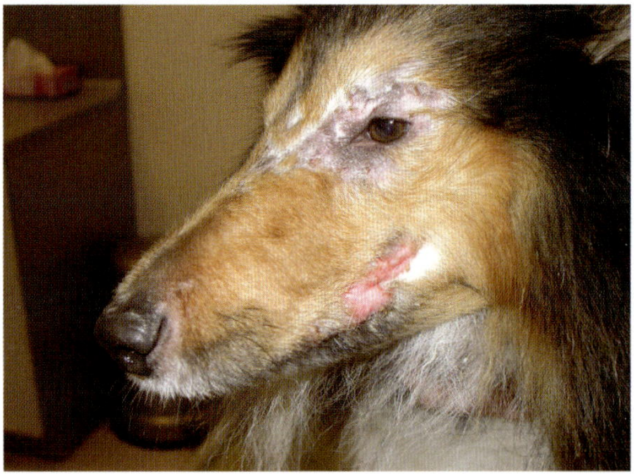

Fig. 3.4.3 Dermatomyositis in a Collie. Alopecia and crusting of periocular skin and lips.

can vary from subtle atrophy of temporal and masseter muscle to generalized muscular atrophy with megaesophagus and lameness (Hargis et al. 1984; Haupt et al. 1985a,b).

Whereas very early lesions may show dystrophic hair follicles (with keratinocyte vacuolation and apoptosis), most biopsies from dermatomyositis patients will reveal marked hair follicle atrophy (Fig. 3.4.4). This is accompanied by a cell-poor often very mild lymphohistiocytic interface dermatitis (rarely with cleft formation) and dermal pallor with rarefied collagen bundles (Gross and Kunkle 1987). Some biopsies may demonstrate evidence of a cell-poor vasculitis and/or evidence of myositis with interstitial inflammation and myofiber degeneration and regeneration (Hargis et al. 1986).

Etiology and pathogenesis of dermatomyositis are not yet known, although inheritance of dermatomyositis in Shetland Sheepdogs has been linked to canine chromosome 35 (Clark et al. 2005). It is most likely that vascular lesions and local ischemia play a central role in disease progress. This can explain the distribution of lesions that occur at pressure points (carpus, tarsus) and areas of low sustained circulation. Therapy of dermatomyositis comprises prevention of trauma and excessive solar exposure, as these factors can worsen the disease. In mild lesions, spontaneous healing is possible. In more severe lesions, patients require systemic therapy. Pentoxifylline (25 mg/kg twice daily) has shown some efficacy in dogs with familial canine dermatomyositis (Rees and Boothe 2003). Other options are prednisone (1 mg/kg daily), vitamin E, or lipid supplements.

3.4.3 Ischemic dermatopathy following vaccine administration in dogs and cats

Ischemic dermatopathy can be the result of vaccine administration to dogs or cats. Vaccine-associated ischemic dermatopathy is usually seen in adult animals (Vitale et al. 1999). It occurs 2–3 months after vaccine administration, but it may even take longer to develop clinically. It can occur as a focal lesion overlying the site of vaccine administration, or it can be widespread. The

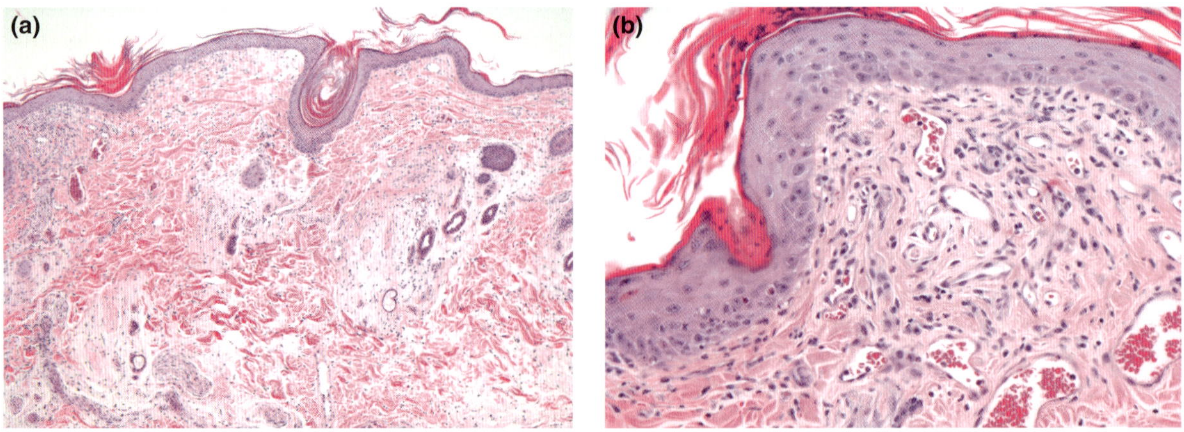

Fig. 3.4.4 Skin histology of canine dermatomyositis. (a) Moderate diffuse inflammation in the dermis and marked atrophy of hair follicles; (b) perivascular lymphoplasmacytic inflammation with scattered apoptotic keratinocytes in the epidermis.

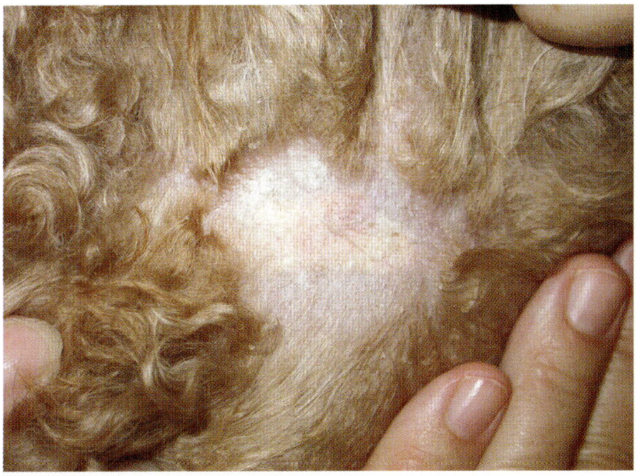

Fig. 3.4.5 Vaccine-induced ischemic dermatopathy in a dog.

local form typically occurs over the shoulders, back, or the posterolateral thighs and represents a firm circular patch of erythema and alopecia. Old lesions will have a shiny appearance with mild scaling (Fig. 3.4.5). The *generalized form* has only been described in the dog so far. Clinically, it mirrors canine dermatomyositis, suggesting that the disease is caused by local ischemia of skin regions that are prone to impaired circulation. The difference is the older age of onset and often a more widespread and more severe form of the disease. Rarely, a similar disease in the Jack Russell Terrier has been described where no history of previous vaccination was evident (Parker and Foster 1996).

Histologically, the localized form of ischemic dermatopathy will show dystrophic and/or atrophic hair follicles and dermal pallor with rarefied collagen bundles. In addition, the panniculus will demonstrate a nodular inflammatory reaction comprising large macrophages and giant cells that surround a central area of necrosis, often with basophilic debris (Hendrick and Dunagan 1991). The basophilic material can also be seen within macrophages and giant cells. Eosinophils may accompany the histiocytic inflammation. Lymphocytes frequently aggregate in nodular lymphoid follicles around blood vessels in the periphery of the necrosis. In ischemic dermatopathy induced by rabies vaccine in dogs (*canine postrabies vaccination panniculitis*), the lesions as described above are accompanied by cell-poor vasculitis of small blood vessels in the panniculus and the deep dermis. Vasculitis may be very subtle. It is most likely associated with deposition of rabies antigen in the vascular wall (Wilcock and Yager 1986). Postrabies vaccination panniculitis is typically a disease of long-haired toy breeds such as Miniature Poodles, Bichon Frises, Shih Tzu, Lhasa Apso, Maltese, Yorkshire Terrier, Silky Terrier, and Chihuahua.

The localized form of ischemic dermatopathy does usually not require therapy. If inflammation is prominent, glucocorticoids may be used. The generalized form of ischemic dermatopathy requires systemic therapy. As for dermatomyositis, pentoxifylline (25 mg/kg twice daily) or prednisone (1 mg/kg daily) can be used. In dogs, dapsone (1 mg/kg 3 times a day) can be used as well. Rarely do patients need more aggressive immunosuppressive therapy with higher doses of prednisone, cyclophosphamide, or azathioprine.

3.4.4 Canine traction alopecia

A severe form of atrophic hair loss has been repeatedly described in long-haired dogs with the use of rubber bands or barrette placement (Rosenkrantz et al. 1989; Ordeix et al. 2001). These grooming devices are used to style hairs, usually on the top of the head. It is assumed that the devices disrupt cutaneous blood flow and thus induce malnutrition of hair follicles. These undergo gradual atrophy that may finally result in a permanent loss of hair follicles and scarring. Histology will show atrophic hair follicles. In late stages, follicles vanish and are completely replaced by bands of fibrous tissue (scar) with only some melanophages labeling the previous site of hair follicles. One report describes a vasculitis that had developed at the site of alopecia (Ordeix et al. 2001).

3.4.5 Feline post-traumatic alopecia

An atrophic form of alopecia on the rump has been described in cats that have experienced traumatic pelvic fracture (Declerq 2004). It is speculated that the trauma disrupts blood supply to the skin and thus is responsible for an ischemic atrophy of cutaneous adnexa. Hair loss is seen within days after trauma and in most cases is permanent, despite a moderate regrowth of hair in the periphery. Alopecia is due to a severe atrophy of hair follicles. This is usually accompanied by some perifollicular fibrosis, fibrosis of the subepidermal dermis, atrophy of sebaceous glands and apocrine glands, and often degeneration of adipocytes in the subcutis. There is no therapy for follicular atrophy. Hair follicles that have undergone atrophy are

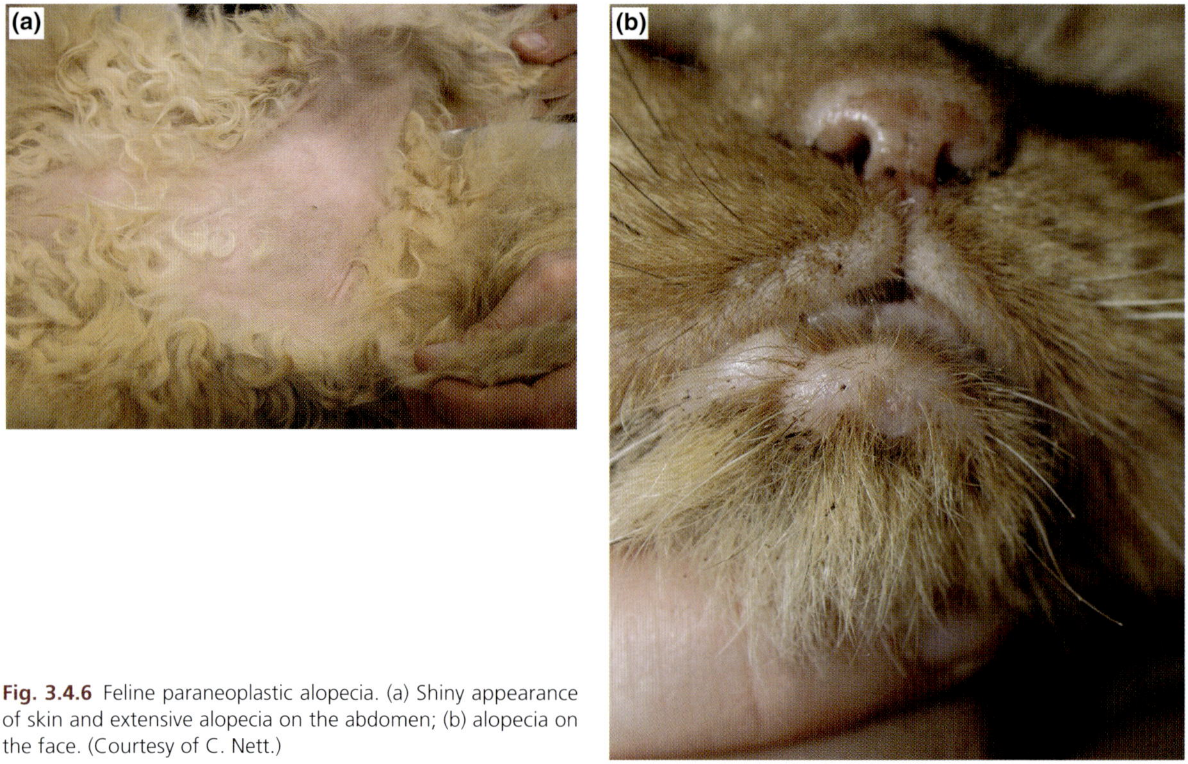

Fig. 3.4.6 Feline paraneoplastic alopecia. (a) Shiny appearance of skin and extensive alopecia on the abdomen; (b) alopecia on the face. (Courtesy of C. Nett.)

permanently lost, as it must be assumed that follicular stem cells have vanished. The prognosis for regrowth therefore is guarded. However, it will represent a mere cosmetic problem.

3.4.6 Feline paraneoplastic alopecia

A form of alopecia associated with internal malignancies occasionally occurs in the old cat (Brooks et al. 1994; Pascal-Tenorio et al. 1997; Godfrey 1998). The vast majority of cases has been presented with pancreatic adenocarcinomas, but it has also been reported in a cat with hepatocellular and cholangiocellular carcinoma (Pascal-Tenorio et al. 1997; Marconato et al. 2007). Alopecia starts on the abdomen and then rapidly spreads to the thorax and extremities, and eventually may become generalized (Fig. 3.4.6). Hairs that are still present may epilate very easily. The alopecic skin has a very characteristic shiny and glistening appearance. Footpads are mostly dry with excessive circular scaling. Most cats show concurrent anorexia and weight loss as a consequence of the pancreatic malignancy that may have already metastasized into the lung and liver. Some patients may show excessive grooming that can further contribute to alopecia. However, the main form of alopecia is a lack of hair fiber growth, not breaking of hair fibers due to grooming. Skin biopsy results show atrophic hair follicles meaning they are smaller than expected in telogen. Anagen hair follicles are lacking. Atrophic hair follicles are characterized by few keratinocytes in the isthmus region that are surrounded by a slightly thickened connective tissue sheath (Fig. 3.4.7). Small, condensed dermal papillae are occasionally found at the bottom of these epithelial strands. Additional characteristic findings are mild acanthosis and excessive desquamation of the stratum corneum that often is parakeratotic. Normal telogen hair follicles with or without hair shafts may be found as well.

The diagnosis is confirmed by histopathology of skin biopsies and demonstration of a pancreatic neoplasm, either by radiography, sonography, computed tomography, or laparotomy. Although cases of remission after successful excision of the neoplasm have

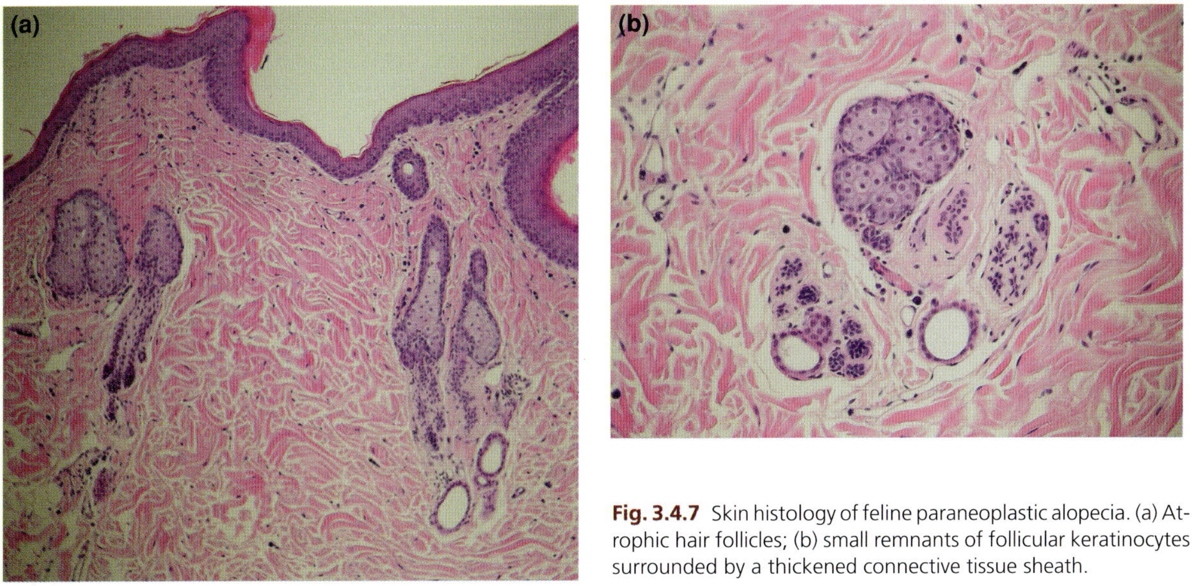

Fig. 3.4.7 Skin histology of feline paraneoplastic alopecia. (a) Atrophic hair follicles; (b) small remnants of follicular keratinocytes surrounded by a thickened connective tissue sheath.

been described (Tasker et al. 1999), most cases are diagnosed much too late for therapy. Most patients are presented with a rapidly deteriorating disease that requests euthanasia within 4 weeks.

References

Amoh Y, Li L, Katsuoka K, Hoffman RM. 2007. Chemotherapy targets the hair-follicle vascular network but not the stem cells. *Journal of Investigative Dermatology* 127(1):11–15.

Brooks DG, Campbell KL, Dennis JS, Dunstan RW. 1994. Pancreatic paraneoplastic alopecia in three cats. *Journal of the American Animal Hospital Association* 30:557.

Chun R, Garrett L, MacEwen IG. 2001. Cancer chemotherapy. In: Withrow SJ, MacEwen EG (eds), *Small Animal Clinical Oncology*, p. 95. Philadelphia: WB Saunders.

Chun R, Garrett L, Vail DM. 2007. Cancer chemotherapy. In: Withrow Stephen J, Vail David M (eds), *Withrow and MacEwen's Small Animal Clinical Oncology*, 4th edn, pp. 163–192. Edinburgh: Elsevier Saunders.

Clark LA, Credille KM, Murphy KE, Rees CA. 2005. Linkage of dermatomyositis in the Shetland sheepdog to chromosome 35. *Veterinary Dermatology* 16:392.

Crounse RC, Van Scott EJ. 1960. Changes in the scalp hair roots as a measure of toxicity from cancer chemotherapeutic drugs. *Journal of Investigative Dermatology* 35:83–90.

Declerq J. 2004. Alopecia and dermatopathy of the lower back following pelvic fractures in three cats. *Veterinary Dermatology* 15:42.

Dunstan RW, Credille KM, Mansell J, Tucker KA, Bloom PJ, Petersen AJ, Nachreiner RF, Davenport GM, Lupton CJ. 2001 April. A common sense approach to the morphology of alopecia: addressing 10 points of follicular confusion. *ISVD Meeting*, Norfolk, VA.

Ferguson EA, Cerundolo R, Lloyd DH, Rest J, Cappello R. 2000. Dermatomyositis in five Shetland sheepdogs in the United Kingdom. *Veterinary Record* 146:214.

Fitzpatrick JE. 2003. Mucocutaneous complications of antimeoplastic therapy. In: Fitzpatrick AZ, Eisen K, Wolff KF, Freedberg IM, Austen KF (eds), *Fitzpatrick's Dermatology in General Medicine*, 6th edn, pp. 1337–1347. New York: McGraw-Hill.

Godfrey DR. 1998. A case of feline paraneoplastic alopecia with secondary *Malassezia*-associated dermatitis. *Journal of Small Animal Practice* 39:394.

Gross TL, Ihrke PJ, Walder EJ, Affolter VK (eds). 2005. *Skin Diseases of the Dog and Cat*, 2nd edn. Ames: Blackwell Publishing.

Gross TL, Kunkle GA. 1987. The cutaneous histology of dermatomyositis in collie dogs. *Veterinary Pathology* 24:11.

Hargis AM, Haupt KH, Hegreberg GA, Prieur DJ, Moore MP. 1984. Familial canine dermatomyositis. Initial characterization of the cutaneous and muscular lesions. *American Journal of Pathology* 116:234.

Hargis AM, Prieur DJ, Haupt KH, Collier LL. 1986. Post-mortem findings in a Shetland sheepdog with dermatomyositis. *American Journal of Pathology* 123:480.

Haupt KH, Prieur DJ, Hargis AM, Cowell RL, McDonald TL, Werner LL, Evermann JF. 1985a. Familial canine dermatomyositis: clinicopathologic, immunologic, and serologic studies. *American Journal of Veterinary Research* 46:1870.

Haupt KH, Prieur DJ, Moore MP, Hargis AM, Hegreberg GA, Gavin PR, Johnson RS. 1985b. Familial canine dermatomyositis: clinical, electrodiagnostic, and genetic studies. *American Journal of Veterinary Research* 46:1861.

Hendrick MJ, Dunagan CA. 1991. Focal necrotizing granulomatous panniculitis associated with subcutaneous injection of rabies vaccine in cats and dogs: 10 cases (1988–1989). *Journal of the American Veterinary Medical Association* 198:304.

Hendrix S, Handjiski B, Peters EM, Paus R. 2005. A guide to assessing damage response pathways of the hair follicle: lessons from cyclosphosphamide-induced alopecia in mice. *Journal of Investigative Dermatology* 125:42–51.

Herzberg JJ. 1966. Cytostatische alopecien einschließlich thallium-alopecien. *Archiv Fur Klinische Und Experimentelle Dermatologie* 227:452–467.
Julie A. Yager, Brian P. Wilcock (eds.) 1994. Color atlas and text of surgical pathology of the dog and cat. Dermatopathology and skin tumors. London: Mosby-Year Book. (ISBN-10: 0815197527, ISBN-13: 978-0815197522).
Kisseberth WC, MacEwen EG. 2001. Complications of cancer and its treatment. In: Withrow SJ, MacEwen EG (eds), *Small Animal Clinical Oncology*, p. 95. Philadelphia: WB Saunders.
Marconato L, Albanese F, Viacava P, Marchetti V, Abramo F. 2007 Aug. Paraneoplastic alopecia associated with hepatocellular carcinoma in a cat. *Veterinary Dermatology* 18(4):267–271.
Ohnemus U, Unalan M, Handjiski B, Paus R. 2004. Topical estrogen accelerates hair regrowth in mice after chemotherapy-induced alopecia by favoring the dystrophic catagen response pathway to damage. *Journal of Investigative Dermatology* 122(1):7–13.
Ordeix L, Fondevila MD, Ferrer L, Fondati A. 2001. Traction alopecia with vasculitis in an Old English sheepdog. *Journal of Small Animal Practice* 42:304.
Parker WM, Foster RA. 1996. Cutaneous vasculitis in five Jack Russell terriers. *Veterinary Dermatology* 7:109.
Pascal-Tenorio A, Olivry T, Gross TL, Atlee BA, Ihrke PJ. 1997. Paraneoplastic alopecia associated with internal malignancies in the cat. *Veterinary Dermatology* 8:47.
Rees CA, Boothe DM. 2003. Therapeutic response to pentoxifylline and its active metabolites in dogs with familial canine dermatomyositis. *Veterinary Therapeutics* 4(3):234–241.
Rosenkrantz WS, Griffith CE, Walder EJ. 1989. Traction alopecia in the canine: four case reports. *California Veterinarian* 43:7.
Selleri S, Seltmann H, Gariboldi S, Shirai YF, Balsari A, Zouboulis CC, Rumio C. 2006. Doxorubicin-induced alopecia is associated with sebaceous gland degeneration. *Journal of Investigative Dermatology* 126(4):711–720.
Sharov AA, Siebenhaar F, Sharova TY, Botchkareva NV, Gilchrest BA, Botchkarev VA. 2004. Fas signaling is involved in the control of hair follicle response to chemotherapy. *Cancer Research* 64(17):6266–6270.
Tasker S, Griffon DJ, Nuttall TJ, Hill PB. 1999. Resolution of paraneoplastic alopecia following surgical removal of a pancreatic carcinoma in a cat. *Journal of Small Animal Practice* 40: 16.
Van Vleet JF, Ferrans VJ. 1980. Clinical observations, cutaneous lesions, and hematologic alterations in chronic adriamycin intoxication in dogs with and without vitamin E and selenium supplementation. *American Journal of Veterinary Research* 41: 691.
Vitale CB, Gross TL, Magro CM. 1999. Vaccine-induced ischemic dermatopathy in the dog. *Veterinary Dermatology* 18 :131.
Wilcock BP, Yager JA. 1986. Focal cutaneous vasculitis and alopecia at sites of rabies vaccination in dogs. *Journal of the American Veterinary Medical Association* 188:1174.
Yun SJ, Kim SJ. 2007. Hair loss pattern due to chemotherapy-induced anagen effluvium: a cross-sectional observation. *Dermatology* 215(1):36–40.

3.5

Traumatic alopecia

Monika Linek

Acquired noninflammatory alopecia can be induced by self-inflicted hair loss. The two main causes for this are pruritus and psychogenic disorders. Whereas the former is recognized in any species to a greater or lesser extent, pure psychogenic alopecia has been almost exclusively described in cats. Both have in common that alopecia is produced by constant licking, rubbing, pulling of hairs, chewing or biting, and excessive grooming. Alopecia is often the only evident alteration, but may be accompanied by inflammation. It is then difficult to determine whether inflammation is a sequela to self-trauma or vice versa.

3.5.1 Feline psychogenic alopecia

3.5.1.1 Etiology and pathogenesis

The primary abnormality in psychogenic alopecia of cats is excessive grooming of easily reached areas, such as the medial aspects of the forelimbs and inner thighs, caudal aspect of the abdomen and the inguinal region (Fig. 3.5.1). Dorsal aspects of the lumbar, sacral, and tail areas are less commonly involved (Scott et al. 2001; Waisglass et al. 2006). However, as these regions are commonly affected by many pruritic diseases, it is very important to keep in mind that the diagnosis of psychogenic alopecia can only be made if other conditions have been ruled out. The true incidence of psychogenic disorders may be overestimated, as a complete workup is often limited by insufficient owner compliance or financial constraints.

3.5.1.2 Diagnosis

The diagnostic approach of feline psychogenic alopecia begins with obtaining a complete history and performing a thorough physical examination. Owners often do not realize that their cat is licking. Therefore, it is advisable to ask for tufts of hair lying in the cats' favorite hiding place or hairs excreted with feces. Since behavioral problems may result from anxiety neurosis, the questionnaire should include any alteration in lifestyle such as moving to a new home, hospitalization, boarding, new surroundings, a new pet or baby in the household, or the loss of a favorite companion. Cats of all ages and both sexes can be affected. There is a predilection for Oriental cat breeds (Scott et al. 2001; Waisglass et al. 2006). The physical examination reveals short stubby hairs. Trichograms are used to distinguish clinically between self-induced alopecia and spontaneous alopecia (see Section 2.1.4.3). In self-induced alopecia, hair shafts show split tips but hair roots reveal normal anagen and telogen bulbs. Hairs are not easily epilated. Minimum additional testing includes cytology, examination of superficial skin scrapings, and submission of hair samples for fungal culture (Werner and Manigot 2002). Evaluation of responses to parasiticidal treatment and feeding an elimination diet for 8–12 weeks are very important in the workup, since clinical response to parasitic treatment, flea bite allergy (FBA), and food adverse reaction made up to 70% of self-induced alopecia in cats (Waisglass et al. 2006). A thorough and intensive ectoparasitic treatment for 4–6 weeks is recommended as a diagnostic trial therapy for parasitic diseases and FBA. In endemic areas for *Demodex gatoi*, a trial therapy with lime sulfur may also be warranted. Hematological and biochemical blood analysis, including evaluation of thyroid gland function, may be necessary to rule out metabolic disorders, such as hyperthyroidism, hyperadrenocorticism, and diabetes mellitus. Urinary tract disease that can cause pain and discomfort is excluded

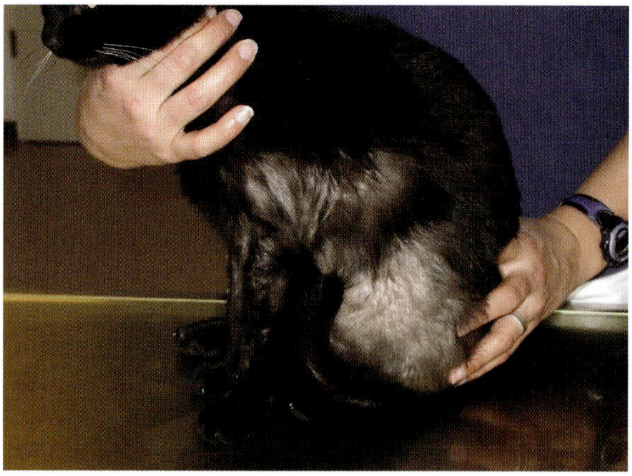

Fig. 3.5.1 Feline self-induced "psychogenic" alopecia. Note extensive incomplete alopecia on abdomen, flanks, and extremities.

by urinalysis (Werner and Manigot 2002). If results of these tests are negative, atopic dermatitis and psychogenic alopecia remain as differentials, as in both the diagnosis is made by excluding all other possible causes of clinical signs. Histological examination of skin biopsies may then be helpful in eliminating a diagnosis of psychogenic alopecia. It has been stated that the presence of even a few eosinophils in the dermis can be used to rule out psychogenic alopecia (Gross et al. 2005; Waisglass et al. 2006), as cats with histologic evidence of inflammation were subsequently found to have a medical condition. The assumption, however, that a lack of inflammatory lesions in skin biopsies can be used to confirm a diagnosis of psychogenic alopecia does not hold true (Waisglass et al. 2006). Treatment with antipruritic doses of glucocorticoids may help to differentiate pruritus from behavioral self-trauma, because glucocorticoids are unlikely to cause any substantial improvement in cats with a compulsive disorder. Specific allergen testing cannot be used to prove atopy as a cause of overgrooming. In fact, at this level there may remain a considerable overlap between the two conditions. Glucocorticoids could have effects on the behavior as described in human patients (Plihal et al. 1996). Serotonin reuptake inhibitors like clomipramine and fluoxetine used to treat psychogenic disorders may have antihistaminic effects. Stressful conditions may potentiate pruritus through a variety of mechanisms, including changes in cytokine and hormone profiles and the release of opioids and serotonin as well as various other vasoactive peptides (Virga 2003), and scratching can induce changes in sensory perception (Yamaoka et al. 2007). Compulsive disorders such as trichotillomania have been identified in humans in association with alopecia. They have no apparent goal, and can be repetitive, exaggerated, and so intense that they might be difficult to interrupt. In dogs acral lick dermatitis and flank or tail sucking have been implicated with compulsive disorders (Scott et al. 2001).

Although the pathophysiology of compulsive disorders is not entirely understood, an underlying alteration in neurotransmitters is a likely factor and pharmacologic intervention is often needed. Alterations in β-endorphins, dopamine, and serotonin have all been implicated in compulsive disorders, primarily on the basis of response to treatment, but abnormal serotonin metabolism has been suggested to be the primary mechanism by which these disorders are induced (Landsberg et al. 2003; Luescher 2003).

3.5.1.3 Therapy

The patient may improve without medical therapy or with only a short course of antianxiety drugs, if an underlying problem can be identified and if this problem can be modified or removed. A behaviorist should always be consulted. If potential stressors cannot be identified or eliminated, long-term therapy may be necessary.

Drugs that inhibit serotonin reuptake such as clomipramine and fluoxetine have been shown to be most effective in the treatment of cats and dogs with compulsive disorders (Hewson et al. 1998; Sawyer et al. 1999; Mertens et al. 2006). Psychogenic alopecia in cats has also been successfully managed with phenobarbital or diazepam, amitriptyline, naloxone, and buspirone (Willemse et al. 1994; Sawyer et al. 1999; Scott et al. 2001). Progestational compounds as megestrol acetate are considered obsolete due to their striking side effects (Scott et al. 2001) (Table 3.5.1).

3.5.2 Pruritus

3.5.2.1 Etiology and pathogenesis

As illustrated in the former chapter, pruritus can elicit alopecia by licking, rubbing, chewing, pulling, and

Table 3.5.1 Treatment options and success rates for psychogenic alopecia in cats

Drug	Dose	Response rate (duration of response)
Clomipramine	1.25–2.5 mg/day, oral	100% (3.6 months); additional environmental changes
Amitriptyline	2.5 mg/day, oral	66% (17–27 months)
Buspirone	5 mg, twice daily, oral	25% (4 months); additional environmental changes

Adapted from Sawyer et al. 1999.

biting. The list of differential diagnoses for animals with alopecia accompanied by marked pruritus and cutaneous inflammation is often lengthy, and a detailed discussion of the approach to this presentation is beyond the scope of this book.

3.5.2.2 Diagnosis

In most pruritic diseases there will be additional cutaneous changes, such as inflammation, seborrhea, hyperkeratosis, erosion, or ulceration. Distinctive distribution patterns may help to establish a ranking list of differential diagnoses (Griffin and DeBoer 2001; Scott et al. 2001). Hypersensitivity reactions, such as food allergy and atopy, present in the dog with erythema, excoriation, and self-induced alopecia periorally, on the forelegs, the distal extremities, the dorsum of the paws, lateral thorax, and ventral abdomen (Fig. 3.5.2). In fleabite allergy the dorsal lumbal and caudal thighs are more commonly affected. Scabies has a similar clinical picture as atopy, but severe crusting of elbows and the tips of the pinnae and a diffuse

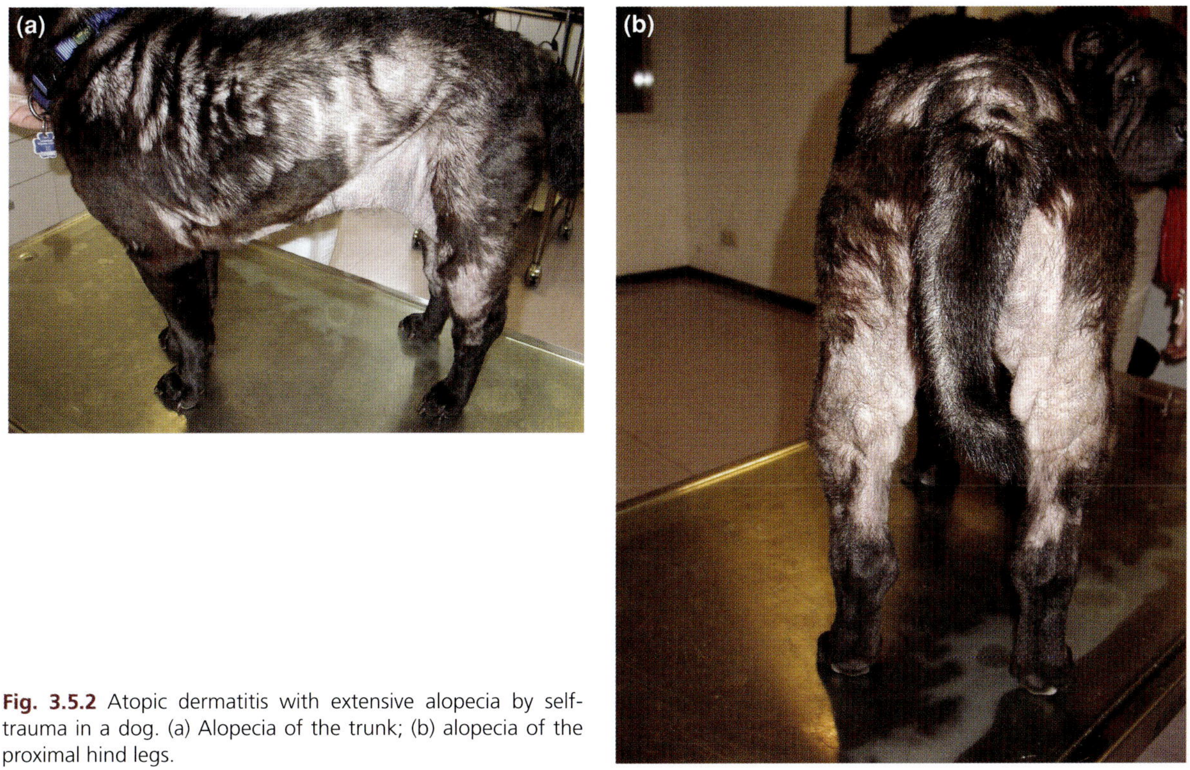

Fig. 3.5.2 Atopic dermatitis with extensive alopecia by self-trauma in a dog. (a) Alopecia of the trunk; (b) alopecia of the proximal hind legs.

maculopapulars rash of the ventral abdomen may predominate. It shall be emphasized that a strict adherence to the clinical approach as outlined earlier (see Chapter 2.1) is mandatory if pruritus is present. Similarly important is the identification and classification of primary and secondary skin lesions and the ability to correlate them to specific skin diseases. Primary skin lesions are macules, papules or plaques, pustules, vesicles or bullae, and nodules. Scales, alopecia, pigmentary abnormalities, comedones, and crusts may be primary or secondary lesions, and lichenification, epidermal collarettes, scars, erosions, ulcers, excoriations, fissures, and callus are all secondary lesions (Scott et al. 2001).

The knowledge of breed, age, and sex predilections and the ability to interpret laboratory and histological reports may help to abbreviate the steps necessary for a final diagnosis (Scott et al. 2001; Gross et al. 2005).

In the dog, there might also be pruritic alopecia without any inflammatory changes, where the animal licks or rubs the pruritic area more gently and alopecia remains the predominate lesion. Common underlying causes are *Malassezia* dermatitis, *Sarcoptes* incognito, *Cheylitiella* infestation, atopy, and food allergy. In these cases it is primarily important to distinguish self-induced alopecia from spontaneous alopecia. If a self-inflicted alopecia has been diagnosed and an underlying cause cannot be found, an aggressive trial therapy for ectoparasites may be still advisable. This would include a minimum of three times of biweekly spot-on application of selamectin or moxidectin with imidacloprid. This trial therapy might be combined with an elimination diet to shorten the workup time. Further workup of atopic dermatitis in dogs and cats is deferred to special textbooks.

References

Griffin CE, DeBoer DJ. 2001. The ACVD task force on canine atopic dermatitis (XIV): clinical manifestations of canine atopic dermatitis. *Veterinary Immunology and Immunopathology* 81:255–269.

Gross TL, Ihrke PJ, Walder EJ, Affolter VK. 2005. *Skin Diseases of the Dog and the Cat*. Oxford: Blackwell Science.

Hewson CJ, Luescher UA, Parent JM, Conlon PD, Ball RO. 1998. Efficacy of clomipramine in the treatment of canine compulsive disorder. *Journal of the American Veterinary Medical Association* 213:1760–1766.

Landsberg GM, Hunthausen W, Ackerman L. 2003. Stereotypic and compulsive disorders. In: von Gary Landsberg. Wayne Hunthausen. Lowell J. Ackerman (eds), *Handbook of Behavior Problems of the Dog and Cat*, pp. 195–225. Edinburgh: WB Saunders.

Luescher AU. 2003. Diagnosis and management of compulsive disorders in dogs and cats. *Veterinary Clinics of North America. Small Animal Practice* 33:253–267, vi.

Mertens PA, Torres S, Jessen C. 2006. The effects of clomipramine hydrochloride in cats with psychogenic alopecia: a prospective study. *Journal of the American Animal Hospital Association* 42:336–343.

Plihal W, Krug R, Pietrowsky R, Fehm HL, Born J. 1996. Corticosteroid receptor mediated effects on mood in humans. *Psychoneuroendocrinology* 21:515–523.

Sawyer LS, Moon-Fanelli AA, Dodman NH. 1999. Psychogenic alopecia in cats: 11 cases (1993–1996). *Journal of the American Veterinary Medical Association* 214:71–74.

Scott DW, Miller WH, Griffin CE. 2001. *Muller and Kirk's Small Animal Dermatology*, pp. 457–476. Philadelphia: WB Saunders.

Virga V. 2003. Behavioral dermatology. *Veterinary Clinics of North America. Small Animal Practice* 33:231–232, vi.

Waisglass SE, Landsberg GM, Yager JA, Hall JA. 2006. Underlying medical conditions in cats with presumptive psychogenic alopecia. *Journal of the American Veterinary Medical Association* 228:1705–1709.

Werner AH, Manigot GA. 2002. Diagnosing and treating psychogenic alopecia. In: Thoday KL, Foil CS, Bond R (eds), *Advances in Veterinary Dermatology*, Vol. 4, pp. 280–281. Oxford, England: Blackwell Science.

Willemse T, Mudde M, Josephy M, Spruijt BM. 1994. The effect of haloperidol and naloxone on excessive grooming behavior of cats. *European Neuropsychopharmacology* 4:39–45.

Yamaoka J, Di ZH, Sun W, Kawana S. 2007. Changes in cutaneous sensory nerve fibers induced by skin-scratching in mice. *Journal of Dermatological Science* 46:41–51.

3.6

Scarring alopecia

Lars Mecklenburg

In man, a very large number of follicular diseases may lead to destruction and replacement of the pilosebaceous unit by scar tissue (Abell 2007). These alopecias are referred to as scarring alopecia or cicatricial alopecia. They comprise diseases such as lichen planopilaris, lupus erythematosus, dissecting folliculitis, acne keloidalis, central centrifugal scarring alopecia, and yet unclassified forms of scarring alopecia including "pseudopelade of Brocq." The latter likely represents the end-stage or clinical variant of various other forms of scarring alopecia (Sperling 2001). Classification of scarring alopecia in human medicine is under continuous debate, and therefore, extrapolations from human to veterinary medicine should be conducted with great caution.

The term "scarring alopecia" is not commonly used in veterinary dermatology although, as in humans, numerous different diseases can lead to follicular destruction, such as physical or chemical trauma (including erythema ab igne), infectious or sterile furunculosis (including juvenile cellulitis), mural folliculitis, or ischemic dermatopathy. Scarring, that is, replacement of the pilosebaceous unit by fibrous tissue, is rarely observed. This phenomenon is yet unexplained, but might result from the comparatively small size of pilosebaceous units in most domestic animals such as the dog. Scarring is represented by a scar tract that extends into the subcutaneous tissue, associated with remnants of the elastic fiber sheath of the damaged hair follicle. Sebaceous glands, apocrine glands, and arrector pili muscles may remain.

In domestic animals, scarring alopecia may be seen as an end stage of lymphocytic mural folliculitis (see Chapter 4.4) or as an end stage of follicular atrophy (see Chapter 3.4). It is per se unspecific and does not allow determination of the underlying pathogenesis, except for those cases where earlier stages of follicular destruction are contained in the biopsy. Clinically, scarring alopecia is associated with a loss of follicular openings (ostia). The skin is usually shiny and smooth with a sharp border between haired and alopecic skin areas. Differential diagnosis such as alopecia areata, follicular atrophy, and mural folliculitis need to be excluded by histopathology. Scarring alopecia is permanent since stem cells, usually located in the bulge area, are lost; hence, there is no treatment for this condition.

Morphea (syn. localized scleroderma) is a distinct but still enigmatic skin disease in humans where dermal connective tissue and cutaneous adnexa are replaced by fibrous tissue of variable degree of organization. It may range from almost normal to a typical scar formation. A similar disease has rarely been described in dogs and cats (Scott 1986; Bensignor et al. 1998). However, neither clinical investigation nor histopathology allows a clear differentiation from cicatricial alopecia (see above). It is therefore questionable whether a distinct disease entity of morphea actually exists in domestic animals. Histopathology may reveal mild dermal inflammation, whereas the clinical appearance is reported as well-demarcated alopecia with a smooth and shiny skin surface.

References

Abell E. 2007. Inflammatory diseases of the epidermal appendages and of cartilage. In: Elder D, Elenitsas R, Jaworsky C, Johnson B. (eds), *Lever's Histopathology of the Skin*, 8th edn, p. 414. Philadelphia: Lippincott-Raven Publishers.

Bensignor E, Carlotti DN, Pin D. 1998. Morphea-like lesion in a cat. *Journal of Small Animal Practice* 39(11):538–540.

Scott DW. 1986. Localized scleroderma (morphea) in two dogs. *Journal of the American Animal Hospital Association* 22:207–211.

Sperling LC. 2001. Scarring alopecia and the dermatopathologist. *Journal of Cutaneous Pathology* 28:333–342.

Part 4

Inflammatory alopecias

4.1

Folliculitis with intraluminal organisms

Monika Linek

In this chapter, inflammation of the hair follicle is discussed, in which inflammatory cell invasion into the follicular lumen is evoked by intraluminal organisms. The inflammatory infiltrate is predominated by polymorphonuclear leukocytes (Gross et al. 1992, 2005; Yager and Wilcock 1994). Attracted by the intraluminal pathogen, cells migrate from the perifollicular vessels to the hair follicle, penetrate the hair follicle wall, and accumulate in the follicular lumen. The pathogen can be located either in the hair shaft (e.g., dermatophytes) or in the follicular lumen (e.g., bacteria, mites, or nematodes). By definition, every luminal folliculitis must have been mural initially, but in mural folliculitis (see Chapter 4.4) the infiltrate will remain in the follicular wall and will not be present in the lumen (Gross et al. 1997). In addition, mural folliculitis is mostly dominated by mononuclear leukocytes instead of polymorphonuclear inflammatory cells. Only in some cases of demodicosis and dermatophytosis, where very low numbers of organisms are present, does the mural pattern of inflammation predominate, which can then be mistaken for an autoimmune mural lymphocytic interface folliculitis such as in lupus erythematosus (Gross et al. 2005).

A *furunculosis* is morphologically defined as a mural and luminal folliculitis, where the entire follicular wall is destroyed by the inflammatory reaction. The inflammatory character then changes to a (pyo)granulomatous infiltrate composed of neutrophils, macrophages, eosinophils, plasma cells, and eventually giant cells. The naked keratin of hair shafts in the dermis then contributes to a foreign body reaction. Severe furunculosis completely destroys the affected pilosebaceous unit, which is replaced by scarring (Gross et al. 2005).

The most common clinical signs of luminal folliculitis in all animals are multifocal areas of alopecia, follicular papules or pustules (Fig. 4.1.1), crusts, and epidermal collarettes that form circular rims of scales (Fig. 4.1.2) (Scott et al. 2001). It can be accompanied by excessive scaling, and scales are often pierced by hairs. Pruritus is variable. The type and length of hair coat may influence the clinical presentation. Short-haired breeds in dogs and horses often present with multiple superficial papules that look similar to urticaria, since the inflammation in and around the follicles causes the hairs to stand more erect (Ihrke 1996; Pilsworth and Knottenbelt 2007). These raised tufts of hair are most striking if viewed against light. They are easily epilated, an important feature that helps to distinguish superficial folliculitis from true urticaria, in which hairs do not epilate easily. When the hairs fall out they leave patches of focal alopecia and give the coat a moth-eaten appearance (Fig. 4.1.3). Foci of hair loss may coalesce to larger areas of alopecia. The underlying skin does not always look inflamed, particularly if it is darkly pigmented. In long-haired animals owners initially report increased shedding and a dull hair coat, subsequently developing scaling, crusts, pustules, and epidermal collarettes (Mason 1993; Scott et al. 2001).

If furunculosis develops, it presents macroscopically as an erythematous nodule in the dermis, often associated with hair loss. Hairs are always easily epilated and exudation of blood or pus is seen, if the nodule is squeezed (Ihrke 1996; Scott et al. 2001). In confluating furuncles (also called “carbuncles”) pain, ulceration, hemorrhagic crusts, bullae, and draining tracts with serosanguinous or purulent exudate may be seen (Fig. 4.1.4). Lichenification and hyperpigmentation

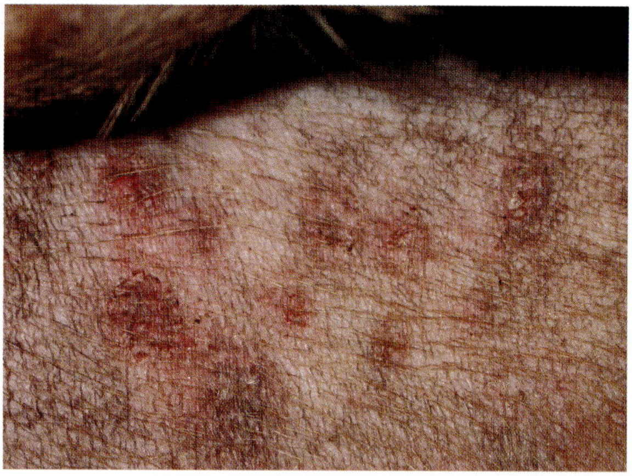

Fig. 4.1.1 Follicular papules and pustules.

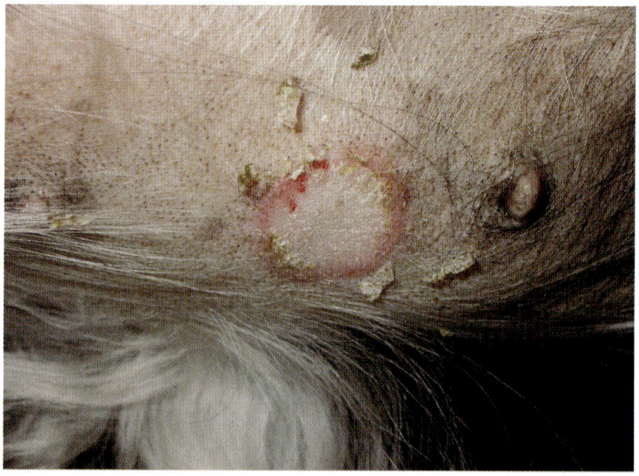

Fig. 4.1.3 Superficial canine pyoderma. Note epidermal collarettes that depict circular rims of scales.

are signs of chronic inflammation, which are completely unspecific.

Since age, breed, history, or clinical picture do not allow a specific diagnosis of the underlying etiology, it is essential to follow the standard dermatological examination protocol and perform cytology, skin scrapings, trichogram, Wood's lamp examination, and a dermatophyte culture. Biopsies might become necessary whenever there is no diagnosis after these tests have been performed. Detailed examination procedures have been explained elsewhere (see Chapter 2.1), and will be briefly mentioned in the next paragraphs, where the main differentials for luminal folliculitis are reviewed in more detail.

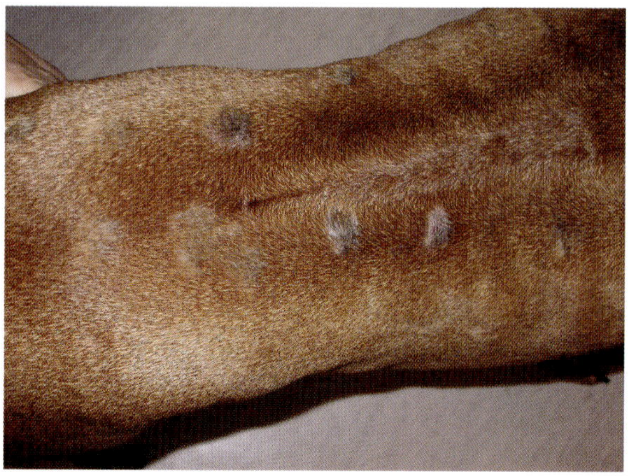

Fig. 4.1.2 Multifocal "moth-eaten" alopecia due to folliculitis.

4.1.1 Bacterial folliculitis

4.1.1.1 Etiology and pathogenesis

Bacterial folliculitis can be classified on the basis of the extent of infection and its etiology, and can be divided into primary or secondary disease (Gross et al. 1997).

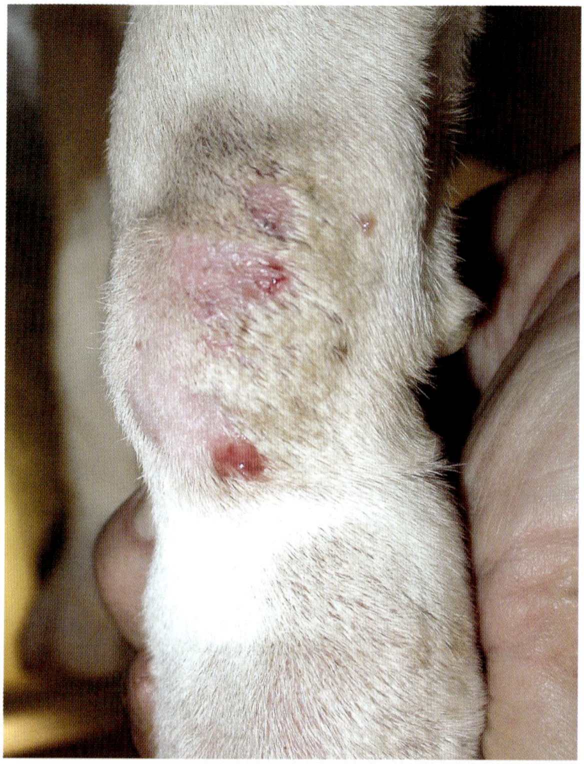

Fig. 4.1.4 Deep canine pyoderma. Note draining tracts with serohemorrhagic to purulent exudate.

Superficial bacterial folliculitis, the most common clinical presentation of pyoderma in dogs, horses, and presumably cats, involves the superficial part of the hair follicle lumen and is characterized by pustules. Intact pustules are erythematous and can be very small. A hair is normally protruding from the center of the pustule and helps to distinguish follicular pustules from pustules of the interfollicular skin (such as impetigo and pemphigus). However, pustules are transient; they easily rupture and eventually result in papules that are covered by crusts.

Deep bacterial folliculitis includes inflammation of the entire hair follicle with or without furunculosis. Deep pyoderma may evolve from more superficial lesions and can coexist with them or may develop autonomously. It is less common, more serious in nature, and usually more painful than superficial pyoderma. One of the typical features of deep folliculitis is alopecia developing as a sequela to follicular inflammation and destruction. Scarring may finally occur (Ihrke 1996; Gross et al. 2005). Alopecia can be accompanied by lichenification, hyperpigmentation, and swelling. Pus or a hemorrhagic exudate and sometimes fragments of hair shafts may extrude upon pressure. Nodules may rupture and form fistules and draining tracts. Erosions and ulcers develop secondary to selftrauma.

Pyoderma is etiologically classified according to the main bacteria involved in the infection. In all species, staphylococci are most frequently associated with pyoderma. However, other bacteria such as *Pseudomonas*, *Escherichia coli*, *Proteus*, and *Corynebacterium* have also been isolated (Heffner et al. 1988; Scott et al. 2001; Pilsworth and Knottenbelt 2007).

Pyoderma is further divided into primary and secondary, depending on whether or not it is triggered by an underlying disease. *Primary pyoderma* occurs in otherwise healthy animals, without an identifiable predisposing cause. Primary pyoderma resolves completely upon appropriate antimicrobial treatment and recurrence is not expected. Development of chronic recurrent superficial or deep primary pyoderma is most often caused by inappropriate antibiotic therapy, that is, failures in dosing, duration of treatment, or selection of the right medication. Another cause for recurrent primary pyoderma is concurrent corticosteroid administration.

Secondary pyoderma is much more common than primary pyoderma, recurs in spite of appropriate therapy, and is due to an underlying disease. Common diseases associated with secondary pyoderma include allergies (flea allergy, atopic dermatitis due to food or environmental allergens), endocrinopathies (hyperadrenocorticism or hypothyroidism), seborrheic conditions (including primary follicular or sebaceous gland diseases), ectoparasitosis (e.g., demodicosis), or anatomic predispositions (e.g., skin folds) (Ihrke 1996; Scott et al. 2001). Any inflammatory, obstructive, atrophic, or degenerative disease of the hair follicle, as discussed in this book, can predispose to secondary bacterial infection of the hair follicle.

Whereas in primary pyoderma trunk, head, and proximal extremities are most often affected, in secondary pyodermas the clinical distribution pattern depends on the underlying disease.

4.1.1.1.1 Canine pyoderma

In the dog, *Staphylococcus intermedius* and *S. aureus* have been reported as the most frequent isolates associated with pyoderma (May 2006). *S. intermedius* is a common resident bacteria in the dog. It is located at mucocutaneous junctions of mouth, nose, and anus and in the external ear canal from which it is transferred to the rest of the skin by grooming (Allaker et al. 1992a,b). Most recently *S. pseudointermedius* (opposed to *S. intermedius*) has been identified by phenotypic speciation to be the most common cause of canine pyoderma (Bannoehr et al. 2007; Sasaki et al. 2007). Other staphylococci, particularly the coagulase-negative species such as *S. epidermidis*, *S. sciuri*, and *S. xylosus*, are generally considered as transient and nonpathogenic (Harvey and Lloyd 1994). However, *S. schleiferi* (both the coagulase-negative subspecies *S. schleiferi*, schleiferi, and the coagulase-positive subspecies *S. schleiferi*, coagulans) has been isolated from pyoderma and otitis in dogs (Frank et al. 2003; May et al. 2005; Morris et al. 2006; Rich et al. 2007). There is yet insufficient information on the incidence of pyoderma caused by these newly reported staphylococcal species, since most veterinary laboratories do not differentiate them routinely (Zdovc et al. 2004).

Other bacteria such as *Pseudomonas spp.*, *Escherichia coli*, and *Proteus* can also cause canine pyoderma and are particularly common in deep pyodermas (Ihrke 1996; Cole et al. 1998; Petersen et al. 2002). *Pseudomonas aeruginosa* has frequently been isolated from post-grooming furunculosis, an acute and painful furunculosis developing after bathing or grooming (Hillier et al. 2003). Shampoos or bathing equipments may be contaminated by *Pseudomonas* and violent, traumatizing grooming may facilitate infection.

The clinical presentation of canine bacterial folliculitis is highly variable, particularly between breeds. Pustules and erythema are often absent in short-haired breeds. These dogs most frequently present with hyperpigmented foci of alopecia, 0.5–2 cm in diameter (Fig. 4.1.3), or firm papules or nodules. Some breeds such as Collies and Shetland Sheepdogs often show diffuse widespread alopecia with mild erythema and epidermal collarettes at the periphery, often mimicking an endocrinopathy. Breeds such as the West Highland White Terrier may develop seborrheic plaques (Scott et al. 2001). In chronic cases of canine bacterial folliculitis, erythematous papules, small pustules, epidermal collarettes, and hyperpigmentation are simultaneously present. Many cases of canine pyoderma are associated with pruritus (Hill and Moriello 1994). Any body area can develop pyoderma, but the glabrous site of the groin and axilla are most commonly affected.

Canine deep pyoderma is less common than superficial bacterial folliculitis, but it is still a relatively common skin disease. It may develop de novo or may progress from superficial folliculitis. The deep follicular inflammation leads to rupture of the hair follicle wall and subsequent development of a granulomatous foreign body response against hair shaft fragments. Canine deep pyoderma commonly presents as firm nodules or poorly defined edematous plaques. Circumscribed, red to dark-blue colored nodules with a fragile surface and hemorrhagic bullae are additional distinctive clinical features (Fig. 4.1.5). Pain or pruritus is common. Focal or even generalized lymphadenopathy may develop. Deep pyodermas with furunculosis may affect any body area but certain areas are preferably involved. Elbows, hocks, and lateral stifles (where callus may preexist) are more prone to deep infections, possibly due to recurrent traumatic follicular irritation.

Acral lick granulomas arise in areas where constant licking results in self-inflicted follicular trauma. Pyotraumatic furunculosis, which occurs predominately at the cheek or neck of Golden Retrievers (and other large breed dogs such as the Newfoundland Dog or the Saint Bernard Dog), is also a clinical manifestation of deep pyoderma (Holm et al. 2004). Interdigital furunculosis is a very common clinical pattern in the dog, and plant awns, fragmented hair shafts, *Demodex* mites, or other foreign bodies play a significant pathogenetic role (Breathnach et al. 2008). Certain subtypes of deep bacterial folliculitis and furunculosis in dogs present with a distinctive clinical picture, but are not further discussed in this chapter, since they are not primarily alopecic.

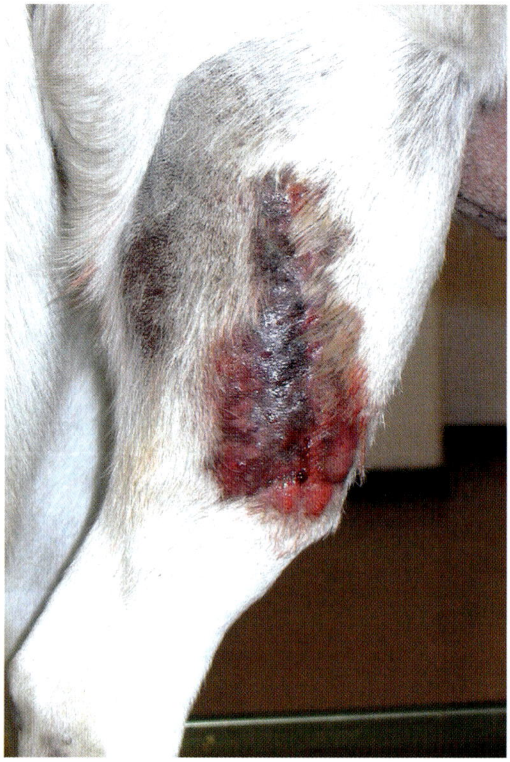

Fig. 4.1.5 Alopecia in canine pyoderma. Note red to dark blue-colored nodules with a fragile surface.

4.1.1.1.2 Feline pyoderma

Bacterial folliculitis and furunculosis in the cat is significantly less frequent than in the dog. Similar to dogs, most cases of primary feline pyoderma are associated with *S. intermedius* and *S. aureus* (May 2006). Less frequently *S. schleiferi*, both coagulase positive and negative species, β-hemolytic streptococci, and *Pasteurella multocida* have been isolated. Deep infections in the cat are most commonly associated with wounds and present as subcutaneous abscesses and nodules, associated with various aerobic and anaerobic organisms. Infections by atypical or opportunistic mycobacteria have been described (Scott et al. 2001; Gross et al. 2005).

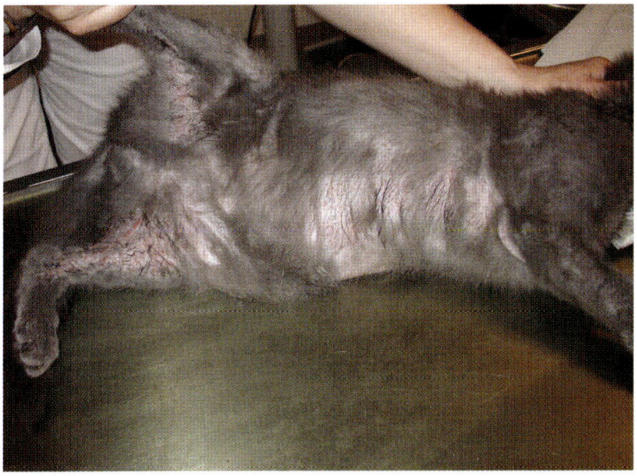

Fig. 4.1.6 Self-induced alopecia in feline eosinophilic plaque. Note extensive hair loss associated with numerous erythematous plaques.

Bacterial folliculitis in cats may be overlooked and underdiagnosed as the most common clinical finding is scaling and crusting. Intact pustules are rarely found (Wildermuth et al. 2006). Superficial pyoderma in the cat can present as a miliary dermatitis, mimicking feline allergy. Feline skin diseases such as eosinophilic granuloma, eosinophilic plaque (Fig. 4.1.6) ulcerative head and neck lesions, or feline lick alopecia are commonly associated with secondary superficial pyoderma. Secondary recurrent nonhealing deep pyoderma in cats can also be associated with systemic diseases such as feline immunodeficiency virus or feline leukemia virus infection.

4.1.1.1.3 Equine pyoderma

In the horse bacterial skin diseases are most often caused by *S. intermedius* and *S. aureus*. In addition, *Staphylococcus hyicus*, *Streptococcus equi*, and *Corynebacterium pseudotuberculosis* have been isolated in equine folliculitis (Pascoe 1984; Heffner et al. 1988; Pilsworth and Knottenbelt 2007). "Heat rash," "summer rash," "summer scub," "sweating eczema," "saddle scab," and "saddle boils" are all common names for pyoderma in the horse and reflect the underlying etiology of excessive sweating, friction, and trauma from track and saddle and/or allergies to insect bites. Clinical signs are as described before. Pustules and erythema are often absent, while crusts and alopecia usually develop in a circular pattern with an exfoliative border (Fig. 4.1.7). Variable pruritus is seen.

Dermatophilus congolensis is one of the most important skin pathogens in the horse. It usually occurs in association with moist environmental conditions (Rosser 1995). Dermatophilosis shows a very characteristic clinical picture with exudation, matted hair, and excessive scab formation (Fig. 4.1.8). Localized or widespread alopecia and crusting with little pruritus are typical. In the short coat of the summer, lesions tend to be smaller and less exudative, leaving a moth-eaten appearance, whereas the thick winter coat becomes severely matted with a purulent exudate and a thick creamy pus adhering to the skin (Rosser 1995). The distribution pattern of the lesions generally reflects the areas that are exposed to excessive moistening by rain or sweating under rugs. In racing horses the cannon region may be solely affected, and a traumatic cause is suspected. Dermatophilosis may be easily diagnosed by cytology, where cocci with a "railroad track"-like growth pattern are found.

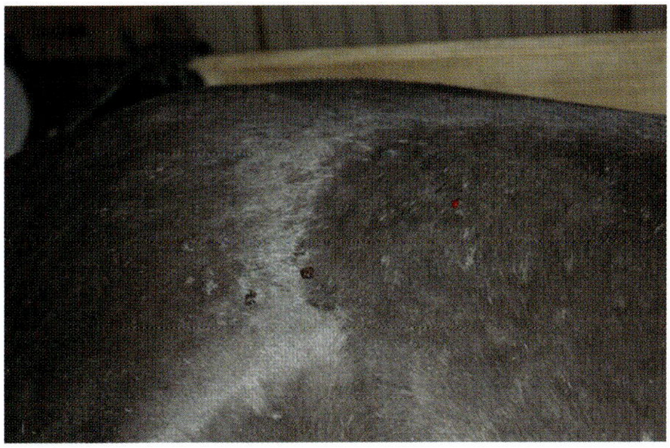

Fig. 4.1.7 Equine pyoderma. Multifocal crusts, alopecia, and exfoliation in a circular pattern with absence of pustules and erythema. (Courtesy of S. Rüfenacht.)

Deep pyoderma is uncommon in the horse. Staphylococcal deep pyoderma can present as a nodular

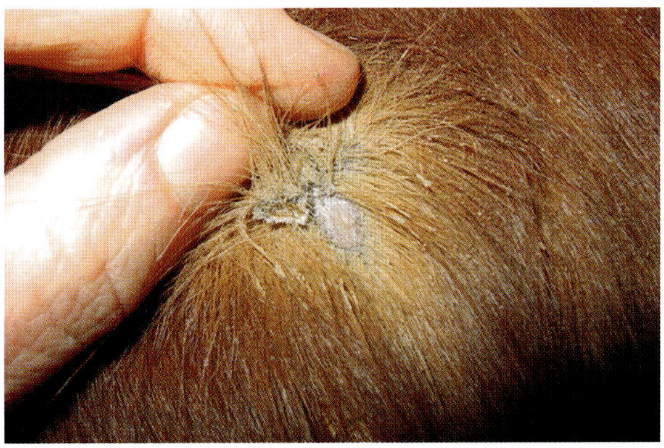

Fig. 4.1.8 Equine dermatophilosis. Matted hair and excessive scab formation with exudation. (Courtesy of S. Rüfenacht.)

disease termed "botryomycosis," which mimics a deep fungal infection. These lesions may require surgical excision as well as long-term antibiotical therapy. Solitary or multiple abscesses are often caused by *Corynebacterium pseudotuberculosis* (Heffner et al. 1988; Farstved et al. 2004).

4.1.1.1.4 Ovine pyoderma

A *facial bacterial folliculitis* in adult sheep is caused by virulent strains of *S. aureus*. Affected animals develop a nonpruritic dermatitis characterized by alopecia, erythema, hyperpigmentation, crusting, superficial ulcers, exudation, and thickening of the skin (Scott et al. 1980; Koutinas et al. 2007).

Sheep fleece rot is another distinct ovine pyoderma characterized by marked exudation and crust formation. It is triggered by poor hygiene such as constant wetting of the skin. *Pseudomonas aeruginosa* seems to be the main causative organism of fleece rot (Salisbury and Barrowman 1984; Norris et al. 2007).

4.1.1.2 Diagnosis

As mentioned before, clinical signs of bacterial folliculitis are variable, and therefore many differential diagnoses have to be considered. Differential diagnoses for superficial folliculitis include demodicosis (see Section 4.1.3), *Malassezia dermatitis*, dermatophytosis (see Section 4.1.2), and other nonfollicular bacterial diseases such as impetigo and superficial spreading pyoderma. Uncommon pustular and crusting diseases such as pemphigus foliaceus (see Section 4.3.1) and in the cat feline exfoliative dermatitis (see Section 4.4.2.1) have to be considered. Clinical differential diagnoses for deep bacterial folliculitis include demodicosis (see Section 4.1.3), dermatophytosis (see Section 4.1.2), cutaneous fungal diseases, protothecosis, mycobacterial infection, and neoplasia (Scott et al. 2001).

Differentiation is primarily based on clinical signs and cytology. Multiple deep skin scrapings are needed to rule out parasitic infections, particularly *Demodex* mites. Wood's lamp examination and dermatophyte cultures should be performed to exclude dermatophytosis. Biopsies and bacterial cultures are needed in many cases to accomplish a final diagnosis (Ihrke 1987, 1996; Gross et al. 2005).

In superficial pyoderma, direct impression smears of intact pustules, epidermal collarettes, or moist erythematous skin underlying crusts reveals large numbers of neutrophils, cocci, rods, or both (Fig. 2.1.10). Neutrophils with intracellular bacteria are considered the cytological hallmark of superficial pyoderma. Furunculosis will reveal a mixed inflammatory infiltrate with neutrophils, macrophages, eosinophils, lymphocytes, and plasma cells, while bacteria are quite sparse. Impression smears of alopecic or scaling skin are less diagnostic, since they may reveal only large numbers of exfoliating keratinocytes with overlying bacteria.

Bacterial culture and susceptibility testing to antibiotics are mandatory in cases of deep pyoderma, recurrent superficial pyoderma, and pyoderma that does not respond to adequate antibacterial therapy. It is also recommended if rods are the predominate infectious agent, since antimicrobial susceptibility of these organisms is rather unpredictable. Accurate test results are most likely to be obtained from intact pustules or deep lesions. Nodular lesions are best cultured from macerated tissue obtained via a sterile biopsy technique (see Section 2.1.4.11).

As mentioned before, any diagnosis of bacterial folliculitis or furunculosis has to be accompanied by a thorough search for an underlying disease that fosters secondary pyoderma.

4.1.1.3 Therapy

4.1.1.3.1 Topical therapy

Focal superficial pyoderma may be treated with topical antibiotics such as 2% mupirocin, 2% fucidinic acid, or silver sulfadiazine cream. Topical neomycin is not recommended, since it may cause contact allergy. Topical bacitracin or polymyxin B are more effective against Gram-negative bacteria than other topical antibiotics but are inactivated with purulent exudates (Ihrke 1996; Scott et al. 2001). Daily shampooing with an antibacterial shampoo as a sole therapy may resolve more widespread superficial pyoderma, but is usually not sufficient for deep pyodermas. Appropriate antibacterial shampoos contain benzoyl peroxide, chlorhexidine, chlorhexidine–miconazole, ethyl lactate, or triclosan. Shampooing will remove bacteria, crusts, and scales, and it will reduce the pruritus and odor associated with pyoderma. Additional clipping of the hair coat is helpful as it prevents accumulation of debris and facilitates bathing and lathering (de Jaham 2003).

4.1.1.3.2 Systemic therapy

The primary treatment of pyoderma is with appropriate antibiotics administered systemically for at least 3–4 weeks. Chronic, recurrent, or deep pyodermas typically require 8–12 weeks or even longer to resolve completely. As a general rule, treatment is continued beyond complete clinical remission for 8 days in superficial and for 14 days in deep pyoderma (Deboer 1990, 1995). Antibiotic treatment of 10–14 days duration is inappropriate for patients with recurrent bacterial skin infections and may favor the emergence of multidrug-resistant strains (Pellerin et al. 1998; Loeffler et al. 2007). Empiric antibiotic therapy is inappropriate except for cases of mild, first-time superficial pyodermas without complicating factors. Any systemic antibacterial therapy should be accompanied by shampooing with an antibacterial substance as mentioned before. Immunomodulatory therapy has been used with variable success rates for the management of idiopathic recurrent pyoderma where no underlying etiology has been found (Deboer 1990; Curtis 1998; Curtis et al. 2006).

The choice of an antibiotic to treat bacterial folliculitis should be based on the chronicity of the disease, microbial isolates, susceptibility testing, and safety. A review of the mechanisms of action and common side effects of antibiotics is beyond the scope of this book but can be found elsewhere (Prescott et al. 2000; Plumb 2005).

β-lactam antibiotics and *tetracylines* are inappropriate choices for treating canine superficial or deep pyodermas, because they are ineffective in 90% of cases (Kim et al. 2005; May 2006). Superficial pyoderma should be treated with β-lactamase-stable antibiotics such as amoxicillin-clavulanic acid, cephalexin, or cefadroxil. These drugs have shown very low occurrence of bacterial resistance so far (Lloyd et al. 1997; Holm et al. 2002; Ganiere et al. 2005; White et al. 2005). There is, however, emerging evidence that with repeated exposure to these antibiotics, methicillin-resistant strains of *S. intermedius* (MRSI) occur (Kania et al. 2004; Loeffler et al. 2007). Methicillin-resistant *S. aureus* (MRSA) has been a major problem in human medicine for more than a decade, and has increasingly been isolated in companion animals. (Boag et al. 2004; Rich 2005; Jones et al. 2007). In most bacteria, methicillin resistance is conferred to a low-affinity penicillin-binding protein 2a that is encoded by the bacterial "*mecA*" gene. Resistance includes all β-lactam antibiotics and cephalosporins, even if in vitro resistance testing has indicated susceptibility. This is extremely important when interpreting results from diagnostic laboratories. In many cases of MRSA or MRSI, drugs such as rifampicin, potentiated sulfonamids, and chloramphenicol need to be used, although they bear a higher risk of adverse effects (Loeffler et al. 2007).

Clindamycin belongs to the lincosamid class and is distributed to fibrous tissue and therefore is a good choice to treat deep infections when based on culture and susceptibility testing (Harvey et al. 1993; Scott et al. 1998; Bloom and Rosser 2001). Clindamycin is bacteriostatic at low doses and bacteriocidal at higher doses. Lincomycin is less commonly used nowadays due to an increased bacterial resistance.

Fluoroquinolone antibiotics such as enrofloxacin, marbofloxacin, ibafloxacin, or orbifloxacin are broad-spectrum antibiotics with activity against Gram-positive and Gram-negative bacteria (Paradis et al. 2001; Ganiere et al. 2004; Horspool et al. 2004, 2006). Fluoroquinolones distribute to most tissues and accumulate in white blood cells, which results in high concentrations at sites where bacteria are present. They are commonly used for their safety and convenience in administration (once daily). However, fluoroquinolones should not be used for empiric therapy and should not represent the first choice antibiotic, even if susceptibility has been demonstrated, because there has been a significant increase of reports on bacterial resistance to fluoroquinolones in the last decade (Lloyd et al. 1999). Pradofloxacin, a new fluoroquinolone antibiotic, can be used in deep pyodermas of dogs, where it has demonstrated similar efficacy as amoxycillin/clavulanic acid (Mueller and Stephan 2007).

Potentiated sulfonamids remain a reasonable choice of antibiotic therapy in small animals, as staphylococci, including methicillin-resistant and coagulase-negative species, are mostly susceptible. However, idiosyncratic adverse effects (hepatotoxicitiy, vasculitis, polyarthritis, and anemia) are quite common. Treatment for a prolonged time period has additionally caused hypothyroidism in the dog (Daminet and Ferguson 2003; Trepanier et al. 2003). In the horse the most commonly used antibiotic for pyoderma is trimethoprim sulfa (30 mg/kg) given orally every 12 h for 2–6 weeks or even longer, if infection is deep. Enrofloxacin (7.5 mg/kg once daily) may be effective in cases of staphylococcal resistance, but should be avoided in horses less than

2 years of age due to possible cartilage damage (Pascoe 1984; Pilsworth and Knottenbelt 2007).

4.1.2 Dermatophytosis

4.1.2.1 Etiology and pathogenesis

Dermatophytosis is a superficial cutaneous infection of hair, skin, and nails with one or more of the fungal species in the keratinophilic genera *Microsporum*, *Trichophyton*, and *Epidermophyton*. The most common *Microsporum* and *Trichophyton* species are usually separated on the basis of host preference and natural habitat. *M. canis* (new nomenclature: Arthroderma otae Gräser et al. 2008) is the most common pathogen in cats and dogs, but is able to infect all species (Foil 1994; Scott et al. 2001; Kerl 2003). *M. gypseum* and *T. mentagrophytes* (subspecies mentagrophytes) are recognized in a wide range of animals, including dogs, cats, cattle, horses, and sheep. *T. verrucosum* is more frequent in cattle, *M. nanum* in pigs, and *T.* and *M. equinum* in horses. Most dermatophytes found in animals represent a group of zoophilic pathogens able to infect people and cause severe human disease (tinea) depending on the immune response of the infected individual (Moriello 2003b).

Infection occurs via direct transmission of fungal spores to a susceptible host. Reservoirs of infection for both, people and animals, include contaminated environments and objects, animals with subclinical or clinical infections, and animals that are mechanical carriers of the spores on their hair coat (Mancianti and Papini 1996; Mancianti et al. 2003; Heinrich et al. 2005). The disease tends to be more common in warm tropical and subtropical climates or where there are large numbers of feral animals.

Any age, sex, or breed of animal is susceptible to infection. However, the disease tends to be more common in young, sick, debilitated, and old animals. Immunodeficient patients, human or animal, are more prone to infection. Long-haired animals, particularly Persian cats, seem to be more susceptible and more difficult to treat, either due to hereditary internal factors or simply due to the fact that the long hairs easily trap fungal spores (Moriello and DeBoer 1995a).

Once infection has been established, dermatophytes invade the keratin of hairs and skin. Fungal arthrospores can produce various enzymes such as proteinases, keratinases, and mannases that facilitate penetration into the keratin. This provokes both a humoral and a cell-mediated immune response.

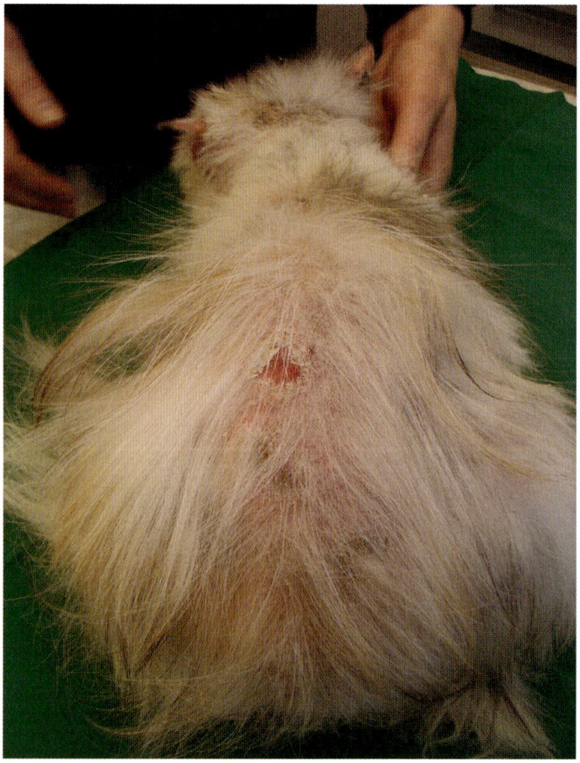

Fig. 4.1.9 Feline dermatophytosis with extensive alopecia, scaling, and crusts on the dorsum.

Clinical lesions consist of any combination of papules, pustules, focal to widespread alopecia, erythema, scaling, and crusting (Fig. 4.1.9). Nodular lesions (kerion) may develop particularly on the face where they mimic areas of deep pyoderma or furunculosis (Fig. 4.1.10). *Trichophyton* and *M. persicolor* are

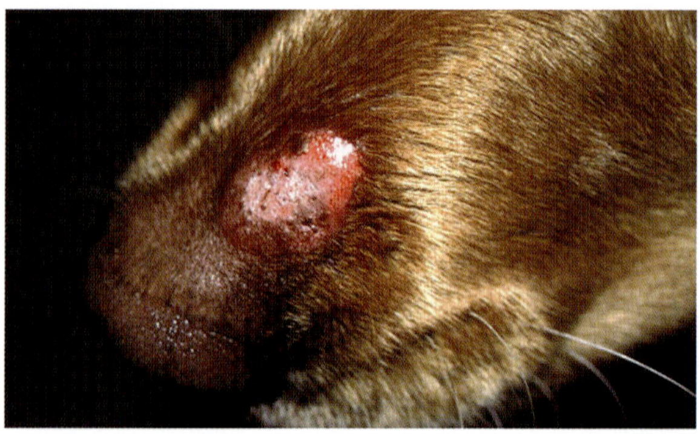

Fig. 4.1.10 Alopecia in canine dermatophytosis. Note nodular lesion (kerion) on the face.

able to induce acantholysis and thus can mimic autoimmune blistering skin diseases (Gross et al. 2005). In cats, lesions may resemble miliary dermatitis.

4.1.2.2 Diagnosis

Diagnostic steps include Wood's lamp investigation, trichograms, and fungal culture (see Section 2.1.4) (Moriello 1995; Moriello 2001). Only *M. canis*-infected hairs fluoresce with Wood's ultraviolet light (Fig. 2.1.8). This examination is a screening tool and is helpful for identification of hairs for direct examination and/or culture; a negative test does not rule out dermatophytosis. Fluorescence due to scales, creams, and crusts may cause false-positive results. Only fluorescence of the hair shafts is indicative of dermatophytosis (see Section 2.1.4.4).

Direct examination of hairs and scales looks for the presence of ekto- or endotrix fungal hyphae and/or spores (Fig. 4.1.11). This procedure can be performed with mineral oil, but is facilitated by the use of clearing agents such as 10% potassium hydroxide or 20% chlorphenolac. A positive result confirms dermatophytosis but does not allow specification of the causative agent.

Definitive diagnosis is achieved by fungal culture on Sabouraud's dextrose agar or dermatophyte test medium (DTM). Both culture media contain broad-spectrum antibiotics to inhibit concurrent bacterial growth. The DTM agar uses phenol as a pH indicator that changes color in the presence of by-products of fungal reproduction. Fungal cultures are best incubated in a dark humid environment and at a temperature of 24–28°C. They should be incubated for up to 4 weeks and need to be examined regularly. Growth characteristics and the presence of macro- or microconidia are documented (Fig. 2.1.9) to determine the fungal species. In general, the clinician needs to be aware of falsely negative and falsely positive cultures, particularly as *T. verrucosum*, for example, does not grow on DTM agar (Moriello 2001).

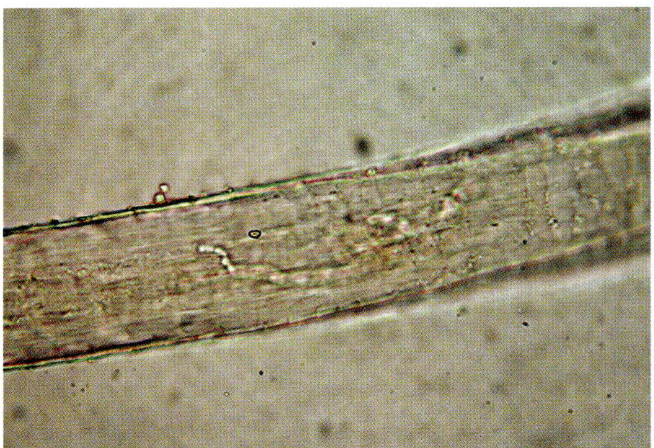

Fig. 4.1.11 Trichogram of dermatophytosis. Note the presence of fungal hyphae and ektotrix spores. (Courtesy of C. Nett.)

Diagnosis via skin biopsy is not as sensitive as a fungal culture. Skin biopsy, however, is helpful for the diagnosis of kerion and granulomatous inflammation when cultures are often negative (Gross et al. 2005).

4.1.2.3 Therapy

In healthy animals, dermatophytosis is generally a self-curing disease that will spontaneously resolve within 3 months (Medleau and Chalmers 1992). Remission occurs when infected hair follicles pass the telogen phase and shed their hair shafts or when a curative inflammatory response is mounted against the fungus. However, treatment is important to limit spreading of spores to other susceptible animals and especially people, and to minimize contamination of the environment. Many treatment protocols have been described in the literature (Moriello and DeBoer 1995a; Moriello and Newbury 2006). Treatment aims at remission of dermatological signs, mycological cure (represented by two consecutive negative cultures), and environmental decontamination. Treatment protocols differ according to the animal species and depend on the animals' husbandry condition.

The most thorough protocol has to be applied in cats, particularly in multicat households, since cats tend to become clinically inapparent carriers. In horses, topical treatment combined with cleaning of the tack is often curative. In cattles, studies have shown that a live-attenuated vaccine to *T. verrucosum* is curative and protective (Gordon and Bond 1996; Bredahl and Gyllensvaan 2000).

Treatment of dermatophytosis in cats and dogs should comprise a combination of topical treatment, systemic treatment, and environmental treatment. This is initiated according to the following algorithm:

1 Perform dermatophyte culture from the suspected animal and from all animals that had contact to it
2 Start systemic therapy for all animals with lesions or positive cultures
3 Apply topical therapy to all infected animals

4 Apply topical therapy to all animals that have contact to infected animals
5 Start decontamination of the environment

4.1.2.3.1 Topical therapy

Topical antifungal treatments for dermatophytosis have been evaluated both in vitro (using isolated infected hairs) and in various in vivo studies (Deboer and Moriello 1995a; Moriello and Deboer 1995b; Paterson 1999; Mason et al. 2000; Sparkes et al. 2000; Hnilica and Medleau 2002; Moriello et al. 2002; Guillot et al. 2002; Perrins and Bond 2003; Moriello et al. 2004b). Topical therapy is always necessary in a multicat or multipet household, in order to avoid spreading of spores. It is also necessary if environmental contamination is a serious risk for people, which includes children, elderly people, immunocompromised people, and people with occupational risk of transmission (contact to many susceptible people such as teachers and health care providers).

Topical therapy is used to complement systemic therapy (Paterson 1999; Sparkes et al. 2000; Perrins and Bond 2003). Only under certain circumstances, lime sulfur without systemic antifungal therapy has been reported to be effective in some experimentally infected cats that were clipped and treated twice weekly (Moriello 2003a). Mycological cure was very slow and was not achieved before 10 weeks of treatment.

Dipping, rinsing, or shampooing is the recommended form of topical application. Topical therapy should not be used locally, since infective spores can occur as far as 10 cm away from the visible lesion. Clipping of the hair coat is still discussed controversially, since minor trauma may facilitate development of pseudomycetomas. However, clipping will facilitate topical treatment and will diminish environmental contamination. Clipping is necessary in long-haired cats, in generalized infection, and if environmental contamination is a serious risk for other cats and people.

Enilconazole

Enilconazole is approved for the treatment of canine and equine dermatophytosis. Only in France it is registered for feline dermatophytosis. Enilconazole is very effective on *M. canis*-infected hair (Moriello 2004). A 0.2% solution is used as a sponge-on and leave-on treatment. Toxicity has been reported in cats and is considered to be related to oral ingestion by grooming. However, the risk is usually low (Hnilica and Medleau 2002), and to prevent grooming an Elizabethan collar is advised until the treated hair coat is thoroughly dry.

Miconazole and chlorhexidine

Miconazole and chlorhexidine are frequently used for topical dermatophyte treatment. A shampoo with 2% miconazole and 2% chlorhexidine is widely used and has demonstrated efficacy as an adjunct treatment to systemic therapy, if applied twice weekly (Paterson 1999; Sparkes et al. 2000). Higher concentrations of miconazole (5.2%) and chlorhexidine (5.9%) demonstrate similar antifungal efficacy as lime sulfur (Moriello and Verbrugge 2007).

Lime sulfur

Lime sulfur is used in a dilution of 1:32 or 1:16. It is one of the most effective topical products (Moriello and Verbrugge 2007). It is very safe even in young animals, but has a bad smell. It should not be ingested, since it can cause vomitus and diarrhea.

4.1.2.3.2 Systemic therapy

Griseofulvin

Griseofulvin is a fungistatic agent that inhibits nucleic acid synthesis and cell mitosis metaphase by interfering with the function of spindle microtubules (Gentles and Barnes 1960). Given with a fatty meal, griseofulvin is well absorbed. It is still a good systemic drug for dermatophytosis, particularly in dogs and horses where in contrast to cats myelotoxicity is not a concern. In the cat, bone marrow suppression with life-threatening and irreversible leukopenia is a severe and unpredictable side effect of griseofulvin therapy. It is more common in cats infected with the feline immunodeficiency virus. Griseofulvin is highly teratogenic and must not be used in pregnant animals (Hill et al. 1995; Moriello and Deboer 1995b).

The daily dose regimen depends on the formulation (microsize versus ultramicrosize) (Moriello 2004). The recommended dose in small animals for microsize griseofulvin is 50 mg/kg once daily and for ultramicrosize griseofulvin it is 10–15 mg/kg/day. Griseofulvin is given orally. When used as the only therapy for feline dermatophytosis, mycological cure is achieved in 63–70 days (Moriello and Deboer 1995b). The efficacy and proper dose of griseofulvin in horses has not been thoroughly researched. However, a dosage of 100 mg/kg daily has been advocated. There are no reports on the necessary treatment duration in horses (Rosser 1995).

Ketoconazole
Griseofulvin therapy is rapidly being replaced by azoles that block ergosterol biosynthesis, a key component of the cytoplasmic membrane of fungi (Vanden Bossche et al. 2003). Ketoconazole is the prototype of azoles. However, it is not approved for the therapy of dermatophytosis in animals and has demonstrated considerable side effects at high doses. Since other azoles are approved for the treatment of dermatophytosis, ketoconazole should no longer be used in animals.

Itraconazole
Itraconazole is an azole derivate with particular accumulation in lung, kidney, liver, bone, muscle, skin, and nails. It is, therefore, ideally suited to treat dermatophytosis. In humans, itraconazole formulated in capsules should be administered with food (Barone et al. 1993). The soluble formulation, however, should be given without food. Concurrent treatment with antacida will diminish absorption. Itraconazole is generally well tolerated. The most common side effects are vomiting, anorexia and elevation of liver enzymes, and in rare cases icterus. In the dog cutaneous vasculitis has been described with dosages higher than 5 mg/kg. Itraconazole is with teratogenic in laboratory animals. Although less prominent than in ketoconazole, it has a known potential for drug–drug interactions, mediated through the effects on the cytochrome P450 3A isoenzyme and the P-glycoprotein system. Thus, the plasma concentration of several important therapeutics such as cyclosporine, digoxin, warfarin, and ivermectin may be increased when given together with itraconazole. Phenobarbitals and phenytoin might increase the metabolism of itraconazole and hence can decrease its plasma levels (Willems et al. 2001). Due to its retention in target sites (skin and nails), it is possible to use intermittent dosing. In cats, a residual effect for up to 2 weeks has been described (Sterkens 1997; Vlaminck and Engelen 2004).

The proposed dosing of itraconazole is a 6-week pulse therapy with 1 week on treatment (daily dosing of 5 mg/kg) and 1 week off. This treatment schedule has been described to achieve clinical cure in 100% of shelter cats and mycological cure within 12 weeks in 85% of them (Cieslicki 2004). When given orally once daily at 5 mg/kg for 28 days, followed by an alternating weekly therapy, a 100% clinical and mycological cure has been achieved after 70 days of treatment (Colombo et al. 2001).

Terbinafine
Similar to azoles, allylamines interfere with ergosterol biosynthesis in the fungal membrane, although at an earlier step in the enzymatic pathway. Allylamines inhibit the fungal enzyme squalene epoxidase. The main compound of the allylamine class is terbinafine. Terbinafine is one of the main treatment options for dermatophyte infections in animals. Compared to griseofulvin, it is more effective and less toxic. There are several studies on the use of terbinafine and various doses have been reported to treat dogs or cats (Mancianti et al. 1999; Chen 2000; Castanon-Olivares et al. 2001; Kotnik et al. 2001; Kotnik 2002; Moriello 2003a). The recommended dose is 30–40 mg/kg orally once a day, but there are additional studies necessary to evaluate short-term cycles or continuous versus pulse therapy. Terbinafine is available in both oral and topical formulations and appears to be well tolerated in dogs and cats. However, terbinafine is not yet approved for the use in veterinary medicine.

Lufenuron
Lufenuron is a benzyl-urea phenol compound that inhibits chitin synthesis and is used as an insecticide. Since chitin is a critical component of the outer cell wall of fungi, chitin inhibition can also have antifungal activity. Its efficacy in the therapy of dermatophytosis in dogs and cats was evaluated in several studies, reporting contradictory results (Ben Ziony and Arzi 2000, 2001; Guillot et al. 2002; Deboer et al. 2003; Moriello 2004; Zur and Elad 2006). Although one retrospective study suggests a strong association with recovery from dermatophytosis (Ben Ziony and Arzi 2000), controlled blinded prospective studies did not confirm these results. Lufenuron did not prevent infection, nor did it alter the course of infection (Deboer et al. 2003; Moriello et al. 2004a; Zur and Elad 2006). Furthermore, the use of lufenuron in conjunction with topical enilconazole in two catteries with dermatophytosis did not result in cure (Guillot et al. 2002). Therefore, lufenuron should not be used for the treatment of dermatophytosis.

4.1.2.3.3 Environmental decontamination
Commercial disinfectants are tested for antifungal actions by observing their effects on suspensions of fungal spores or fungal mycelium in vitro. In

dermatophytosis, however, the dermatophytes grow in or along hair fibers, and these may protect the fungus from the action of disinfectants. Studies that mimic the actual conditions in isolated infected hair demonstrated that most consistent fungicidal activity is provided by lime sulfur (1:33), enilconazole, and 1:10 bleach. Lime sulfur and enilconazole are 100% fungicidal, even if the recommended concentration is diluted 1:4 (Moriello et al. 2004b; Moriello and Newbury 2006). Recently, the efficacy of benzalkonium chloride, a quaternary ammonium compound, and Virkon-S was tested against *M. canis* (Marchetti et al. 2006) and showed approximately 90% efficacy. In contrast, chlorhexidine solutions, phenolic disinfectants, and other quaternary ammonium compounds have no effects (Moriello et al. 2004b).

4.1.2.3.4 Vaccination

Vaccination against dermatophytosis with life-attenuated *T. verrucosum* has proven efficacy in cattle. Large-scale vaccination programs initiated during the past 30 years in eastern Europe and some Scandinavian countries have reduced the prevalence of dermatophytosis in cattle to less than 1% of all herds (Gordon and Bond 1996; Bredahl and Gyllensvaan 2000). Similar results were obtained in farmed foxes with a combination of a life vaccine and an inactivated vaccine for *M. canis* (Bredahl et al. 2000). In cats and horses, however, commercially available inactivated vaccines did neither prevent infection nor did they provide a faster mycological cure when compared to nonvaccinated controls (Deboer and Moriello 1995b; DeBoer et al. 2002; Karle et al. 2002). No studies on dermatophyte vaccination have been performed in dogs so far.

4.1.3 Demodicosis

4.1.3.1 Etiology and pathogenesis

Demodicosis is a common and often serious skin disease of the dog. It is less common in cats and very rarely reported in horses and farm animals. *Demodex* mites are thought to be normal inhabitants of the pilosebaceous unit in humans and most animals. In the dog, it is known that *Demodex canis* mites are transmitted to neonates from the bitch within the first few days after birth. They feed on skin cells, sebum, and epidermal debris and spend their entire life cycle on the host. Although normal inhabitants, it is difficult to demonstrate mites in healthy animals since their number is very low (Scott et al. 2001). The life cycle of *D. canis* lasts 3–4 weeks and consists of four stages: a fusiform egg, a six-legged larva, an eight-legged nymph, and an eight-legged cigar-shaped adult (Scott et al. 2001).

Many mammals may host more than one species of *Demodex* mites, but so far proof of distinctive different species is lacking. In the dog, a short-bodied *D. cornei* has been reported to coinfect the skin with *D. canis* and resides in the stratum corneum rather than the hair follicle (Chesney 1999; Tamura et al. 2001). *D. injai* is a long-bodied mite with about twice the length of *D. canis* (Desch and Hillier 2003). These mites prefer the dorsal trunk and cause excessive greasiness more than alopecia. Terrier breeds and their crosses were overrepresented in one study.

In the dog, infections with *Demodex* mites can be divided into juvenile and adult onset and can be described as localized or generalized. Localized demodicosis in young dogs can occur in any breed and is frequently self-limiting. Generalized juvenile demodicosis by contrast is a severe disease that is more common in purebred dogs. A hereditary predisposition is likely and an autosomal recessive mode has been proposed. Studies in dogs with generalized demodicosis have demonstrated a decrease in lymphoblastogenesis and a reduction in interleukin-2 and its receptor expression, most likely associated with a mite-specific reduction in Th-1 response (Lemarié and Horohov 1996). However, puppies with demodicosis do not seem to suffer from immune dysfunction, and unspecific immunostimulation does not change the course of the disease (Mueller 2004). On the basis of the heritability of demodicosis, dogs with generalized demodicosis and their parents should be excluded from further breeding.

Adult onset demodicosis in most cases develops due to an immunosuppressing disease or therapy, and a thorough clinical work-up for any underlying disease is warranted.

In the cat, the equivalent to *D. canis* is *D. felis* that harbors the hair follicle (Desch and Nutting 1979; Chesney 1989). Cats, however, do not develop a juvenile onset of demodicosis, but rather develop adult onset disease secondary to immunosuppression caused by feline immunodeficiency virus, feline leukemia virus, or diabetes mellitus (Ackerman 1984; Scott et al. 2001; Lowenstein et al. 2005). Cats can also be infected by a short-bodied mite, *D. gatoi* (Desch and

Stewart 1999). It is a stubby and small mite that lives in the stratum corneum rather than the hair follicle. Infection causes severe pruritus (Beale 1998). Its worldwide distribution differs with most reports from the United States and very few reports so far from Europe or Japan.

4.1.3.2 Diagnosis

4.1.3.2.1 Clinical presentation of canine demodicosis

Localized demodicosis usually consists of one or several small erythematous or hyperpigmented alopecic and slightly scaly lesions. Follicular plugging, comedones, or follicular casts may be present. The face, lip commissures, periocular area, and forelegs are the most common sites. In general, lesions are not symmetric and bilaterally periocular alopecia, although often cited, is not pathognomonic for canine demodicosis. Pruritus is variable. There are no uniformly accepted criteria for differentiating the localized from the generalized form. In general, localized forms are considered less than 6–8 focal lesions with less than 3 cm in diameter and no involvement of the feet (Gortel 2006). Most cases occur in young otherwise healthy dogs and resolve without treatment. Progression to generalized disease is rare and cannot be avoided by local treatment.

Generalized demodicosis is a severe and potentially life-threatening skin disease. It involves more than six spots, one entire body region, or at least two feet. It can be divided into juvenile onset and adult onset (Lemarié and Horohov 1996). The former usually starts in dogs less than 18 months of age and the lesions may be similar to those of localized demodicosis, but are often complicated by secondary pyoderma. Pruritus can become severe with secondary skin infections. Cutaneous changes include extensive hair loss, papules, and pustules that coalesce to crusted plaques and sometimes nodular lesions with deep folliculitis and furunculosis due to secondary infections. Comedones and follicular casts are common features. Peripheral lymphadenopathy is always present and some dogs develop fever, pain, and septicemia. In contrast to short-coated breeds, some long-coated breeds and some terriers (e.g., West Highland White Terrier, Scottish Terrier) do not develop extensive alopecia, but present with extensive scaling, exfoliation, and especially severe follicular casts (Scott et al. 2001).

Head, trunk, and legs are most frequently affected. Involvement of the paws may occur in conjunction with generalized demodicosis or alone and is marked by severe swelling, erythema, and interdigital hemorrhagic bullae (Fig. 4.1.12). Infections by *D. injai* may present with oily seborrhea over the back as the only clinical sign (Hillier and Desch 2002).

Purebred dogs and short-haired breeds such as Doberman Pinscher, Pit Bull Terrier, Pug, Boxer, English Bulldog, Boston Terrier, Great Dane, Chinese Shar-Pei, American Staffordshire Terrier, and Dalmatian seem to be at increased risk for developing demodicosis. There might be a familiar accumulation in certain litters. Commonly affected medium-haired breeds include the West Highland White Terrier,

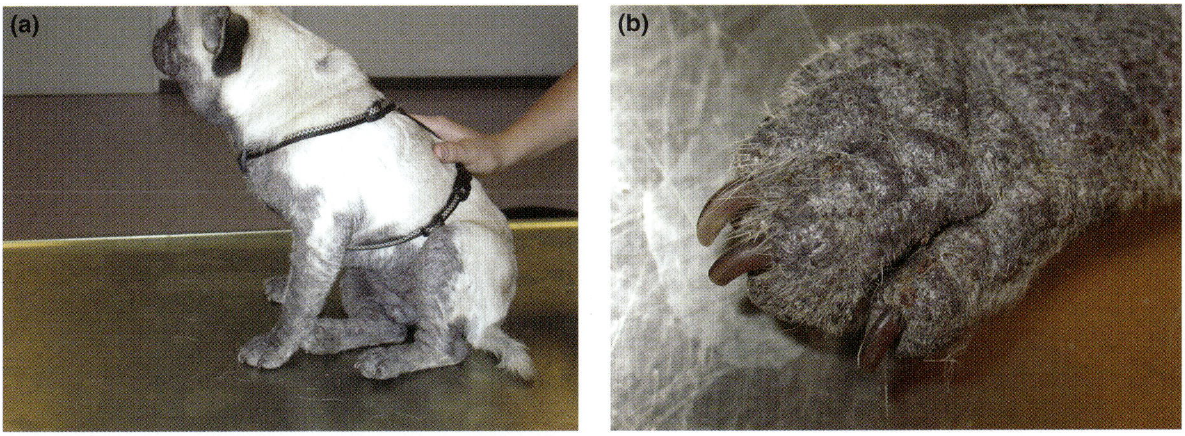

Fig. 4.1.12 Generalized demodicosis in a Pug. (a) Extensive alopecia, furunculosis, and lichenification of the ventral trunk and extremities; (b) severe involvement of the paws.

Scottish Terrier and Airedale Terrier. Long-haired breeds at increased risk are the German Shepherd Dog, Collie, Old English Sheepdog, and Afghan Hound (Gross et al. 2005).

Adult onset generalized demodicosis is often seen in conjunction with immunosuppressive drugs such as corticosteroids or cytotoxic drugs, or immunosuppressive diseases such as hyperadrenocorticism, lymphoma or other neoplasias, leishmaniasis, and hypothyroidism (Scott et al. 2001). A thorough clinical work-up for any underlying disease is recommended, but not always can an immunosuppression be documented.

4.1.3.2.2 Clinical presentation of feline demodicosis

In the cat, infection with *D. cati* is often localized to the head, periocular regions, and neck. Lesions consist of patches or plaques of erythema, ulceration, crusts, and alopecia. Generalized demodicosis affects the neck, trunk, and limbs and reveals variable pruritus. Lesions range from generalized alopecia with scaling and seborrhea (Fig. 4.1.13) to erythema, hyperpigmentation, and crusting. *D. cati* infections in the cat can also present simply with a ceruminous otitis externa (Scott et al. 2001).

Feline demodicosis caused by the short-bodied *D. gatoi* in most cases is very pruritic and therefore resembles clinically allergic skin diseases or feline scabies. Alopecia, excoriation, crusts, and multifocal erythema are concentrated at the head, neck, and limbs. In some cases alopecia of the abdomen mimics feline hypersensitivity reactions or psychogenic alopecia. The infection with *D. gatoi* is thought to be contagious.

4.1.3.2.3 Diagnostic tests

To diagnose demodicosis due to *Demodex* mites that harbor the hair follicle or sebaceous glands, a deep skin scraping is evaluated under the microscope (see Section 2.1.4.6) (Hall and Keirstead 2005; Gortel 2006). In most patients, both adult and immature vital mites and eggs are found at the initial presentation (Fig. 2.1.3). It is necessary to differentiate between immature and adult mites, since a continuous high proportion of immature mites suggests treatment failure. Trichograms can also be useful for the diagnosis of

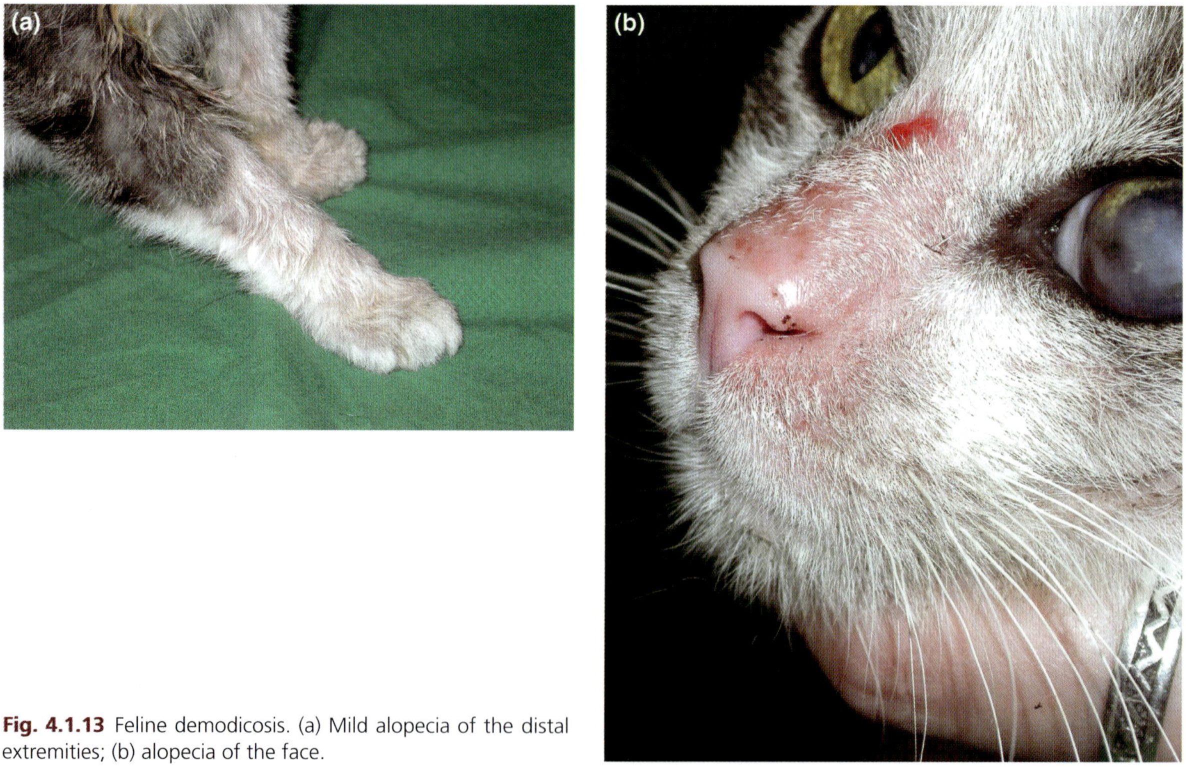

Fig. 4.1.13 Feline demodicosis. (a) Mild alopecia of the distal extremities; (b) alopecia of the face.

demodicosis, especially in areas where skin scrapings are difficult to obtain (Saridomichelakis et al. 2007). Negative trichograms, however, do not rule out the disease. Since *Demodex* mites are part of the normal cutaneous fauna, occasionally a single mite may be found on skin scrapings of normal patients. In questionable cases, additional scrapings should be obtained. In contrast to the mites living in hair follicles, the short-bodied mites such as *D. gatoi* are localized superficially in the stratum corneum, and can be found in superficial skin scrapings, although they may easily be overlooked due to their small size.

Biopsies may be needed to diagnose demodicosis in some breeds such as the Shar-Pei, in some areas of the body such as the feet, or in cases with chronic scarring lesions (Gross et al. 2005). Histopathology will reveal a lymphocytic perifolliculitis and mural folliculitis. Intraluminal mites and a nodular granulomatous dermatitis with fragments of mites are diagnostic for demodicosis (Figure 4.1.14a,b) (Caswell et al. 1997).

4.1.3.3 Therapy

4.1.3.3.1 Therapy of canine demodicosis

Localized demodicosis resolves spontaneously in most cases. Treatment may comprise topical benzoyl shampoo (or benzoyl gel) or systemic antibiotics for secondary pyoderma. Miticidal therapy should not be performed, since otherwise neither spontaneous regression nor generalization of the disease can be determined. The latter, however, would suggest breeding restrictions.

Generalized demodicosis is a serious disease, and treatment of this condition is lengthy and expensive. The general health status should be assessed and concurrent underlying diseases should be treated (Mueller 2004; Gortel 2006). Immunosuppressive drugs should be discontinued whenever possible. Most dogs with generalized demodicosis suffer from secondary superficial or deep pyoderma, requiring a 4–6 week course of antibiotics (see Section 4.1.1.3.2).

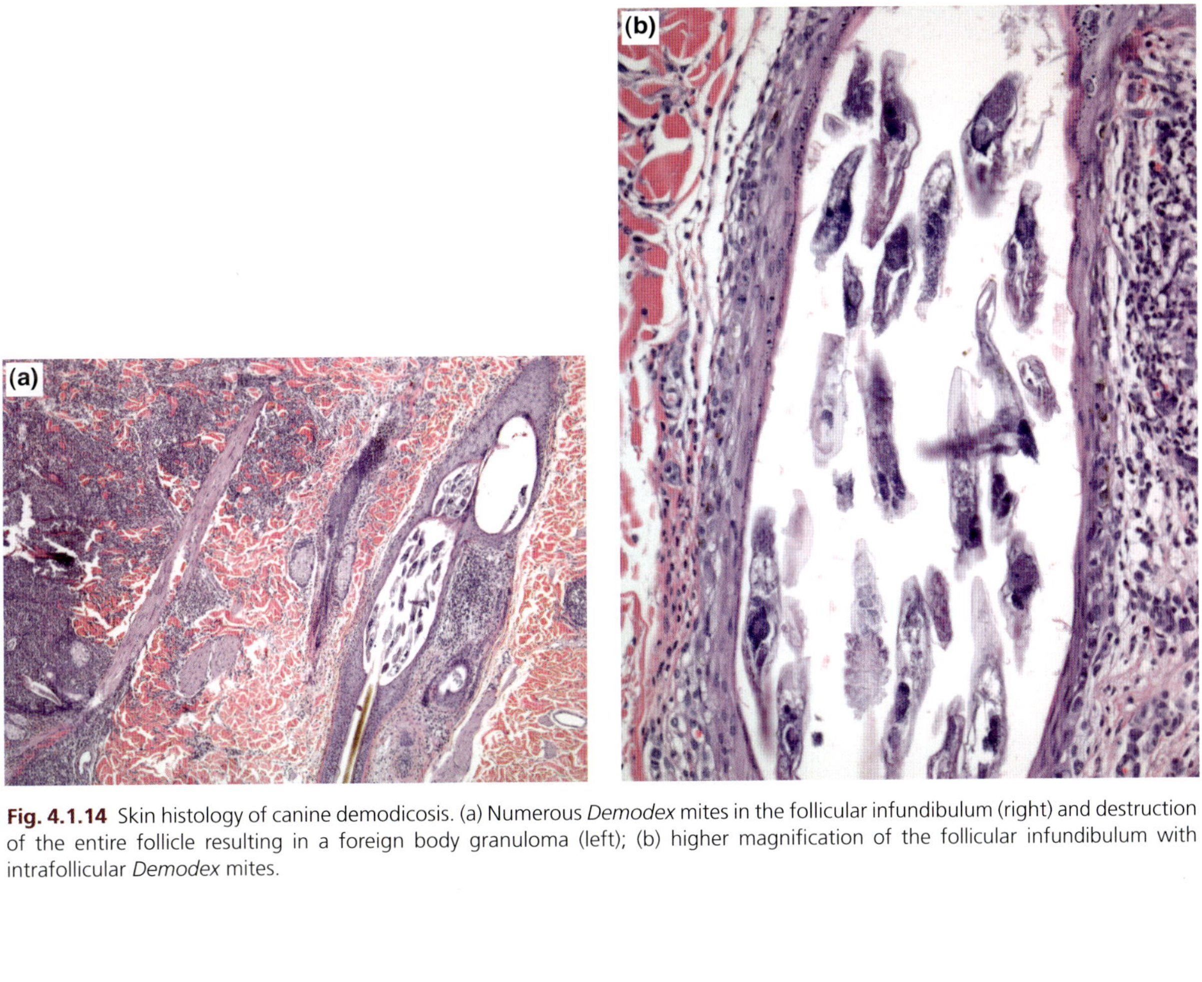

Fig. 4.1.14 Skin histology of canine demodicosis. (a) Numerous *Demodex* mites in the follicular infundibulum (right) and destruction of the entire follicle resulting in a foreign body granuloma (left); (b) higher magnification of the follicular infundibulum with intrafollicular *Demodex* mites.

Treatment of demodicosis has to be monitored by clinical and parasitological responses. Skin scrapings from previously affected areas are collected every 4 weeks regardless of the clinical assessment. Skin scrapings are negative if only dead mites or mite segments are present. Treatment should be continued until at least two consecutive skin scrapings are negative. A patient can be considered cured, if there has been no relapse within 12 months after cessation of therapy.

Amitraz

The only approved, highly efficacious acaricide for the treatment of generalized demodicosis is amitraz. Amitraz inhibits monoamine oxidase and prostaglandin synthesis and is an α2-adrenergic agonist (Hugnet et al. 1996). Amitraz is applied topically as a weekly or fortnightly rinse at a concentration of 0.025–0.05%. To maximize skin contact, clipping of the hair coat in medium- and long-haired dogs is essential. The use of a bactericidal shampoo to remove crusts and bacteria is recommended before applying amitraz. To avoid rinsing off the medication, dogs should not be wetted in between treatments. Although higher concentrations of amitraz (up to 1.25%) or a higher frequency of rinses may result in a higher success rate, this off-label use is also associated with more side effects (Hugnet et al. 2001). Even with the standard therapy, adverse effects are common and include depression, bradycardia, ataxia, hyperglycemia, and gastrointestinal disturbance. A premedication with Atipamezol (0.1 mg/kg i.m.) or Yohimbin (0.1 mg/kg p.o.) has been used to counteract and prevent side effects in higher concentrations. Rinsing with Amitraz should be performed in a well-ventilated room, and protective clothing (gloves) should be worn, since adverse effects such as respiratory problems have been observed in humans (Scott et al. 2001). Amitraz may interact with other monoamine oxidase inhibitors and therefore sedatives should be avoided.

Avermectins

Systemic macrocyclic lactones such as avermectins (e.g., ivermectin, doramectin) and milbemycins (milbemycin oxime and moxidectin) are broad-spectrum antiparasitic agents. Their efficacy in the treatment of generalized demodicosis has been demonstrated in a number of studies (Mueller 2004).

Macrocyclic lactones potentiate glutamate-gated chloride channels or gamma-aminobutyric acid (GABA)-gated chloride channels of the nervous system of mites and insects. This results in an increased cell permeability to chloride ions, resulting in neuromuscular blockage, paralysis, and death of the mite. Mammals lack glutamate-gated chloride channels and GABA-gated chloride channels in the peripheral nervous system. Since macrocyclic lactones do not cross the blood–brain barrier, they are regarded as safe in mammals (Campbell 1981, 1993).

Ivermectin given orally at daily doses of 300–600 μg/kg has demonstrated efficacy in several studies (Mueller 2004). Adverse effects are rare and include mydriasis, lethargy, and ataxia. A gradually increasing dose starting at 50 μg/kg followed by addition of another 50 μg/kg until a dose of 400 μg/kg is achieved improves the safety profile. However, adverse reactions can still occur up to 10 weeks into treatment. Owners should be instructed to observe their pet closely during the entire treatment period.

Collies, their crossbreeds, and other herding breeds (Shetland Sheepdog, Australian Shepherd, White Swiss Shepherd, Border Collie, McNab, Silken Windhound, Long-haired Whippet) are at increased risk for severe life-threatening neurotoxicity (Geyer et al. 2005a,b, 2007). In these breeds, a mutation of the multidrug resistance (mdr1) gene has been found. This gene encodes for P-glycoprotein, a transporter molecule that transports drugs from the brain back into the blood (Fromm 2000). Dogs that are homozygous for the mutation show an increased ivermectin sensitivity. Toxicity comprises ataxia, stupor, paralysis, coma, and death. There is no antidote. In many countries, a commercial test for detecting the mutation is now available and should be considered if dogs with increased risk or unknown pedigree have to be treated (Geyer et al. 2005b). Ivermectin is not approved for the treatment of demodicosis in dogs or cats.

Milbemycin

Milbemycin oxime is approved in most countries for preventing infection with heartworms and intestinal parasites. An evidence-based review of the literature describes efficacy of milbemycin in demodicosis at a daily dose of 2 mg/kg. This dose is well tolerated and can even be applied in ivermectin-sensitive dogs, as Collies only showed signs of toxicity at 5 mg/kg (Tranquilli et al. 1991). One disadvantage of milbemycin oxime, however, is its high cost.

Moxidectin is another milbemycin that has shown good efficacy in generalized demodicosis at a dose of 400 μg/kg per day. Similar side effects as with ivermectin may occur, but are less common (Paul et al. 2000; Geyer et al. 2005a). Moxidectin has recently been launched as a topical 1% spot-on solution combined with imidacloprid. It is approved and marketed for the treatment of demodicosis. In mild cases the response rate is comparable to what is reported for other treatments. However, the outcome for more severely affected patients in unsatisfactory (Mueller et al. 2008).

4.1.3.3.2 Therapy of feline demodicosis

There are only few reports on the treatment of feline demodicosis. Weekly dips with 2% lime sulfur are recommended. Weekly rinses with 0.0125–0.025% amitraz have been effective but adverse effects are numerous in the cat (Mueller 2004). Ivermectin (400 μg/kg/day p.o.) has been used in a few cases with good success. Adverse effects include mydriasis, blindness, ataxia and Heinz body anemia (from the glycol vehicle). As the short bodied mite is thought to be contagious, all cats in the household should be treated.

4.1.4 Rhabditic folliculitis

Pelodera (syn. *Rhabditis*) *strongyloides* is a free-living saprophytic nematode whose natural habitat is decaying organic material. *Pelodera* can be very numerous in damped straw, hay, soil, or marshes. Its third-stage larvae are able to invade mammalian skin that comes into contact with contaminated soil or straw (Scott et al. 2001). It is therefore not surprising that rhabditic folliculitis has been reported in many mammalian species including dogs and humans. Domestic animals are generally considered as aberrant hosts to *P. strongyloides* (Willers 1970; Farrington et al. 1976; Pasyk 1978; Clark et al. 1989; Ramos et al. 1996; Saari and Nikander 2006).

Rhabditic folliculitis is a rare skin disease in domestic animals, particularly with increasing indoor housing of pet animals. Most reports originate from Central Europe and the Midwestern United States, but recently 11 cases from Finland were described. Hunting dogs and dogs with short-hair coat are overrepresented (Saari and Nikander 2006).

Clinical features of *Pelodera dermatitis* are quite severe pruritus, alopecia, and an erythematous and crusting dermatitis affecting body sites in contact with the ground (Scott et al. 2001). Differential diagnoses of rhabditic folliculitis include demodicosis, dirofilariosis, strongyloides stercoralis infection, *Straelensia* infection, hookworm dermatitis, contact dermatitis, and superficial bacterial folliculitis.

The fastest and easiest way to confirm the diagnosis is to demonstrate typical larvae in skin scrapings, where the relatively small (approximately 650 μm in length) motile larvae are found. In uncertain cases, skin biopsies are diagnostic and will reveal an eosinophil-rich perifolliculitis, folliculitis, and furunculosis with similarity to demodicosis (Gross et al. 2005). Fragments of nematodes are found within the follicular infundibulum. If confirmation of the parasite is requested, nematodes can be cultured from skin scrapings on an ordinary blood agar.

Therapy mainly consists of a complete removal of the moist bedding, as the infection is self-limiting if the source of infection is abandoned. Various ectoparasiticides are reported to be effective such as organophosphate dips, selamectin and ivermectin. Antibiotic therapy is supportive if a concomitant pyoderma exists.

4.1.5 Straelensiosis

Straelensia cynotis belongs to the Leeuwenhoekiidae, a family close to Trombiculidae. A distinctive nodular dermatitis in dogs, induced by the larvae of *Straelensia cynotis*, was first reported in 1999 (Le Net et al. 1999). Since then there have been several cases reported from the south of France and one case from Portugal (Bourdeau et al. 2000; Le Net et al. 2002; Seixas et al. 2006). All affected dogs lived in rural areas either as hunting dogs or outdoor dogs with free access to wildlife.

Nymphs and adults from the families Trombiculidae and Leeuwenhoekiidae are free-living, whereas the larvae primarily parasitize wild mammals, birds, and reptiles and only rarely parasitize domestic animals and humans (Scott et al. 2001). For *Straelensia cynotis* it was postulated that the natural host was the fox, whereas the dog is only an incidental host. *Straelensia cynotis* infections in dogs are not contagious.

The most striking clinical feature of strealensiosis is a very sudden onset and a rapid development of numerous nodules, papules, and crusts with a central crater, sometimes accompanied by scales and erythema. Lesions are not regional as in trombiculosis but are rather multifocal or generalized. Main localizations are the head, the neck, and the dorsum, often associated with lesions on the front legs and tail. Severely affected dogs may show pruritus and pain accompanied by lethargy and anorexia.

Since mites are firmly attached to the hair follicle wall by their chelicerae, skin scrapings will not reveal any parasites. Histopathology is the diagnostic tool of choice and will demonstrate dermal nodules composed of a dilated follicular ostium that contains a well-preserved larval arthropod with oval shape and a length of approximately 800 μm. In addition, there is a severe irregular hyperplasia of the infundibular epithelium and a perifollicular mucinosis that can almost be considered pathognomonic for this condition. The inflammatory infiltrate mainly consists of neutrophils and plasma cells, in some cases developing into a suppurative folliculitis and furunculosis. Diagnosis can be confirmed by dissection of biopsies in ethanol and investigation of the larval mite.

The clinical response to topical ectoparasitic therapy is minimal, except for amitraz used twice a week (0.5–1%). Systemic ivermectin has demonstrated some efficacy. Spontaneous cure has been observed after several months.

References

Ackerman L. 1984. Demodicosis in cats. *Modern Veterinary Practice* 65:751–752

Allaker RP, Lloyd DH, Bailey RM. 1992a. Population sizes and frequency of staphylococci at mucocutaneous sites on healthy dogs. *Veterinary Record* 130:303–304

Allaker RP, Lloyd DH, Simpson AI. 1992b. Occurrence of *Staphylococcus intermedius* on the hair and skin of normal dogs. *Research in Veterinary Science* 52:174–176.

Bannoehr J, Ben Zakour NL, Waller AS, Guardabassi L, Thoday K, Van Den Broek AHM, Fitzgeraldi R. 2007. Population genetic structure of the *Staphylococcus intermedius* group: insights into *agr* diversification and the emergence of methicillin-resistant strains. *Journal of Bacteriology* 189(23):8685–8692.

Barone JA, Koh JG, Bierman RH, Colaizzi JL, Swanson KA, Gaffar MC, Moskovitz BL, Mechlinski W, Van de Velde V. 1993. Food interaction and steady-state pharmacokinetics of itraconazole capsules in healthy male volunteers. *Antimicrobial Agents and Chemotherapy* 37:778–784.

Beale KM. 1998. Contagion and occult demodicosis in a family of 2 cats. *Proceedings of the 14th AAVD/ACVD Meeting*, San Antonio, p. 99.

Ben Ziony Y, Arzi B. 2000. Use of lufenuron for treating fungal infections of dogs and cats: 297 cases (1997–1999). *Journal of the American Veterinary Medical Association* 217:1510–1513.

Ben Ziony Y, Arzi B. 2001. Updated information for treatment of fungal infections in cats and dogs. *Journal of the American Veterinary Medical Association* 218:1718.

Bloom PB, Rosser EJ. 2001. Efficacy of once-daily clindamycin hydrochloride in the treatment of superficial bacterial pyoderma in dogs. *Journal of the American Animal Hospital Association* 37:537–542.

Boag A, Loeffler A, Lloyd DH. 2004. Methicillin-resistant *Staphylococcus aureus* isolates from companion animals. *Veterinary Record* 154:411.

Bourdeau P, Degorce-Rubiales F, Breton C, Poujade Deverdier A. 2000. Newly recognized cutaneous manifestation of acariosis associated with epithelial encystment of probable follicular origin in the dog. *Veterinary Dermatology* 11(1 Suppl):14–40.

Breathnach RM, Fanning S, Mulcahy G, Bassett, Jones BR. 2008. Canine pododermatitis and idiopathic disease. *Veterinary Journal* 176(2):146–157.

Bredahl L, Gyllensvaan C. 2000. Incidence and control of cattle ringworm in Scandinavia. *Mycoses* 43(1 Suppl):8–10.

Bredahl LK, Bratberg AM, Solbakk IT. 2000. Efficacy of an experimental *Microsporum canis* vaccine in farmed foxes. *Veterinary Dermatology* 12(1 Suppl):39.

Campbell WC. 1981. An introduction to the avermectins. *New Zealand Veterinary Journal* 29:174–178.

Campbell WC. 1993. Ivermectin, an antiparasitic agent. *Medicinal Research Reviews* 13:61–79.

Castanon-Olivares LR, Manzano-Gayosso P, Lopez-Martinez R, De la Rosa-Velazquez IA, Soto-Reyes-Solis E. 2001. Effectiveness of terbinafine in the eradication of *Microsporum canis* from laboratory cats. *Mycoses* 44:95–97.

Caswell JL, Yager JA, Parker WM, Moore PF. 1997. A prospective study of the immunophenotype and temporal changes in the histologic lesions of canine demodicosis. *Veterinary Pathology* 34:279–287.

Chen C. 2000. The use of terbinafine for the treatment of dermatophytosis. *Veterinary Dermatology* 12(1 Suppl):41.

Chesney CJ. 1989. Demodicosis in the cat. *Journal of Small Animal Practice* 30:689–695.

Chesney CJ. 1999. Short form of *Demodex* species mite in the dog: occurrence and measurements. *Journal of Small Animal Practice* 40:58–61.

Cieslicki M. 2004. Itrafungol, a new oral antimycotic drug for the therapy of *Microsporum canis* infections in the cat. *Der Praktische Tierarzt. Zeitschrift für fortschrittliche Tiermedizin* 85:548–554.

Clark EG, Griffin S, Goodall P. 1989. Saskatchewan. Pelodera dermatitis in a dog. *Canadian Veterinary Journal* 30:970.

Cole LK, Kwochka KW, Kowalski JJ, Hillier A. 1998. Microbial flora and antimicrobial susceptibility patterns of isolated pathogens from the horizontal ear canal and middle ear in dogs with otitis media. *Journal of the American Veterinary Medical Association* 212:534–538.

Colombo S, Cornegliani L, Vercelli A. 2001. Efficacy of itraconazole as a combined continuous/pulse therapy in feline dermatophytosis: preliminary results in nine cases. *Veterinary Dermatology* 12:347–350.

Curtis C. 1998. Canine idiopathic recurrent superficial pyoderma. *Veterinary Record* 143:344.

Curtis CF, Lamport AI, Lloyd DH. 2006. Masked, controlled study to investigate the efficacy of a *Staphylococcus intermedius* autogenous bacterin for the control of canine idiopathic recurrent superficial pyoderma. *Veterinary Dermatology* 17:163–168.

Daminet S, Ferguson DC. 2003. Influence of drugs on thyroid function in dogs. *Journal of Veterinary Internal Medicine* 17:463–472.

de Jaham C. 2003. Effects of an ethyl lactate shampoo in conjunction with a systemic antibiotic in the treatment of canine superficial bacterial pyoderma in an open-label, nonplacebo-controlled study. *Veterinary Therapeutics* 4:94–100.

Deboer DJ. 1990. Strategies for management of recurrent pyoderma in dogs. *Veterinary Clinics of North America. Small Animal Practice* 20:1509–1524.

Deboer DJ. 1995. Management of chronic and recurrent pyoderma in the dog. In: Bonagura JD (ed), *Kirk's Current Veterinary Therapy XII*, pp. 611–617. Philadelphia: WB Saunders.

Deboer DJ, Moriello KA. 1995a. Inability of two topical treatments to influence the course of experimentally induced

dermatophytosis in cats. *Journal of the American Veterinary Medical Association* 207:52–57.
Deboer DJ, Moriello KA. 1995b. Investigations of a killed dermatophyte cell-wall vaccine against infection with *Microsporum canis* in cats. *Research in Veterinary Science* 59:110–113.
Deboer DJ, Moriello KA, Blum JL, Volk LM. 2003. Effects of lufenuron treatment in cats on the establishment and course of *Microsporum canis* infection following exposure to infected cats. *Journal of the American Veterinary Medical Association* 222:1216–1220.
DeBoer DJ, Moriello KA, Blum JL, Volk LM, Bredahl LK. 2002. Safety and immunologic effects after inoculation of inactivated and combined live-inactivated dermatophytosis vaccines in cats. *American Journal of Veterinary Research* 63:1532–1537.
Desch C, Nutting WB. 1979. *Demodex cati* Hirst 1919: a redescription. *Cornell Veterinarian* 69:280–285.
Desch CE, Hillier A. 2003. *Demodex injai*: a new species of hair follicle mite (Acari: Demodecidae) from the domestic dog (Canidae). *Journal of Medical Entomology* 40:146–149.
Desch CE, Stewart TB. 1999. *Demodex gatoi*: new species of hair follicle mite (Acari: Demodecidae) from the domestic cat (Carnivora: Felidae). *Journal of Medical Entomology* 36:167–170.
Farrington DO, Lundvall RL, Greve JH. 1976. *Pelodera strongyloides* dermatitis in a horse in Iowa. *Veterinary Medicine, Small Animal Clinician* 71:1199–1202.
Farstvedt EG, Hendrickson DA, Dickenson CE, Spier SJ. 2004. Treatment of suppurative facial cellulitis and panniculitis caused by *Corynebacterium pseudotuberculosis* in two horses. *Journal of the American Veterinary Medical Association* 224(7):1139–1142, 1112.
Foil CS. 1994. Fungal diseases. *Clinics in Dermatology* 12:529–542.
Frank LA, Kania SA, Hnilica KA, Wilkes RP, Bemis DA. 2003. Isolation of *Staphylococcus schleiferi* from dogs with pyoderma. *Journal of the American Veterinary Medical Association* 222:451–454.
Fromm MF. 2000. P-glycoprotein: a defense mechanism limiting oral bioavailability and CNS accumulation of drugs. *International Journal of Clinical Pharmacology and Therapeutics* 38:69–74.
Ganiere JP, Medaille C, Etore F. 2004. In vitro antimicrobial activity of orbifloxacin against *Staphylococcus intermedius* isolates from canine skin and ear infections. *Research in Veterinary Science* 77:67–71.
Ganiere JP, Medaille C, Mangion C. 2005. Antimicrobial drug susceptibility of *Staphylococcus intermedius* clinical isolates from canine pyoderma. *Journal of Veterinary Medicine. Part B: Infectious Diseases and Veterinary Public Health* 52:25–31.
Gentles JC, Barnes MJ. 1960. A report on animal experiments with griseofulvin. The griseofulvin content of hair. *Archives of Dermatology* 81:703–708.
Geyer J, Doring B, Godoy JR, Leidolf R, Moritz A, Petzinger E. 2005a. Frequency of the nt230 (del4) MDR1 mutation in collies and related dog breeds in Germany. *Journal of Veterinary Pharmacology and Therapeutics* 28:545–551.
Geyer J, Doring B, Godoy JR, Moritz A, Petzinger E. 2005b. Development of a PCR-based diagnostic test detecting a nt230(del4) MDR1 mutation in dogs: verification in a moxidectin-sensitive Australian shepherd. *Journal of Veterinary Pharmacology and Therapeutics* 28:95–99.
Geyer J, Klintzsch S, Meerkamp K, Wohlke A, Distl O, Moritz A, Petzinger E. 2007. Detection of the nt230(del4) MDR1 mutation in white Swiss shepherd dogs: case reports of doramectin toxicosis, breed predisposition, and microsatellite analysis. *Journal of Veterinary Pharmacology and Therapeutics* 30:482–485.
Gordon PJ, Bond R. 1996. Efficacy of a live attenuated *Trichophyton verrucosum* vaccine for control of bovine dermatophytosis. *Veterinary Record* 139:395–396.
Gortel K. 2006. Update on canine demodicosis. *Veterinary Clinics of North America. Small Animal Practice* 36:229–41, ix.
Graeser Y, Scott J, Summerbell R. 2008. The new species concept in dermatophytosis-a polyphasic approach. *Mycopathologia* 166:239–256.
Gross TL, Ihrke PJ, Walder EJ. 1992. *Veterinary Dermatopathology: A Macroscopic and Microscopic Evaluation of Canine and Feline Skin Disease.* St. Louis: Mosby Year Book.
Gross TL, Ihrke PJ, Walder EJ, Affolter VK. 2005. *Skin Diseases of the Dog and the Cat.* Oxford: Blackwell Science.
Gross TL, Stannard AA, Yaeger JA. 1997. An anatomical classification of folliculitis. *Veterinary Dermatology* 8:147–156.
Guillot J, Malandain E, Jankowski F, Rojzner K, Fournier C, Touati F, Chermette R, Seewald W, Schenker R. 2002. Evaluation of the efficacy of oral lufenuron combined with topical enilconazole for the management of dermatophytosis in catteries. *Veterinary Record* 150:714–718.
Hall JA, Keirstead N. 2005. Diagnostic dermatology. Demodicosis. *Canadian Veterinary Journal* 46:949–950, 952.
Harvey RG, Lloyd DH. 1994. The distribution of *Staphylococcus intermedius* and coagulase-negative staphylococci on the hair, skin surface, within the hair follicles and on the mucous membranes of dogs. *Veterinary Dermatology* 5:75–78.
Harvey RG, Noble WC, Ferguson EA. 1993. A comparison of lincomycin hydrochloride and clindamycin hydrochloride in the treatment of superficial pyoderma in dogs. *Veterinary Record* 132:351–353.
Heffner KA, White SD, Frevert CW, Jakowski R. 1988. *Corynebacterium* folliculitis in a horse. *Journal of the American Veterinary Medical Association* 193:89–90.
Heinrich K, Newbury S, Verbrugge M. 2005. Detection of environmental contamination in homes exposed to *Microsporum canis* arthrospores and efficacy of the triple cleaning technique (abstract). *Veterinary Dermatology* 16:192.
Hill PB, Moriello KA. 1994. Canine pyoderma. *Journal of the American Veterinary Medical Association* 204:334–340.
Hill PB, Moriello KA, Shaw SE. 1995. Systemic antifungal drugs. *Veterinary Dermatology* 6:59–66.
Hillier A, Alcorn JR, Cole LK et al. 2003. Pyoderma due to *Pseudomonas aeruginosa* infection in dogs: 15 cases. *Proceedings of the 18th AAVD/ACVD Meeting,* Monterey, p. 222.
Hillier A, Desch CE. 2002. Large-bodied *Demodex* mite infestation in 4 dogs. *Journal of the American Veterinary Medical Association* 220:623–627, 613.
Hnilica KA, Medleau L. 2002. Evaluation of topically applied enilconazole for the treatment of dermatophytosis in a Persian cattery. *Veterinary Dermatology* 13:23–28.
Holm BR, Petersson U, Morner A, Bergstrom K, Franklin A, Greko C. 2002. Antimicrobial resistance in staphylococci from canine pyoderma: a prospective study of first-time and recurrent cases in Sweden. *Veterinary Record* 151:600–605.
Holm BR, Rest JR, Seewald W. 2004. A prospective study of the clinical findings, treatment and histopathology of 44 cases of pyotraumatic dermatitis. *Veterinary Dermatology* 15: 369–376.
Horspool LJ, van Laar P, Van Den BR, Mawhinney I. 2004. Treatment of canine pyoderma with ibafloxacin and marbofloxacin–fluoroquinolones with different pharmacokinetic profiles. *Journal of Veterinary Pharmacology and Therapeutics* 27: 147–153.
Horspool LJ, van Laar P, Van Den BR, Mawhinney IC. 2006. Clinical efficacy of two ibafloxacin formulations in the treatment of canine pyoderma. *Veterinary Record* 158:236–237.
Hugnet C, Bruchon-Hugnet C, Royer H, Bourdoiseau G. 2001. Efficacy of 1.25% amitraz solution in the treatment of generalized demodicosis (eight cases) and sarcoptic mange (five cases) in dogs. *Veterinary Dermatology* 12:89–92.

Hugnet C, Buronrosse F, Pineau X, Cadore JL, Lorgue G, Berny PJ. 1996. Toxicity and kinetics of amitraz in dogs. *American Journal of Veterinary Research* 57:1506–1510.

Ihrke PJ. 1987. An overview of bacterial skin disease in the dog. *British Veterinary Journal* 143:112–118.

Ihrke PJ. 1996. Bacterial skin diseases in the dog: a guide to canine pyoderma. *Veterinary Learning Systems, Conference Proceeding*, Trenton, pp. 1–97.

Jones RD, Kania SA, Rohrbach BW, Frank LA, Bemis DA. 2007. Prevalence of oxacillin- and multidrug-resistant staphylococci in clinical samples from dogs: 1,772 samples (2001–2005). *Journal of the American Veterinary Medical Association* 230:221–227.

Kania SA, Williamson NL, Frank LA, Wilkes RP, Jones RD, Bemis DA. 2004. Methicillin resistance of staphylococci isolated from the skin of dogs with pyoderma. *American Journal of Veterinary Research* 65:1265–1268.

Karle J, Steller U, Fenner A. 2002. Controlled blind study to prove the efficacy of the inactivated vaccine Insol Dermatophyton in artificially infected horses. *Pferdeheilkunde* 18:625–628.

Kerl ME. 2003. Update on canine and feline fungal diseases. *Veterinary Clinics of North America. Small Animal Practice* 33:721–747.

Kim TJ, Na YR, Lee JI. 2005. Investigations into the basis of chloramphenicol and tetracycline resistance in *Staphylococcus intermedius* isolates from cases of pyoderma in dogs. *Journal of Veterinary Medicine. Part B: Infectious Diseases and Veterinary Public Health* 52:119–124.

Kotnik T. 2002. Drug efficacy of terbinafine hydrochloride (Lamisil) during oral treatment of cats, experimentally infected with *Microsporum canis. Journal of Veterinary Medicine. Part B: Infectious Diseases and Veterinary Public Health* 49:120–122.

Kotnik T, Kozuh EN, Kuzner J, Drobnic-Kosorok M. 2001. Terbinafine hydrochloride treatment of *Microsporum canis* experimentally induced ringworm in cats. *Veterinary Microbiology* 83:161–168.

Koutinas AF, Saridomichelakis MN, Argyroudis S, Koutinas CK, Karatzanos P, Giadinis N. 2007. Clinical, histopathological and therapeutic considerations in a flock of sheep with facial staphylococcal-associated dermatitis. *Veterinary Dermatology* 18:211–216.

Lemarié SL, Horohov DW. 1996. Evaluation of interleukin-2 production and interleukin-2 receptor expression in dogs with generalised demodicosis. *Veterinary Dermatology* 7:213–219.

Le Net J-L, Fain A, George C et al. 1999. Dermatitis in dogs induced by larval mite (Acari) of the genus *Straelensia* (Prostigmata: Leeuwenhoekiidae) in France. *Proceedings of the 24th World Small Animal Veterinary Association Congress*, Lyon, France.

Le Net JL, Fain A, George C, Rousselle S, Theau V, Longeart L. 2002. Straelensiosis in dogs: a newly described nodular dermatitis induced by *Straelensia cynotis. Veterinary Record* 150:205–209.

Lloyd DH, Carlotti DN, Koch HJ, Van Den Broek AH. 1997. Treatment of canine pyoderma with co-amoxyclav: a comparison of two dose rates. *Veterinary Record* 141:439–441.

Lloyd DH, Lamport AI, Noble WC, Howell SA. 1999. Fluoroquinolone resistance in *Staphylococcus intermedius. Veterinary Dermatology* 10:249–251.

Loeffler A, Linek M, Moodley A, Guardabassi L, Sung JM, Winkler M, Weiss R, Lloyd DH. 2007. First report of multiresistant, mecA-positive *Staphylococcus intermedius* in Europe: 12 cases from a veterinary dermatology referral clinic in Germany. *Veterinary Dermatology* 18:412–421.

Lowenstein C, Beck W, Bessmann K, Mueller RS. 2005. Feline demodicosis caused by concurrent infestation with *Demodex cati* and an unnamed species of mite. *Veterinary Record* 157:290–292.

Mancianti F, Nardoni S, Corazza M, D'Achille P, Ponticelli C. 2003. Environmental detection of *Microsporum canis* arthrospores in the households of infected cats and dogs. *Journal of Feline Medicine & Surgery* 5:323–328.

Mancianti F, Papini R. 1996. Isolation of keratinophilic fungi from the floors of private veterinary clinics in Italy. *Veterinary Research Communications* 20(2):161–166.

Mancianti F, Pedonese F, Millanta F, Guarnieri L. 1999. Efficacy of oral terbinafine in feline dermatophytosis due to *Microsporum canis. Journal of Feline Medicine & Surgery* 1:37–41.

Marchetti V, Mancianti F, Cardini G, Luchetti E. 2006. Evaluation of fungicidal efficacy of benzalkonium chloride (Steramina G u.v.) and Virkon-S against *Microsporum canis* for environmental disinfection. *Veterinary Research Communications* 30:255–261.

Mason I. 1993. Pustules and crusted papules. In: Locke PH, Harvey RG, Mason I (eds), *Manual of Small Animal Dermatology*, pp. 60–64. Gloucestershire: BSAVA.

Mason K, Frost A, O'Boyle D, Connole MD. 2000. Treatment of a *Microsporum canis* infection in a colony of Persian cats with griseofulvin and a shampoo containing 2% miconazole, 2% chlorhexidine, 2% miconazole and 2% chlorhexidine or placebo. *Veterinary Dermatology* 12(1 Suppl):55.

May ER. 2006. Bacterial skin diseases: current thoughts on pathogenesis and management. *Veterinary Clinics of North America. Small Animal Practice* 36:185–202.

May ER, Hnilica KA, Frank LA, Jones RD, Bemis DA. 2005. Isolation of *Staphylococcus schleiferi* from healthy dogs and dogs with otitis, pyoderma, or both. *Journal of the American Veterinary Medical Association* 227:928–931.

Medleau L, Chalmers SA. 1992. Resolution of generalized dermatophytosis without treatment in dogs. *Journal of the American Veterinary Medical Association* 201:1891–1892.

Moriello K. 1995. Diagnostic testing. In: Moriello K, Mason IS (eds), *Handbook of Small Animal Dermatology*, pp. 19–44. Oxford: Pergamon.

Moriello KA. 2001. Diagnostic techniques for dermatophytosis. *Clinical Techniques in Small Animal Practice* 16:219–224.

Moriello KA. 2003a. Feline dermatophytosis: topical and systemic treatment recommendations. *Veterinary Medicine* 98:877–884.

Moriello KA. 2003b. Zoonotic skin diseases of dogs and cats. *Animal Health Research Review* 4:157–168.

Moriello KA. 2004. Treatment of dermatophytosis in dogs and cats: review of published studies. *Veterinary Dermatology* 15:99–107.

Moriello KA, DeBoer DJ. 1995a. Feline dermatophytosis: recent advances and recommendations for therapy. In: Kunkle GA (ed), *Feline Dermatology*, pp. 901–922. Philadelphia: WB Saunders.

Moriello KA, Deboer DJ. 1995b. Efficacy of griseofulvin and itraconazole in the treatment of experimentally induced dermatophytosis in cats. *Journal of the American Veterinary Medical Association* 207:439–444.

Moriello KA, Deboer DJ, Schenker R, Blum JL, Volk LM. 2004a. Efficacy of pre-treatment with lufenuron for the prevention of *Microsporum canis* infection in a feline direct topical challenge model. *Veterinary Dermatology* 15:357–362.

Moriello KA, DeBoer DJ, Volk L. 2002. Determination of strain variability of *Microsporum canis* to disinfectants (abstract). *Veterinary Dermatology* 13:225.

Moriello KA, Deboer DJ, Volk LM, Sparkes A, Robinson A. 2004b. Development of an in vitro, isolated, infected spore testing model for disinfectant testing of *Microsporum canis* isolates. *Veterinary Dermatology* 15:175–180.

Moriello KA, Newbury S. 2006. Recommendations for the management and treatment of dermatophytosis in animal shelters. *Veterinary Clinics of North America. Small Animal Practice* 36:89–114.

Moriello KA, Verbrugge M. 2007. Use of isolated infected spores to determine the sporocidal efficacy of two commercial antifungal rinses against *Microsporum canis. Veterinary Dermatology* 18:55–58.

Morris DO, Rook KA, Shofer FS, Rankin SC. 2006. Screening of *Staphylococcus aureus*, *Staphylococcus intermedius*, and *Staphylococcus schleiferi* isolates obtained from small companion animals for antimicrobial resistance: a retrospective review of 749 isolates (2003–2004). *Veterinary Dermatology* 17:332–337.

Mueller RS. 2004. Treatment protocols for demodicosis: an evidence-based review. *Veterinary Dermatology* 15:75–89.

Mueller RS, Stephan B. 2007. Pradofloxacin in the treatment of canine deep pyoderma: a multicentred, blinded, randomized parallel trial. *Veterinary Dermatology* 18:144–151.

Mueller RS, Meyer U, Bensignor E. 2008. Treatment of canine generalised demodicosis with a 'spot-on' formulation containing 10% moxidectin and 2.5% imidacloprid (Advokate, Bayer). *Veterinary Dermatology* 19(1 Suppl. 1):12.

Norris BJ, Colditz IG, Dixon TJ. 2007. Fleece rot and dermatophilosis in sheep. *Veterinary Microbiology* 128:217–230.

Paradis M, Abbey L, Baker B, Coyne M, Hannigan M, Joffe D, Pukay B, Trettien A, Waisglass S, Wellington J. 2001. Evaluation of the clinical efficacy of marbofloxacin (Zeniquin) tablets for the treatment of canine pyoderma: an open clinical trial. *Veterinary Dermatology* 12:163–169.

Pascoe RR. 1984. Infectious skin diseases of horses. *Veterinary Clinics of North America. Large Animal Practice* 6:27–46.

Pasyk K. 1978. Dermatitis rhabditidosa in an 11-year-old girl: a new cutaneous parasitic disease of man. *British Journal of Dermatology* 98:107–112.

Paterson S. 1999. Miconazole/chlorhexidine shampoo as an adjunct to systemic therapy in controlling dermatophytosis in cats. *Journal of Small Animal Practice* 40:163–166.

Paul AJ, Tranquilli WJ, Hutchens DE. 2000. Safety of moxidectin in avermectin-sensitive collies. *American Journal of Veterinary Research* 61:482–483.

Pellerin JL, Bourdeau P, Sebbag H, Person JM. 1998. Epidemiosurveillance of antimicrobial compound resistance of *Staphylococcus intermedius* clinical isolates from canine pyodermas. *Comparative Immunology, Microbiology and Infectious Diseases* 21:115–133.

Perrins N, Bond R. 2003. Synergistic inhibition of the growth in vitro of *Microsporum canis* by miconazole and chlorhexidine. *Veterinary Dermatology* 14:99–102.

Petersen AD, Walker RD, Bowman MM, Schott HC, Rosser EJ Jr. 2002. Frequency of isolation and antimicrobial susceptibility patterns of *Staphylococcus intermedius* and *Pseudomonas aeruginosa* isolates from canine skin and ear samples over a 6-year period (1992–1997). *Journal of the American Animal Hospital Association* 38:407–413.

Pilsworth RC, Knottenbelt D. 2007. Staphylococcal pyoderma and furunculosis. *Equine Veterinary Education* 19:88–89.

Plumb DC 2005. *Plumb's Veterinary Drug Handbook*, 5th edn. London: Wiley-Blackwell.

Prescott JF, Baqqot JD, Walker RD, Dowling PM. 2000. *Antimicrobial Therapy in Veterinary Medicine*, 4th edn. Oxford: Iowa State Press.

Ramos JJ, Luco DF, Verde MT, Lucientes J, Fernandez A. 1996. Pelodera dermatitis in sheep. *Veterinary Record* 138:474–475.

Rich M. 2005. Staphylococci in animals: prevalence, identification and antimicrobial susceptibility, with an emphasis on methicillin-resistant *Staphylococcus aureus. British Journal of Biomedical Science* 62:98–105.

Rich M, Roberts L, Jones M, Young V. 2007. *Staphylococcus schleiferi* subspecies coagulans in companion animals. *Veterinary Record* 161:107.

Rosser EJ Jr. 1995. Infectious crusting dermatoses. *Veterinary Clinics of North America. Equine Practice* 11(1):53–59.

Saari SA, Nikander SE. 2006. *Pelodera* (syn. *Rhabditis*) *strongyloides* as a cause of dermatitis—a report of 11 dogs from Finland. *Acta Veterinaria Scandinavica* 48:18.

Salisbury RH, Barrowman PR. 1984. Fleece-rot: the epidemiology and significance of the disease in sheep. *Journal of the South African Veterinary Association* 55:147–151.

Saridomichelakis MN, Koutinas AF, Farmaki R, Leontides LS, Kasabalis D. 2007. Relative sensitivity of hair pluckings and exudate microscopy for the diagnosis of canine demodicosis. *Veterinary Dermatology* 18:138–141.

Sasaki T, Kikuchi K, Tanaka Y, Takahashi N, Kamata S, Hiramatsu K. 2007. Reclassification of phenotypically identified *Staphylococcus intermedius* strains. *Journal of Clinical Microbiology* 45(9):2770–2778.

Scott DW, Beningo KE, Miller WH Jr, Rothstein E. 1998. Efficacy of clindamycin hydrochloride capsules for the treatment of deep pyoderma due to *Staphylococcus intermedius* infection in dogs. *Canadian Veterinary Journal* 39:753–756.

Scott DW, Miller WH, Griffin CE. 2001. *Muller and Kirk's Small Animal Dermatology.* Philadelphia: WB Saunders.

Scott FM, Fraser J, Martin WB. 1980. Staphylococcal dermatitis of sheep. *Veterinary Record* 107:572–574.

Seixas F, Travassos PJ, Pinto ML, Correia J, Pires MA. 2006. Dermatitis in a dog induced by *Straelensia cynotis*: a case report and review of the literature. *Veterinary Dermatology* 17:81–84.

Sparkes AH, Robinson A, MacKay AD, Shaw SE. 2000. A study of the efficacy of topical and systemic therapy for the treatment of feline *Microsporum canis* infection. *Journal of Feline Medicine & Surgery* 2:135–142.

Sterkens P. 1997. Pharmacokinetics of itraconazol and hydroxyitraconazol in cats treated orally at 5 mg/kg/day following the proposed treatment schedule. Janssen Research Foundation, Report No. FK 1855.

Tamura Y, Kawamura Y, Inoue I, Ishino S. 2001. Scanning electron microscopy description of a new species of *Demodex canis* spp. *Veterinary Dermatology* 12:275–278.

Tranquilli WJ, Paul AJ, Todd KS. 1991. Assessment of toxicosis induced by high-dose administration of milbemycin oxime in collies. *American Journal of Veterinary Research* 52:1170–1172.

Trepanier LA, Danhof R, Toll J, Watrous D. 2003. Clinical findings in 40 dogs with hypersensitivity associated with administration of potentiated sulfonamides. *Journal of Veterinary Internal Medicine* 17:647–652.

Vanden Bossche H, Engelen M, Rochette F. 2003. Antifungal agents of use in animal health—chemical, biochemical and pharmacological aspects. *Journal of Veterinary Pharmacology and Therapeutics* 26:5–29.

Vlaminck KMJA, Engelen MACM. 2004. Itraconazole: a treatment with pharmacokinetic foundations. *Veterinary Dermatology* 15(1 Suppl):8.

White SD, Brown AE, Chapman PL, Jang SS, Ihrke PJ. 2005. Evaluation of aerobic bacteriologic culture of epidermal collarette specimens in dogs with superficial pyoderma. *Journal of the American Veterinary Medical Association* 226:904–908.

Wildermuth BE, Griffin CE, Rosenkrantz WS. 2006. Feline pyoderma therapy. *Clinical Techniques in Small Animal Practice* 21:150–156.

Willems L, Van Der GR, de Beule K. 2001. Itraconazole oral solution and intravenous formulations: a review of pharmacokinetics and pharmacodynamics. *Journal of Clinical Pharmacy and Therapeutics* 26:159–169.

Willers WB. 1970. *Pelodera strongyloides* in association with canine dermatitis in Wisconsin. *Journal of the American Veterinary Medical Association* 156:319–320.

Yager JA, Wilcock BP. 1994. *Colour Atlas and Text of Surgical Pathology of the Cat and Dog*. London: Wolfe Publishing.

Zdovc I, Ocepek M, Pirs T, Krt B, Pinter L. 2004. Microbiological features of *Staphylococcus schleiferi* subsp. coagulans, isolated from dogs and possible misidentification with other canine coagulase-positive staphylococci. *Journal of Veterinary Medicine. Part B: Infectious Diseases and Veterinary Public Health* 51:449–454.

Zur G, Elad D. 2006. In vitro and in vivo effects of lufenuron on dermatophytes isolated from cases of canine and feline dermatophytoses. *Journal of Veterinary Medicine. Part B: Infectious Diseases and Veterinary Public Health* 53:122–125.

4.2

Eosinophilic folliculitis

Monika Linek

Some alopecic diseases are histologically characterized by an eosinophil-predominated, folliculocentric inflammation. Many of these diseases may look alike, although multiple etiological triggers are able to initiate an eosinophilic reaction pattern. Intrafollicular parasites such as *Demodex* mites or *nematodes* can induce follicular inflammation rich in eosinophils. In these diseases, however, the inflammatory infiltrate is quite heterogeneous and mostly parasites can be detected within the lesion. The eosinophilic folliculitis mentioned in this chapter does not show any pathogens and is characterized by a striking predominance of eosinophils that not only center around hair follicles but also accumulate within the follicular wall and the follicular lumen. The high number of infiltrating eosinophils is frequently coupled with peripheral eosinophilia and often responds to immunosuppressive dosages of glucocorticoids (Scott et al. 2001; Gross et al. 2005). A subgroup of lymphocytic mural folliculitis in dogs may be associated with large numbers of perifollicular eosinophils. This canine disease is named "eosinophilic mucinotic mural folliculitis" (see Section 4.4.2.5), since mucin deposition within the follicular wall is a striking feature. However, since any infiltration of eosinophils can be associated with mucin deposition, mucin alone cannot be used to distinguish the diseases reliably. As the striking clinical picture in eosinophilic folliculitis is not alopecia, we provide the reader only with a brief review of these diseases.

4.2.1 Canine facial eosinophilic furunculosis

Facial eosinophilic furunculosis is a rare skin disease of the dog. The etiology and pathomechanism are still unclear although a hypersensitivity response to arthropod venoms from stinging insects is proposed by most authors (Gross 1993; Curtis et al. 1995; Guaguere et al. 1996). Most of the dogs develop lesions in the warm season and after an outdoor activity, but a direct documentation of arthropod insults is rare. The hypothesis of arthropod hypersensitivity is contradicted by reports of cases in cold seasons and the fact that recurrence or repetitive lesions have not been reported except in one case (Linek and Mecklenburg 2002; Scott et al. 2001). There is a clinically and histologically similar disease in humans where an autoimmune reaction to sebaceous glands, microorganisms, or *Demodex* mites has been discussed (Basarab 1997; Magro and Crowson 1994; Mengesha and Bennett 2002; Ofuji et al. 1970; Spira et al. 1986).

Eosinophilic furunculosis is characterized by the rapid development of bilateral pruritic papular, pustular, and ulcerative lesions in the face, predominantly on the bridge of the nose, the lateral muzzle, and the periorbital region (Fig. 4.2.1). Lesions may also develop on the pinnae, the extremities, and the glabrous skin of the axilla and abdomen (Gross 1993; Scott et al. 2001). The disease starts with papules, pustules, or nodules accompanied by severe pruritus and self-trauma. These first lesions rapidly ulcerate forming draining tracts and crusts. The severity is variable. In more destructive and widespread cases fever and anorexia develop. Blood eosinophilia may be present. There is no sex predilection. Affected dogs are mostly young and belong to large or moderately large breeds. However, the author has seen the disease in the Dachshund and the West Highland White Terrier.

Clinical differential diagnoses include nasal deep bacterial folliculitis, severe demodicosis or dermatophytosis, and a facially-oriented pemphigus foliaceus. A hallmark of eosinophilic furunculosis, however,

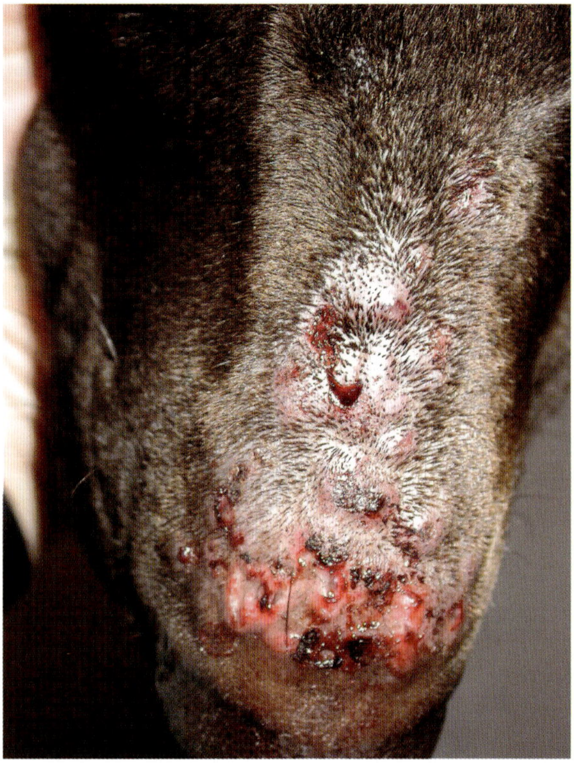

Fig. 4.2.1 Canine facial eosinophilic furunculosis. Alopecia on the nose with marked erythema, papules, ulceration, and crusts.

is that none of these differential diagnoses develop lesions as fulminant as in eosinophilic facial furunculosis.

Diagnosis is made by history, clinical picture, cytology, and biopsy. A deep skin scrape and a dermatophyte culture to exclude demodicosis and dermatophytosis are advisable. Cytology reveals predominately eosinophils. It is, however, important to sample acute not self-traumatized or ulcerated lesions, since in the latter neutrophils with intracellular bacteria may become more numerous. Biopsies should also be taken from intact nodules and papules or edematous swollen areas, whereas ulcerated lesions should be avoided. Histopathology may vary due to severity of the disease, but demonstrates a nodular perifollicular eosinophilic inflammation in all cases. Eosinophils infiltrate the hair follicle wall and accumulate both intramurally and intraluminally. Follicular rupture with subsequent foreign body granuloma and numerous eosinophils are common (Fig. 4.2.2). Eosinophilic degranulation may focus around collagen fibers and may cause "flame figures." A severe dermal edema and some dermal mucin deposition are frequently seen. Heavy inflammation may be accompanied by fibrinoid vasculitis and hemorrhage.

In mild cases, the course of the disease is self-limiting and most cases respond excellently to short courses of immunosuppressive doses of prednisolon (1–2 mg/kg/day) given for 8–14 days, tapering down as soon as the lesions disappear (Gross 1993; Guaguere et al. 1996). Glucocorticoids are combined with oral antibiotics such as cefalosporines, if secondary pyoderma exists.

4.2.2 Feline mosquito bite hypersensitivity

Feline mosquito bite hypersensitivity has some similarities to canine eosinophilic furunculosis of the face (see Section 4.2.1). It is an uncommon seasonal skin disease in cats where lesions develop in the summer and regress in autumn and winter. The face and ear pinnae are predominantly affected as is dark and sparsely haired skin (Nagata and Ishida 1997).

According to its name, the disease is thought to represent a hypersensitivity reaction to mosquito bites (Mason and Evans 1991). However, since its frequency of occurrence is highly variable in different geographic regions, it is assumed that only some mosquito species may induce hypersensitivity. The disease can be prevented by insect repellents and sting protection such as indoor confinement (Mason and Evans 1991). Challenges with mosquito bites induce typical lesions at the sites of the bite (Nagata and Ishida 1997). Intradermal allergy testing with mosquito antigen and positive Prausnitz–Küster testing indicate that a type I hypersensitivity reaction is involved in the pathogenesis. In addition, the clinical and histological reaction pattern suggests a concomitant delayed type IV hypersensitivity reaction (Gross et al. 2005).

The clinical picture is visually distinctive. Lesions are usually found bilaterally on the bridge of the nose (Fig. 4.2.3), the convex and less commonly the concave surface of the pinnae, and rarely the eyelids. The nasal planum and philtrum can be involved. Very rarely can the disease become more widespread affecting the flexor surface of carpi, footpads, and adjacent skin (Power and Ihrke 1995). Feline mosquito bite hypersensitivity may resemble miliary dermatitis, especially when the pinnae are affected. Early lesions are

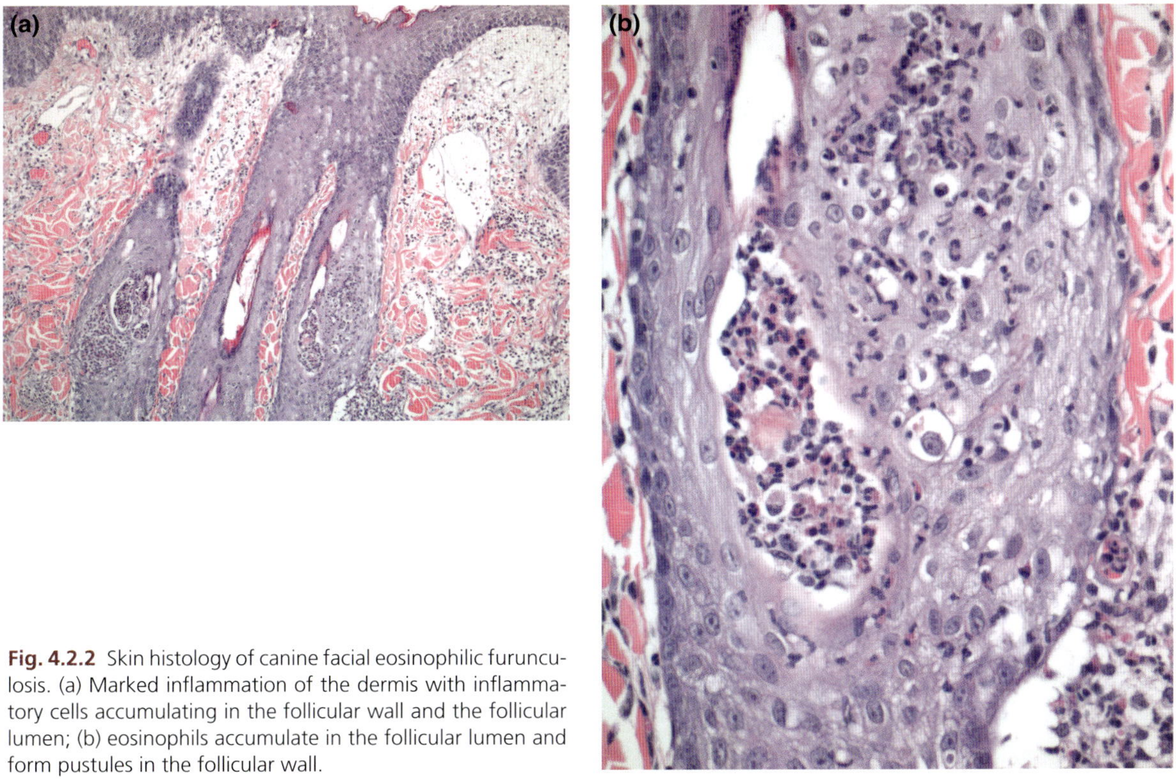

Fig. 4.2.2 Skin histology of canine facial eosinophilic furunculosis. (a) Marked inflammation of the dermis with inflammatory cells accumulating in the follicular wall and the follicular lumen; (b) eosinophils accumulate in the follicular lumen and form pustules in the follicular wall.

characterized by erythematous papules or nodules, whereas later stages show well demarcated ulcers, crusts, and necrotic lesions. Concurrent hyperpigmentation or hypopigmentation or alopecic nodules may be seen (Scott et al. 2001). Pruritus is present, but its severity is variable. Regional lymphadenopathy is common.

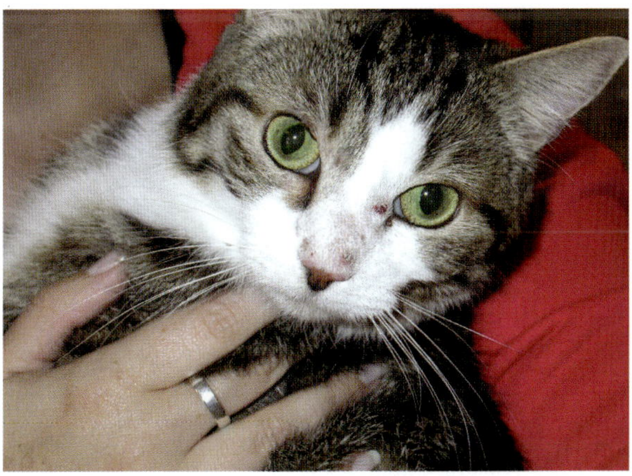

Fig. 4.2.3 Feline mosquito bite hypersensitivity. Note focal alopecia and erythema on the bridge of the nose.

Differential diagnoses include herpesvirus-induced dermatitis (see Section 4.6.1), pemphigus foliaceus (see Section 4.3.1), food hypersensitivity and atopy, in early cases, dermatophytosis (see Section 4.1.2) and demodicosis (see Section 4.1.3). Some severe ulcerative cases may resemble squamous cell carcinoma or pox virus infection (see Section 4.6.2). Cytology reveals predominately eosinophils. Peripheral eosinophilia and hypergammaglobulinemia have been reported commonly in one large study (Nagata and Ishida 1997).

Histopathology will reveal a strikingly eosinophil-rich inflammatory infiltrate that spreads from the superficial to the deep dermis. Hypereosinophilic collagen bundles ("flame figures") and mural eosinophilic folliculitis and furunculosis are frequently found. These findings, however, are not diagnostic, since similar histopathological changes occur in cats with other allergic diseases. Herpesvirus ulcerative dermatitis (see Section 4.6.1) may be indistinguishable from mosquito bite hypersensitivity, if inclusion bodies cannot be identified (Gross et al. 2005). Immunohistochemistry or polymerase chain reaction tests may be necessary to rule out feline herpesvirus infection. A history of mosquito bites and disease regression upon strict avoidance of mosquito bites allow a final diagnosis.

Avoidance of mosquito bites is the treatment and prophylactic measure of choice. This might involve confinement to indoors during the peak mosquito feeding time, and appliance of repellents such as permethrin, diethyltoluamid, or iciridin. Good immediate response is usually seen to short courses of glucocorticoids.

4.2.3 Equine culicoides hypersensitivity

Culicoides hypersensitivity or insect bite hypersensitivity in horses is also known under the names "sweet itch," "Queensland itch," "summer eczema," or "allergic urticaria."

Equine culicoides hypersensitivity is a chronic, recurrent, and seasonal dermatitis of horses caused by an allergic reaction to the bites of mosquitos of the genus *Culicoides* (Brostrom et al. 1987). It is by far the most common allergic dermatitis in horses with striking geographical variations in its prevalence (van Grevenhof et al. 2007).

A genetic predisposition has been assumed as some horse breeds are particularly sensitive, such as Shire, Iceland, and Welsh Ponies. Icelandic horses living in Iceland do not have insect bite hypersensitivity due to the absence of relevant insects, but acquire it at high frequency after being imported to mainland Europe (Brostrom et al. 1987). The sensitivity in Icelandic horses born outside of Iceland is not significantly different from the disease prevalence in other horse breeds (Bjornsdottir et al. 2006; Hamza et al. 2007). Therefore, the existence of a genetic predisposition needs further proof.

Most horses become affected by the age of 4–5 years and the disease usually progresses with age. There is no sex or hair/skin color predilection. The disease is characterized by intense irritation, scratching, and rubbing, leading to self-inflicted trauma, exfoliation, serous exudation, and alopecia. The species of *Culicoides* dictates the location of the clinical distribution

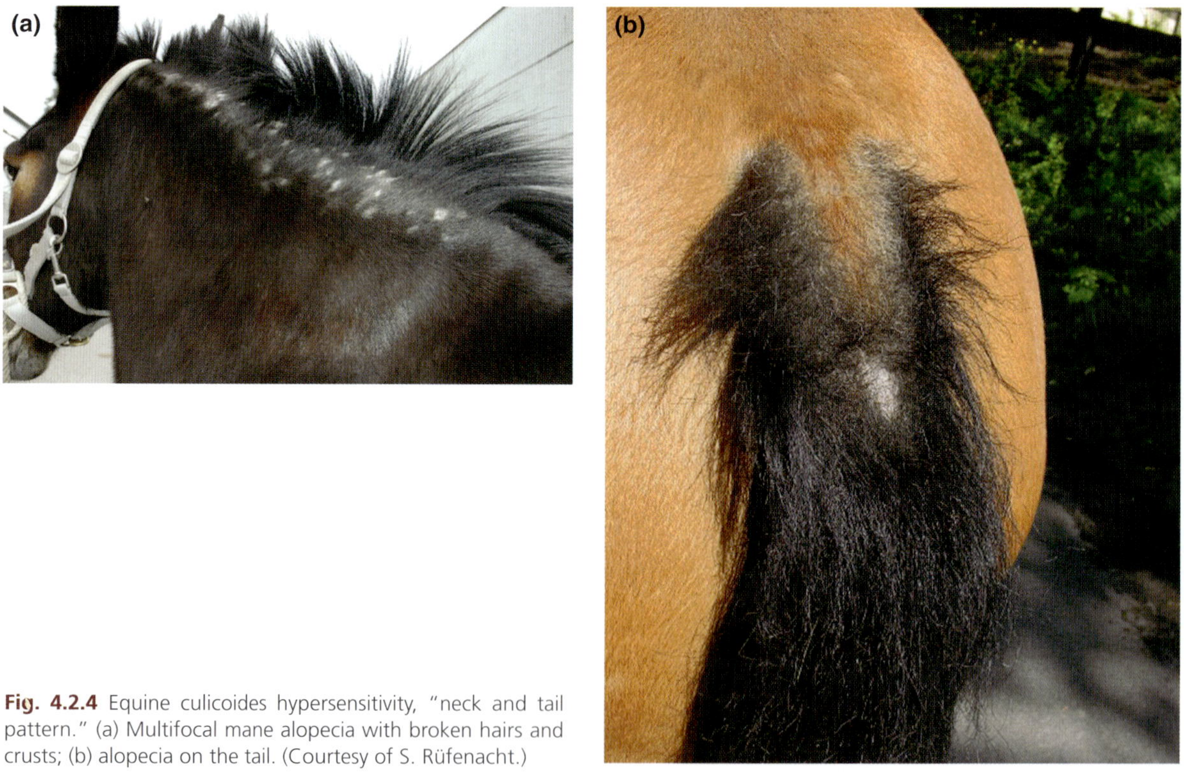

Fig. 4.2.4 Equine culicoides hypersensitivity, "neck and tail pattern." (a) Multifocal mane alopecia with broken hairs and crusts; (b) alopecia on the tail. (Courtesy of S. Rüfenacht.)

pattern. The "neck and tail pattern" is the most common one with sparse and broken tail and mane hairs (Fig. 4.2.4). In chronic cases thickening of the skin, formation of hyperkeratotic rugae, severe hair loss, and coarse hair develop. A "ventral pattern" of the disease is rarely found.

Although the clinical picture is visually striking, the list of differential diagnoses is long and includes parasitic infestations such as lice, *Chorioptes* and *Psoroptes* mites, *Oxyuris equi*, fly bites, ticks, and onchocercal dermatitis. Dermatophytosis and dermatophilosis have to be considered as well as more rare dermatoses such as unilateral papular dermatitis, alopecia areata (mane and tail dystrophy) (see Section 4.7.3), and chemical irritation.

Diagnosis is based on characteristic clinical signs, seasonality, and elimination of all other ectoparasitic diseases. A discussion about different tests for allergen-specific IgE and IgG in horses and the sensitivity and specificity of skin tests and in vitro tests is beyond the scope of this book and is sufficiently summarized in the literature (Fadok and Greiner 1990; Ferroglio et al. 2006; Wagner et al. 2006).

Biopsies are needed to differentiate equine culicoides hypersensitivity from mane and tail dystrophy or unilateral papular dermatitis. Biopsies of equine culicoides hypersensitivity will show an eosinophilic folliculitis and dermatitis.

The most important part of therapy is protection of the horse from further insect bites. The armamentarium comprises stabling of the horse at the peak biting time, installation of very fine screen mesh at all windows and doors, and installation of fans. Horses should be treated with repellents. Fenvalerate and permethrin have been claimed to be effective when used regularly and intensively. Covering the horse with a face mask, blankets, and newly developed nose-to-tail protection blankets may be considered. Acute cases can be treated with short courses of oral or intramuscular glucocorticoids, but prolonged usage is not advisable due to the risk of significant side effects. Response to antihistamines is weak and variable. Allergen-specific immunotherapy is still a matter of controversy.

References

Basarab T. 1997. HIV-associated eosinophilic pustular folliculitis. *Journal of the American Academy of Dermatology* 37:670–671.

Bjornsdottir S, Sigvaldadottir J, Brostrom H, Langvad B, Sigurdsson A. 2006. Summer eczema in exported Icelandic horses: influence of environmental and genetic factors. *Acta Veterinaria Scandinavica* 48(1):3.

Brostrom H, Larsson A, Troedsson M. 1987. Allergic dermatitis (sweet itch) of Icelandic horses in Sweden: an epidemiological study. *Equine Veterinary Journal* 19:229–236.

Curtis CF, Bond R, Blunden AS, Thomson DG, McNeil PE, Whitbread TW. 1995. Canine eosinophilic folliculitis and furunculosis in three cases. *Journal of Small Animal Practice* 36:119–123.

Fadok VA and Greiner EC. 1990. Equine insect hypersensitivity: skin test and biopsy results correlated with clinical data. *Equine Veterinary Journal* 22:236–240.

Ferroglio E, Pregel P, Accossato A, Taricco I, Bollo E, Rossi L, Trisciuoglio A. 2006. Equine culicoides hypersensitivity: evaluation of a skin test and of humoral response. *Journal of Veterinary Medicine, A. Physiology Pathology Clinical Medicine* 53:30–33.

Gross TL. 1993. Canine eosinophilic furunculosis of the face. In: Ihrke PJ, Mason IS, White SD (eds), *Advances in Veterinary Dermatology*, Vol. 3, pp. 239–246. Boston: Butherworth Heinemann.

Gross TL, Ihrke PJ, Walder EJ, Affolter VK. 2005. *Skin Diseases of the Dog and the Cat*. Oxford: Blackwell Science.

Guaguere E, Prelaud P, Peyronnet L, Delverdier-Poujade A, Magnol J-P. 1996. Furonculose eosinophilique chez le chien: étude retrospectivede 12 cas. *Pratique Medicale et Chirurgicale de l'Animal de Compagnie*, 31(5):413–419.

Hamza E, Doherr MG, Bertoni G, Jungi TW, Marti E. 2007. Modulation of allergy incidence in Icelandic horses is associated with a change in IL-4-producing T cells. *International Archives of Allergy and Immunology* 144:325–337.

Linek M, Mecklenburg L. 2002. Die Eosinophile pustulöse Follikulitis des Hundes: Eine Beschreibung von drei Fällen. *Praktischer Tierarzt, Zeitschrift für fortschrittliche Veterinärmedizin* 83:946–950.

Magro CM, Crowson AN. 1994. Eosinophilic pustular follicular reaction: a paradigm of immune dysregulation. *International Journal of Dermatology* 33(3):172–178.

Mason KV, Evans AG. 1991. Mosquito bite-caused eosinophilic dermatitis in cats. *Journal of the American Veterinary Medical Association* 198: 2086–2088.

Mengesha YM, Bennett ML. 2002. Pustular skin disorders: diagnosis and treatment. *American Journal of Clinical Dermatology* 3(6):389–400.

Nagata M, Ishida T. 1997. Cutaneous reactivity to mosquito bites and its antigens in cats. *Veterinary Dermatology* 8:19–26.

Ofuji S, Ogino A, Horio T, Oseko T, Uehara M. 1970. Eosinophilic pustular folliculitis. *Acta Dermato Venereologica* 50(3):195–203.

Power HT, Ihrke PJ. 1995. Selected feline eosinophilic skin diseases. *Veterinary Clinics of North America Small Animal Practice* 25:833–850.

Scott DW, Miller WH, Griffin CE. 2001. *Muller and Kirk's Small Animal Dermatology*. Philadelphia: WB Saunders.

Spira I, Simon M Jr, Keller J. 1986. Sterile eosinophilic pustulosis. *Der Hautarzt* 37:222–225.

van Grevenhof EM, Ducro B, Heuven HC, Bijma P. 2007. Identification of environmental factors affecting the prevalence of insect bite hypersensitivity in Shetland ponies and Friesian horses in The Netherlands. *Equine Veterinary Journal* 39:69–73.

Wagner B, Miller WH, Morgan EE, Hillegas JM, Erb HN, Leibold W, Antczak DF. 2006. IgE and IgG antibodies in skin allergy of the horse. *Veterinary Research* 37:813–825.

Wilson AD, Harwood LJ, Bjornsdottir S, Marti E, Day MJ. 2001. Detection of IgG and IgE serum antibodies to culicoides salivary gland antigens in horses with insect dermal hypersensitivity (sweet itch). *Equine Veterinary Journal* 33(7):707–713.

4.3

Pustular folliculitis

Monika Welle

Pustular mural folliculitis describes pustule formation within the infundibular epithelium of the hair follicle. This pattern is usually associated with a pustular dermatitis of the interfollicular epidermis. Since these diseases are extensively described in other textbooks, not all aspects of them are discussed in this chapter.

4.3.1 Pemphigus foliaceus

The pemphigus complex is a group of diseases that is characterized by the formation of pustules or vesicles, developing due to the loss of cohesion between keratinocytes (i.e., acantholysis). Acantholysis is immunologically accompanied by the presence of autoantibodies to components of the keratinocyte desmosomes. Pemphigus foliaceus (PF) has been reported in dogs, cats, horses, and goats (Scott et al. 1987; Scott 1988; Valdez et al. 1995; Scott et al. 2001; Vandenabeele et al. 2004; Gross et al. 2005; Ginn et al. 2007), and all aspects of this disease have been extensively reviewed recently (Olivry 2006). In this review it was suggested that canine PF may not be a single disease but a clinicopathological syndrome which is clinically, histologically, and immunologically heterogeneous. Whether feline, equine, and caprine PF are immunologically heterogeneous currently remains unknown.

Autoantigens and the pathogenicity of circulating autoantibodies in feline, equine, and caprine PF have not been investigated until now, whereas in the dog autoantigens have been studied for many years. For a long time a 14 kDa and a 160 kDa antigen, both binding to serum IgG autoantibodies, were suspected to represent different glycosylation forms of canine desmoglein-1 (dsg1). Dsg1 is the major PF antigen in humans. However, in recent years it turned out that recombinant canine dsg1 is recognized by sera from human patients with PF, but not by IgG from any of the tested canine PF sera (Iwasaki and Olivry 2004; Yabuzoe et al. 2006). In addition, only five of 83 canine PF sera (6%) recognized canine dsg1-transfected human cells. Therefore, dsg1 is most likely only a minor autoantigen in canine PF, with the major autoantigen still being unknown.

In dogs, PF is a disease of the middle age and may occur as a sequela of chronic or ongoing inflammatory skin diseases (Pascal et al. 1995). Various drugs (antibiotics, methimazol) have been reported to cause PF in dogs. In some cases withdrawal of the drug leads to complete remission of the disease (PF-like drug reaction), whereas in others the disease continues (drug-induced PF). In both forms, clinical signs develop rapidly after drug administration (White et al. 2002; Olivry et al. 2004; Gross et al. 2005).

Clinical signs of PF appear to be similar in all domestic animal species. PF is characterized by transient large and sometimes confluent pustules that rapidly evolve into erosions and crusts. In rare occasions, pustules, erosions, and crusts are grouped in a unique annular or polycyclic pattern. Alopecia and generalized exfoliative erythroderma follow. Pruritus is present in less than 50% of the patients and systemic symptoms such as anorexia, depression, fever, and weight loss are usually only encountered in patients with widespread erosive skin lesions.

In most dogs, the disease begins with bilateral lesions on the face, namely on the dorsal muzzle, nasal planum, periocular skin, and ears. Lesions progress and can become generalized within 3–12 months. Only rarely the disease begins with generalized skin lesions. A remarkable finding of canine PF is the predilection of lesions for the footpads. These are involved in one third of all cases. Some canine patients may even show skin lesions that are restricted to the footpads (Ihrke et al. 1985; Mueller et al. 2006). Mucosal lesions have only been seen in approximately 2% of canine PF patients (Mueller et al. 2006). One canine case with PF lesions confined to the claws has been reported (Guaguere and Degorce-Rubiales 2004).

In cats, pustules are more transient and thus the clinical phenotype is dominated by erosions and yellowish crusts on the face, ears, and the feet. Pedal lesions, consisting of suppuration or crusts, can be seen on or around the footpads or the nail beds. Feline PF is usually mild and fairly localized, but generalized lesions are possible (Preziosi et al. 2003). Dogs and cats with widespread lesions are often febrile, anorectic, and depressed.

Horses with PF usually present with multifocal to generalized crusting, scaling, and alopecia affecting the face, neck, trunk, and extremities (Fig. 4.3.1). Pustules are observed rarely, and whenever present, they are transient. A remarkable ventral edema is seen in many horses with PF. Systemic symptoms such as depression and lethargy were noticed in 50% of the horses with PF in one study. Lesions of equine PF are occasionally painful and pruritic (Vandenabeele et al. 2004; Zabel et al. 2005).

In goats, pustules, crusts, scales, and alopecia are seen on the face, ventral abdomen, limbs, perineum, and tail. In female animals, lesions may affect the udder and teats (Jackson et al. 1984; Scott et al. 1984a; Valdez et al. 1995).

Cytology is a useful screening test to differentiate PF from superficial pyoderma (see Section 4.1.1). Classical PF pustules reveal mainly nondegenerated neutrophils (rarely eosinophils) and clusters of acantholytic keratinocytes. Superficial pyoderma in contrast is characterized by abundant degenerated neutrophils with intracellular bacteria, some macrophages, and only rare acantholytic cells. However, the diagnosis needs to be confirmed by histopathology, as there is some cytological overlap between PF, superficial pyoderma, and dermatophytosis.

Histopathology is until now the most important tool to diagnose PF since serological tests are only useful in those cases where the major autoantigen is known. Biopsy findings are similar in all species. It is described that in very early lesions epidermal vesicles with acantholytic keratinocytes and scarce neutrophils can be seen (Olivry 2006). However, the major histological findings are intragranular or subcorneal pustules with isolated or clustered acantholytic cells and many well-preserved neutrophils. Variable numbers of eosinophils may be found. Similar pustules are also seen in the infundibular epithelium of the hair follicle (Fig. 4.3.2). In general, the pustules are large and span

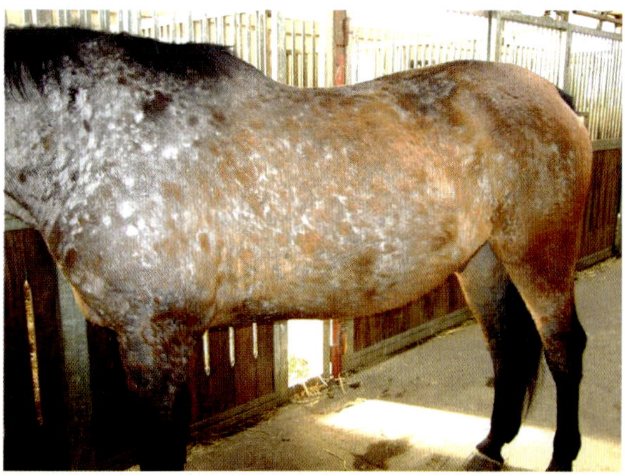

Fig. 4.3.1 Equine pemphigus foliaceus. Multifocal to generalized crusting, scaling, and alopecia affecting face, neck, trunk, and extremities. (Courtesy of M. Linek.)

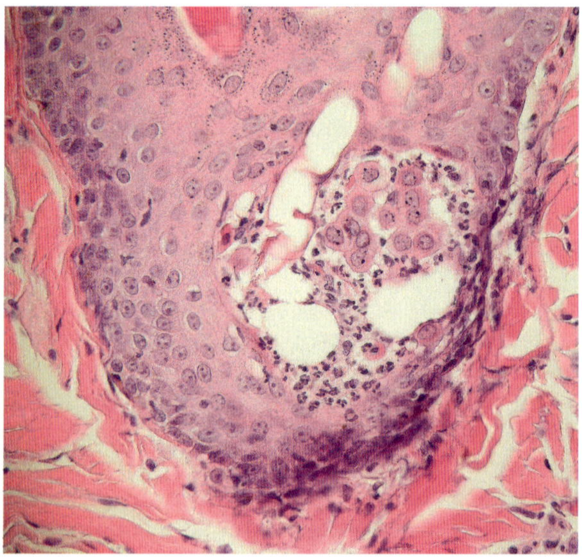

Fig. 4.3.2 Skin histology of pemphigus foliaceus. Pustules with well-preserved neutrophils and acantholytic keratinocytes are found in the infundibular epithelium of the hair follicle.

the length of multiple follicular ostia, a finding that differentiates PF from bacterial folliculitis or superficial dermatophytosis. Furthermore, a newly formed stratum corneum at the base of neutrophilic pustules and nonspongiotic detachment of keratinocytes are more suggestive of PF than bacterial folliculitis and dermatophytosis. Apoptotic keratinocytes are often seen in the epidermis of dogs with PF, but are not considered a marker for an underlying drug reaction (Scott et al. 2001; Gross et al. 2005).

Immune suppression with oral glucocorticoids, such as prednisone or prednisolone, at daily dosages varying from 2 to 6.6 mg/kg divided into one or two administrations per day are the treatment of choice (Ihrke et al. 1985; Scott et al. 1987; Rosenkrantz 2004; Mueller et al 2006). If the response is good, dose or administration frequency should be reduced (Ihrke et al. 1985; Rosenkrantz 2004). In canine patients, where glucocorticoids alone are insufficient, cytotoxic drugs such as azathioprine (2–2.5 mg/kg, orally, once daily), cyclophosphamide (25 mg/kg, orally, once daily), or chlorambucil (0.2 mg/kg every 24–48 h) have been used (Ihrke et al. 1985; Scott et al. 1987; Rosenkrantz 2004). In one study additional antibiotic treatment during the induction of immunosuppression was associated with a significant improvement of the survival rate (Gomez et al. 2004). In cats with PF, glucocorticoid monotherapy with oral prednisolone is often sufficient (Graham-Mize and Rosser 2005). If response to treatment is insufficient, prednisolone or chlorambucil (0.2 mg/kg, orally, once daily) can be used in addition (Helton-Rhodes and Shoulberg 1992; Preziosi et al. 2003). Similar to dogs and cats, lesions of PF in horses and goats can be treated successfully with either prednisolone or dexamethasone alone or in combination with aurothioglucose (Scott et al. 1987; Valdez et al. 1995; Vandenabeele et al. 2004). Careful monitoring depending on the combination of treatments is necessary.

4.3.2 Pemphigus erythematosus

The clinical, histopathological, and immunological characteristics of pemphigus erythematosus (PE) in dogs and cats have first been described by Scott et al. (1980). Although still controversially discussed, most dermatologists consider PE a rare variant of PF, with a more local, that is, facial distribution pattern (Olivry 2006).

Clinical signs of PE are similar to PF but less severe. Pustules, erosions, and crusts are localized on the face and the ear pinnae. Depigmentation, erythema, erosion, and ulceration of the nasal planum and the dorsal muzzle are seen in addition (Scott et al. 1980; Faircloth and Montgomery 1982; Kaufman and Blakemore 1984; Scott et al. 1984b; Bennett et al. 1985; Olivry 1986; Scott et al. 1987; Griffies et al. 2004; Gonsalves-Hubers 2005). Only rare patients exhibit nonfacial lesions (Scott et al. 1987).

Skin biopsies from dogs and cats with PE will reveal similar findings to PF, that is, intragranular to subcorneal epidermal and infundibular pustules filled with neutrophils, eosinophils, and acantholytic cells. In contrast to PF, a mild interface dermatitis occurs in the superficial dermis that resembles discoid lupus erythematosus (Scott et al. 1980; Faircloth and Montgomery 1982; Kaufman and Blakemore 1984; Scott et al. 1984b; Bennett et al. 1985; Olivry 1986; Scott et al. 1987; Griffies et al. 2004; Gonsalves-Hubers 2005).

PE lesions in dogs and cats respond well to the same immunosuppressive therapy as is used in PF (Scott et al. 1987). One of two dogs with PE treated with tetracycline and niacinamide showed a partial response (White et al. 1992). The use of sun-avoidance and sunscreens or topical treatment with 0.1% tacrolimus ointment has been reported to be of benefit (Scott et al. 1987; Griffies et al. 2004).

4.3.3 Canine idiopathic linear pustular acantholytic dermatosis

The first case of this disease has been described in a young Brittany Spaniel in 2001 (Beningo and Scott 2001) and the same author reported a second case in a young Australian Shepherd dog in 2003 (Scott 2003). Since then, to the authors' knowledge, no further cases have been described. The etiology of this disease is still unknown. In the two described cases, contact dermatitis, self-trauma, vasculitis, and lymphangitis were ruled out (Beningo and Scott 2001; Scott 2003).

Idiopathic linear pustular acantholytic dermatosis is characterized by coalescent annular papules, pustules, and crusts. Mild erythema and scaling are also present. Alopecia develops later on. Histology is characterized by a predominant eosinophilic and to a lesser extent neutrophilic pustular mural folliculitis with marked acantholysis. Many of the acantholytic keratinocytes contain keratohyalin granules, suggesting they derive from the stratum granulosum of the follicular infundibulum. The surface epidermis and the hair follicle infundibulum show a marked regular or irregular hyperplasia, a mild to moderate orthokeratotic or parakeratotic hyperkeratosis, and focally intense areas of intercellular edema associated with exocytosis of eosinophils. In the dermis, a superficial perivascular to interstitial infiltrate composed of eosinophils with smaller numbers of neutrophils, plasma cells, and lymphocytes is seen.

Both described cases of canine idiopathic linear pustular acantholytic dermatosis responded well to an immunosuppressive dose of prednisolone (1.6 mg/kg once daily, orally). Treatment was slowly tapered and eventually stopped. In the second reported case, lesions reoccurred several times and regressed spontaneously without treatment (Scott 2003).

References

Beningo KE, Scott DW. 2001. Idiopathic linear pustular acantholytic dermatosis in a young Brittany spaniel dog. *Veterinary Dermatology* 12:209–213.

Bennett D, Kelly DF, Kirkham D. 1985. Two cases of pemphigus erythematosus (the Senear–Usher syndrome) in the dog. *Journal of Small Animal Practice* 26:219–227.

Faircloth JC, Montgomery JK. 1982. A practitioner case report: pemphigus erythematosus in a cat. *Feline Practice* 12:31–33.

Ginn PE, Mansell JEKL, Rakich PM. 2007. Skin and appendages. In: Maxie MG (ed.), *Jubb, Kennedy and Palmer's Pathology of Domestic Animals*, pp. 553–781. Edinborough, Scotland: Elsevier Saunders.

Gomez SM, Morris DO, Rosenbaum MR, Goldschmidt MH. 2004. Outcome and complications associated with treatment of pemphigus foliaceus in dogs: 43 cases (1994–2000). *Journal of the American Veterinary Medical Association* 224(8):1312–1316.

Gonsalves-Hubers T. 2005. Pemphigus erythematosus in a chow chow. *Canadian Veterinary Journal* 46:925–927.

Graham-Mize CA, Rosser EJ. 2005. Absorption, bioavailability and activity of prednisone and prednisolone in cats. In: Hillier A, Foster AP, Kwochka KW (eds.) *Advances in Veterinary Dermatology*, pp. 152–158. Oxford, UK: Blackwell Publishing.

Griffies JD, Mendelsohn DL, Rosenkrantz WS. 2004. Topical 0.1% tacrolimus for the treatment of discoid lupus erythematosus and pemphigus erythematosus in dogs. *Journal of the American Animal Hospital Association* 40:29–41.

Gross TL, Ihrke PJ, Walder EJ, Affolter VK. 2005. *Skin Diseases of the Dog and Cat: Clinical and Histopathological Diagnosis*. Oxford: Blackwell Science.

Guaguere E, Degorce-Rubiales F. 2004. Pemphigus foliaceus confined to the nails in a Hungarian short-haired pointer (Abstract). *Veterinary Dermatology* 15(1 Suppl):56.

Helton-Rhodes K, Shoulberg N. 1992. Chlorambucil: effective therapeutic options for the treatment of feline immune-mediated dermatoses. *Feline Practice* 20:5–8.

Ihrke PJ, Stannard AA, Ardans AA, Griffin CE. 1985. Pemphigus foliaceus in dogs: a review of 37 cases. *Journal of the American Veterinary Medical Association* 186:59–66.

Iwasaki T, Olivry T. 2004. Spontaneous canine model of pemphigus foliaceus. In: Chan LS (ed.), *Animal Models of Human Inflammatory Skin Diseases*, pp. 309–319. Boca Raton, FL: CRC Press.

Jackson PPG, Lloyd S, Jeffries AR. 1984. Pemphigus foliaceus in a goat. *Veterinary Record* 114:479.

Kaufman GM, Blakemore JC. 1984. Facial dermatitis in a dog. *Compendium on Continuing Education for the Practicing Veterinarian* 6:109–112.

Mueller RS, Krebs I, Power HT, Fieseler KV. 2006. Pemphigus foliaceus in 91 dogs. *Journal of the American Animal Hospital Association* 42:189–196.

Olivry T. 1986. Les dermatoses auto-immunes du chien et du chat. Université Paul-Sabatier, Toulouse.

Olivry T. 2006. A review of autoimmune skin diseases in domestic animals: I—superficial pemphigus. *Veterinary Dermatology* 17:291–305.

Olivry T, Bergvall KE, Atlee BA. 2004. Prolonged remission after immunosuppressive therapy in six dogs with pemphigus foliaceus. *Veterinary Dermatology* 15(4):245–252.

Pascal A, Scheibert J, Ihrke PJ. 1995. Seasonality and environmental risk factors for pemphigus foliaceus in animals: a retrospective study of 83 cases presented to the Veterinary Medical Teaching Hospital, University of California, Davis from 1976–1994. *Proceedings of the 11th AAVD/ACVD Meeting*, Santa Fe, pp. 24–25.

Preziosi DE, Goldschmidt MH, Greek JS, Jeffers JG, Shanley KS, Drobatz K, Mauldin EA. 2003. Feline pemphigus foliaceus: a retrospective analysis of 57 cases. *Veterinary Dermatology* 14:313–321.

Rosenkrantz WS. 2004. Pemphigus: current therapy. *Veterinary Dermatology* 15:90–98.

Scott DW. 1988. *Large Animal Dermatology*. Philadelphia: WB Saunders.

Scott DW. 2003. Canine idiopathic linear pustular acantholytic dermatosis: a second case. *Veterinary Dermatology* 14:275.

Scott DW, Miller WH, Griffin CE. 2001. *Muller and Kirk's Small Animal Dermatology*. Philadelphia: WB Saunders.

Scott DW, Miller WH, Lewis RM. 1980. Pemphigus erythematosus in the dog and the cat. *Journal of the American Animal Hospital Association* 16:815–823.

Scott DW, Smith MC, Smith CA. 1984a. Pemphigus foliaceus in a goat. *Agri-Practice* 5:38–45.

Scott DW, Walton DK, Slater MR. 1987. Immune-mediated dermatoses in domestic animals: ten years after—part I. *Compendium on Continuing Education for the Practicing Veterinarian* 9:424–435.

Scott DW, Walton DK, Smith CA. 1984b. Unusual findings in canine pemphigus erythematosus and discoid lupus erythematosus. *Journal of the American Animal Hospital Association* 20:579–584.

Valdez RA, Gelberg HB, Morin DE. 1995. Use of corticosteroids and aurothioglucose in a pygmy goat with pemphigus foliaceus. *Journal of the American Veterinary Medical Association* 207:761–765.

Vandenabeele SI, White SD, Affolter VK, Kass PH, Ihrke PJ. 2004. Pemphigus foliaceus in the horse: a retrospective study of 20 cases. *Veterinary Dermatology* 15:381–388.

White SD, Carlotti DN, Pin D, Bonenberger T, Ihrke PJ, Monet E, Nishifuji K, Iwasaki T, Papich MG. 2002. Putative drug-related pemphigus foliaceus in four dogs. *Veterinary Dermatology* 13(4): 195–202.

White SD, Rosychuk RAW, Reinke SI, Paradis M. 1992. Use of tetracycline and niacinamide for treatment of autoimmune skin disease in 31 dogs. *Journal of the American Veterinary Medical Association* 200:1497–1500.

Yabuzoe A, Nishifuji K, Shimizu A. 2006. Ultrastructural localization of binding site of serum antibodies in pemphigus foliaceus by post-embedding immunoelectron microscopy in one dog. *Veterinary Dermatology* 17:220.

Zabel S, Mueller RS, Fieseler KV, Bettenay SV, Littlewood JD, Wagner R. 2005. Review of 15 cases of pemphigus foliaceus in horses and a survey of the literature. *Veterinary Record* 157:505–509.

4.4

Lymphocytic mural folliculitis

Monika Welle

Mural folliculitis with predominately lymphocytes can occur in association with similar epidermal lesions or as an autonomous disease without epidermal involvement. Lymphocytic mural folliculitis can further be subdivided into an infiltrative type of lesion where lymphocytes infiltrate the follicular wall without evidence of keratinocyte degeneration and into an interface type of lesion where the lymphocytic infiltrate is associated with vacuolar degeneration and/or apoptosis of outer root sheath keratinocytes, just as in an interface dermatitis.

4.4.1 Lymphocytic mural folliculitis as a bystander of similar epidermal lesions

Lymphocytic mural folliculitis can occur in association with a lymphocytic dermatitis affecting the interfollicular epidermis. These cases are not primarily associated with alopecia, although hair loss can develop when the disease progresses and in rare cases can be the dominant clinical sign. Since these diseases are extensively described in other textbooks (Scott et al. 2001; Gross et al. 2005), not all aspects of them are discussed here.

4.4.1.1 Epitheliotropic T-cell lymphoma

Epitheliotropic T-cell lymphoma is not a dermatitis and mural folliculitis in the strict sense, but a progressive disease characterized by the infiltration of neoplastic T-cells into the epidermis and the adnexal epithelium. However, as it often mimics an inflammatory disease, it is included under the heading of mural folliculitis.

Epitheliotropic T-cell lymphoma is also known as "mycosis fungoides" (MF) and is uncommon in the dog and rare in cats, horses, and cattle (Caciolo et al. 1984; Baker and Scott 1989; Beale and Bolon 1992; Moore and Olivry 1994; Affolter and Moore 2000; Affolter 2007).

4.4.1.1.1 Etiology and pathogenesis

Epitheliotropic T-cell lymphomas are composed of memory (CD45RA−, CD4+, CD8+; 80%) or double negative (CD4−, CD8−; 20%) T-cells that express β1-integrin (Moore et al. 1994; Affolter and Moore 2000; Gross et al. 2005; Affolter 2007). Whereas "pagetoid reticulosis" in humans is composed of γ/δ T-cells, classic MF may be either of γ/δ T-cell or of α/β T-cell origin.

Some studies in man and dogs suggest that MF occurs often in patients that have previously been diagnosed with atopic dermatitis (Winkelmann and Rajka 1983; Abel et al. 1986; Lange-Vejlsgaard et al. 1989; Haselen et al. 1999; Pielop et al. 2001; Fletcher et al. 2004; Santoro et al. 2007). This is in concordance with the observation that MF often develops in areas where atopic dermatitis manifests. However, whether MF is directly linked to atopic dermatitis or whether it might be a consequence of immunomodulatory therapy or other factors is yet unknown. Nevertheless, the simultaneous occurrence of these two diseases might support the hypothesis that chronic antigen stimulation may be an initiator of a clonal neoplastic T-cell population in the skin.

In dogs, the age of onset ranges from 6 to 14 years with a mean age of 11 years. There is no apparent breed or sex predilection. The course of the disease varies from a few months up to 2 years and the lesions may extend to lymph nodes and other organs. Like in the dog, no apparent breed or sex predilection exists in cats and horses where most patients are also of advanced age.

4.4.1.1.2 Clinical presentation

Clinically five different presentations of MF are known that can mimic various other skin diseases (Moore and Olivry 1994; Scott et al. 2001; Gross et al. 2005; Affolter 2007). These forms may occur separately or in any combination and they will merge with chronicity.

1 *Exfoliative erythroderma* is characterized by exfoliative erythema, depigmentation, and alopecia, most often on the head and trunk (Fig. 4.4.1). Lesions may be bilateral and symmetric or may become generalized. In exfoliative erythroderma no palpable mass is present, but patches, plaques, and nodules may appear with progression of the disease. Pruritus varies from mild to severe. This form histologically often presents as pagetoid reticulosis and sometimes as Sézary syndrome (see below).
2 *Mucocutaneous lesions* are characterized by erythema, erosion, ulceration, depigmentation, and alopecia mostly on the facial mucocutaneous junctions such as lips, nasal planum, and eyelids. They may also be seen on the anorectal junction, the vulva, and the prepuce. This form histologically presents as pagetoid reticulosis (see below).
3 The third form is characterized by *solitary or multiple erythematous and scaly plaques or nodules* which may coalesce during progression and become eroded and ulcerated. Lymphadenopathy may be present. In most cases, histology will reveal classical features of MF (see below).
4 The *ulcerative form* of the disease is seen in the oral mucosa. Ulceration varies from mild to severe.
5 In *Sézary syndrome* the cutaneous lesions are associated with concurrent involvement of lymph nodes and peripheral blood. Circulating neoplastic lymphocytes may have hyperchromatic, folded, and grooved nuclei (Sézary cells).

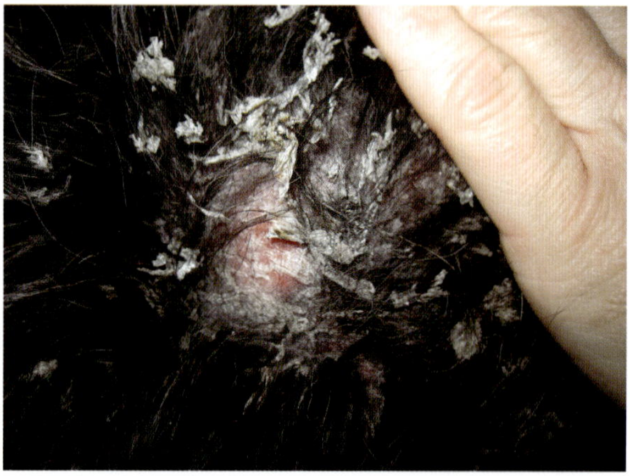

Fig. 4.4.1 Epitheliotropic lymphoma in a dog. Focal alopecia with erythema and exfoliation. (Courtesy of M. Linek.)

4.4.1.1.3 Histopathology

The key diagnostic feature is epitheliotropism of neoplastic lymphocytes. The infiltrate may be diffuse and is most pronounced in the lower level of the epidermis and the follicular infundibulum. It forms so-called Pautrier's micro aggregates in the epithelium. Tropism to adnexal structures including apocrine sweat glands is common. Accompanying mucinosis is possible. Dermal involvement and cytologic features vary among the different forms. Small lymphocytes, medium-sized lymphocytes, euchromatic or hyperchromatic nuclei, nuclei with an irregular contour, and small to moderate amounts of cytoplasm may be seen. MF with cellular features of well-differentiated lymphocytes is hard to distinguish from nonneoplastic interface dermatosis. Tumor-stage lesions are often characterized by larger neoplastic cells, which may have large and often folded or cleaved nuclei. Mitotic activity varies. Histologically, three different patterns can be distinguished.

1 The "classical form" is characterized by neoplastic infiltrates in the epidermis and the adnexal epithelium (Fig. 4.4.2). In the patch and plaque stage the dermal infiltrate is limited to the superficial dermis; in the tumor stage the infiltration is diffuse and involves the deep dermis and subcutis. In the cat, patch and plaque lesions are common, whereas the tumor stage appears to be less prevalent than in the dog.
2 The "d'emblée form" is characterized by tumor formation without previous patch and plaque stages. Keratinocyte apoptosis and confluent epidermal necrosis and ulceration may be seen (Fig. 4.4.3). Reactive dermal infiltrates include small lymphocytes, plasma cells, eosinophils, and neutrophils.
3 In "pagetoid reticulosis" the neoplastic infiltrate is mostly confined to the epidermis and the follicular epithelium (Fig. 4.4.4). Apoptotic keratinocytes

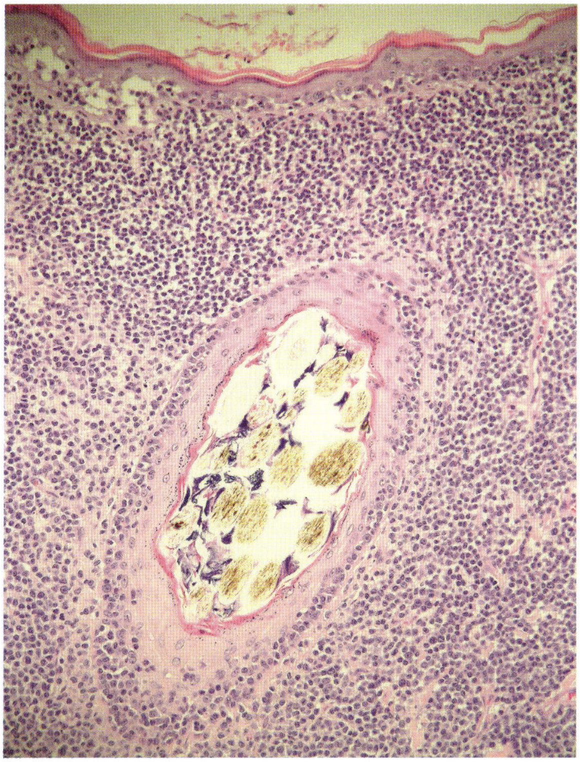

Fig. 4.4.2 Skin histology of epitheliotropic lymphoma, classical form. Diffuse epitheliotropic infiltrate of neoplastic lymphocytes, most pronounced in the lower level of the epidermis and the follicular infundibulum.

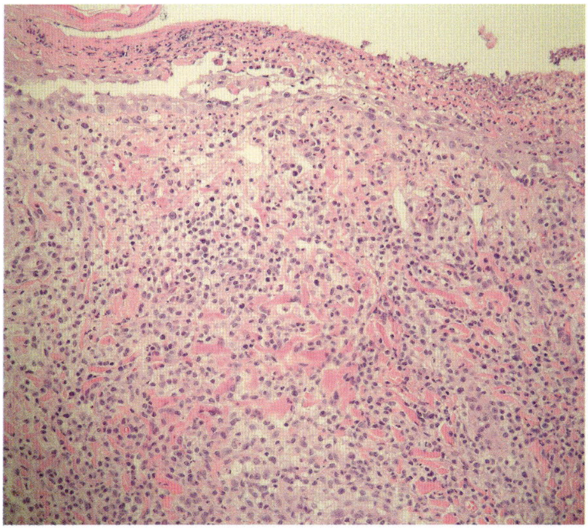

Fig. 4.4.3 Skin histology of epitheliotropic lymphoma, "d'emblée" form. Tumor formation with keratinocyte apoptosis and confluent epidermal necrosis and ulceration.

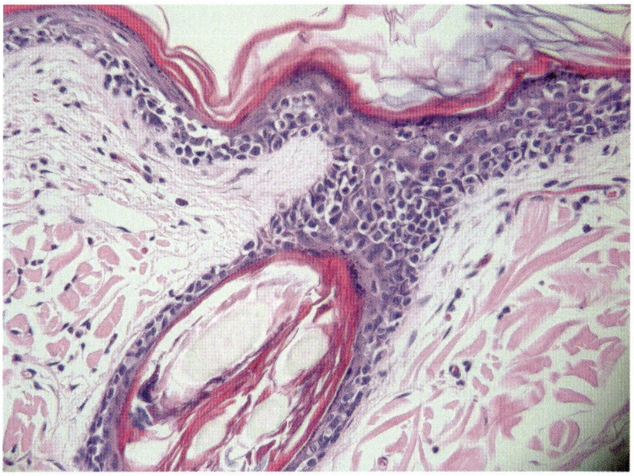

Fig. 4.4.4 Skin histology of epitheliotropic lymphoma, "pagetoid reticulosis" form. The neoplastic infiltrate is mostly confined to the epidermis and the follicular epithelium.

may be observed in conjunction with the lymphocytic infiltrate. The neoplastic cells are often small lymphocytes. The superficial dermis may contain a pleocellular reactive infiltrate. With disease progression the lesions extend into the dermis.

4.4.1.1.4 Therapy

Several chemotherapy protocols have been used in the dog with little success. A concise update on the management of canine epitheliotropic cutaneous T-cell lymphoma has recently been published (de Lorimier 2006). Retinoids or topical nitrogen mustard may be a helpful approach in early lesions. However, due to its carcinogenic potential and its potential for other adverse skin reactions, topical nitrogen mustard is rarely recommended. In more advanced disease, lomustine has shown complete response for more than 511 days in 15% of cases and partial response for 80 days in 57% of cases (Risbon et al. 2006). Careful monitoring is necessary with this therapy due to numerous side effects such as myelosuppression and hepatotoxicity; the reader is referred to oncology textbooks for more detailed information (Withrow and Vail 2006). Surgery or radiation therapy (30 Gray) is an option in small or localized lesions (Withrow and Vail 2006; Rüfenacht et al. 2007).

4.4.1.2 Systemic and discoid lupus erythematosus

Lupus erythematosus is divided into *systemic lupus erythematosus* (SLE), *discoid lupus erythematosus*

(DLE) and in the dog the rather newly described entities *vesicular lupus erythematosus* (see Section 4.4.1.3) and *exfoliative cutaneous lupus* (see Section 4.4.1.4).

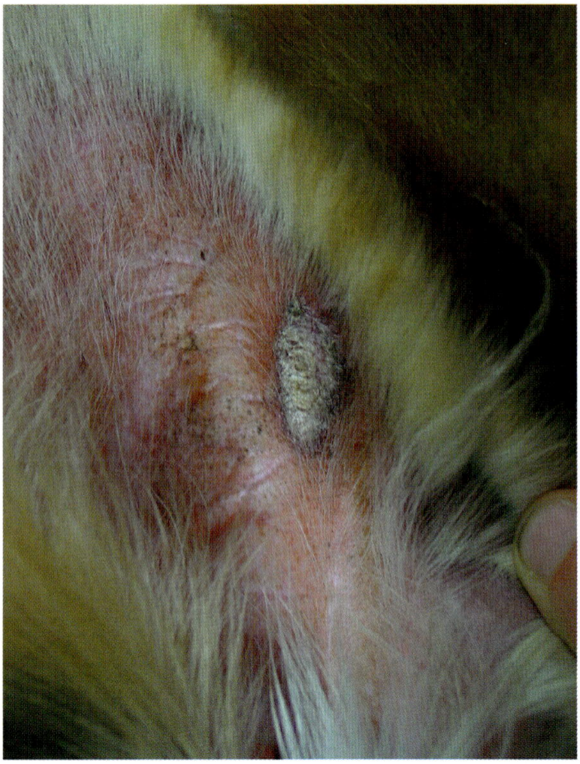

Fig. 4.4.5 Systemic lupus erythematosus in a dog. Mild scaling, erythema, and alopecia. (Courtesy of Section of Clinical Dermatology, Vetsuisse Faculty, University of Berne.)

4.4.1.2.1 Etiology and pathogenesis

Although the term lupus erythematosus encompasses a group of diseases that have different clinical syndromes and are still not fully understood, the main characteristics in the skin are damaged keratinocytes accompanied by a lymphohistiocytic infiltrate in the basement membrane zone of the epidermis and the follicular wall. It is most likely that damaged keratinocytes expressed formerly nuclear and cytoplasmic antigens and these lead to the formation of autoantibodies and immunocomplexes. Antinuclear antibody (ANA) titers are positive in SLE and mostly negative in DLE. The organ-specific and non-organ-specific circulating autoantibodies are directed against a wide variety of tissue antigens such as double-stranded DNA, RNA, nucleoproteins, and histones. Ultraviolet radiation (UVR) damage seems to contribute to the pathogenesis of both SLE and DLE, and it has been demonstrated that cutaneous lesions can be induced by ultraviolet light exposure in previously unexposed skin (Bennion and Norris 1997). The exact pathogenesis of UVR damage is not clear, but it is known that UVA and UVB can induce cell damage and cytokine release possibly leading to the exposure of novel intracellular antigens on the surface of keratinocytes.

4.4.1.2.2 Diagnosis

SLE occurs in horses, dogs, and cats without clear age or sex predilection. Poodle, Collie, Shetland Sheepdog, German Shepherd dog, Spitz, and Siamese, Persian, and Himalayan cats are apparently predisposed. SLE is a severe multisystemic autoimmune disease with different organ involvement and only 20–50% of cases may be associated with cutaneous signs (Scott et al. 2001; Gross et al. 2005; Ginn et al. 2007). SLE has been reported rarely in cats and horses and is uncommon in dogs. DLE is rather benign and restricted to the skin.

4.4.1.2.3 Clinical cutaneous presentation

Skin lesions tend to occur in areas exposed to sunlight, such as the face, ears, nose, lips, and lightly pigmented, sparsely haired areas of other body regions. Clinically, skin lesions are highly variable and may range from mild scaling, erythema, and alopecia to a severe ulcerative dermatitis (Fig. 4.4.5). Ulcers may be the consequence of ruptured bullae in the skin, mucocutaneous junctions, and mucous membranes. Generalized exfoliative dermatitis, ulcers of footpads, and panniculitis have been seen. In horses the clinical lesions of SLE are characterized by rather sharply demarcated areas of depigmentation around the eyes, lips, nostrils, genitalia, and skin of the perianal and perineal regions. Onset may be gradual or rapid. The clinical signs may wax and wane.

DLE occurs without age or sex predilection. Collie, Shetland Sheepdog, German Shepherd dog, and Siberian Husky appear to be predisposed. The disease presents initially with depigmentation, erythema, scaling, and loss of the normal cobblestone-like architecture of the nasal planum. With chronicity, lesions may involve the bridge of the nose. Subsequently erosions, ulcerations, and crusts are seen. Lesions may be observed, though less frequently, on the dorsum of the muzzle, the lips, in periocular regions, on the pinnae, the genitals, and rarely in the oral cavity (Angarano

1989; Gross et al. 2005). Like in SLE, cutaneous lesions are at least photoaggrevated if not photoinduced, and tend to be more severe under intense UV light exposure.

4.4.1.2.4 Histopathology

The classical histological findings in both DLE and SLE are an either cell-poor (hydropic) or cell-rich interface dermatitis with basal cell vacuolation and apoptosis of basal cells. The band-like inflammatory component is rather mild in SLE and more severe in DLE. The cellular infiltrate is composed of lymphocytes and to a lesser extent of plasma cells. However, on mucocutaneous junctions the infiltrate may be plasma cell rich, and it is a challenge for the dermatopathologist to distinguish DLE from mucocutaneous pyoderma. Basal cell vacuolation may lead to dermal–epidermal separation and ulceration. The outer root sheath of the hair follicles to the level of the isthmus may be equally involved. Additional findings are a lymphocytic and plasma cellular perivascular infiltrate, pigmentary incontinence, and focal basement membrane thickening (Yager and Wilcock 1994; Scott et al. 2001; Wiemelt et al. 2004; Gross et al. 2005). The epidermis is usually hyperplastic but may have focal areas of atrophy (Gross et al. 2005). Dermal and epidermal mucinosis may be present (Gross et al. 2005).

4.4.1.2.5 Therapy

Treatment of systemic lupus erythematosus depends on the severity of lesions and the organs involved, and consists of a variety of immunosuppressive and immunomodulating treatment options. These options are described in detail in other textbooks. Discoid lupus erythematosus often responds to topically applied glucocorticoids or 0.1% tacrolimus and sun avoidance (Griffies et al. 2004). In more severe cases a combination of tetracycline and niacinamide has been successful (White et al. 1992).

4.4.1.3 Canine vesicular cutaneous lupus erythematosus

This disease occurs exclusively in adult rough Collies, Shetland Sheepdogs, and their crosses, and was formerly described as *suppurative hidradenitis* (Schwartzman and Maguire 1969; Reedy et al. 1973), *bullous pemphigoid* (White et al. 1981; Scott et al. 1982), and finally *ulcerative dermatitis* of Shetland Sheepdogs and rough Collies (Ihrke and Gross 1995). In the latter description it was thought to represent a subgroup of dermatomyositis (see Section 3.4.2). Since it has clinical and histological similarities to the photosensitive vesicular form of subacute cutaneous lupus erythematosus in humans (Kovacs and Kovacs 1998), it was renamed in 2001 to vesicular cutaneous lupus erythematosus (Jackson and Olivry 2001).

The breed specificity of this disease supports a hereditary predisposition. Immunological studies support an autoimmune pathogenesis (Jackson et al. 2004). In the majority of dogs, deposition of immunoglobulin was found at the dermoepidermal junction. A similar finding is seen in the so-called lupus band in humans. The onset of clinical signs in the summer months and the distribution of the lesions over sparsely haired areas support a pathogenetic role of UV light. This is further supported by the detection of autoantibodies against RO/SSA; these are small ribonucleoprotein complexes that are translocated from the nucleus to the cytoplasm and the cell membrane after UV radiation (Sibilia 1998; Jackson et al. 2004).

Characteristically middle aged and older dogs with a mean age of 5 years are affected. In the majority of the described cases the onset of the disease is during the summer months and remission during the winter month is possible (Jackson 2004). Clinical findings in early lesions are transient vesicles or bullae that rupture easily. Thus, the major clinical findings are annular, polycyclic, and serpiginous erosions and ulcerations distributed over sparsely haired areas of the body such as the ventral abdomen, groin, axillae, and medial thighs. They may progress and involve the mucocutaneous junctions of the eyes, mouth, external genitalia, and anus, the oral cavity, concave aspects of the pinnae, and footpads. Ulcerative lesions may be painful. Secondary pyoderma occurs. A myositis has been documented by electromyography in several dogs. Nevertheless consistent abnormalities on physical examination other than the dermatological lesions are not noted (Ihrke and Gross 1995).

Skin biopsies are characterized by an interface dermatitis and a mural interface folliculitis. Vacuolation and basal cell apoptosis may be severe in the epidermis and the hair follicle to the level of the isthmus. Coalescing vacuolation of the basal keratinocytes may result in vesiculation at the dermal–epidermal junction. Apoptotic cells may be seen in the basal cell layer and in the lower level of the stratum spinosum. The superficial dermis contains a band-like subepidermal mixed mononuclear infiltrate that invades the basal cell layer of the epidermis and the outer root sheath of the hair follicle and obscures the dermo-epidermal junction. The infiltrate is composed mainly of CD3+ T-lymphocytes expressing CD4 in acute and CD8 in older lesions. In addition, in epidermis and dermis, CD1+ and MHCII-expressing antigen presenting cells are present (Jackson et al. 2004). In areas of ulceration neutrophils are prominent. Superficial dermal edema and congestion of the vessels may be present in variable severity.

Vesicular cutaneous lupus erythematosus in the rough Collie and Shetland Sheepdog is best managed with aggressive immunosuppressive therapy such as oral administration of short-acting glucocorticoids alone or in combination with azathioprine. The prognosis is guarded for complete remission, but clinical signs can be controlled with adequate therapy. Since 100% remission is not achieved in most cases, intermittent topical or systemic antibacterial therapy during the course of treatment may be necessary. Sun avoidance or the use of sunscreens is also important in the management of the disease (Jackson 2004). Recently it was also reported that orally administered cyclosporin A successfully controlled vesicular cutaneous lupus erythematosus for more than 18 months (Jackson 2006).

4.4.1.4 *Exfoliative cutaneous lupus erythematosus in the German Short-haired Pointer*

This uncommon disease was originally reported as *hereditary lupoid dermatosis of the German Short-haired Pointer* (Gross et al. 1992) and has been seen in dogs from Europe, North America, and Australia (Gross et al. 1992; Theaker and Rest 1992; Vroom et al. 1995; White and Gross 1995; Vercelli and Schiavi 1996; Olivry et al. 1999; Bryden and Burrows 2004). Since these dogs histologically have a lymphocytic interface dermatitis similar to lupus-specific dermatoses of humans, it has been proposed to rename this syndrome exfoliative cutaneous lupus erythematosus (ECLE) (Olivry et al. 1999).

The pathogenesis of ECLE is poorly understood but the recognition of this disease exclusively in the German Short-haired Pointer and its familial incidence strongly suggest a hereditary origin (Olivry et al. 1999).

Dogs clinically affected with this skin disease are young adults between 6 months and 2.75 years at the age of onset (Vroom et al. 1995; Bryden and Burrows 2004). The most prominent clinical features are adherent scales, crusts, and alopecia, which are typically seen on the muzzle, the pinnae, and the dorsal trunk. Lesions may progress and involve the limbs and ventral trunk or become generalized. In the generalized cases pressure points and the scrotum are severely involved. Follicular casts may be present. Secondary pyoderma and *Malassezia* dermatitis may be present. Peripheral lymphadenopathy and, less often, pyrexia have been reported. Systemic signs of pain and lameness are seen. Anemia and intermittent episodes of thrombocytopenia may occur. Severity of the disease may wax and wane.

Histological examination reveals a severe vacuolar degeneration of the basal cell layer. Apoptotic keratinocytes throughout the epidermis are seen in most cases and may become focally confluent. Lymphocytic exocytosis throughout the epidermis is moderate to marked. A moderate to marked discontinuous or continuous subepidermal band-like infiltrate composed of lymphocytes in the superficial dermis may be seen. Comparable to the epidermal lesions a lymphocytic interface mural folliculitis to the level of the isthmus is present. In one study the epitheliotropic lymphocytes were identified as CD8+ T cells (Olivry et al. 1999). In addition to the interface changes, the epidermis is moderately hyperplastic and a moderate, diffuse predominantly orthokeratotic but multifocally also parakeratotic hyperkeratosis is present. A lymphocytic sweat gland infiltrate and absence of sebaceous glands are observed in approximately 50% of the cases.

Treatment of ECLE with topical antiseborrheic shampoo and humectants, oral fatty acid supplementation, and oral tetracycline and niacinamide administration have all produced transient improvement but have failed to achieve long-term remission. Treatment response to immunosuppressive therapy using either prednisolone, cyclosporine, or leflunomide was both reported to be successful and unsuccessful (Bryden and Burrows 2004).

4.4.1.5 *Erythema multiforme*

Erythema multiforme (EM) is a rare condition reported in dogs, cats, horses, and cows. It is thought to be a host-specific T-cell mediated reaction pattern directed toward various triggering agents such as drugs or infectious agents (Fabbri and Panconesi 1993; Fritsch and Elias 1993). No age or sex predilections have been documented in most studies. A human classification system (Bastuji-Garin et al. 1993) has been adapted to veterinary medicine (Hinn et al. 1998) and according to this, *EM minor* is reserved for patients with "target" lesions. In these patients no more than one mucosal surface and less than 10% of the body surface are affected. In *EM major*, more than one mucosal surface and between 10 and 50% of the body surface are involved. Epithelial detachment has to be less than 10%. *Stevens–Johnson syndrome* (SJS) is reserved for those patients where more than 50% of the body surface is affected and epidermal detachment ranges from 10 to 30%. *Toxic epidermal necrolysis* (TEN), which has a completely different histological picture, is used for patients with generalized disease and more than 30% epithelial detachment. A SJS/TEN overlap syndrome is recognized.

4.4.1.5.1 Etiology and pathogenesis

EM may be elicited by a wide array of triggering factors, and its pathogenesis is incompletely understood (Huff et al. 1983; Ledesma and McCormack 1986; Goldberg 1987; Fabbri and Panconesi 1993; Fritsch and Elias 1993; Scott et al. 1995a; Gross et al. 2005). One recent study suggests that in canine EM phenotypic changes in keratinocytes (e.g., upregulation of ICAM-1, MHCII, CD1a, and CD44) might be a primary factor in disease pathogenesis (Affolter et al. 1998).

In one study the majority of canine cases (59%) and all cases in cats were associated with administration of drugs. Antibiotics such as trimethoprim-sulfadiazine, chloramphenicol, and enrofloxacin are frequently found as triggering factors in drug-induced cases. However, other drugs such as antiparasitics have been associated with EM as well. In one study in which the human classification system (Bastuji-Garin et al. 1993) was adapted for animals (Hinn et al. 1998), drugs were found to be causative in only 19% of the EM minor and major cases, but were associated with 92% of SJS and SJS/TEN cases.

Infections (viral, fungal, or bacterial) are other possible triggering factors for EM. In one case canine parvovirus was identified to be the triggering factor (Favrot et al. 2000). In five puppies with EM-compatible skin lesions, canine distemper virus, canine parvovirus, and canine herpesvirus were demonstrated. Feline EM has been associated with feline herpes virus (Scott et al. 2001; Gross et al. 2005).

EM has also been associated with underlying neoplasia (Ginn et al. 2007) and with adverse reactions to ingested beef and soy (Scott and Miller 1999). However, in numerous cases the triggering agent could not be identified. The various triggers for EM in cats and dogs are nicely summarized in two reviews (Hinn et al. 1998; Scott and Miller 1999).

4.4.1.5.2 Diagnosis

In the dog, EM is a vesiculobullous and/or ulcerative disease. Occasionally maculopapular eruptions are seen. Lesions develop mostly in the axillary and groin region, on mucocutaneous junctions, the oral cavity, the pinnae, and the footpads. Lesions may be mildly to moderately painful and are rarely pruritic. Target lesions (i.e., lesions that appear as concentric rings), Nikolsky's sign (i.e., the top layers of the skin slip away from the lower layers when slightly rubbed), and pitting edema (i.e., edema that retains for a time the indentation produced by pressure) of the distal limbs are occasionally seen. Affected dogs frequently show systemic signs of illness such as depression, lethargy, anorexia, and pyrexia. Hemograms, serum biochemistry profiles, and urinalyses are usually unremarkable.

Clinical lesions in the cat are predominantly vesicular bullous or ulcerative (Scott and Miller 1999), but generalized exfoliative lesions have also been described (Gross et al. 2005). Presumably drug-associated EM occurs after 1–2 weeks of treatment and markedly improves within 1–2 weeks of discontinuation of the offending drug (Huff et al. 1983; Scott et al. 1983; Hees et al. 1985; Mason 1990; Medleau et al. 1990; Delmage and Payne-Johnson 1991; Bond and Brownlie 1992; Fritsch and Elias 1993; Rosenkrantz 1993; Keck et al. 1995; Noli et al. 1995; Ihrke 1997; Scott and Miller 1999; Scott et al. 2001).

Skin and mucocutaneous biopsy specimens are characterized by an interface dermatitis. The epidermis typically is mildly to moderately hyperplastic with multifocal areas of hydropic degeneration of basal keratinocytes, lymphocytic exocytosis, and apoptotic keratinocytes in all layers of the epidermis. Mild to moderate numbers of lymphocytes and histiocytes are present directly underneath the epidermis and may obscure the dermoepidermal junction. Similar findings are usually observed in the infundibular

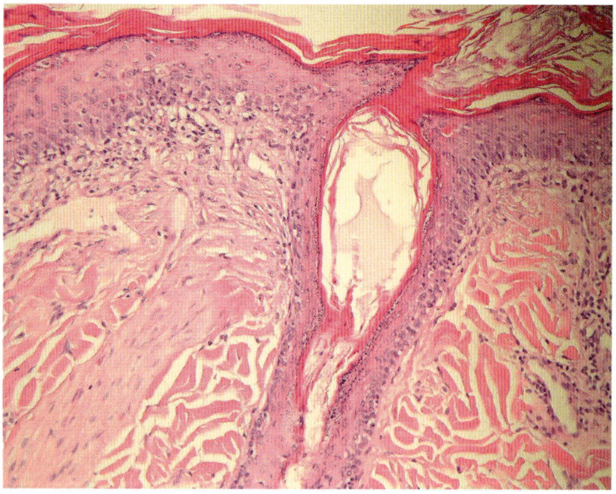

Fig. 4.4.6 Skin histology of erythema multiforma in a dog. Scattered apoptotic keratinocytes in the epidermis and the infundibular epithelium of hair follicles.

hair follicle epithelium (Fig. 4.4.6). Satellitosis and segmental areas of epidermal necrosis are frequently found. Occasionally, full-thickness epidermal necrosis may result in dermoepidermal separation. Pigmentary incontinence is frequent. Small numbers of plasma cells, neutrophils, and eosinophils infiltrate the dermis. Neutrophils and plasma cells are numerous in areas of ulceration and/or secondary bacterial infection. No apparent histopathological differences between cases with suspected triggers and those without (i.e., idiopathic) could be defined so far.

4.4.1.5.3 Therapy

The most important aspects in the therapy of EM are recognition and elimination of triggering factors (Huff et al. 1983; Ledesma and McCormack 1986; Goldberg 1987; Fritsch and Elias 1993; Scott et al. 2001). When the triggering factor can be eliminated, EM usually resolves within 1–2 weeks (Huff et al. 1983; Scott et al. 1983; Hees et al. 1985; Mason 1990; Medleau et al. 1990; Delmage and Payne-Johnson 1991; Bond and Brownlie 1992; Fritsch and Elias 1993; Rosenkrantz 1993; Keck et al. 1995; Noli et al. 1995; Ihrke 1997; Scott and Miller 1999; Scott et al. 2001). In dogs with infection- or diet-associated EM, it may take up to 4 weeks until clinical signs improve.

In human medicine, the use of immunosuppressive drugs, especially glucocorticoids, is still controversially discussed (Huff et al. 1983; Ledesma and McCormack 1986; Goldberg 1987; Fabbri and Panconesi 1993; Fritsch and Elias 1993). In a study presented by Scott and Miller (1999), 4 dogs with idiopathic EM clearly benefited from treatment with large doses of glucocorticoids or with azathioprine. These dogs went into complete remission while being treated, and relapsed each time therapy was stopped (Scott and Miller 1999).

4.4.2 Autonomous lymphocytic mural folliculitis

Lymphocytic mural folliculitis can be associated with (interface type) or without (infiltrative type) significant degeneration of keratinocytes. It again needs to be emphasized that "mural folliculitis" is an anatomic pathologic term and not a disease diagnosis (see Section 2.2.3.7). Numerous diseases can present with this morphology, among others dermatophytosis (see Section 4.1.2) and demodicosis (see Section 4.1.3).

4.4.2.1 Feline exfoliative dermatitis with lymphocytic mural folliculitis

4.4.2.1.1 Etiology and pathogenesis

Exfoliative dermatitis with either interface or infiltrative lymphocytic mural folliculitis is a rather newly described group of skin diseases in cats that cannot be associated with one single etiology. Disease names associated with this group of skin diseases are feline thymoma-associated exfoliative dermatitis, feline idiopathic mural folliculitis, and feline sebaceous adenitis. Various causative factors have been identified in recent years. The most well-documented cause is thymoma (Loveday 1959; Carpenter and Holzworth 1982; Scott et al. 1995b; Forster-Van Hijfte et al. 1997; Turek 2003; Rottenberg et al. 2004). Other cases of feline mural lymphocytic folliculitis and exfoliative dermatitis have been associated with other neoplasms (Pascal-Tenorio et al. 1997), drug administration (Scott et al. 2001; Gross et al. 2005), a lupus erythematosus-like disease (Wilhelm et al. 2005), nutritional factors (Declercq 2000), and seasonal influences (Marignac et al. 2003). However in most cases an underlying etiology cannot be determined (Declercq 1995, 2000; Pascal-Tenorio et al. 1997; Wendlberger 1999; Marignac et al. 2003; Foster 2004; Wilhelm et al. 2005).

In cases where a thymoma has been identified the disease is named "thymoma-associated exfoliative dermatitis." It is an uncommon disease in the cat and has also been reported in one rabbit (Florizoone 2005). The pathogenesis is unknown, but the lymphocytic interface nature of the follicular and epidermal inflammation suggests a cell-mediated autoimmunity caused by the thymic tumor (Scott et al. 1995b). Autoreactive cells, however, have not been demonstrated yet. Since cases with unknown etiology but a similar clinical or histological picture are seen, it is most likely that feline lymphocytic mural folliculitis with exfoliative dermatitis is an immune-mediated T-cell-associated reaction pattern.

4.4.2.1.2 Diagnosis

Clinical presentation

Cats with thymoma-associated exfoliative dermatitis are usually middle-aged to aged and may show signs of systemic illness such as lethargy. Extensive exfoliation with sheets of tightly adherent scales is a clinical hallmark of this paraneoplastic syndrome. The head, trunk, and limbs are most commonly affected before the lesions become generalized. The hair coat is often raised by the thick scales or crusts that adhere to the skin. Alopecia is noted secondary to severe exfoliative erythroderma (Fig. 4.4.7). The ear canals may be plugged with crusty debris. Brown, waxy, keratosebaceous debris may also accumulate in the interdigital skin around the nail beds. Ulceration may be seen (Scott et al. 1995b). Pruritus is usually not present but was reported in conjunction with secondary overgrowth of Malassezia (Forster-Van Hijfte et al. 1997; Mauldin et al. 2002).

In cats where no thymoma can be detected and the etiology remains unknown, similar clinical features may be seen. One diet-related case was described where erosions on the lips and eyelids predominated. In this case, footpads were dry and scaly (Declercq 2000).

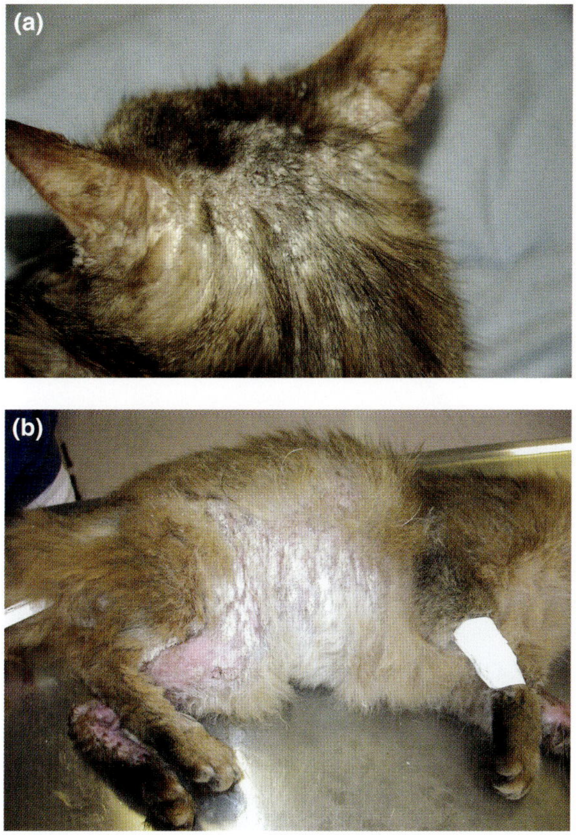

Fig. 4.4.7 Feline exfoliative dermatitis and mural folliculitis associated with a thymoma. (a) Alopecia on the neck (Courtesy of Section of Clinical Dermatology, Vetsuisse Faculty, University of Berne); (b) Alopecia on the abdomen associated with severe exfoliative erythroderma. (Courtesy of M. Linek.)

Histopathology

Histopathological features of feline lymphocytic mural folliculitis with exfoliative dermatitis are best described in thymoma-associated cases. The disease presents with an interface mural folliculitis where lymphocytes and few histiocytes target the follicular isthmus and the infundibulum (Fig. 4.4.8) (Gross et al. 1997; Power 1998; Declercq 2000; Scott et al. 2001). The lymphocytic infiltrate may also be present in the sebaceous glands and a complete loss of sebaceous glands (as in canine sebaceous adenitis) may occur (Rottenberg et al. 2004). In addition, a mild to moderate interface dermatitis with apoptotic cells in all layers of the epidermis is present. Exfoliation is reflected by a moderate to severe laminar orthokeratic hyperkeratosis. Variable serocellular crusting may be seen. As mentioned before, cases with an identical histological picture but no thymoma have been reported. However, detailed studies on morphological and clinical differences between cats with and without thymoma have not been conducted so far. It is not known, for example, whether higher severity of exfoliation is associated with a higher severity grade of interface dermatitis. It seems that cases of the so-called idiopathic feline mural folliculitis (Declercq 1995; Gross et al. 1997; Scott et al. 2001) and feline sebaceous adenitis (Gross et al.

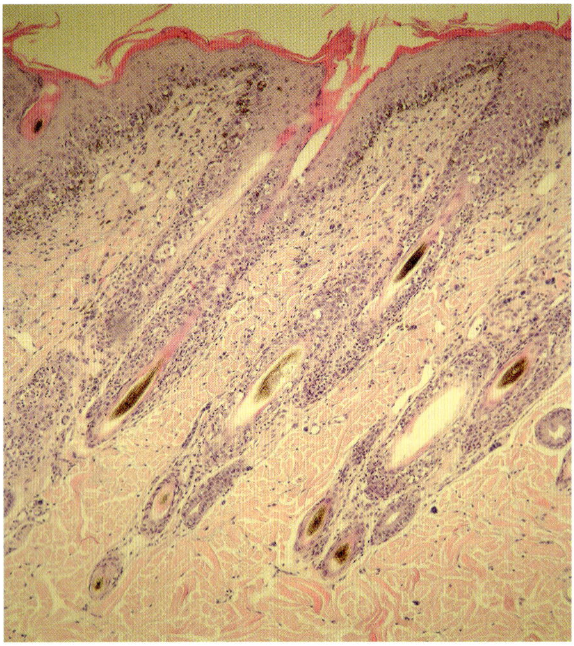

Fig. 4.4.8 Skin histology of feline exfoliative dermatitis and mural folliculitis associated with a thymoma. Lymphocytes and histiocytes targeting the follicular isthmus and the infundibulum.

2005) show a similar clinical and histopathological presentation as thymoma-related cases, but without interface changes in the epidermis or the hair follicle wall. These cases may be particularly difficult to separate histopathologically from pseudopelade-like isthmic folliculitis (see Section 4.4.2.2). Other differential diagnoses of feline lymphocytic mural folliculitis with exfoliative dermatitis are dermatophytosis (see Section 4.1.2) and epitheliotropic T-cell lymphoma (see Section 4.4.1.1).

4.4.2.1.3 Therapy

As already pointed out, patients should be carefully evaluated for any underlying disease. If a thymoma is present, surgical resection is the treatment of choice. Tumors that are noninvasive and easily excisable tumors have a good prognosis with a median survival time of almost 2 years (Withrow 2001). Cats with invasive tumors, however, representing approximately 15% of cases, often do not survive the perioperative period (Withrow 2001). Cats without a thymoma or any other neoplasm are difficult to treat. Cases have both responded and failed to respond to glucocorticoids and retinoids (Declercq 1995; Power 1998). Cyclosporine has been used with success in two cats (Wilhelm et al. 2005). Some cases of idiopathic feline mural folliculitis resolved spontaneously (Declercq 1995, Marignac et al. 2003).

4.4.2.2 Canine and feline isthmic lymphocytic mural folliculitis (pseudopelade-like folliculitis)

Isthmic mural folliculitis can be observed in conjunction with demodicosis (see Section 4.1.3), dermatophytosis (see Section 4.1.2), and canine sebaceous adenitis (see Chapter 4.8). However, it has also been described independent of the above-mentioned diseases. Lymphocytic mural folliculitis in dogs and cats has been named "pseudopelade" because it bears some clinical and morphological similarities to "pseudopelade of Brocq" that describes a slowly progressive cicatricial (scarring) alopecia in humans. The name refers to the clinical similarity (pseudo) to alopecia areata (pelade) on casual clinical inspection. However, since "pseudopelade" in humans represents the end stage of several diseases and thus is an ill-defined term, the canine and feline disease should rather be summarized under the descriptive term "lymphocytic mural folliculitis of the isthmus," which clearly separates it from *nonisthmic lymphocytic mural folliculitis.*

Isthmic lymphocytic mural folliculitis has been reported in cats and dogs and is apparently a very rare disease (Gross et al. 2000; Olivry et al. 2000).

4.4.2.2.1 Etiology and pathogenesis

Lymphocytic mural folliculitis of the isthmus is considered an immune-mediated disease. Folliculotropic lymphocytes exhibit most commonly CD3 and CD8 and thus represent cytotoxic T-cells. Autoantibodies specific for the lower hair follicle were detected in the serum of affected patients. Immunoblotting demonstrated binding of these antibodies to multiple follicular keratinocyte proteins, including hair keratins and trichohyalin. However, as with alopecia areata, it is unknown whether the occurrence of autoantibodies to keratinocyte proteins is a primary or a secondary event in the pathogenesis of this disease.

4.4.2.2.2 Diagnosis

Clinically, the disease is characterized by focal or multifocal well-demarcated patches of alopecia that do not show any signs of primary inflammation (Fig. 4.4.9).

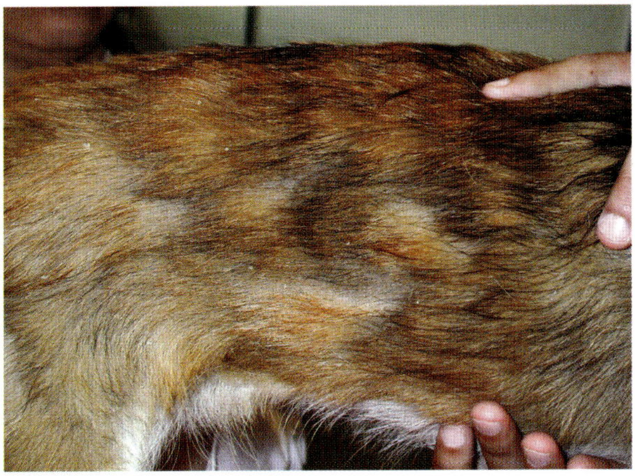

Fig. 4.4.9 Isthmic mural folliculitis (pseudopelade) in a dog. Multifocal well-demarcated patches of alopecia that do not show any signs of primary inflammation. (Courtesy of K. Bergvall.)

Scales and hyperpigmentation may be present. Hair loss progresses gradually. Whereas hair regrowth has not been reported in human "pseuopelade," some hair regrowth has been observed in dogs and cats. This might be a result of the different localization of follicular stem cells in different species. So far neither a breed nor a sex predilection has been noted in cats and dogs. Pruritus or systemic signs have not been reported. In the single case report of a cat with lymphocytic mural folliculitis of the isthmus, alopecic lesions were similar to the canine cases, but onychorrhexis and onychomadesis were seen in addition.

The major histological finding in dogs is a mainly lymphocytic infiltration that targets more or less exclusively the follicular isthmus. Mural inflammation may be mild to severe. Follicular keratinocytes may be swollen or degenerated. Occasionally, inflammation extends above and below the follicular isthmus but does not involve the hair bulb or the epidermis. A perifollicular infiltrate composed of lymphocytes, plasma cells, and histiocytes is present around the isthmus. In late-stage lesions, severe follicular atrophy and variable atrophy of sebaceous glands is seen and inflammation is rather sparse. The epidermis is mildly hyperplastic. Histological findings in the single reported feline case are similar.

4.4.2.2.3 Therapy

Due to the small number of cases that have been described in the scientific literature, there is no established therapy for isthmic mural folliculitis in cats and dogs.

4.4.2.3 Equine linear alopecia

Equine linear alopecia is primarily seen in quarter horses, but can also occur in other horse breeds (Fadok 1995).

4.4.2.3.1 Etiology and pathogenesis

Etiology and pathogenesis of equine linear alopecia are not yet understood. A localized keratinization disorder was once suggested (Scott 1988), but nowadays a T-cell-mediated immunological reaction against follicular keratinocytes is favored. The cause of this immune reaction is unknown, and an etiologic agent has not been identified (Tscharner et al. 2000). Because of the vertical orientation of the lesions, it was suggested that an external factor "dripping" down the skin may be involved. However, no such factor has been documented so far.

4.4.2.3.2 Diagnosis

Lesions may already be observed shortly after birth, but most frequently occur between 1 and 5 years of age. They are slowly progressive. Skin lesions consist of one or more vertically orientated linear areas of alopecia with varying degrees of scaling or crusting (Fig. 4.4.10). They are usually 2–10 mm wide and vary in length from a few centimeters to more than a meter. In some horses multiple hyperkeratotic and alopecic papules coalesce into linear bands. Anecdotal reports describe variants in quarter horses that are characterized by circular spots of alopecia rather than linear ones. Circular and linear lesions may coexist in the same horse. Common sites are the neck and lateral aspects of the thorax. Skin lesions are usually not associated with pruritus. Since in some patients alopecia predominates whereas in others hyperkeratosis is the most prominent clinical finding, it has been suggested that equine linear alopecia may actually represent two separate disease entities (Fadok 1995).

The primary histopathological lesion is an infiltrative lymphocytic mural folliculitis with subsequent damage of the follicular wall. Variable degrees of edema in the follicular wall may be present. In older (or more well-developed) lesions epithelioid macrophages and giant cells may be seen infiltrating the outer root sheath of the affected follicles, thus

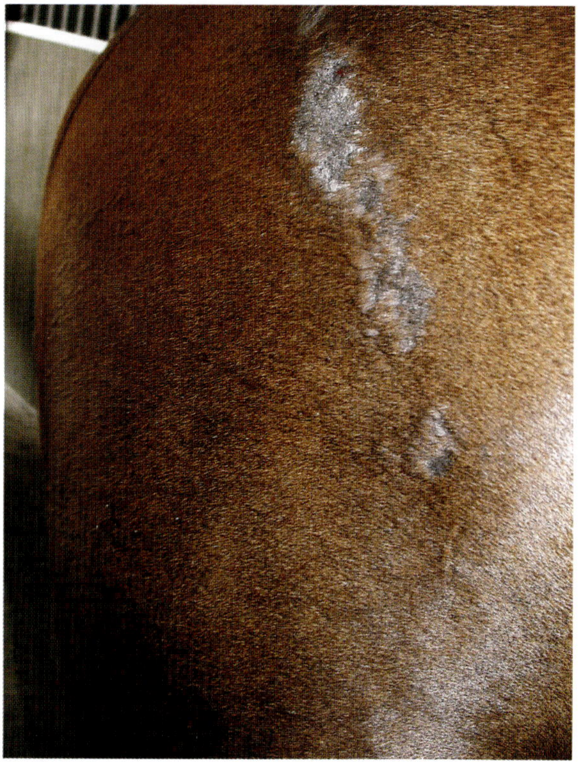

Fig. 4.4.10 Equine linear alopecia with vertically orientated linear areas of alopecia, scaling, and crusting. (Courtesy of K. Bergvall.)

representing a more histiocytic or granulomatous type of mural folliculitis (see Chapter 4.5). The end stage of the process may result in complete follicular destruction and permanent nonreversible alopecia. Sebaceous glands may be involved in the inflammatory process and may eventually undergo atrophy.

Other histological findings are a regular or irregular epidermal hyperplasia with a mild to severe orthokeratotic hyperkeratosis. In some but not all cases, striking epidermal lesions resembling erythema multiforme are found. These are represented by apoptotic keratinocytes and lymphocytic satellitosis. Other epidermal lesions include diffuse spongiosis and exocytosis. Parakeratosis may be seen. Varying degrees of perivascular eosinophilic dermatitis may also be present.

4.4.2.3.3 Therapy

Skin lesions are persistent and do not regress spontaneously. The owner should be informed that with our present knowledge of the disease, cure is impossible. Corticosteroid therapy (either topically or systemically) may slow down the progression of lesions; rarely resolution may be achieved. In cases with significant scaling and crusting any of the keratolytic shampoos can be used on a regular basis (every 3–4 days).

4.4.2.4 Canine and feline follicular mucinosis

4.4.2.4.1 Etiology and pathogenesis

Follicular mucinosis is a very rare skin disease of the dog and cat (Scott et al. 1987; Bell and Oliver 1995; Gross et al. 2005). In humans with a morphologically similar disease, follicular mucinosis is associated with immunological dysfunction, lymphoma, leukemia, or hematological disease (Mehregan et al. 1991; Cerroni and Kerl 2004). About 50% of the cases are associated with infiltration of a monoclonal population of T-lymphocytes.

4.4.2.4.2 Diagnosis

Two cases of follicular mucinosis have been reported *in cats*. In both cases, skin problems developed without associated internal lesions, and finally progressed to epitheliotropic lymphoma (Scott et al. 1987). The disease presents with a well-demarcated alopecia with fine scaling on the head, ears, and neck (Scott et al. 2001).

Three cases of follicular mucinosis have been reported *in dogs*. All three cases occurred in older retrievers. In one case, association with an epitheliotropic lymphoma was discussed, but could not be confirmed after euthanasia (Walder et al. 2007). The two other dogs have been described without further clinical abnormalities (Gross et al. 2001). In dogs lesions are patchy to diffuse, widespread, scaly, and alopecic. The head, trunk, and legs are most severely affected (Bell and Oliver 1995). Hyperpigmentation may be seen.

In all canine cases a perifollicular and intrafollicular infiltrate composed of plasma cells and lymphocytes was observed. Lymphocytes infiltrating the follicular and sebaceous epithelium did not show any evidence of atypia. Perifollicular and mural deposition of mucin is found, associated with epithelial degeneration and cystic mucin-filled intraepithelial spaces. Lymphocytic infiltrates and mucin deposition affect both isthmus and infundibulum. Follicular lesions in cats are similar with moderate to severe epidermal hyperplasia.

In one canine case, an interface dermatitis has been described in addition to the follicular lesions (Bell and Oliver 1995). The interface dermatitis was composed of a scant exocytosis of benign lymphocytes, associated with a compact orthokeratotic hyperkeratosis overlying a mildly hyperplastic epidermis with basal cell vacuolation and rare apoptotic cells.

4.4.2.4.3 Therapy

In humans follicular mucinosis can progress to a chronic condition or may resolve spontaneously (Mehregan et al. 1991). In dogs and cats, both prognosis and therapy are insufficiently documented.

4.4.2.5 Canine eosinophilic mucinotic mural folliculitis

Eosinophilic mucinotic mural folliculitis has so far only been described in dogs. It shares clinically and histologically some similarities with canine follicular mucinosis (see Section 4.4.2.4), and it cannot be ruled out that these two diseases actually represent one disease entity (Gross et al. 2005). The clinical picture of both diseases is similar. The histological differentiation between canine follicular mucinosis and eosinophilic mucinotic mural folliculitis is based on the fact that in the latter perifollicular inflammation shows numerous eosinophils (not seen in follicular mucinosis). Furthermore, mucin deposition in eosinophilic mucinotic mural folliculitis is less abundant and more perifollicular than intrafollicular (Gross et al. 2005). It therefore needs to be differentiated from eosinophilic folliculitis (see Chapter 4.2).

In the dog one case of eosinophilic mucinotic mural folliculitis was observed in conjunction with a T-cell lymphoma (Gross et al. 2005). Histopathology of other cases revealed a small number of *Demodex* mites or mite fragments, suggesting that this disease might represent a reaction pattern to a persistent parasitic stimulus.

The clinical picture of eosinophilic mucinotic mural folliculitis is predominated by alopecia, but may be highly variable in extension. Alopecia can be patchy, partial, or generalized. It is moderately well demarcated and erythema, crusting, hyperpigmentation, and greasiness of the hair coat have been noted (Gross et al. 2005). In severe cases ulceration may be seen within alopecic areas. Despite the numerous eosinophils, pruritus is inconsistently found. Retrievers and their crossbreeds appear to be overrepresented. There is no sex or age predilection (Gross et al. 2005). Clinical differential diagnoses depend on the extent of the alopecia and include demodicosis (see Section 4.1.3), dermatophytosis (see Section 4.1.2), alopecia areata (see Chapter 4.7), follicular mucinosis (see Section 4.4.2.4), and lymphocytic mural folliculitis of the isthmus (see Section 4.4.2.2).

Skin scrapings and dermatophyte cultures are mandatory for excluding demodicosis and dermatophytosis. Cytology in solely alopecic lesions is not feasible. In crusted lesions an eosinophil-dominated inflammatory infiltrate is seen. Skin biopsies are required for diagnosis and reveal perifollicular and intrafollicular inflammation composed of lymphocytes, histiocytes, and eosinophils. Mural folliculitis primarily affects the isthmic region of the hair follicle and is accompanied by intrafollicular and perifollicular mucinosis.

References

Abel EA, Nickoloff BJ, Shelby DM. 1986. Tumor stage mycosis fungoides in a patient treated with long-term corticosteroids for asthma and atopic-like dermatitis. *Journal of Dermatologic Surgery and Oncology* 12:1089–1093.

Affolter VK. 2007. Round cell tumors. *ESVD Workshop on Skin Oncology*, Berne, pp. 70–72.

Affolter VK, Moore PF. 2000. Lymphoid proliferations of the skin. *Workshop on Skin Immunology*, St. Paul de Vence.

Affolter VK, Moore PF, Sandmaier BM. 1998. Immunohistochemical characterization of canine acute graft-versus-host disease and erythema multiforme. In: Kwochka EW, Willemse T, von Tscharner C (eds), *Advances in Veterinary Dermatology*, pp. 103–115. Boston: Butterworth-Heinemann.

Angarano DW. 1989. Dermatoses of the nose and the footpads in dogs and cats. In: Kirk RW (ed.), *Kirk's Current Veterinary Therapy X*, pp. 616–621. Philadelphia: WB Saunders.

Baker JL, Scott DW. 1989. Mycosis fungoides in two cats. *Journal of the American Animal Hospital Association* 25:97–101.

Bastuji-Garin S, Rzany B, Stern RS, Shear NH, Naldi L, Roujeau JC. 1993. Clinical classification of cases of toxic epidermal necrolysis, Stevens–Johnson syndrome, and erythema multiforme. *Archives of Dermatology* 129:92–96.

Beale KM, Bolon B. 1992. Canine cutaneous lymphosarcoma: epitheliotropic and nonepitheliotropic, a retrospective study. In: Ihrke PJ, Mason IS, White SD (eds), *Advances in Veterinary Dermatology*, pp. 273–284. Oxford: Pergamon Press.

Bell A, Oliver F. 1995. Alopecia mucinosa (follicular mucinosis) in a dog. *Veterinary Dermatology* 6:221–226.

Bennion SD, Norris DA. 1997. Ultraviolet light modulation of autoantigens, epidermal cytokines and adhesion molecules as contributing factors of the pathogenesis of cutaneous LE. *Lupus* 6:181–192.

Bond R, Brownlie SE. 1992. Drug eruption resembling erythema multiforme major in a dog. *Veterinary Dermatology* 14:50–53.

Bryden SL, Burrows AK. 2004. Successful management of exfoliative cutaneous lupus erythematosus in three German shorthaired pointer siblings. *Veterinary Dermatology* 14:253.

Caciolo PL, Nesbitt GH, Patnaik AK, Hayes AA. 1984. Cutaneous lymphosarcoma in the cat; a report of nine cases. *American Journal of the Animal Hospital Association* 20:491–496.

Carpenter JL, Holzworth J. 1982. Thymoma in 11 cats. *Journal of the American Veterinary Medical Association* 181:248–251.

Cerroni L, Kerl H. 2004. Primary follicular mucinosis and association with mycosis fungoides and other cutaneous T-cell lymphomas. *Journal of the American Academy of Dermatology* 51:146–147.

de Lorimier LP. 2006. Updates on the management of canine epitheliotropic cutaneous T-cell lymphoma. *Veterinary Clinics of North America. Small Animal Practice* 36(1):213–218.

Declercq J. 1995. Lymphocytic mural folliculitis in two cats. *Vlaams Diergeneeskundig Tijdschrift* 64:177.

Declercq J. 2000. A case of diet-related lymphocytic mural folliculitis in a cat. *Veterinary Dermatology* 11:75–80.

Delmage DA, Payne-Johnson CE. 1991. Erythema multiforme in a doberman on trimethoprim-sulphamethoxazole therapy. *Journal of Small Animal Practice* 32:635–639.

Fabbri P, Panconesi E. 1993. Erythema multiforme ("minus" and "maius") and drug intake. *Clinics in Dermatology* 11:479–489.

Fadok VA. 1995. Update on four unusual equine dermatoses. *Veterinary Clinics of North America: Equine Practice* 11:105–110.

Favrot C, Olivry T, Dunston SM, Degorce-Rubiales F, Guy JS. 2000. Parvovirus infection of keratinocytes as a cause of canine erythema multiforme. *Veterinary Pathology* 37:647–649.

Fletcher CL, Orchard GE, Whittaker SJ. 2004. CD30+ cutaneous lymphoma in association with atopic eczema. *Archives of Dermatology* 140:449–454.

Florizoone K. 2005. Thymoma-associated exfoliative dermatitis in a rabbit. *Veterinary Dermatology* 16:281–284.

Forster-Van Hijfte MA, Curtis CF, White RN. 1997. Resolution of exfoliative dermatitis and Malassezia pachydermatis overgrowth in a cat after surgical thymoma resection. *Journal of Small Animal Practice* 38:451–454.

Foster AP. 2004. Mural folliculitis (MF). *5th World Congress of Veterinary Dermatology*, Vienna, pp. 56–57.

Fritsch PO, Elias PM. 1993. Erythema multiforme and toxic epidermal necrolysis. In: Fitzpatrick TB, Eisen AZ, Wolff K, Freedberg IM, Austen KF (eds), *Dermatology in General Medicine*, 4th edn, pp. 585–600. New York: McGraw-Hill.

Ginn PE, Mansell JEKL, Rakich PM. 2007. Skin and appendages. In: *Ginn, Kennedy's and Palmers Pathology of Domestic Animals.* Edinburg: Elsevier Saunders.

Goldberg GN. 1987. Erythema multiforme controversies and recent advances. *Advances in Dermatology* 2:73–90.

Griffies JD, Mendelsohn DL, Rosenkrantz WS. 2004. Topical 0.1% tacrolimus for the treatment of discoid lupus erythematosus and pemphigus erythematosus in dogs. *Journal of the American Animal Hospital Association* 40(1):29–41.

Gross TL, Ihrke PJ, Walder EJ. 1992. Hereditary lupoid dermatosis of the German shorthaired pointer. In: *Veterinary Dermatopathology: A Macroscopic and Microscopic Evaluation of Canine and Feline Skin Diseases.* St. Louis: Mosby Elsevier Health Science.

Gross TL, Ihrke PJ, Walder EJ, Affolter VK. 2005. *Skin Diseases of the Dog and Cat: Clinical and Histopathological Diagnosis.* Oxford: Blackwell Science.

Gross TL, Olivry T, Tobin DJ. 2000. Morphologic and immunologic characterization of a canine isthmus mural folliculitis resembling pseudopelade of humans. *Veterinary Dermatology* 11:17–24.

Gross TL, Olivry T, Vitale CB, Power HT. 2001. Degenerative mucinotic mural folliculitis in cats. *Veterinary Dermatology* 12:279–283.

Gross TL, Stannard AA, Yager JA. 1997. Review article: an anatomical classification of folliculitis. *Veterinary Dermatology* 8:147–156.

Haselen CWV, Toonstra J, Preesman AH. 1999. Sezary syndrome in a young man with severe atopic dermatitis. *British Journal of Dermatology* 140:704–707.

Hees JV, Mason KV, Gross TL, Burren VS. 1985. Levamisole-induced drug eruptions in the dog. *Journal of the American Animal Hospital Association* 21:255–260.

Hinn AC, Olivry T, Luther PB, Cannon AG, Yager JA. 1998. Erythema multiforme, Stevens–Johnson syndrome, and toxic epidermal necrolysis in the dog. Clinical classification, drug exposure, and histopathological correlations. *Journal of Veterinary Allergy and Clinical Immunology* 6:13–20.

Huff JC, Weston WL, Tonneson MG. 1983. Erythema multiforme: a critical review of characteristic diagnostic criteria and causes. *Journal of the American Academy of Dermatology* 8:763–773.

Ihrke PJ. 1997. Cutaneous adverse drug reactions. *Compendium of Continuing Education* 19(Suppl):87–92.

Ihrke PJ, Gross TL. 1995. Ulcerative dermatosis of Shetland Sheepdogs and Collies. In: Bonagura JD (ed.), *Kirk's Current Veterinary Therapy XII (Small Animal Practice)*, pp. 639–640. Philadelphia: WB Saunders.

Jackson HA. 2004. Eleven cases of vesicular cutaneous lupus erythematosus in Shetland sheepdogs and rough collies: clinical management and prognosis. *Veterinary Dermatology* 15:37–41.

Jackson HA. 2006. Vesicular cutaneous lupus. *Veterinary Clinics of North America* 36:251–255.

Jackson HA, Olivry T. 2001. Ulcerative dermatosis of the Shetland sheepdog and rough collie dog may represent a novel vesicular variant of cutaneous lupus erythematosus. *Veterinary Dermatology* 12:19–27.

Jackson HA, Olivry T, Berget F, Dunston SM, Bonnefont C, Chabanne L. 2004. Immunopathology of vesicular cutaneous lupus erythematosus in the rough collie and Shetland sheepdog: a canine homologue of subacute cutaneous lupus erythematosus in humans. *Veterinary Dermatology* 15:230–239.

Keck G, Nash L, Buronfosse F, Peroux F. 1995. Accident cutané médicamenteux évoquant un érythème polymorphe de type Steven–Johnson chez un berger allemand. *Point Vétérinaire* 27:81–83.

Kovacs SO, Kovacs SC. 1998. Dermatomyositis. *Journal of the American Academy of Dermatology* 39:899–920.

Lange-Vejlsgaard G, Ralfkiaer E, Larsen JK. 1989. Fatal cutaneous T cell lymphoma in a child with atopic dermatitis. *Journal of the American Academy of Dermatology* 20:954–958.

Ledesma GN, McCormack PC. 1986. Erythema multiforme. *Clinics in Dermatology* 4:70–80.

Loveday RK. 1959. Thymoma in a Siamese cat. *Journal of South African Veterinary Medical Association* 30:33–34.

Marignac GL, Barlerin L, Guillot J, Mialot M, Delisles F, Scott DW. 2003. A case of seasonal lymphocytic mural folliculitis with spontaneous resolution in a cat. *Veterinary Dermatology* 14:247.

Mason KV. 1990. Cutaneous drug eruptions. *Veterinary Clinics of North America* 20:1633–1653.

Mauldin EA, Morris DO, Goldschmidt MH. 2002. Retrospective study: the presence of Malassezia in feline skin biopsies. A clinicopathological study. *Veterinary Dermatology* 13:7–13.

Medleau L, Shanley KJ, Rakich PM, Goldschmidt MH. 1990. Trimethoprim-sulfonamide-associated drug eruptions in dogs. *Journal of the American Animal Hospital Association* 26:305–311.

Mehregan DA, Gibson LE, Muller SA. 1991. Follicular mucinosis: histopathologic review of 33 cases. *Mayo Clinic Proceedings* 66:387–390.

Moore PF, Olivry T. 1994. Cutaneous lymphomas in companion animals. *Clinics in Dermatology* 12:499–505.

Moore PF, Olivry T, Naydan D. 1994. Canine cutaneous epitheliotropic lymphoma (mycosis fungoides) is a proliferative disorder of CD8+ T cells. *American Journal of Pathology* 144:421–429.

Noli C, Koeman JP, Willemse T. 1995. A retrospective evaluation of adverse reactions to trimethoprim-sulphonamide combinations in dogs and cats. *Veterinary Quarterly* 17:123–128.

Olivry T, Luther PB, Dunston SM, Moore PF. 1999. Interface dermatitis and sebaceous adenitis in exfoliative cutaneous lupus erythematosus ("Lupoid Dermatosis") of German short-haired pointer. *Proceedings of the 15th Meeting Academy of Veterinary Dermatology*, Maui.

Olivry T, Power HT, Woo JC, Moore PF, Tobin DJ. 2000. Anti-isthmus autoimmunity in a novel feline acquired alopecia resembling pseudopelade of humans. *Veterinary Dermatology* 11:261–270.

Pascal-Tenorio A, Olivry T, Gross TL, Atlee BA, Ihrke PJ. 1997. Paraneoplastic alopecia associated with internal malignancies in the cat. *Veterinary Dermatology* 8:47–52.

Pielop JA, Jones D, Duvic M. 2001. Transient CD30+ nodal transformation of cutaneous T-cell lymphoma associated with cyclosporine treatment. *International Journal of Dermatology* 40:505–511.

Power HT. 1998. Newly recognized feline skin diseases. *Proceedings of the 14th Meeting of the American Academy of Veterinary Dermatology*, San Antonio.

Reedy LM, Mallett R, Freeman RG. 1973. Hidradenitis suppurativa in a female Shetland sheepdog. *Veterinary Medicine, Small Animal Clinician* 68:1262.

Risbon RE, de Lorimier LP, Skorupski K, Burgess KE, Bergman PJ, Carreras J, Hahn K, LeBlanc A, Turek M, Impellizeri J, Fred R III, Wojcieszyn JW, Drobatz K, Clifford CA. 2006. Response of canine cutaneous epitheliotropic lymphoma to lomustine (CCNU): a retrospective study of 46 cases (1999–2004). *Journal of Veterinary Internal Medicine* 20(6):1389–1397.

Rosenkrantz WS. 1993. Pemphigus foliaceus. In: Griffin CE, Kwochka KW, MacDonald JM (eds), *Current Veterinary Dermatology*, pp. 154–164. St. Louis: Mosby Year Book.

Rottenberg S, von Tscharner C, Roosje PJ. 2004. Thymoma-associated exfoliative dermatitis in cats. *Veterinary Pathology* 41:429–433.

Rüfenacht S, Ruess-Melzer K, Bley CR. 2007. Clinical and therapeutic aspects of skin tumors. *ESVD Workshop on Skin Oncology*, Bern, pp. 33–48.

Santoro D, Marsella R, Hernandez J. 2007. Investigation on the association between atopic dermatitis and the development of mycosis fungoides in dogs: a retrospective case-control study. *Veterinary Dermatology* 18:101–106.

Schwartzman RM, Maguire HG. 1969. Staphylococcal apocrine gland infections in the dog (canine hidradenitis suppurativa). *British Veterinary Journal* 125:121–127.

Scott DW. 1988. *Large Animal Dermatology*. Philadelphia: WB Saunders.

Scott DW, Manning TO, Lewis RM. 1982. Linear IgA dermatoses in the dog: bullous pemphigoid, discoid lupus erythematosus and a subcorneal pustular dermatitis. *Cornell Veterinarian* 72:394–402.

Scott DW, Miller WH, Griffin CE. 1995a. *Muller and Kirk's Small Animal Dermatology*, 5th edn. Philadelphia: WB Saunders.

Scott DW, Miller WH, Griffin CE. 2001. *Muller and Kirk's Small Animal Dermatology*, 6th edn. Philadelphia: WB Saunders.

Scott DW, Miller WHJ, Goldschmidt MH. 1983. Erythema multiforme in the dog. *Journal of the American Animal Hospital Association* 19:453–459.

Scott DW, Miller WHM. 1999. Erythema multiforme in dogs and cats: literature review and case material from the Cornell University College of Veterinary Medicine (1988–1996). *Veterinary Dermatology* 10:297–309.

Scott DW, Walton DK, Slater MR. 1987. Immune-mediated dermatoses in domestic animals: ten years after. Part I. *Compendium Continuing Education for the Practicing Veterinarian* 9:424–435.

Scott DW, Yager JA, Johnston KM. 1995b. Exfoliative dermatitis in association with thymoma in three cats. *Feline Practice* 23:8–13.

Sibilia J. 1998. Ro(SS-A) and anti-Ro(SS-A): an update. *Revue du Rhumatisme (English Edition)* 65:45–57.

Theaker AJ, Rest JR. 1992. Lupoid dermatosis in a German short-haired pointer. *Veterinary Record* 131:495.

Tscharner Cv, Kunkle G, Yager J. 2000. Linear alopecia (linear keratosis). *Veterinary Dermatology* 11:193–195.

Turek MM. 2003. Cutaneous paraneoplastic syndromes in dogs and cats: a review of the literature. *Veterinary Dermatology* 14:279–296.

Vercelli A, Schiavi S. 1996. A case report of lupoid dermatosis in a German short-haired pointer. In: Kwochka KW, Willemse T, Tscharner C. Von. (eds), *Advances in Veterinary Dermatology*, Vol. 3, pp. 466–467. Oxford: Butterworth-Heinemann Ltd.

Vroom MW, Theaker MJ, Rest JR. 1995. Lupoid dermatosis in five German short-haired pointers. *Veterinary Dermatology* 6:93–98.

Walder EJ, Affolter VK, Moore PF. 2007. Short communication V: A case of alopecia mucinosa in a dog. Is this mycosis fungoides? *Annual Meeting of the International Society of Veterinary Dermatology ISVD*, Lihue, Kauai.

Wendlberger U. 1999. Sebaceous adenitis in a cat. *Kleintierpraxis* 44:293–298.

White SD, Gross TL. 1995. Hereditary lupoid dermatosis of the German shorthaired pointer. In: Kirk RW, Bonagura JD (eds), *Current Veterinary Therapy Small Animal Practice*, pp. 605–606. Philadelphia: WB Saunders.

White SD, Rosser EJJ, Ihrke PJ. 1981. Bullous pemphigoid in a dog: treatment with six-mercaptopurine. *Journal of the American Veterinary Medical Association* 185:683–685.

White SD, Rosychuk RAW, Reinke SI, Paradis M. 1992. Use of tetracycline and niacinamide for treatment of autoimmune skin disease in 31 dogs. *Journal of the American Veterinary Medical Association* 200:1497–1500.

Wiemelt SP, Goldschmidt MH, Greek JS, Jeffers JG, Wiemelt AP, Mauldin EA. 2004. A retrospective study comparing the histopathological features and response to treatment in two canine nasal dermatoses, DLE and MCP. *Veterinary Dermatology* 15:341–348.

Wilhelm S, Grest P, Favrot C. 2005. Zwei Fälle exfoliativer Dermatitis und Follikulitis bei Katzen mit histologischen Eigenschaften eines kutanen Lupus erythematodes. *Tierärztliche Praxis Kleintiere* 33:364–369.

Winkelmann RK, Rajka G. 1983. Atopic dermatitis and Hodgkin's disease. *Acta Dermato-Venereologica* 63:176–177.

Withrow SJ. 2001. Thymoma. In: Withrow SJ, MacEwen EG (eds), *Small Animal Clinical Oncology* pp. 646–651. Philadelphia: WB Saunders.

Withrow SJ, Vail DM. 2006. *Withrow and MacEwen's Small Animal Clinical Oncology*. Philadelphia: Elsevier Health Sciences Division.

Yager JA, Wilcock BP. 1994. *Color Atlas and Text of Surgical Pathology of the Dog and Cat: Dermatopathology and Skin Tumors*, Vol. 1, 1st edn. London: Mosby Year Book, Wolfe Publishing.

4.5

Histiocytic or granulomatous mural folliculitis

Monika Welle and Lars Mecklenburg

Inflammation that focuses and invades hair follicle walls at or below the isthmus is often dominated by lymphocytes (see Chapter 4.4). Lymphocyte infiltration into the follicular wall does not necessarily result in destruction of the hair follicle, and it is most easily diagnosed in its early stage. There are some rare forms of mural inflammation that are associated with a significant infiltration of histiocytes, occasionally even forming giant cells. Those forms of mural infiltrative folliculitis are mostly destructive and therefore can easily be confused with a furunculosis caused by a luminal folliculitis.

Histiocytic mural folliculitis is a very rare finding in domestic animals and is yet ill defined. It rather represents a reaction pattern than one disease with a defined etiology. In the scientific literature, cases of destructive lymphohistiocytic mural folliculitis are described in cats, dogs, and deer only, but there are anecdotal (unpublished) reports of further cases affecting horses, cattle, and goats.

4.5.1 Canine granulomatous degenerative mural folliculitis

Granulomatous mural folliculitis is very rarely reported in dogs. There is only one case reported in the scientific literature (Scott 1999) and few additional ones are mentioned in textbooks or abstracts (Gross and Schick 1993; Scott et al. 2001; Gross et al. 2005). The lack of sufficient data does not allow further subclassification of this disease entity in the dog, but it is likely that etiology, pathogenesis, and prognosis vary between individual cases. Some published cases have been associated with adverse drug reactions to amitraz, cefadroxil, L-thyroxin, and various topical agents (Scott et al. 2001).

The clinical picture of canine granulomatous folliculitis is very variable. The main clinical feature is well-circumscribed multifocal to coalescing alopecia on the face, the trunk, and the proximal extremities, eventually spreading over the whole body (Fig. 4.5.1). Some cases show surprisingly rapid progression of the disease with generalized alopecia developing within less than 6 months. Besides pelage hair follicles, alopecia may involve eyelashes as well. The alopecic skin is usually mildly erythemic with some degree of scaling. Advanced cases will reveal a very shiny smooth alopecic skin with variable degrees of hypopigmentation (Fig. 4.5.2).

Histopathology reveals a lymphohistiocytic infiltrate that tightly surrounds hair follicles. It strikingly centers around the follicular isthmus and the inferior segment, but may extend into the bulb and/or the infundibulum (Fig. 4.5.3). Histiocytes and lymphocytes infiltrate into the follicular wall and accumulate between the inner and the outer root sheath. In early lesions, inflammatory cells are not located within the hair canal, whereas later lesions may show disruption of the follicular wall and luminal folliculitis, merging into furunculosis. Intramural histiocytes are mainly composed of large epithelioid cells, and occasionally multinucleated giant cells can be found within the follicular wall (Fig. 4.5.4). The inflammation extends into the perifollicular mesenchyme and frequently obliterates sebaceous glands. Additional changes that may be found in cases of canine granulomatous mural folliculitis are perifollicular pyogranulomas, lupus-like interface dermatitis, erosions, and ulceration.

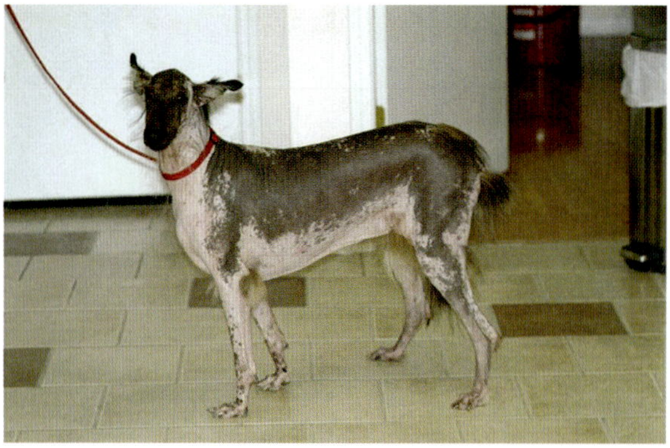

Fig. 4.5.1 Canine granulomatous folliculitis in a Collie. Rapidly developing generalized alopecia. (Courtesy of P. White.)

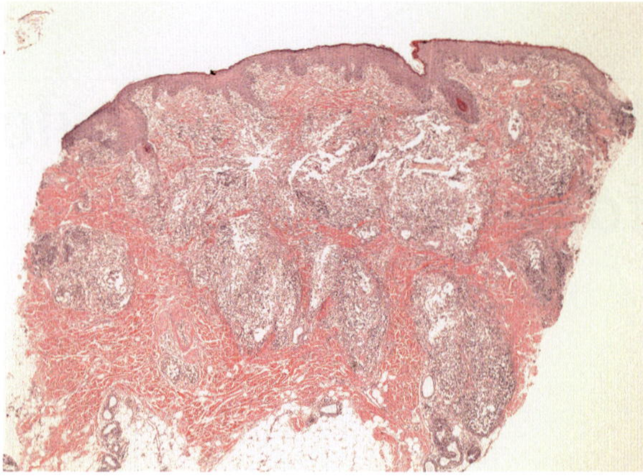

Fig. 4.5.3 Skin histology of canine granulomatous folliculitis. Extensive inflammation targeting the hair follicles.

Canine granulomatous mural folliculitis is considered an immune-mediated disease and thus is best treated with immunosuppressive or immunomodulatory drugs. Cyclophosphamide and prednisone have been described to be effective. Many cases, however, will result in follicular atrophy and permanent loss of adnexal structures.

4.5.2 Feline lymphohistiocytic degenerative mural folliculitis with intrafollicular mucinosis

A distinct alopecic disease in cats has been named feline degenerative mucinotic mural folliculitis (Gross

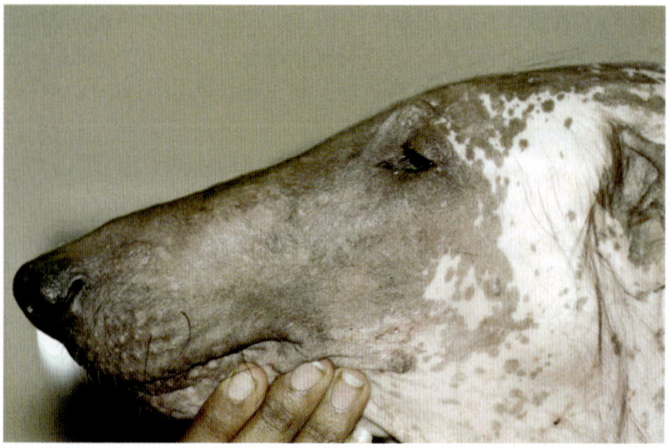

Fig. 4.5.2 Canine granulomatous folliculitis in a Collie. Complete alopecia of the head, including eye lashes. (Courtesy of P. White.)

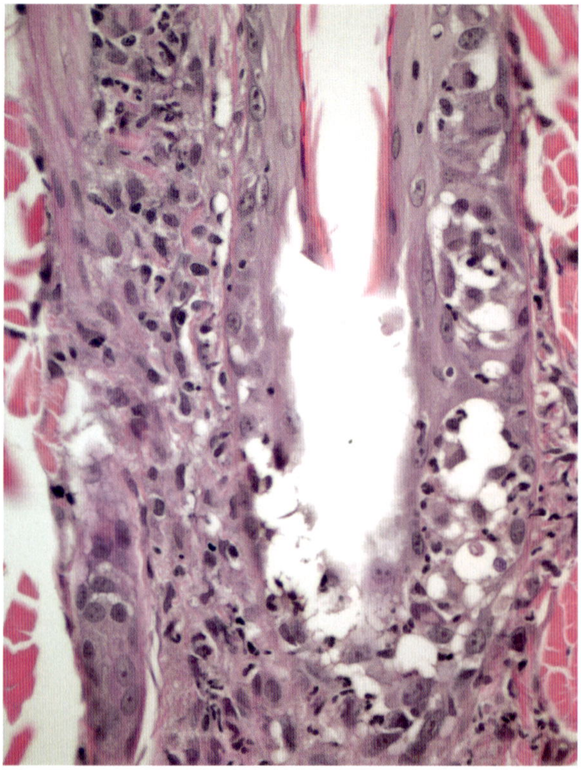

Fig. 4.5.4 Skin histology of canine granulomatous folliculitis. Inflammation starts with histiocytes infiltrating into the follicular wall.

et al. 2001). In contrast to follicular mucinosis (see Section 4.4.2.4), no epitheliotropic lymphoma is associated with this entity. Etiology and pathogenesis of feline degenerative mucinotic mural folliculitis have not been clarified yet. Some cats had antibodies to feline immunodeficiency virus and none has shown antibodies against feline leukemia virus.

The main clinical feature of this disease is alopecia. Alopecia starts around the muzzle, is often symmetric, and expands to involve the entire face. Progression of alopecia can be very variable with rare cases progressing within a few months and others progressing within 1–2 years. Alopecia can spread to neck, shoulders, trunk, and extremities. The alopecic skin is shiny and feels rubbery. Occasional scaling may be seen. A characteristic feature of most cases is a marked swelling of the facial skin including the eyelids, resulting in blepharospasm (Fig. 4.5.5). Most cases show some degree of lethargy, suggesting an underlying internal disease. However, no consistent disease process could be identified to be associated with degenerative mucinotic folliculitis so far.

Histopathology reveals a perifollicular and intramural infiltrate of histiocytes and lymphocytes. These are variably accompanied by plasma cells and neutrophils (Fig. 4.5.6). Giant cells are usually not found in this disease, but may occur in granulomas once

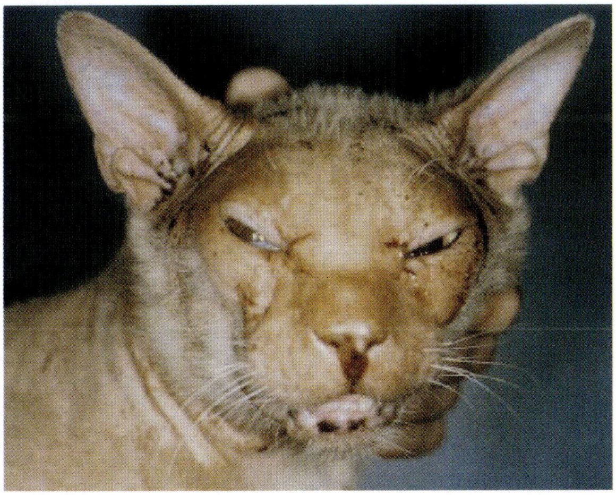

Fig. 4.5.5 Feline lymphohistiocytic degenerative mural folliculitis with intrafollicular mucinosis. Severe generalized alopecia and swelling of the face. (Reprinted with permission from Gross et al. (2001).)

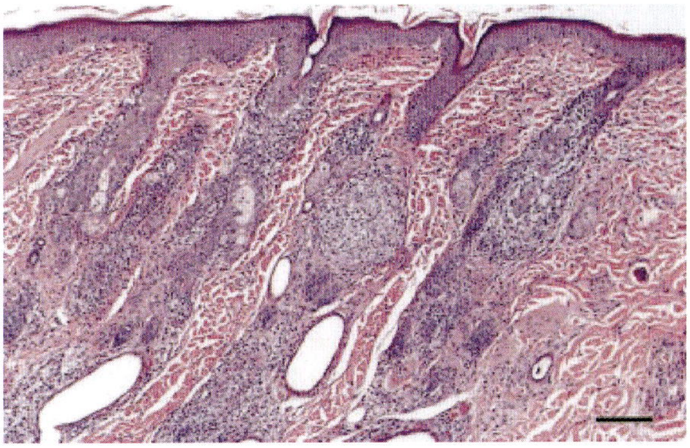

Fig. 4.5.6 Skin histology of feline lymphohistiocytic degenerative mural folliculitis with intrafollicular mucinosis. Lymphohistiocytic inflammation effacing the isthmus of two hair follicles. Note degeneration of follicle at right. (Reprinted with permission from Gross et al. (2001).)

severely affected hair follicles have degenerated. Inflammation centers around the isthmus and upper inferior segment of hair follicles, but may also involve the infundibulum. A characteristic feature of the disease is intramural mucinosis that can occur in variable degrees but is not pathognomonic (see Section 4.4.2.4). Mixed inflammation may be observed in the superficial dermis, and the epidermis may show acanthosis and spongiosis. Chronic cases will show hair follicle atrophy.

Most cases that have been described in the literature have not responded adequately to immunosuppressive doses of corticosteroids, or other medications such as antihistamines and medicated shampoos. Prognosis is guarded, particularly if lethargy and weight loss occur concurrently with alopecia. Many affected cats have been euthanized for progressive hair loss and lethargy within 2–8 weeks after diagnosis. However, since sporadically patients have responded, a therapeutic trial with aggressive immunomodulatory or immunosuppressive therapy is warranted in any case.

4.5.3 Granulomatous degenerative mural folliculitis in other species

Sporadic cases of granulomatous mural folliculitis in species other than cat and dog have been reported, but none are published in the scientific literature. The authors have seen two cases of granulomatous mural folliculitis with degeneration of the hair follicle wall in goats. One case has been observed in a 3-year-old female dwarf goat. Alopecia occurred very rapidly, affecting more than 50% of the body surface within one day. Within less than a week, alopecia was generalized. The entire body surface was covered with thick dry adherent scales, and the patient developed lethargy and laminitis. No pathogen was found, and PCR (polymerase chain reaction) from skin biopsies for caprine herpesvirus-2 (see below) was negative. Histopathology revealed a mild mural infiltrate in the follicular infundibulum and a moderate infiltration in the isthmus. The infiltrate was lymphohistiocytic with a moderate amount of multinucleated giant cells. Intramural pustules were seen in the isthmus. Apoptotic keratinocytes were present in the infundibular wall. The moderate perifollicular infiltrate was also lymphohistiocytic. The other case occurred in a single 1.5-year-old Spanish goat from a herd in Texas, United States, that showed multifocal alopecia beginning on the back. Alopecia progressed quickly and involved more than 50% of the entire body surface within 6 weeks. It finally involved the entire trunk, face, and extremities (Fig. 4.5.7). In addition to alopecia, a severe dry hyperkeratosis with multifocal secondary pyoderma was present. Histopathology revealed a severe perifollicular lymphohistiocytic infiltrate that centered around the isthmus and the inferior segment of all hair follicles. Lymphocytes and macrophages infiltrated the follicular wall with occasional multinucleated giant cells and epithelioid macrophages accumulating between the outer and inner root sheath (Fig. 4.5.8). The goat was euthanized at the owner's request without further postmortem analysis.

A histopathologically similar disease was described in two sika deer from a zoo in Florida that were infected with caprine herpesvirus-2 (caprine malignant catarrhal fever virus, distinct from ovine herpesvirus-2). The animals presented with slowly progressive generalized alopecia and a granulomatous mural folliculitis comprising epithelioid macrophages and giant cells. In addition to skin lesions, both deer showed perivascular lymphohistiocytic inflammation consistent with malignant catarrhal fever in internal organs such as kidney or reticulum (Crawford et al. 2002). Despite the demonstration of viral DNA and histopathological findings consistent with malignant catarrhal fever, it is yet unknown whether the granulomatous mural folliculitis in these two animals was indeed caused by caprine herpesvirus-2.

Chronic lesions of linear alopecia in the horse (see Section 4.4.2.3) may present with epithelioid cells and giant cells infiltrating the follicular wall and need to be differentiated from primary histiocytic or granulomatous folliculitis.

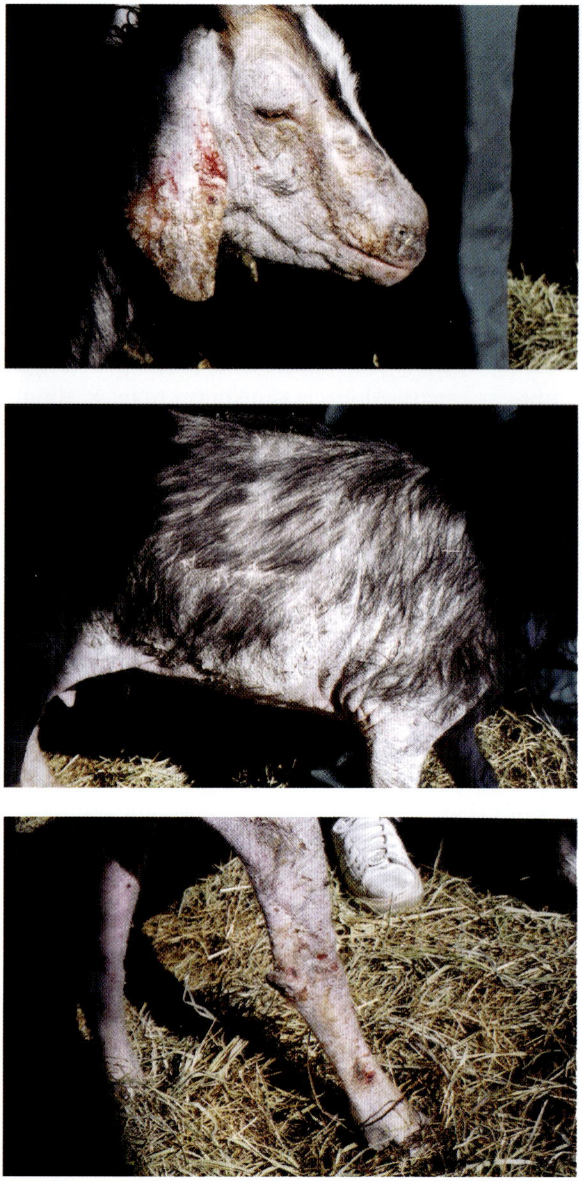

Fig. 4.5.7 Granulomatous folliculitis in a goat. Extensive alopecia affecting head, trunk, and extremities. (Courtesy of R. Judd.)

References

Crawford TB, Li H, Rosenburg SR, Norhausen RW, Garner MM. 2002. Mural folliculitis and alopecia caused by infection with goat-associated malignant catarrhal fever virus in two sika deer. *Journal of the American Veterinary Medical Association* 221:843–847.

Gross TL, Ihrke PJ, Walder EJ, Affolter VK. 2005. Skin diseases of the dog and cat. In: Gross TL, Ihrke PJ (eds.), *Clinical and Histopathologic Diagnosis*, pp. 474–477. Oxford: Blackwell Science.

Gross TL, Olivry T, Vitale CB, Power HT. 2001. Degenerative mucinotic mural folliculitis in cats. *Veterinary Dermatology* 12:279–283.

Gross TL, Schick RO. 1993. Dermatopathology of newly described diseases. In: Ihrke PJ, Mason IS, White SD (eds), *Advances in Veterinary Dermatology*, Vol. 2, pp. 417–420. Oxford: Pergamon Press.

Scott DW. 1999. Folliculite murale granulomateuse chez le chien: manifestation d'un accident médicamenteux cutené? *Medecin Veterinaire du Quebec* 29:154–156.

Scott DW, Miller WH, Griffin CE. 2001. *Muller and Kirk's Small Animal Dermatology*, 6th edn, Philadelphia: WB Saunders.

4.6

Necrotizing mural folliculitis

Monika Linek and Lars Mecklenburg

Both feline herpesvirus and poxvirus infections in the cat can be associated with massive necrosis of epithelial cells, including the epidermis and the upper follicular epithelium. Both diseases are, however, not primarily alopecic but rather ulcerative and nodular, respectively.

4.6.1 Feline herpesvirus infection

Feline herpesvirus-1 usually targets the upper respiratory tract and causes rhinotracheitis and conjunctivitis. It most likely persists in the trigeminal ganglia where it can be reactivated by immunosuppression. Skin lesions associated with feline herpesvirus are uncommon. Cats will present with alopecia, ulceration, and crusts at the muzzle, often in conjunction with similar lesions at the periorbital skin and at the nasal planum (Fig. 4.6.1). In rare cases, other body regions can be affected as well. A coexisting stomatitis has been described infrequently (Hargis et al. 1999; Hargis and Ginn 1999).

Histologically, feline herpesvirus-induced skin lesions are characterized by ulceration with marked eosinophilic and neutrophilic inflammation and crust formation. The epidermis adjacent to ulcers is mostly hyperplastic and spongiotic. Necrotic keratinocytes may be found in these areas as well as in the infundibular epithelium of hair follicles. In proximity to necrotic keratinocytes of the epidermis, hair follicle, or sebaceous gland, viable cells with intranuclear inclusion bodies may be found and will confirm the diagnosis (Fig. 4.6.2). In cases where inclusion bodies cannot be demonstrated, immunohistochemistry or PCR (polymerase chain reaction) allow further confirmation.

Spontaneous regression of mild lesions may occur. Good success has been achieved with interferon-omega therapy in three cats (Gutzwiller et al. 2007). So far antiviral therapy like acyclovir was not very effective in cats and caused severe side effects (Caney 2005). Most recently famciclovir (20 mg/kg every other day), the oral form of penciclovir, has shown efficacy in nine cats with feline herpesvirus-1 infection and no adverse effects have been reported (Beccati and Peano 2007). The authors of this chapter have successfully used famciclovir in three cases of herpesvirus-induced dermatitis.

4.6.2 Feline cowpox virus infection

Outdoor cats that have contact with rodents may rarely become infected with the cowpox virus that is mainly found in Europe, particularly in the United Kingdom (Finn 1989). Outdoor cats may contract the virus from bites of woodland rodents, particularly voles.

The infected sites present with plaques or nodules, eventually showing ulceration and crusts. The forelegs, head, and neck are most commonly affected (Fig. 4.6.3). Ulcerative stomatitis has been described, and in rare cases does the virus spread to the upper respiratory tract (Godfrey et al. 2004; Schöniger et al. 2007).

Histopathology shows massive necrosis of epidermal and outer root sheath keratinocytes. Many cells demonstrate large eosinophilic intracytoplasmic viral inclusion bodies of variable size and shape (Fig. 4.6.4). The dermal inflammation is dominated by neutrophils.

Feline cowpox virus-infected lesions can heal without therapeutic intervention within weeks of initial infection. Response rates to specific antiviral therapies such as interferons are not reported. Secondary bacterial infections should be treated appropriately. In

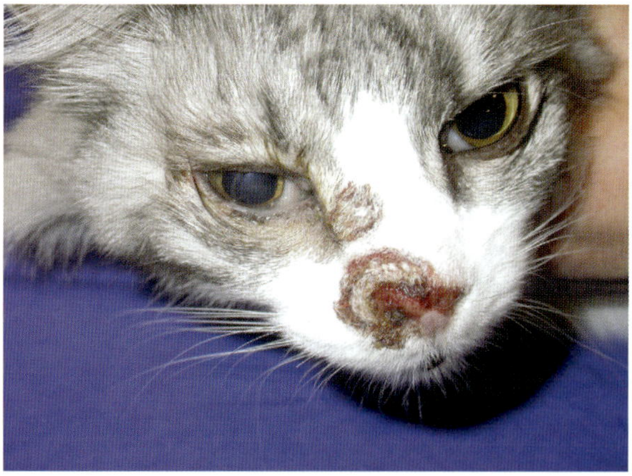

Fig. 4.6.1 Feline herpesvirus-1-induced dermatitis. Alopecia and crusts on the nose.

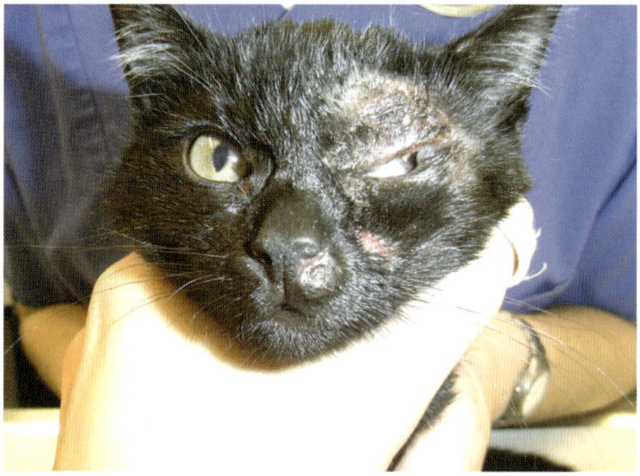

Fig. 4.6.3 Feline cowpox virus-induced dermatitis. Alopecia, ulceration, and crusts on the face.

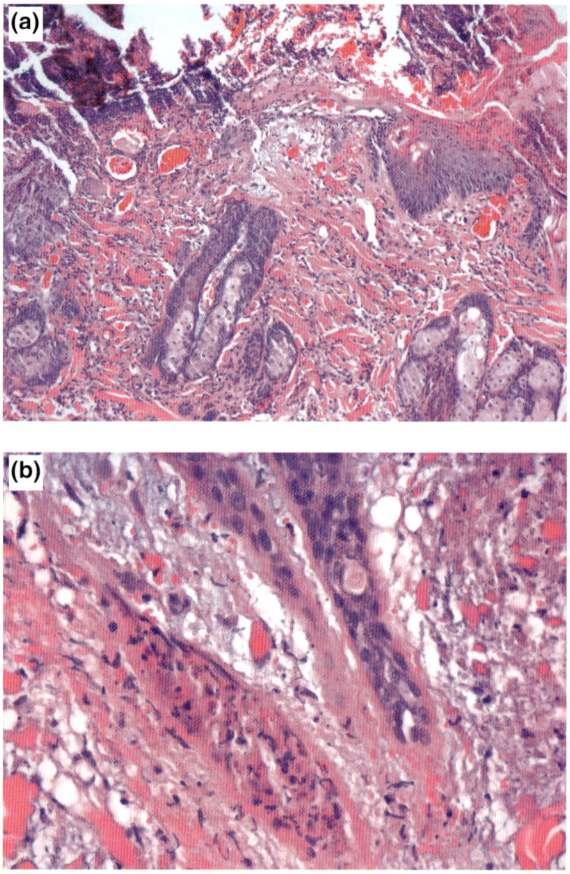

Fig. 4.6.2 Skin histology of feline ulcerative dermatitis caused by feline herpesvirus-1. (a) Ulceration with diffuse eosinophilic and neutrophilic dermatitis; (b) extensive epithelial necrosis.

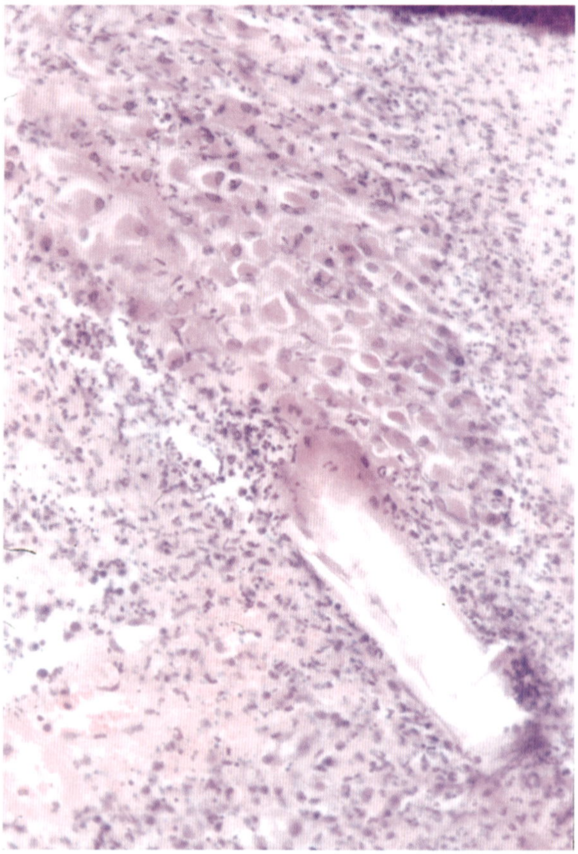

Fig. 4.6.4 Skin histology of feline cowpox virus-induced dermatitis. Necrotizing folliculitis with eosinophilic intracytoplasmic inclusion bodies in follicular keratinocytes.

cases where skin lesions are associated with respiratory disease, the prognosis is guarded. Any stress and immunosuppression are to be avoided.

It is very important to inform the owners about the zoonotic potential of cowpox virus (Schulze et al. 2007). Nowadays, most humans become infected from cats, not cows (what originally gave the virus its name). Symptoms of cowpox virus infection in humans are pustules on the hands. In very rare cases, however, the virus can spread and become generalized, representing a serious threat to immunocompromised people.

References

Beccati M, Peano A. 2007. Investigation of the efficacy of famciclovir in the treatment of feline herpesvirus-1 infection. *Veterinary Dermatology* 18:381.

Caney S. 2005. Antiviral therapy in cats: current rationale and recommendations. *In Practice* 27:454–457.

Finn JP. 1989. Cowpox in cats. *Veterinary Record* 125(16):426.

Godfrey DR, Blundell CJ, Essbauer S, Pfeffer M, Shearer DH, Rest JR, Baker JF. 2004. Unusual presentations of cowpox infection in cats. *Journal of Small Animal Practice* 45(4):202–205.

Gutzwiller ML, Brachelente C, Taglinger K, Suter MM, Wiessenböck H, Roosje P. 2007. Feline herpes dermatitis treated with interferon omega. *Veterinary Dermatology* 18:50–54.

Hargis AM, Ginn PE. 1999. Feline herpesvirus 1-associated facial and nasal dermatitis and stomatitis in domestic cats. *Veterinary Clinics of North America* 29:1281–1289.

Hargis AM, Ginn PE, Mansell JEKL, Garber RL. 1999. Ulcerative facial and nasal dermatitis and stomatitis in cats associated with feline herpesvirus 1. *Veterinary Dermatology* 10:267–274.

Schöniger S, Chan DL, Hollinshead M, Humm K, Smith GL, Beard PM. 2007. Cowpox virus pneumonia in a domestic cat in Great Britain. *Veterinary Record* 160(15):522–523.

Schulze C, Alex M, Schirrmeier H, Hlinak A, Engelhardt A, Koschinski B, Beyreiss B, Hoffmann M, Czerny CP. 2007. Generalized fatal cowpox virus infection in a cat with transmission to a human contact case. *Zoonoses Public Health* 54(1):31–37.

4.7

Alopecia areata

Desmond J. Tobin

Alopecia areata (AA) represents one of the most enigmatic of the common dermatoses, affecting approximately 2% of the general human population (Safavi et al. 1995), and is also not uncommon in several nonhuman mammalian species (McElwee et al. 1998b; Tobin and Olivry 2004). However, it is likely that incidence in both humans, and possibly also nonhuman mammals, is much greater as minor forms will often go unnoticed (e.g., especially in humans and animals with overlapping layers of long hair). Common to all subtypes of AA in all species is the selective, largely reversible damage to the anagen hair follicle (Van Scott 1958; Messenger and Bleehen 1984; Messenger et al. 1986; Tobin et al. 1990, 1997a).

AA-like disease has been reported in nonhuman mammals including cats (Conroy 1979), horses (Conroy 1979; Scott 1988; Middleton and Church 1994; Affolter and Cannon 1998; Tobin et al. 1998; Colombo et al. 2004), cows (Paradis et al. 1988; Scott 1988; Scott and Guard 1988), dogs (Olivry et al. 1996; Tobin et al. 1996, 2003; Tobin and Olivry 2004), and in nonhuman primates (Conroy 1979; Eichberg and De Villez 1984; Beardi et al. 2007). However, the poor characterization of many of these cases prevents assessment of their scientific or clinical value. Still, animal models, including outbred animals, are likely to be valuable for the dissection of the common pathways underlying the pathogenesis of AA and for the development and evaluation of therapies for AA. Indeed, much of the recent progress in AA research has emerged not from studies on human cases, but is instead due to the development of animal models for human AA. The best characterized of these include the inbred rodent models of the C3H/HeJ mouse (Sundberg et al. 1994) and the DEBR rat (Michie et al. 1991). Both models have provided useful data not only on the complex genetics of AA-like hair loss but also on its associated immune perturbations (Michie et al. 1990; Tobin et al. 1997b; McElwee et al. 1998a, 2002, 2003, 2005b; Sundberg et al. 2003; Freyschmidt-Paul et al. 2004) and assessment of various treatment modalities (Shapiro et al. 1999; Freyschmidt-Paul et al. 2000, 2001, 2004; Tang et al. 2003a,b, 2004; Verma et al. 2004). There has also been some progress on the assessment of the immune status of other nonhuman mammals with AA-like disease, particularly in dogs (Olivry et al. 1996; Tobin 1996, 2003; Tobin and Olivry 2004) and horses (Tobin et al. 1998; Colombo et al. 2004).

The striking clinical, immunohistopathologic, antigenic, and treatment response similarities associated with AA-like hair loss in humans, nonhuman primates, rodents, dogs, and horses support the view that this form of hair loss may have a common etiology in these mammalian species. Indeed, antibodies to anagen hair follicles in rats, mice, dogs, and horses appear to be not only similar but also cross-reactive with tissues from different species (McElwee et al. 1998b). This observation is likely to reflect a high level of antigen conservation in the hair follicles of many mammalian species.

4.7.1 Etiology and pathogenesis

In humans, AA can present with a broad phenotypic spectrum affecting predominantly the anagen-rich areas of skin, for example, the scalp (Fig. 4.7.1a and b). However, any hair-bearing region of the body can be affected. Mild forms manifest as patchy hair loss (so-called patchy AA) that may resolve spontaneously, remain as patchy disease, or progress to complete loss of all scalp hair (alopecia totalis) or all head and body hair (alopecia universalis) (Fig. 4.7.1).

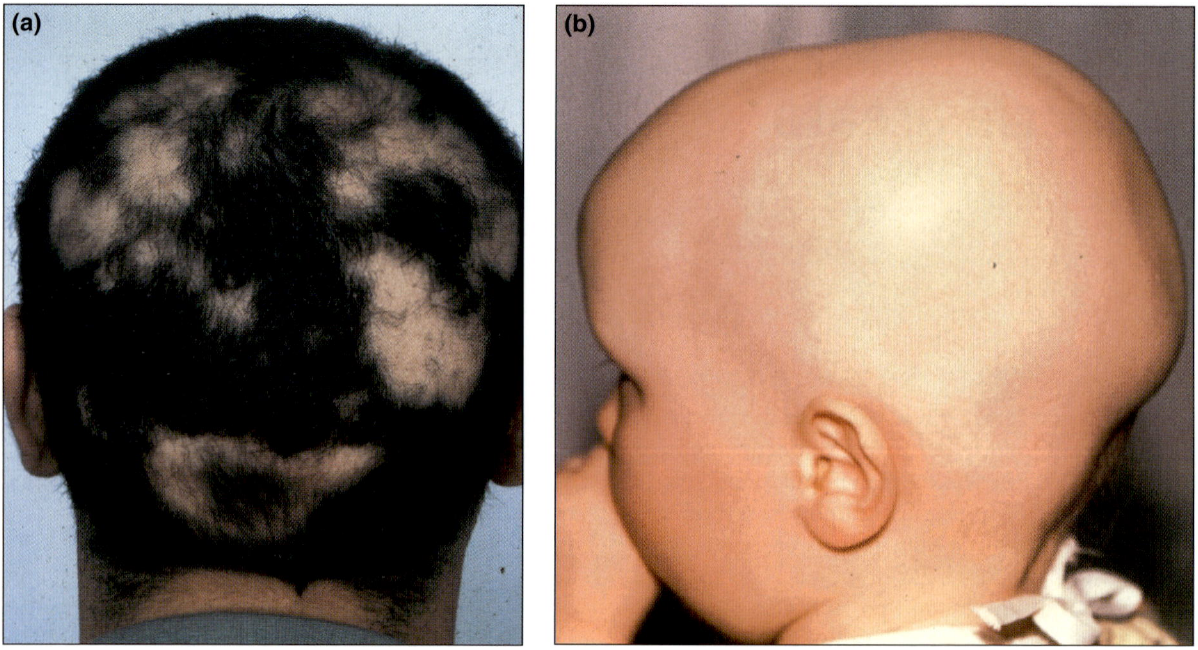

Fig. 4.7.1 Phenotypic variation in human alopecia areata. (a) Common patchy alopecia areata variant affecting scalp of an adult male (Courtesy of Dr. D.A. Fenton); (b) less common alopecia areata totalis variant affecting scalp of a young child (Courtesy of Upjohn Company.)

It is the view of this author that newcomers to AA research should be issued with a disclaimer to interpret the pre-1990s AA literature with considerable caution because of its highly confusing and contradictory nature. This situation emerged in large part due to inconsistency in study design and execution. Specifically, much of the earlier data was based on small numbers of patients, poorly or uncontrolled studies, on differences whose significance were not analyzed statistically, and on results that are often contradictory. However, part of this apparent confusion may be due to the possibility that not all cases of AA represent manifestations of the same disease entity.

Increasing evidence, especially from powerful genetics data, suggests that AA may represent several etiologic entities with multiple confounding epigenetic factors. For example, higher occurrence in identical twins, siblings, as well as high kindred expression over several generations all point to some contribution of inherited factors. Still, with a positive family history of AA of less than 50%, other factors are clearly also involved.

Despite the sometimes strident claims to the contrary in both the clinical and scientific literature, the etiology and indeed precise pathogenesis of AA remains unresolved. An immune-mediated pathogenesis is clear and AA is associated with a number of immune abnormalities (Tobin and Bystryn 1995, 2000). Some of these are nonselective, while others are more specific and point to an immune abnormality selectively targeting a component of the hair follicle when in the anagen phase of the hair growth cycle. There are indications of possible organ-specific autoimmunity in some individuals (Tobin et al. 1994; McElwee et al. 1999b; Kalish and Gilhar 2003; Gilhar and Kalish 2006), though nails and eyes are also commonly targeted. Despite this, most recent research supports the view that the disease process is executed predominantly by CD8+ lymphocytes as part of a pathomechanism driven by CD4+ lymphocytes. This folliculotrophic lymphocytic infiltration appears to respond to an interferon-γ-induced upregulation of MHC class I and II in the lower hair follicle during stages of early hair growth that are coincident with the reconstruction of its pigmentary unit. It has been

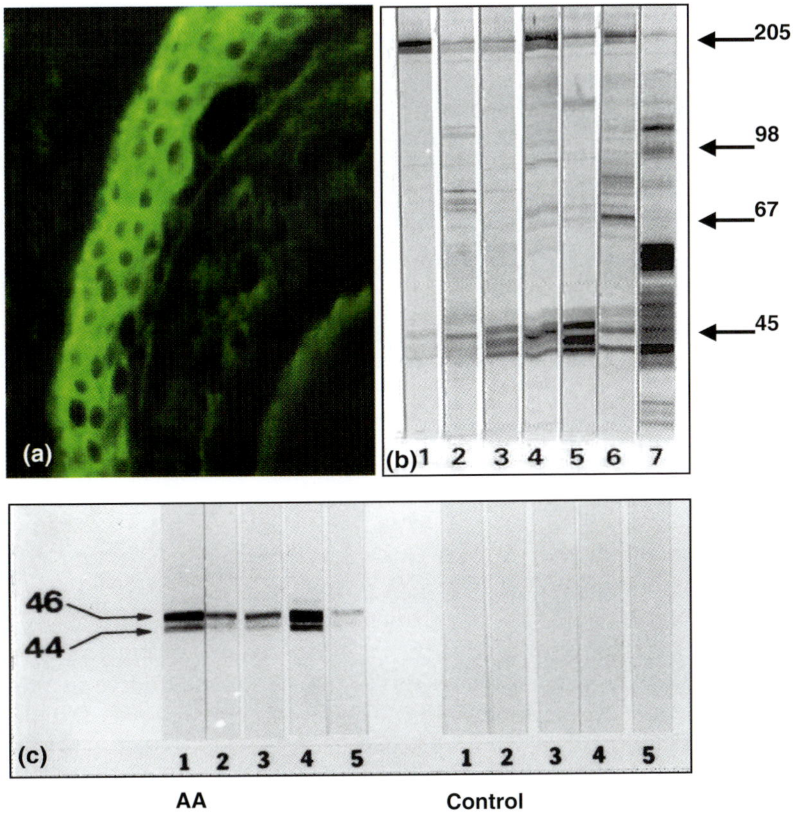

Fig. 4.7.2 Antibodies to hair follicles in human alopecia areata. (a) Indirect immunofluorescence analysis of circulating serum IgG antibodies to outer root sheath keratinocytes of an anagen scalp hair follicle; (b) immunoblotting analysis of circulating serum IgG antibodies to 6 M urea-extracted proteins from scalp hair follicles; (c) target antigen identification in human alopecia areata; hair follicle-specific keratin (44/46 kDa) was immunoprecipitated with five AA sera, separated by SDS-PAGE and immunoblotted with a monoclonal antibody (AE13) raised to hair follicle-specific keratin; five control sera from normal healthy subjects.

proposed that this reflects a disease-associated collapse of "immune privilege" in the lower anagen hair follicle (Gilhar et al. 2007) (see Section 1.2.4). Thus, in immunogenetically predisposed individuals the hair follicle may be attacked by an immune system (stimulated by an unknown trigger/response to autoantigen) where hair follicle anagen-associated antigens having lost the cover of their former immunoprivilege are now targeted by a full-blown anti-hair follicle immune response. This vulnerability to immune attack may be further heightened if the production or function of local immunosuppressive cytokines and neurohormones (e.g., α-MSH) is deficient. A further neuroimmunological link in the pathogenesis of this common hair loss disorder was suggested by increased substance P-positive fibers in early AA lesions. Moreover, substance P itself triggered a transit of hair follicles from anagen to catagen with associated activated CD8+ T-cells (Siebenhaar et al. 2007).

Circulating antibodies (IgG) to hair follicles are also a prominent feature of AA in humans (Tobin et al. 1994; Tobin 1997, 2003), where they can be found at titers far higher than in patients with other disorders of the hair follicle, including scarring alopecia (Fig. 4.7.2a and b). Several hair follicle-associated antigens have been identified in the serum from patients including hair follicle-specific keratins (44/46 kDa) (Fig. 4.7.2) and trichohyalin, and these have been localized to the keratogenous zone of the growing hair follicle. However, it is not clear which, if any, of these targeted hair follicle antigens are immunodominant in the precipitating stage of the disease. It is not yet known whether or not these have any pathogenic potential, as has been demonstrated for bullous pemphigoid. Thus, the role played by circulating antibodies to hair follicle-specific antigens remains to be resolved.

The treatment of AA remains very difficult (Ross and Shapiro 2005). There is no cure, and still no approved medication. Despite this, a broad range of treatment modalities can be used, including topical, systemic, and intralesional corticosteroids; topical immunotherapy; topical minoxidil; anthralin; and

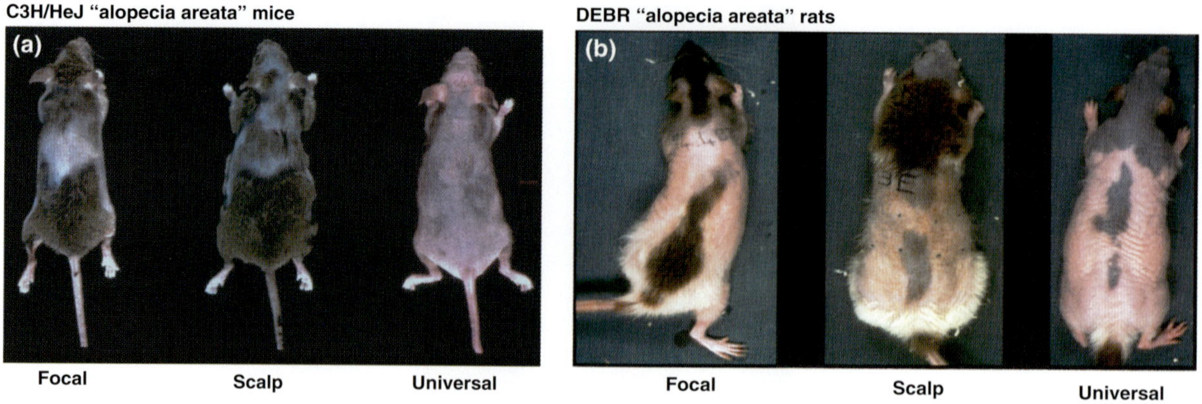

Fig. 4.7.3 Phenotypic variation in rodent alopecia areata. (a) Focal, scalp, and universal hair loss in C3H/H3J mice; (b) hair loss in DEBR rats. (Courtesy of Dr K. McElwee.)

psoralen plus ultraviolet A (PUVA). Despite several studies it remains difficult to separate targeted effects from spontaneous recovery, which usually occurs within 1 year of an AA episode.

Much of AA research today is conducted on inbred rodent models, in particular the C3H/HeJ mouse and to a lesser extent the Dundee experimental bald rat (DEBR) (Fig. 4.7.3). Both models exhibit striking phenotypic similarity with AA in humans and other mammals. As with most other species examined to date, AA first appears usually on the head and face, and progresses to the flanks and back. Spontaneous hair loss appears both earlier and more commonly in female mice than in males. Two substrains of the DEBR rat exist (black and brown hooded) and both show similar AA phenotype in about 40% of animals. Like in affected humans, nail abnormalities can be detected in about 15% of affected females and about 5% in affected males (McElwee 2004). A hair-pull test will reveal the presence of pathognomonic "exclamation mark" hairs in both models. Importantly for a human AA model, both rodent models exhibit similar and characteristic AA histopathology, that is, peri- and intrabulbar lymphocytic infiltration of anagen hair follicles (Fig. 4.7.4). Indeed, the immunophenotype of AA-like hair loss reported in these models, including for both cell-mediated and humoral factors, is very similar to that in human AA (McElwee et al. 1998b, 2005b). A particularly interesting finding is that AA can be experimentally induced in C3H/HeJ mice by grafting lesional skin from an affected mouse to a histocompatible recipient (McElwee et al. 1998a).

The main immune-associated findings in the C3H/HeJ AA mouse model include the observations that depletion of CD4+ or CD8+ T-cells using monoclonal antibodies permit hair regrowth, demonstrating that these T-cell subsets are required to maintain the AA (McElwee et al. 2005a), and that removal of either CD4+ or CD8+ T-cells enables hair regrowth (McElwee et al. 1996b, 1999a; Carroll et al. 2002). The rodent models of AA also exhibit an abnormal autoantibody response to the hair follicle (Fig. 4.7.5) (McElwee et al. 1996a). Importantly, in many cases the presence of antibodies to hair follicles appears before the onset of clinically apparent hair loss. Thus, these may not be produced as a secondary response to hair follicle damage in AA, as is generally considered most likely. Some of the antibodies in both C3H/HeJ mice and humans with alopecia areat react to antigens of 44/46 kDa, which were identified as hair follicle-specific keratins (Tobin and Bystryn 1996) (Fig. 4.7.5d).

4.7.2 Canine alopecia areata

It is difficult to accurately estimate the frequency of AA in dogs due to the very limited number of case reports (most reporting just single cases) on spontaneous AA-like hair loss in dogs in the literature. Moreover, as many conditions can lead to loss of hair, it is not always clear if the diagnosis was unequivocally that of AA. Differential diagnosis for canine AA includes mural lymphocytic folliculitis of the isthmus (see Section 4.4.2.2), demodicosis (see Section 4.1.3), dermatophytosis (see Section 4.1.2),

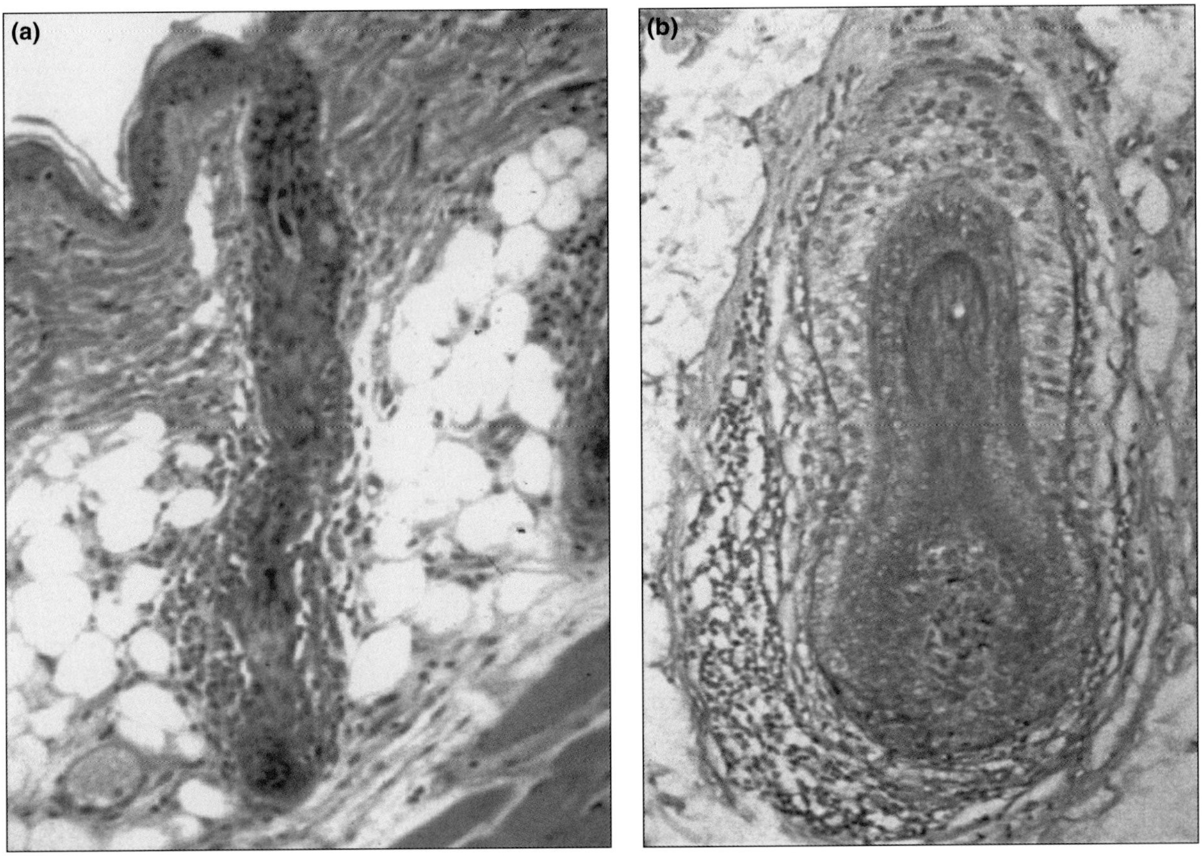

Fig. 4.7.4 Histology of alopecia areata. (a) Peri- and intrafollicular mononuclear cell infiltrates in C3H/HeJ mice (Courtesy of Dr J. Sundberg); (b) cell infiltrates in human alopecia areata (Courtesy of Upjohn Company.)

staphylococcal folliculitis (see Section 4.1.1), and ischemic alopecias such as dermatomyositis (see Section 3.4.2) and rabies vaccine-associated alopecia (see Section 3.4.3). AA-like hair loss has been reported in several breeds including Bernese mountain dog (Scarff 1993), Dachshund (Conroy 1968, 1979; Muller et al. 1983; Gross et al. 1992), Doberman Pinscher (Scarff 1993; Noli and Toma 2006), German Shepherd dog (Olivry et al. 1996), Magyar Vizsla (Conroy 1979), Miniature Poodle (Conroy 1979), English Setter (Alhaidari 2003), and in several mixed-breed dogs (Guernsey 1985; Yager and Wilcock 1994; Scott et al. 1995; Olivry et al. 1996; Tobin et al. 1996).

There is only a single large-scale study in the literature (Tobin et al. 2003) where AA-like hair loss in 25 client-owned dogs was systematically assessed using agreed AA-associated clinical, histological, and immunological criteria (Olsen et al. 1999, 2004). Hair loss onset was highly variable ranging from 1 to 11 years (median: 5 years), with a minority of dogs (the Dachshunds) developing AA in young adulthood (i.e., by 2 years of age). The male-to-female ratio was 0.79, mimicking the female bias in other AA-affected species, and most subjects had been either castrated or spayed. Spontaneous and complete hair regrowth occurred, however, only in the majority of subjects. Interestingly, such regrowth was commonly of white hair, a feature also seen in humans and rodents with AA (Messenger and Bleehen 1984). Nineteen of the 25 dogs with AA were reported as purebred and included four German Shepherd and crosses, three Dachshunds, two Beagles, two Setters, and two Labrador Retriever crosses. The remaining subjects represented crossbreeds. Although reference populations were not available for comparison, the Dachshund breed may appear predisposed to develop AA, as this breed seems

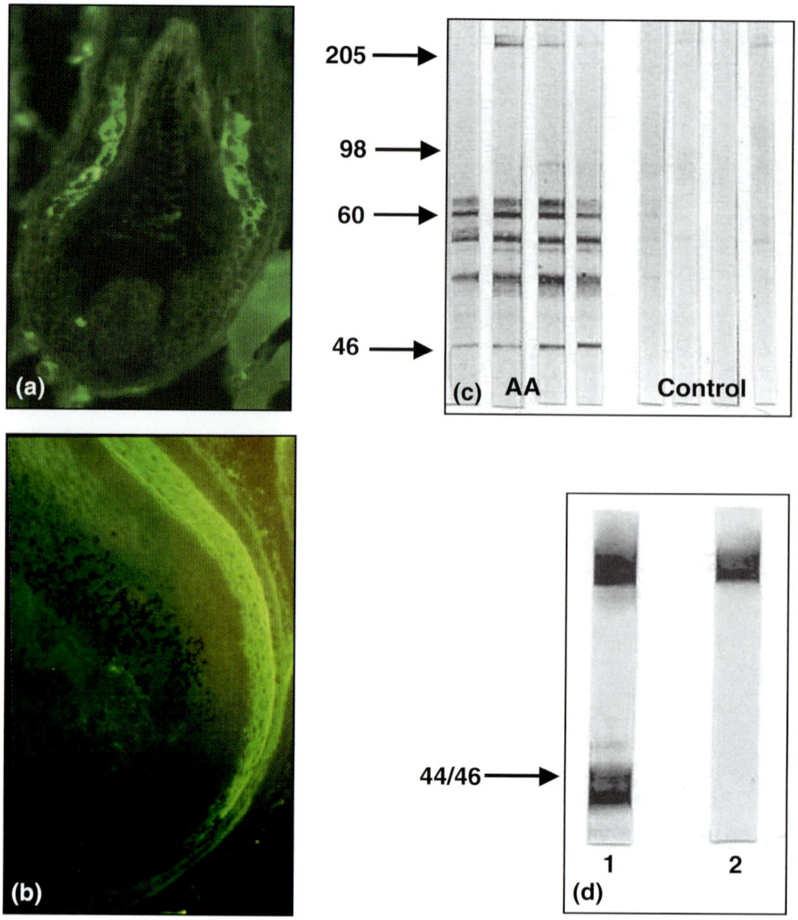

Fig. 4.7.5 Antibodies to hair follicles in rodent alopecia areata. (a) Indirect immunofluorescence analysis of circulating C3H/HeJ AA serum IgG antibodies to inner root sheath keratinocytes of an anagen mouse hair follicle; (b) indirect immunofluorescence analysis of circulating DEBR rat serum IgG antibodies to outer root sheath keratinocytes of an anagen rat hair follicle (courtesy of Dr K. McElwee); (c) immunoblotting analysis of circulating C3H/HeJ serum IgG antibodies to 6 M urea-extracted proteins from mouse hair follicles; (d) target antigen identification in rodent alopecia areata; hair follicle-specific keratin (44/46 kDa) was immunoprecipitated with C3H/HeJ AA sera, separated by SDS-PAGE and immunoblotted with a monoclonal antibody (AE13) raised to hair follicle-specific keratin; (1) AA serum immunoprecipitate, upper band represents mouse IgG; (2) fetal bovine serum immunoprecipitate (control).

overrepresented when all cases reported previously are examined altogether.

4.7.2.1 Diagnosis

Canine AA lesions usually consist of spontaneously arising and well-demarcated alopecic patches at the time of diagnosis (Fig. 4.7.6). Lesions usually develop first on the face and head (muzzle, chin, forehead, periocular, ears), in common with the bias toward scalp and beard in human AA. Facial lesions usually exhibit a bilateral symmetry. Hair loss may also be seen on the legs and in some cases hair loss can progress to a more generalized distribution. In a minority of cases the growth of white hair (i.e., leukotrichia) may precede the first alopecic lesion and supports the growing belief that the hair bulb melanocyte is a target cell population in AA (Messenger and Bleehen 1984; Tobin et al. 1990; Gilhar et al. 2001). Similarly, in subjects with variable coat color, hair loss usually occurs first in dark brown or black areas, again presumed to correlate with the preferential targeting of pigmented hair and the relative sparing of nonpigmented hair in humans with AA (Messenger and Bleehen 1984; Tobin et al. 1990).

Laboratory assessment of the immune status of some of these dogs has been carried out using assays similar to those applied to human and rodent AA research, and include histopathologic and immunopathologic examinations. The histologic hallmark of AA is the so-called "swarm of bees" mononuclear cell infiltrate focused more or less in and around the anagen hair bulb (Van Scott 1958) (Fig. 4.7.7a). Canine AA skin biopsy specimens reveal a raised telogen count, mimicking the high telogen counts in human AA. Marked inflammation of the hair bulb is observed

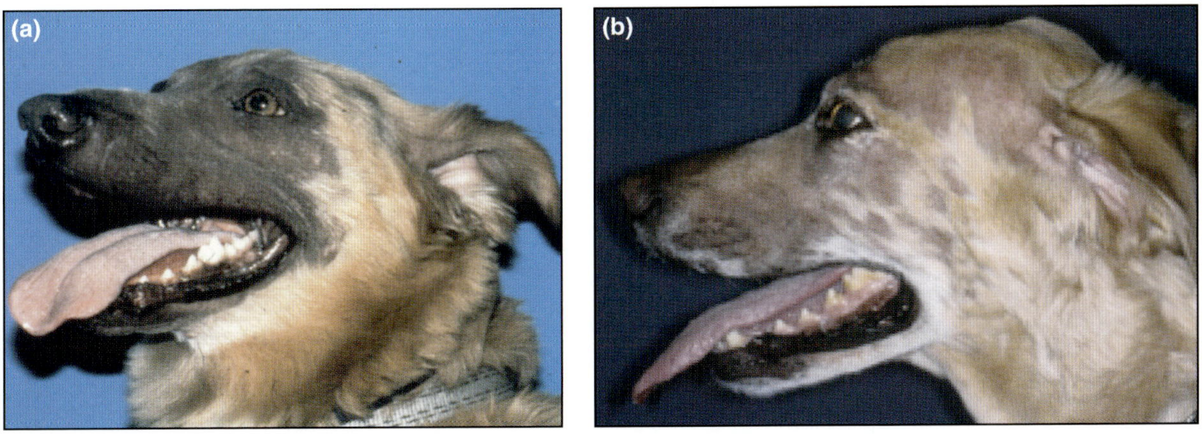

Fig. 4.7.6 Phenotypic variation in canine alopecia areata. Focal scalp and face hair loss in Labrador crossbreed dog. (a) Dog with pigmented skin; (b) dog with non-pigmented skin. (Courtesy of Dr T. Olivry.)

in a majority (though not in all) of lesional anagen hair follicles. In our recent large-scale study (Tobin et al. 2003) the extent of the mononuclear cell infiltrate was graded as mild in about 50% of hair follicles, moderate in 10%, and severe in 3% of hair follicles. Similarly, peribulbitis was seen in around 44% of hair follicles, and was graded as mild in 33%, moderate in 10%, and severe in 1% of hair follicles. Distorted dystrophic hair shafts were a feature in about a quarter of the affected dogs examined. In lymphocytic mural folliculitis of the isthmus (see Section 4.4.2.2) by contrast, lymphocyte epidermotropism targets the mid hair follicle sections, with involution of lower hair follicle segments. The skin of AA affected dogs reveals a predominantly T-lymphocyte infiltration, with T-cell numbers increasing proximally from the isthmus (in about 50% of dogs) to the inferior hair follicle segment (in most dogs) to the hair bulb (in all dogs). The severity of infiltration can be mild to severe in hair bulbs and around the lower hair follicle. To date, only limited lymphocyte immunophenotyping has been performed on lesional canine AA skin (Olivry et al. 1996), and the CD4+ to CD8+ T-cell ratio appears to be 1:3 to 1:4, respectively (McElwee et al., 1998b) (Fig. 4.7.7c and d). As with AA in humans, T-cells that infiltrate the hair bulb epithelium itself are more commonly CD8+, while CD4+ cells predominate in the peribulbar T-cell infiltrates. These lymphocytes expressed the α/β T-cell receptor.

Like in the human and rodent disease, canine AA is associated with the deposition of both immunoglobulin (antibodies) and complement around hair follicles, and the presence of circulating antibodies (IgM and IgG) to hair follicle-specific antigens. IgG deposits are especially found at the edge of active lesions (Fig. 4.7.8) (Tobin and Bystryn 1995; Tobin et al. 2003), where they usually bind to the lower hair follicle glassy membrane and connective tissue sheath, but also within the follicular papilla, medulla, outer root sheath or hair matrix, as well as dermal plasma cells. In a study of dogs with progressive, nonscarring, AA-like hair loss, we reported that sera of four affected dogs contained IgG antibodies (some with titers of up to 2,560) that reacted with components of the lower anagen hair follicle, especially the inner root sheath, outer root sheath, and medulla (Fig. 4.7.9a and b) (Tobin et al. 1996). Anti-hair follicle antibody reactivity was not detected in normal healthy dogs, nor in the sera taken from dogs with inflammatory skin disease due to demodicosis. Interestingly, anti-hair follicle antibody reactivity in canine AA sera was similar when incubated against either normal human or murine skin, indicating the conservation of AA target antigens across different mammalian species. Furthermore, in a larger study of 14 dogs with AA-like hair loss (Tobin et al. 2003), AA sera contained high titer antibodies (>1:500) to multiple hair follicle structures including inner root sheath, outer root sheath, matrix, and precortex.

While immunofluorescence provides detailed information of the histologic localization of target antigens, greater characterization (e.g., molecular weight) of these antigens can be achieved by immunoblotting analysis (Tobin et al. 1994). Using sera from four AA-affected dogs, we found IgG antibodies that

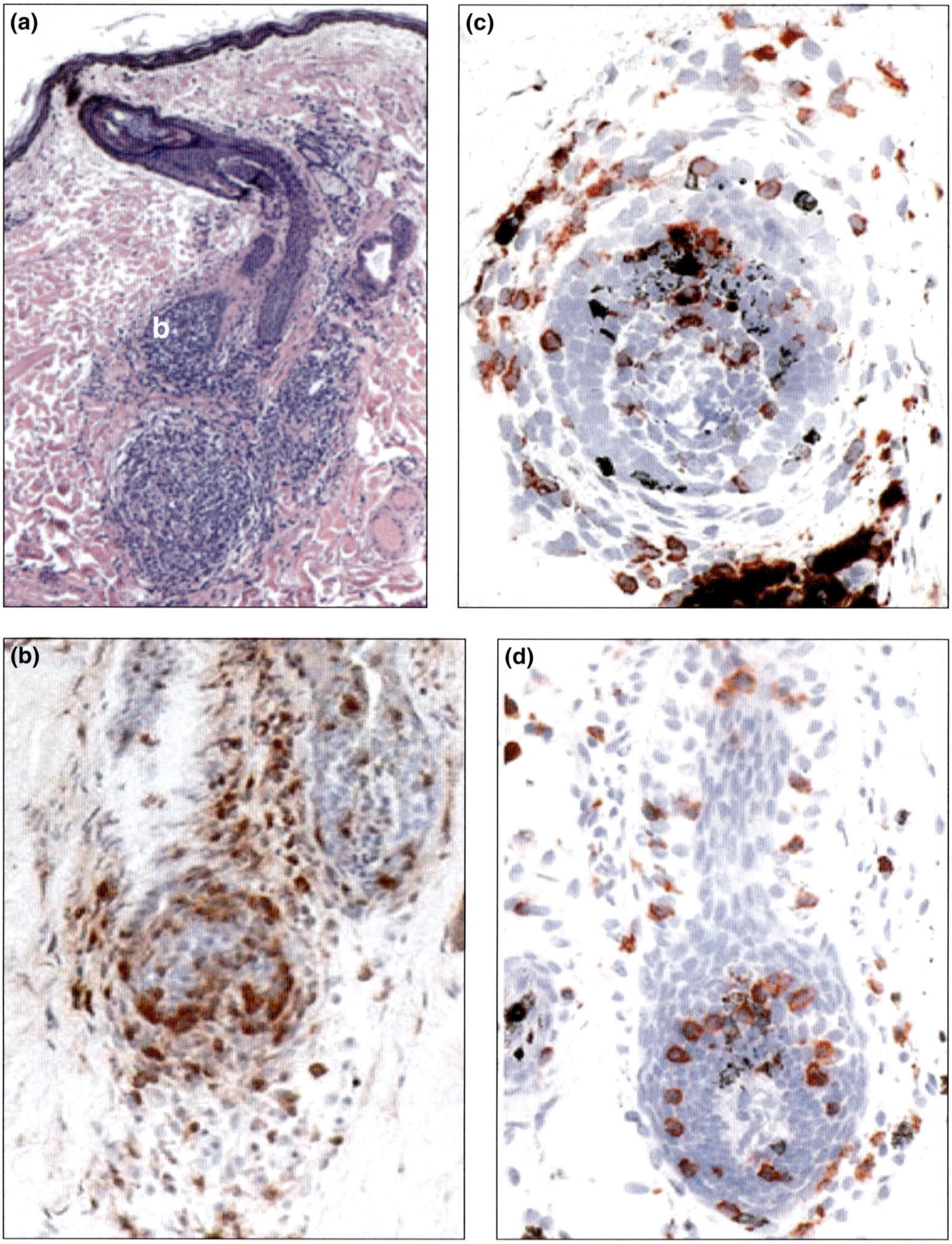

Fig. 4.7.7 Histopathology and immunohistopathology of canine alopecia areata. (a) Peri- and intrafollicular mononuclear cell infiltrates with associated disrupted follicular angle; (b) peri- and intrafollicular CD3-positive lymphocytes (pan-T cell); (c) peri- and intrafollicular CD4-positive lymphocytes; (d) peri- and intrafollicular CD8-positive lymphocytes. (Modified from Tobin DJ, et al. (2003).)

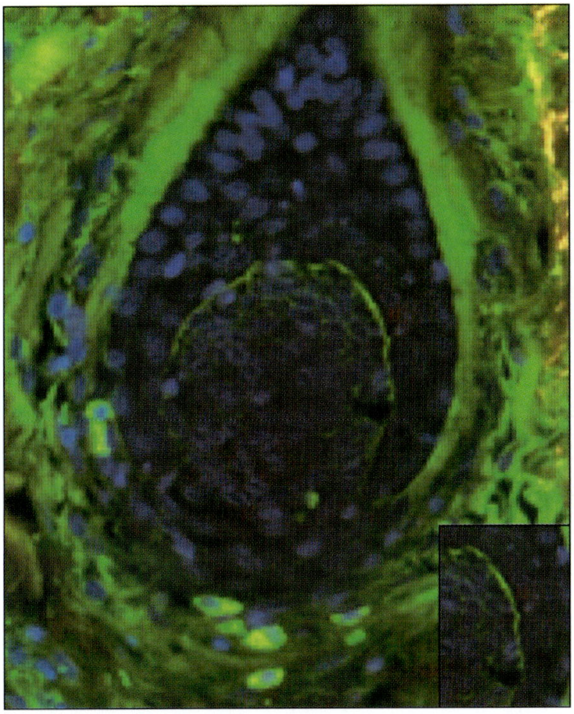

Fig. 4.7.8 Direct immunofluorescence analysis of IgG antibody deposition in anagen hair bulb, decorating the basal lamina separating the follicular dermal papilla from the hair bulb matrix. Note the perifollicular distribution of IgG-positive plasma cells. Inset: higher magnification of basal lamina. (Modified from Tobin DJ, et al. (2003).)

reacted intensely with hair follicle proteins of 200–220 kDa and also with multiple antigens in the 50–60 kDa range (Fig. 4.7.9c and d). Comigration immunoblotting studies suggested that the reactivity to a 200–220 kDa doublet represented binding to the inner root sheath and medulla-rich protein trichohyalin (Tobin et al. 1996), while some of the other targeted proteins in the 50–60 kDa range were likely to represent keratins. We expanded this study to assess anti-hair follicle antibody reactivity in a large number of dogs affected with AA-like hair loss (Tobin et al. 2003), where the analysis again revealed a strong and heterogeneous pattern of anti-hair follicle reactivity in canine AA serum IgG to multiple antigens between 40 and 60 kDa and to a 200–220 kDa doublet. Some of these targeted hair follicle antigens were identified by selective immunoprecipitation assay, in which canine circulating antibodies immunoprecipitate specific target antigens (Tobin et al. 1996, 2003). To date, we have determined that canine AA serum IgG antibodies can selectively immunoprecipitate the trichohyalin protein (200–220 kDa) from crude extracts of total hair follicle protein (Fig. 4.7.9d). The involvement of trichohyalin as a target autoantigen in many species with AA-like hair loss is a particular note. Trichohyalin is an intermediate filament-associated protein family and in the hair follicle is believed to be necessary for correct alignment of keratin filaments of the inner root sheath and medulla (O'Guin et al. 1992). It is likely that defects of inner root sheath differentiation (an anagen-specific event) may result in defective hair shaft formation.

Unlike autoantibodies in pemphigus vulgaris and myasthenia gravis, the pathogenic potential of anti-hair follicle autoantibodies in canine AA remains unclear. However, as they may occur prior to the onset of clinical hair loss, it is possible that they are not the result of a secondary event in response to a preexisting immune insult that was itself cell mediated. We have attempted to assess the pathogenic potential of anti-hair follicle antibodies in canine sera via their passive transfer into anagen skin of naïve mice (Tobin et al. 2003). High titer anti-hair follicle IgG was purified from the sera of AA-affected dogs and twice weekly administered intradermally into anagen III back skin of four C57BL/10scsn mice. While both IgG from AA and normal dogs delayed regrowth of hair in and around the site of IgG administration, administration of "AA" IgG appeared to result in an up to 2 week increased delay of anagen reentry compared to mice administered with control normal IgG (Tobin, unpublished data). However, passive transfer of human AA serum failed to inhibit hair growth when administered to human scalp transplants to nude mice (Gilhar et al. 1992).

4.7.2.2 Therapy

As in humans and rodents with AA, hair regrowth is most commonly spontaneous in canine AA. In resistant cases, however, treatment with oral glucocorticoids or cyclosporine can be attempted. Like in their human correlates, immunosuppressive therapy is successful in stimulating hair regrowth in dogs, including in those not showing spontaneous regrowth. In a large case series (Tobin et al. 2003) treatment with immunosuppressive doses of prednisone (1–2 mg/kg/day) or cyclosporine (5–10 mg/kg/day) was reported to lead to remission of clinical signs. Specifically, the utility of cyclosporine in Pincher dogs with AA has been

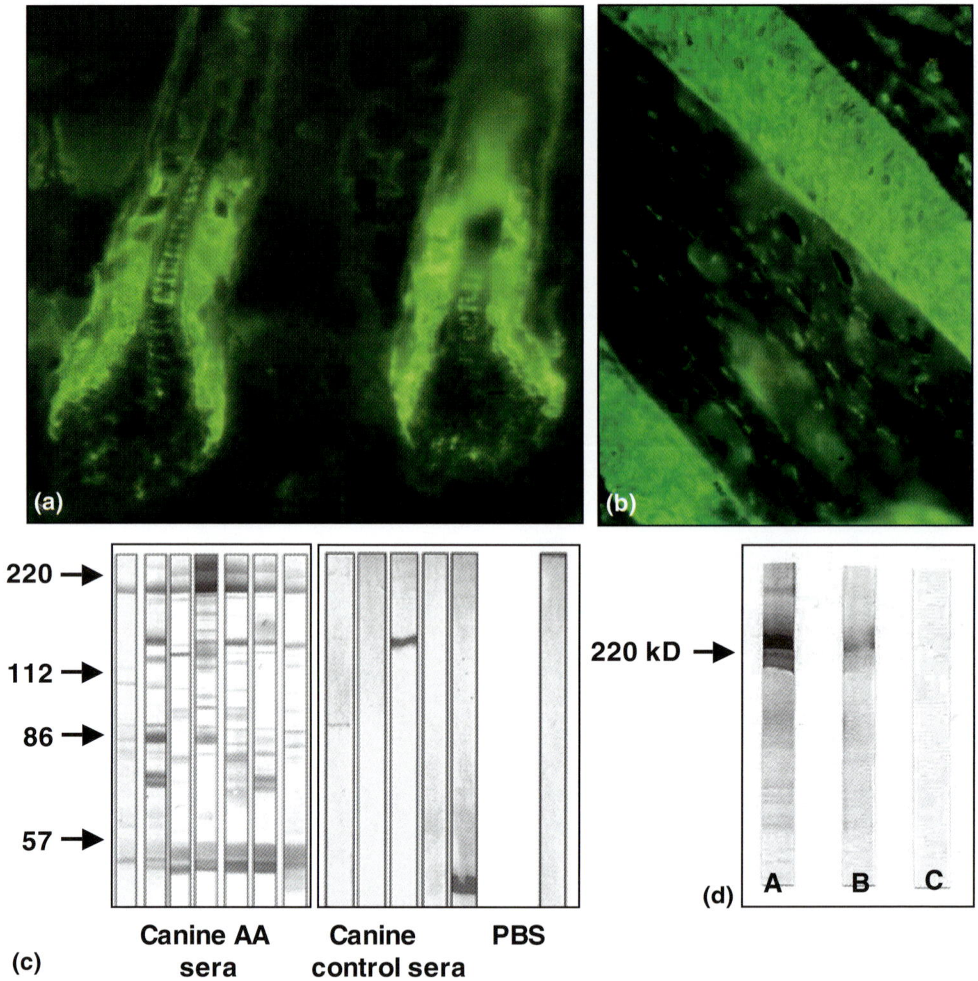

Fig. 4.7.9 Antibodies to hair follicles in canine alopecia areata. Indirect immunofluorescence analysis of circulating canine serum IgG antibodies to (a) inner root sheath keratinocytes of an anagen mouse hair follicle; (b) outer root sheath of a human scalp hair follicle; (c) immunoblotting analysis of circulating canine serum IgG antibodies to 6 M urea-extracted proteins from human hair follicles; (d) target antigen identification in canine alopecia areata. Hair follicle-specific trichohyalin (200–220 kDa) was immunoprecipitated with AE15 antitrichohyalin antibody, separated by SDS-PAGE and immunoblotted. Lane A shows the positive control, lane B the canine AA serum immunoprecipitate, and lane C fetal bovine serum as negative control.

confirmed recently (Noli and Toma 2006). For some dogs, in the latter study, treatment could be discontinued after a few months without relapse, though permanent hair loss in untreated cases is also rare. Interestingly, regrowing white hair occurs in the majority of canine AA cases examined to date, resembling human AA, and confirming the involvement of melanogenic melanocytes located in the anagen hair bulb in this disorder (Messenger and Bleehen 1984; Tobin et al. 1990; Gilhar et al. 2001). Thus, the AA target cell(s) and the antigens therein are likely to be conserved in nature. However, the melanocyte defect may be more severe/long lasting in canine AA (Tobin et al. 2003) compared to other species, as hair may fail to repigment even after several molts. This observation is particularly interesting as melanocyte stem cells are thought to reside in the hair bulge (Nishimura et al. 2002), a site not thought to be targeted in AA as evidenced by the ability of the hair follicle to reenter successive cycles (Tobin et al. 1999).

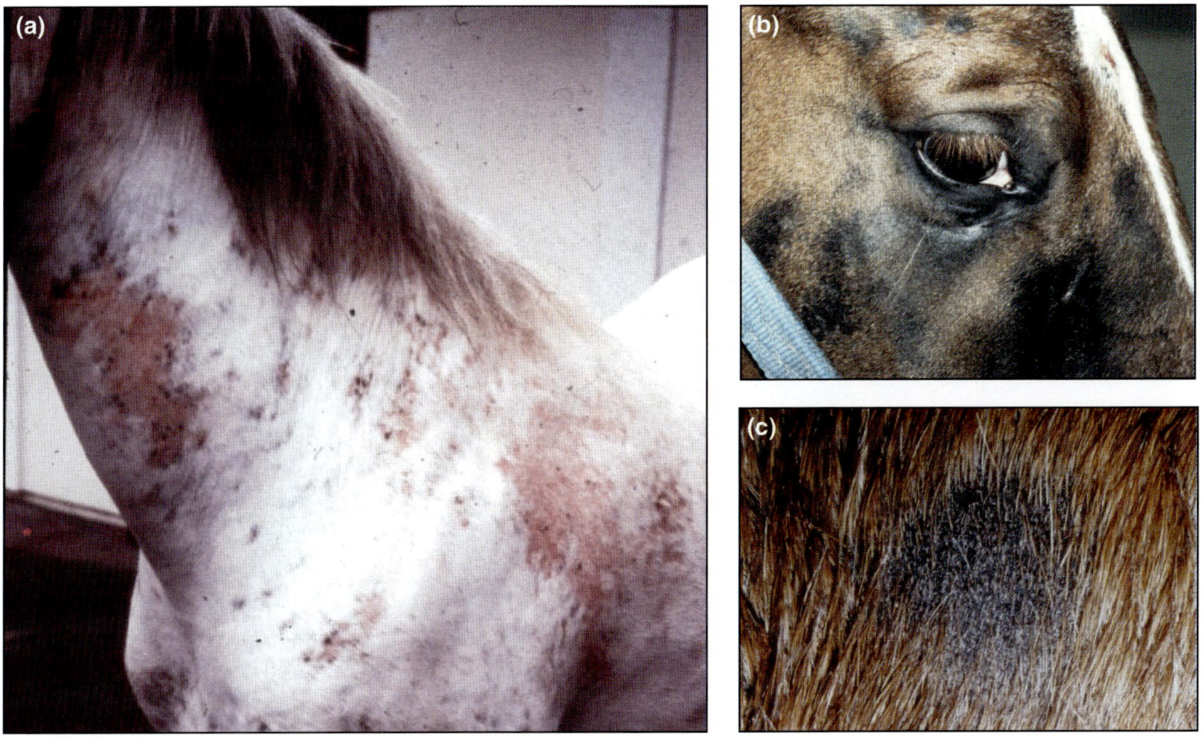

Fig. 4.7.10 Phenotypic variation in equine alopecia areata. (a) Body; (b) facial; (c) focal hair loss in horses with alopecia areata. (Courtesy of Dr Z. Alhaidari.)

4.7.3 Equine alopecia areata

The literature contains just a handful of reports of AA in horses (Middleton and Church 1994; Affolter and Cannon 1998; Tobin et al. 1998; Black et al. 2001; Colombo et al. 2004). Still, there are striking similarities between equine AA and AA-like disease in humans, rodents, and dogs. It is generally reported that AA begins on the head and face (Fig. 4.7.10), though it may also be restricted in horses, affecting just the mane and tail. As in other species, the clinical course of AA in horses is extremely variable (Stannard 2000). Skin biopsies from recently developed areas of alopecia will reveal the typical lymphocytic bulbitis (Fig. 4.7.11a), with the degree of inflammation varying from follicle to follicle. In chronic lesions, however, bulbitis may be very difficult to demonstrate. In fact, the presence of apoptotic cells within the hair follicle matrix, the presence of dysplastic hair shafts, or the presence of a subtle increase in peribulbar fibrous tissue warrant the request for further sections or even additional biopsies in order to verify AA (Stannard 2000).

A recent case describes an AA-like disorder in a 13-year-old chestnut thoroughbred with an 8-year history of alopecia that was described as multifocal, noninflammatory, and nonpruritic (Colombo et al. 2004). In this case the mane and tail were also severely affected, and it was the view of the authors that the clinical entity termed “mane and tail dystrophy” may indeed be a variant of AA. Importantly, hair follicles in the gluteal region of this animal exhibited classical peri- and intrabulbar lymphocyte infiltration (Fig. 4.7.11b). Another case of equine AA-like hair loss has been described by Conroy and colleagues (Conroy 1979) in a palomino horse with broadly similar clinical and histopathologic findings. We have reported on the immunopathologic features of a 13-year-old male Appaloosa horse in which alopecia started 2 years prior to initial visit to the veterinarian (Tobin et al. 1998). Hair loss was first observed on the cheek, extending to the intermandibular area, face, lateral aspects of the neck, and shoulders. Although the hair grew back spontaneously after 18 months, it fell out again after 2 months (at which time biopsies were taken). The hair

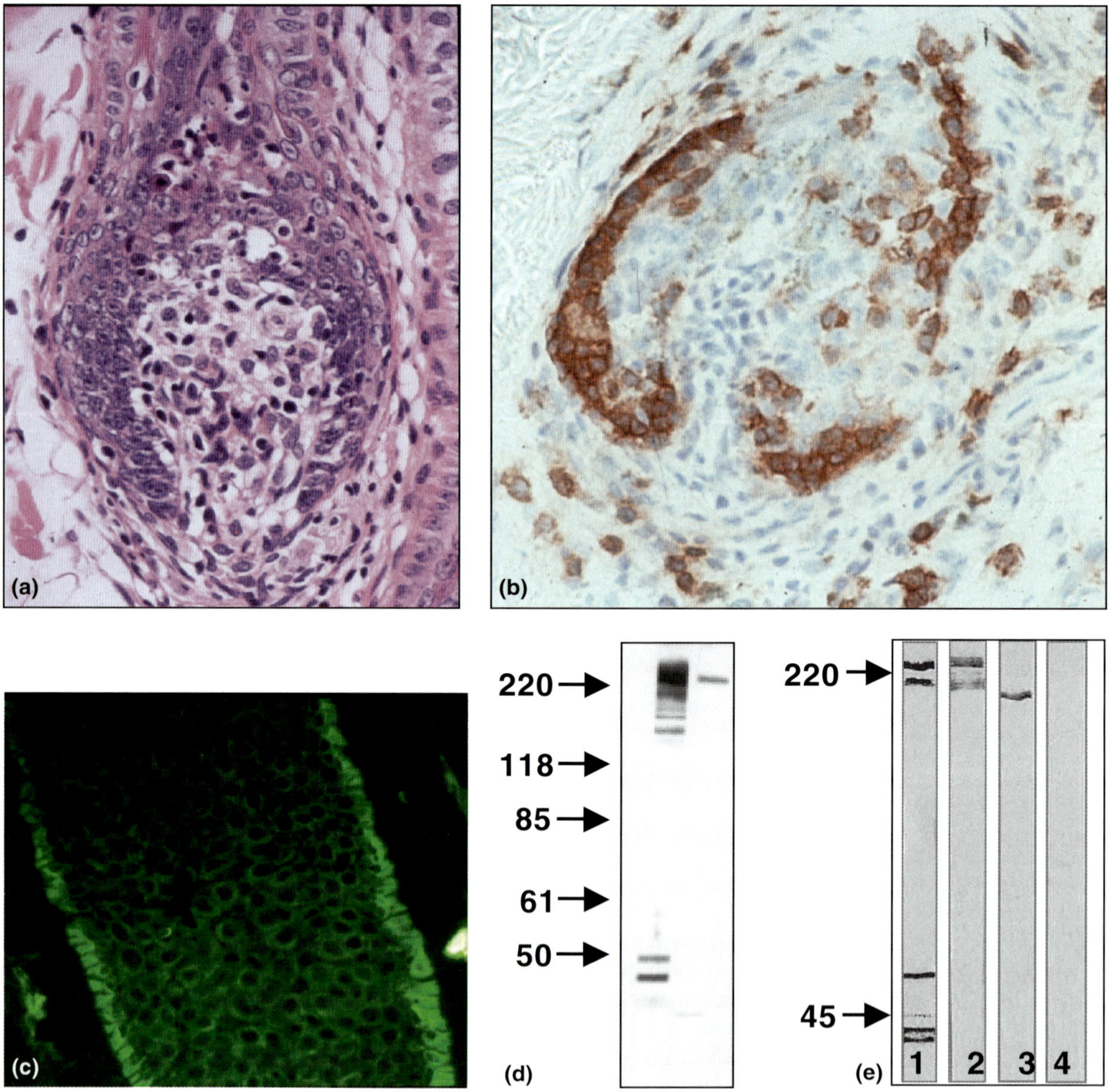

Fig. 4.7.11 Histopathology, immunohistopathology, indirect immunofluorescence and immunoblot analysis of equine alopecia areata. (a) Peri- and intrafollicular mononuclear cell infiltrates; (b) peri- and intrafollicular CD3-positive lymphocytes (pan-T cell); (c) indirect immunofluorescence analysis of circulating equine serum IgG antibodies to outer root sheath of a human scalp hair follicle; (d) immunoblotting analysis of circulating equine serum IgG antibodies from two affected horses to 6 M urea-extracted proteins from human hair follicles; (e) target antigen identification in equine alopecia areata. Immunoblot analysis of 6 M urea-extractable hair follicle antigens with whole equine AA serum (1), or with AE15 antitrichohyalin antibody (2); 6 M urea-extractable hair follicle antigens were immunoprecipitated with whole equine AA serum (3), or with whole equine normal serum (4), and then separated by SDS-PAGE and immunoblotted with AE15 antitrichohyalin antibody. (Modified from Tobin DJ, et al. (1998).)

regrew spontaneously over the body 4 months after the veterinary consultation, but started to fall out again a year later. Indirect immunofluorescence analysis indicated that the equine AA serum reacted intensely with the hair follicle inner root sheath, outer root sheath, and precortex of equine hair follicle, not unlike AA in other species assessed to date (Fig. 4.7.11c). Moreover, immunoblotting analysis revealed antibodies to a 200–220 kDa doublet (presumptive trichohyalin antigen) and to antigens of 40–60 kDa (Fig. 4.7.11d,e). The former doublet could be immunoprecipitated by the serum and was successfully identified as trichohyalin. Moreover, IgG fractions of serum obtained from this horse appeared to retard hair regrowth in an area around the administration site of treated mice, even 13 weeks after the first administration. Surprisingly, the treated skin contained telogen hair follicles often without associated shafts, despite the presence of anagen hair follicles in the remaining dorsum skin.

While the above equine AA study remains preliminary, it demonstrates that antibodies to hair follicle antigens are a feature of AA-like hair loss in horses, and also that some reactivities (e.g., against trichohyalin) are similar to those previously observed in canine AA. Further, this pilot study provided preliminary evidence that such antibodies may disrupt hair regrowth when passively transferred into C57BL/6 mice, supporting the view that anti-hair follicle antibodies in AA may have some pathogenic potential.

Treatment of equine AA is difficult and reports on its efficacy are limited. Systemic corticosteroids have produced minimal response only. Since spontaneous remission can occur, it is most often recommended not to treat affected horses (Stannard 2000).

4.7.4 Bovine alopecia areata

AA is rare in cattle (although it may be seen with a higher incidence in some specific cattle breeds). Very few cases are described in the literature. One includes a case in a Holstein cow (Paradis et al. 1988) that was characterized as an asymptomatic multifocal, noninflammatory alopecia. The diagnosis of AA was confirmed by skin biopsies. The latter revealed peribulbar lymphocyte infiltrates that affected the anagen hair follicles only. Like in other species, AA-like disease in cows is described to appear spontaneously and then wax and wane. It may also involve the eyelashes with spontaneous regrowth (which can be white).

References

Affolter VK, Cannon AG. 1998. Alopecia universalis in a horse. *Proceedings of the 14th AAVD and ACVD Meeting*, San Antonio, Texas, pp. 91–92.

Alhaidari Z. 2003. Alopecia areata in a mixed breed 9-year-old English setter. *Annales de Dermatologie et de Venereologie* 130(4): 416.

Beardi B, Wanert F, Zöller M, Freyschmidt-Paul P, Bodemer W, Kaup FJ. 2007. Alopecia areata in a rhesus monkey (*Macaca mulatta*). *Journal of Medical Primatology* 36(3):124–130.

Black SS, Rashmir-Raven AM, Williams S. 2001. Equine clinical snapshot #4. *Compendium on Continuing Education for the Practicing Veterinarian* 23:758.

Carroll JM, McElwee KJ, King LE, Byrne MC, Sundberg JP. 2002. Gene array profiling and immunomodulation studies define a cell-mediated immune response underlying the pathogenesis of alopecia areata in a mouse model and humans. *Journal of Investigative Dermatology* 119(2):392–402.

Colombo S, Keen JA, Brownstein DG, Rhind SM, McGorum BC, Hill PB. 2004. Alopecia areata with lymphocytic mural folliculitis affecting the isthmus in a thoroughbred mare. *Veterinary Dermatology* 15(4):260–265.

Conroy JD. 1968. Alopecia in dogs and cats. *Journal of the American Animal Hospital Association* 4:200–209.

Conroy JD. 1979. Alopecia areata. In: Andrews EJ, Ward BC, Altman NH (eds), *Spontaneous Animal Model of Human Disease*, pp. 30–31. New York: Academic Press.

Eichberg JW, De Villez RL. 1984. Alopecia totalis in a chimpanzee. *Journal of Medical Primatology* 13(2):81–88.

Freyschmidt-Paul P, Happle R, Hoffman R. 2004. Alopecia areata in animal models–new insights into pathogenesis and treatment of a T-cell-mediated autoimmune disorder. *Journal der Deutschen Dermatologischen Gesellschaft* 2(4):260–273.

Freyschmidt-Paul P, Seiter S, Zoller M, Konig A, Ziegler A, Sundberg JP, Happle R, Hoffmann R. 2000. Treatment with an anti-CD44v10-specific antibody inhibits the onset of alopecia areata in C3H/HeJ mice. *Journal of Investigative Dermatology* 115(4):653–657.

Freyschmidt-Paul P, Ziegler A, McElwee KJ, Happle R, Kissling S, Sundberg JP, Hoffmann R. 2001. Treatment of alopecia areata in C3H/HeJ mice with the topical immunosuppressant FK506 (Tacrolimus). *European Journal of Dermatology* 11:405–409.

Gilhar A, Kalish RS. 2006. Alopecia areata: a tissue specific autoimmune disease of the hair follicle. *Autoimmunity Reviews* 5(1):64–69.

Gilhar A, Landau M, Assy B, Shalaginov R, Serafimovich S, Kalish RS. 2001. Melanocyte-associated T-cell epitopes can function as autoantigens for transfer of alopecia areata to human scalp explants on Prkdc(scid) mice. *Journal of Investigative Dermatology* 117:1357–1362.

Gilhar A, Paus R, Kalish RS. 2007. Lymphocytes, neuropeptides, and genes involved in alopecia areata.*Clinical Investigation* 117(8):2019–2027.

Gilhar A, Pillar T, Assay B, David M. 1992. Failure of passive transfer of serum from patients with alopecia areata and alopecia universalis to inhibit hair growth in transplants of human scalp skin grafted on to nude mice. *British Journal of Dermatology* 126:166–171.

Gross TL, Ihrke PJ, Walder EJ. 1992. Alopecia areata. In: Gross TL, Irhke PJ, Walder EJ (eds), *Veterinary Dermatopathology—A Macroscopic and Microscopic Evaluation of Canine and Feline Skin Disease*, pp. 291–292. St. Louis: Mosby Year Book.

Guernsey GE. 1985. Alopecia areata in a dog. *Canadian Veterinary Journal* 26:403.

Kalish RS, Gilhar A. 2003. Alopecia areata: autoimmunity-the evidence is compelling. *Journal of Investigative Dermatology. Symposium Proceedings* 8(2):164–167.
McElwee KJ. 2004. Spontaneous rat model of alopecia areata in the Dundee Experimental Bald Rat (DEBR). In: Chan LS (ed), *Animal Models of Inflammatory Skin Diseases*, pp. 451–467. Boca Raton: CRC Press.
McElwee KJ, Boggess D, King LE Jr, Sundberg JP. 1998a. Experimental induction of alopecia areata-like hair loss in C3H/HeJ mice using full-thickness skin grafts. *Journal of Investigative Dermatology* 111:797–803.
McElwee KJ, Boggess D, Olivry T, Oliver RF, Whiting D, Tobin DJ, Bystryn J-C, King LE, Sundberg JP. 1998b. Comparison of alopecia areata in human and non-human mammalian species. *Pathobiology* 66:90–107.
McElwee KJ, Freyschmidt-Paul P, Hoffmann R, Kissling S, Hummel S, Vitacolonna M, Zöller M. 2005a. Transfer of CD8+ cells induces localized hair loss whereas CD4+/CD25− cells promote systemic alopecia areata and CD4+/CD25+ cells blockade disease onset in the C3H/HeJ mouse model. *Journal of Investigative Dermatology* 124:947–957.
McElwee KJ, Hoffmann R, Freyschmidt-Paul P, Wenzel E, Kissling S, Sundberg JP, Zoller M. 2002. Resistance to alopecia areata in C3H/HeJ mice is associated with increased expression of regulatory cytokines and a failure to recruit CD4+ and CD8+ cells. *Journal of Investigative Dermatology* 119(6):1426–1433.
McElwee KJ, Niiyama S, Freyschmidt-Paul P, Wenzel E, Kissling S, Sundberg JP, Hoffmann R. 2003. Dietary soy oil content and soy-derived phytoestrogen genistein increase resistance to alopecia areata onset in C3H/HeJ mice. *Experimental Dermatology* 12(1):30–36.
McElwee KJ, Pickett P, Oliver RF. 1996a. The DEBR rat, alopecia areata and autoantibodies to the hair follicle. *British Journal of Dermatology* 134(1):55–63.
McElwee KJ, Spiers EM, Oliver RF. 1996b. In vivo depletion of CD8+ T-cells restores hair growth in the DEBR model for alopecia areata. *British Journal of Dermatology* 135(2):211–217.
McElwee KJ, Spiers EM, Oliver RF. 1999a. Partial restoration of hair growth in the DEBR model for alopecia areata after in vivo depletion of CD4+ T-cells. *British Journal of Dermatology* 140(3):432–437.
McElwee KJ, Tobin DJ, Bystryn J-C, King LE, Sundberg JP. 1999b. Alopecia areata: an autoimmune disease? *Experimental Dermatology* 8(5):371–379.
McElwee KJ, Yu M, Park SW, Ross EK, Finner A, Shapiro J. 2005b. What can we learn from animal models of alopecia areata? *Dermatology* 211(1):47–53.
Messenger AG, Bleehen SS. 1984. Alopecia areata: light and electron microscopic pathology of the regrowing white hair. *British Journal of Dermatology* 110:155–162.
Messenger AG, Slater DN, Bleehen SS. 1986. Alopecia areata: alterations in the hair growth cycle and correlation with follicular pathology. *British Journal of Dermatology* 114:337–347.
Michie HJ, Jahoda CA, Oliver RF, Johnson BE. 1991. The DEBR rat: an animal model of human alopecia areata. *British Journal of Dermatology* 125:94–100.
Michie HJ, Jahoda CA, Oliver RF, Poulton TA. 1990. Immunobiological studies on the alopecic (DEBR) rat. *British Journal of Dermatology* 123:557–567.
Middleton DJ, Church S. 1994. Alopecia universalis in a horse. *Veterinary Dermatology* 67:67–79.
Muller GH, Kirk RW, Scott DW. 1983. *Small Animal Dermatology.* Philadelphia: WB Saunders.
Nishimura EK, Jordan SA, Oshima H, Yoshida H, Osawa M, Moriyama M, Jackson IJ, Barrandon Y, Miyachi Y, Nishikawa S. 2002. Dominant role of the niche in melanocyte stem-cell fate determination. *Nature* 416(6883):854–860.
Noli C, Toma S. 2006. Three cases of immune-mediated adnexal skin disease treated with cyclosporin. *Veterinary Dermatology* 17(1):85–92.
O'Guin WM, Sun TT, Manabe M. 1992. Interaction of trichohyalin with intermediate filaments: three immunologically defined stages of trichohyalin maturation. *Journal of Investigative Dermatology* 98:24–32.
Olivry T, Moore PF, Naydan DK, Puget BJ, Affolter VK, Kline AE. 1996. Antifollicular cell-mediated and humoral immunity in canine alopecia areata. *Veterinary Dermatology* 7:67–79.
Olsen E, Hordinsky M, McDonald-Hull S, Price V, Roberts J, Shapiro J, Stenn K. 1999. Alopecia areata investigational assessment guidelines. National Alopecia Areata Foundation. *Journal of the American Academy of Dermatology* 40(2 Pt 1):242–246.
Olsen EA, Hordinsky MK, Price VH, Roberts JL, Shapiro J, Canfield D, Duvic M, King LE Jr, McMichael AJ, Randall VR, Turner ML, Sperling L, Whiting DA, Norris D, National Alopecia Areata Foundation. 2004. Alopecia areata investigational assessment guidelines–Part II. National Alopecia Areata Foundation. *Journal of the American Academy of Dermatology* 51(3):440–447.
Paradis M, Fecteau G, Scott DW. 1988. Alopecia areata (Pelade) in a cow. *Canadian Veterinary Journal* 29(9):727–729.
Ross EK, Shapiro J. 2005. Management of hair loss. *Dermatologic Clinics* 23(2):227–243.
Safavi, KH, Muller SA, Suman VJ, Moshell AN, Melton LJ. 1995. Incidence of alopecia areata in Olmsted County, Minnesota, 1975–1989. *Mayo Clinic Proceedings* 70:628–633.
Scarff DH. 1993. Disorders of pigmentation, Chapter 3. In: Locke PH, Harvey RG, Mason IS (eds), *Manual of Small Animal Dermatology*, pp. 83–89. British Small Animal Veterinary Association: Cheltenham, Glouchestershire, UK.
Scott DW. 1988. *Large Animal Dermatology.* Philadelphia: WB Saunders.
Scott DW, Guard CLG. 1988. Alopecia areata in a cow. *Agri-Practice* 9:16–19.
Scott DW, Miller WH, Griffin CE. 1995. *Small Animal Dermatology*, 5th edn, pp. 611–613. Philadelphia: WB Saunders.
Shapiro J, Sundberg JP, Bissonnette R, McElwee KJ, McLean DI, Carroll JM, Oliver RF, Tang L, Lui H. 1999. Alopecia areata-like hair loss in C3H/HeJ mice and DEBR rats can be reversed using topical diphencyprone. *Journal of Investigative Dermatology. Symposium Proceedings* 4(3):239.
Siebenhaar F, Sharov AA, Peters EM, Sharova TY, Syska W, Mardaryev AN, Freyschmidt-Paul P, Sundberg JP, Maurer M, Botchkarev VA. 2007. Substance P as an immunomodulatory neuropeptide in a mouse model for autoimmune hair loss (alopecia areata). *Journal of Investigative Dermatology* 127:1489–1497.
Stannard AA. 2000. Alopecia in the horse—an overview. *Veterinary Dermatology* 11(3):191–203.
Sundberg JP, Boggess D, Silva KA, McElwee KJ, King LE, Li R, Churchill G, Cox GA. 2003. Major locus on mouse chromosome 17 and minor locus on chromosome 9 are linked with alopecia areata in C3H/HeJ mice. *Journal of Investigative Dermatology* 120(5):771–775.
Sundberg JP, Cordy WR, King LE. 1994. Alopecia areata in aging C3H/HeJ mice. *Journal of Investigative Dermatology* 102:847–856.
Tang L, Cao L, Sundberg JP, Lui H, Shapiro J. 2004. Restoration of hair growth in mice with an alopecia areata-like disease using topical anthralin. *Experimental Dermatology* 13(1):5–10.
Tang L, Lui H, Sundberg JP, Bissonnette R, I McLean D, Shapiro J. 2003a. Restoration of hair growth with topical diphencyprone in

mouse and rat models of alopecia areata. *Journal of the American Academy of Dermatology* 49(6):1013–1019.
Tang L, Sundberg JP, Lui H, Shapiro J. 2003b. Old wine in new bottles: reviving old therapies for alopecia areata using rodent models. *Journal of Investigative Dermatology. Symposium Proceedings* 8(2):212–216.
Tobin DJ. 1997. Morphological analysis of hair follicles in alopecia areata. *Microscopy Research and Technique* 38:443–451.
Tobin DJ. 2003. Characterization of hair follicle antigens targeted by the anti-hair follicle immune response in alopecia areata. *Journal of Investigative Dermatology. Symposium Proceedings* 8(2):176–181.
Tobin DJ, Alhaidari Z, Olivry T. 1998. Equine alopecia areata autoantibodies target multiple hair follicle antigens and may alter hair growth in passive transfer studies. *Experimental Dermatology* 7:289–297.
Tobin DJ, Bystryn J-C. 1995. Immunity to hair follicles in alopecia areata. *Journal of Investigative Dermatology* 104(5 Suppl):13S–14S.
Tobin DJ, Bystryn J-C. 1996. Alopecia areata is associated with antibodies to hair follicle-specific antigens located predominantly in the proliferative region of hair follicles. In: Neste DJJ, Randall VA (eds), *Hair Research for the Next Millennium*, pp. 237–241. Amsterdam: Elsevier Science.
Tobin DJ, Bystryn J-C. 2000. Immunology of alopecia areata. In: Camacho FM, Randall VA, Price V (eds), *Hair and Hair Disorders: Research, Pathology and Management*, pp. 187–201. London: Martin Dunitz.
Tobin DJ, Fenton DA, Kendall MD. 1990. Ultrastructural observations on the hair bulb melanocytes and melanosomes in acute alopecia areata. *Journal of Investigative Dermatology* 94: 803–807.
Tobin DJ, Gardner SH, Luther PB, Dunston SM, Lindsey NJ, Olivry T. 2003. A natural canine homologue of alopecia areata in humans. *British Journal of Dermatology* 149(5):938–950.
Tobin DJ, Hann SK, Song MS, Bystryn J-C. 1997a. Hair follicle structures targeted by antibodies in patients with alopecia areata. *Archives of Dermatology* 133(1):57–61.
Tobin DJ, Olivry T. 2004. Spontaneous canine model of alopecia areata. In: Chan LS (ed.), *Animal Models of Human Inflammatory Skin Disease*, pp. 469–482. Boca Raton: CRC Press.
Tobin DJ, Olivry T, Bystryn J-C. 1996. Anti-trichohyalin antibodies in canine alopecia areata. In: Kwochka KW, Willemse T, von Tscharner C (eds), *Advances in Veterinary Dermatology*, pp. 355–364. Boston: Butterworth Heinemann.
Tobin DJ, Orentreich N, Fenton DA, Bystryn J-C. 1994. Antibodies to hair follicles in alopecia areata. *Journal of Investigative Dermatology* 102:721–724.
Tobin DJ, Slominski A, Botchkarev V, Paus R. 1999. The fate of hair follicle melanocytes during the hair growth cycle. *Journal of Investigative Dermatology. Symposium Proceedings* 4(3):323–332.
Tobin DJ, Sundberg JP, King Jr LE, Boggess D, Bystryn J-C. 1997b. Autoantibodies to hair follicles in C3H/HeJ mice with alopecia areata-like hair loss. *Journal of Investigative Dermatology* 109:329–333.
Van Scott EJ. 1958. Morphologic changes in pilosebaceous units and anagen hairs in alopecia areata. *Journal of Investigative Dermatology* 31:35–45.
Verma DD, Verma S, McElwee KJ, Freyschmidt-Paul P, Hoffman R, Fahr A. 2004. Treatment of alopecia areata in the DEBR model using cyclosporin A lipid vesicles. *European Journal of Dermatology* 14(5):332–338.
Yager J, Wilcock BP. 1994. Lymphocytic folliculitis resembling human alopecia areata and universalis. In: *Color Atlas and Text of Surgical Pathology of the Dog and Cat*, pp. 196–197. Mosby Year Book Europe Limited (Wolfe).

4.8

Sebaceous adenitis

Monika Linek

Sebaceous adenitis is an uncommon skin disease that has most extensively been described in the dog (Rosser 1992; Dunstan and Hargis 1995; Mueller et al. 2001; Scott et al. 2001). It has also been reported to occur in cats and rabbits, although it is not yet clear whether the disease and its etiology and pathogenesis are in fact identical in all species (Scott 1989; Baer et al. 1993; Bellangeon and Theau 2000; White et al. 2001). The common feature of the disease is an inflammatory infiltration affecting the sebaceous glands and finally resulting in their destruction. Alopecia in this disease occurs by hair shafts that break easily, most likely due to a decreased amount of sebum produced from the sebaceous glands.

Feline SA is presented with multifocal annular alopecia and adherent scales. One report describes a similar condition in domestic rabbits.

4.8.1 Canine sebaceous adenitis

4.8.1.1 Etiology and pathogenesis

Sebaceous adenitis (SA), in senso stricto, is a rare idiopathic skin disease. It is most commonly identified in Standard Poodles and Akitas where an autosomal recessive mode of inheritance has been proposed (Rosser et al. 1987; Hargis 1991; Scarff 2000; Reichler et al. 2001). It is also seen in Vizslas, German Shepherd Dogs, English Springer Spaniels and Hovawarts, and has been diagnosed in various other breeds and mongrel dogs (Carothers et al. 1991; Stewart et al. 1991; Mueller et al. 2001; Tevell et al. 2008). The exact pathogenesis is still unknown. A primary structural defect within the sebaceous gland and its duct or abnormalities in lipid metabolism have been proposed but have not been proven yet (Dunstan and Hargis 1995; Scott et al. 2001). It is most likely that SA is an autoimmune disease, particularly since immunohistochemical studies have shown that the major cell populations in SA are MHC class II positive dendritic cells and CD4+, CD8+ T cells. These are effector cells in cell-mediated autoimmune diseases (Rybnicek et al. 1998; Linek et al. 2005). B cells and autoantibodies against sebaceous glands have not been detected. The hypothesis that SA is a cell-mediated autoimmune disease is further supported by the decrease in T cells and macrophages during immunomodulating therapy with cyclosporin A (Linek et al. 2005).

Secondary sebaceous gland destruction with similar clinical hyperkeratosis can occur with generalized demodicosis (see Section 4.1.3), leishmaniasis, severe granulomatous and histiocytic folliculitis (see Chapter 4.5), and other rare diseases (Gross et al. 2005).

4.8.1.2 Diagnosis

4.8.1.2.1 Clinical presentation

Young adult to middle-aged dogs are most commonly affected and no sex predilection has been reported.

The clinical features, distribution, and severity of SA vary among different breeds and dogs. However, silvery white dandruff and scales that adhere to the hair shafts ("follicular casts") are the common key feature. Follicular casts are most likely the result of the lack of sebum in the infundibular part of the hair follicle where epidermis-like keratinization and desquamation occurs (Sousa 2006).

In long-coated dogs (with Standard Poodles, Akitas, and Samoyeds being the most extensively studied examples) the first sign of disease is a frond-like follicular cast protruding from the hair follicle that ensheathes the hair shaft with tenacious keratinaceous

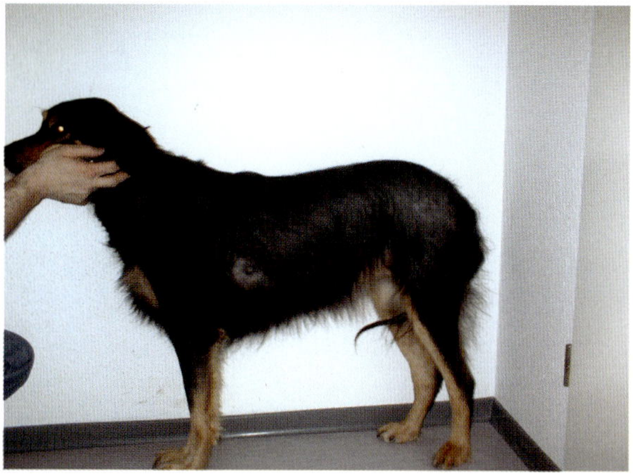

Fig. 4.8.1 Sebaceous adenitis in a Hovawart. Note the dull and brittle hair coat associated with extensive symmetric multifocal alopecia caused by broken hair shafts.

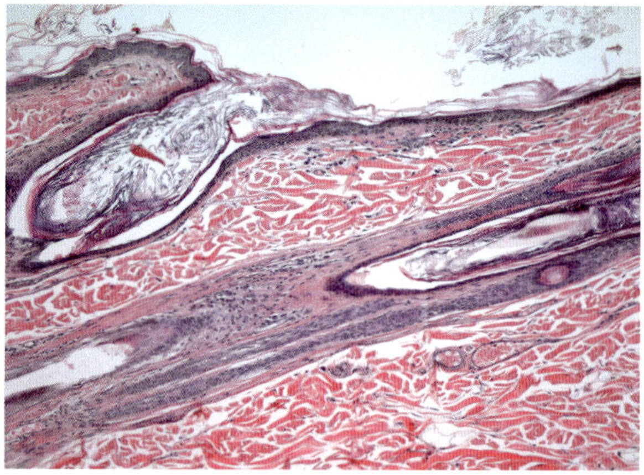

Fig. 4.8.2 Skin histology of canine sebaceous adenitis. Note sparse perifollicular inflammatory cells at the isthmus level of the hair follicles and loss of sebaceous glands.

debris. When epilated, the follicular casts typically surround the root of the hair. In Standard Poodles the disease starts most often on the dorsal muzzle and temporal region, spreading to the dorsal neck and thorax. In Akitas and Hovawarts a more extensive symmetric and multifocal alopecia occurs (Reichler et al. 2001). It is characterized by broken hair shafts and is associated with a dull and brittle hair coat (Fig. 4.8.1). As the disease progresses, it may generalize, and secondary bacterial folliculitis with pruritus and malodor is common at this stage.

Short-coated dogs such as Vizslas have a strikingly different clinical presentation (Carothers et al. 1991; Stewart et al. 1991). Lesions tend to be nodular with arciform and coalescing areas of alopecia giving the coat a moth-eaten appearance and fine nonadherent scaling predominately on the trunk. As additionally cyclical edematous facial swellings occur, some authors suggest that this form of SA is a separate disease (Gross et al. 2005).

The differential diagnoses include not only primary seborrhea and seborrheic dermatitis, vitamin A-responsive dermatitis and ichthyosis, but also generalized demodicosis (see Section 4.1.3) and dermatophytosis (see Section 4.1.2). Bacterial folliculitis and furunculosis could be considered in nodular disease.

4.8.1.2.2 Histology

The histopathological abnormalities in dogs with SA are variable, and their character changes in association with chronicity of the disease. In the early phase, discrete perifollicular inflammatory cells are present at the isthmus level of hair follicles (Yager and Willcock 1994; Gross et al. 2005). Later on, the most common finding is a nodular, granulomatous to pyogranulomatous inflammatory reaction around the sebaceous glands. Sebocytes are destroyed and may no longer be detectable in histological sections. However, hair follicles themselves and the apocrine sweat glands are not affected by the inflammation. The inflammatory infiltrate consists of histiocytes, lymphocytes, and neutrophils (Gross et al. 2005; Linek et al. 2005). In long-coated breeds, a marked orthokeratotic hyperkeratosis and follicular plugging are detectable within the follicular infundibulum, whereas in short-coated breeds, the hyperkeratotic changes tend to be milder (Gross et al. 2005). In advanced stages of the disease, the sebaceous glands are completely destroyed and the inflammatory reaction may vanish (Fig. 4.8.2). Telogenization of hair follicles or follicular atrophy may occur. If a secondary staphylococcal infection is present, suppurative folliculitis or furunculosis will be found.

4.8.1.3 Therapy

Considering that SA is a skin disease that has no impact on the general health status and life expectancy of the patient (except for secondary pyoderma), treating

SA needs to take into account owner compliance, handling, safety, and costs. The main goal of treatment is both restoration of the barrier function of the skin and restoration of hair coat quality. In general, SA cannot be cured and long-term management therapy is required. A variety of treatment protocols have been published (Kwochka 1989; White et al. 1995; Rosser 2000; Linek et al. 2005).

4.8.1.3.1 Topical therapy

A high success rate is achieved with the regular use of antiseborrheic shampoos followed by topical oil soaks and application of humectant sprays. One study used cyclosporin once daily as a topical solution mixing an oral micro-emulsified solution with water 1:10 (Patterson 2005).

4.8.1.3.2 Systemic therapy

Various systemic treatments have been explored to stop the inflammatory destruction of sebaceous glands and to permanently restore their function. Administration of corticosteroids at anti-inflammatory or immunosuppressive doses has been reported to be effective in some short-coated dogs but had no effect in others (Rosser et al. 1987; Carothers et al. 1991). Synthetic retinoids have been used for their anti-inflammatory properties, their effects on keratinocyte differentiation, and their effect on sebaceous glands. They have also been reported to be effective in Vizslas, but achieve lower success rates in other breeds (Kwochka 1989; White et al. 1995). Synthetic retinoids are given at a dose of 1 mg/kg orally once or twice a day, and improvement should be seen within 6 weeks. Thereafter, the administration frequency can be decreased. Oral supplementation of vitamin A at 10,000–30,000 IU twice daily has been studied in one report to produce clinical improvement within 3 months (Sousa 2006). Oral administration of essential fatty acids can also ameliorate clinical signs (Marshall and Williams 1990). Oral treatment with cyclosporin A (5 mg/kg once a day) has been reported to be effective as well (Carothers et al. 1991; Linek et al. 2005). Cyclosporin successfully reduces inflammation and increases the percentage of hair follicles with sebaceous glands, suggesting some sebaceous gland recovery. It seems that treatment in the early phase of the disease (i.e., when there is still considerable inflammation) is more efficient than in chronic cases. Life-long treatment is necessary since discontinuation of cyclosporin A has been observed to be associated with relapse of the disease (Linek et al. 2005). Larger clinical trials comparing the efficacy of different treatment options for SA, however, are still outstanding.

References

Baer K, Soulberg N, Helton K. 1993. Sebaceous adenitis-like disease in two cats. *Veterinary Pathology* 30:437.

Bellangeon M, Theau V. 2000. Adénité sébacée chez un lapin. *Pratique Medicale et Chirurgicale de l'Animal* 35:697–699.

Carothers MA, Kwochka KW, Rojko JL. 1991. Cyclosporine-responsive granulomatous sebaceous adenitis in a dog. *Journal of the American Veterinary Medical Association* 198:1645–1648.

Dunstan RW, Hargis AM. 1995. The diagnosis of sebaceous adenitis in standard poodle dogs. In: Bonagura JD (ed.), *Kirk's Current Veterinary Therapy XII*, pp. 619–622. Philadelphia: WB Saunders.

Gross TL, Ihrke PJ, Walder EL, Affolter VK. 2005. Sebaceous adenitis. In: Gross TL, Ihrke PJ (eds), *Skin Diseases of the Dog and Cat*, 2nd edn, pp. 186–188. Oxford: Blackwell Science.

Hargis A. 1991. Sebaceous adenitis. *Proceedings of the 7th Annual Meeting American Academy of Veterinary Dermatology/American College of Veterinary Dermatology*, pp. 87–88.

Kwochka KW. 1989. Retinoids in dermatology. In: Kirk RW (ed.), *Kirk's Current Veterinary Therapy X*, pp. 553–560. Philadelphia: WB Saunders.

Linek M, Boss C, Haemmerling R, Hewicker-Trautwein M, Mecklenburg L. 2005. Effects of cyclosporine A on clinical and histologic abnormalities in dogs with sebaceous adenitis. *Journal of the American Veterinary Medical Association* 226(1):59–64.

Marshall C, Williams J. 1990. Re-establishment of hair growth, skin pliability and apparent resistance to bacterial infection after dosing fish oil in a dog with sebaceous adenitis. In: Tscharner VC, Halliwell REW (eds), *Advances in Veterinary Dermatology*, Vol. 1, pp. 446–447. London: Bailliere Tindall.

Mueller RS, Bettenay SV, Vogelnest LJ. 2001. Sebaceous adenitis in three German Shepherd dogs. *Australian Veterinary Practice* 31:110–114.

Patterson S. 2005. Topical cyclosporine in sebaceous adenitis. In: Kwochka KW, Rosenkrantz WS (eds), *Shampoos and topical therapy* p. 382. Oxford: Blackwell.

Reichler IM, Hauser B, Schiller I, Dunstan RW, Credille KM, Binder H, Glaus T, Arnold S. 2001. Sebaceous adenitis in the Akita: clinical observations, histopathology and heredity. *Veterinary Dermatology* 12:243–253.

Rosser EJ. 1992. Sebaceous adenitis. In: Bonagura JD, Kirk RW (eds), *Kirk's Current Veterinary Therapy XI*, pp. 534–536. Philadelphia: WB Saunders.

Rosser EJ. 2000. Therapy for sebaceous adenitis. In: Bonagura JD, Kirk RW (eds), *Kirk's Current Veterinary Therapy XIII*, pp. 572–573. Philadelphia: WB Saunders.

Rosser EJ, Dunstan RW, Brenn PT. 1987. Sebaceous adenitis with hyperkeratosis in the standard poodle: a discussion of 10 cases. *Journal of the American Animal Hospital Association* 23:341–345.

Rybnicek J, Affolter VK, Moore PF. 1998. Sebaceous adenitis: an immunohistological examination. In: Kwochka KW, Willemse T,

Tscharner VC (eds), *Advances in Veterinary Dermatology*, Vol. 3, pp. 539–540. Oxford: Butterworth Heinemann.

Scarff DH. 2000. Sebaceous adenitis in standard poodles. *Veterinary Record* 146:476.

Scott DW. 1989. Adénité sébacée granulomateuse chez un chat. *Le Pointe Vétérinaire* 21:107–111.

Scott DW, Miller WH Jr, Griffin CE (eds.) 2001. Small animal dermatology. In: *Muller and Kirk's Small Animal Dermatology*, 6th edn., pp. 738–742. Philadelphia: WB Saunders.

Sousa CA. 2006. Sebaceous adenitis. *Veterinary Clinics of North America, Small Animal Practice* 1:243–249.

Stewart LJ, White SD, Carpenter JL. 1991. Isotretinoin in the treatment of sebaceous adenitis in two vizslas. *Journal of the American Animal Hospital Association* 27:65–71.

Tevell EH, Bergvall K, Egenvall A. 2008. Sebaceous adenitis in Swedish dogs, a retrospective study of 104 cases. *Acta Veterinaria Scandinavica* 50:11.

White SD, Linder KE, Schultheiss P, Scott KV, Garnett P, Taylor M, Best SJ, Walder EJ, Rosenkrantz W, Yaeger JA. 2001. Sebaceous adenitis in four domestic rabbits (*Oryctolagus cuniculus*) . *Veterinary Dermatology* 11(1):53–60.

White SD, Rosychuk RA, Scott KV, Hargis AM, Jonas L, Trettien A. 1995. Sebaceous adenitis in dogs and results of treatment with isotretinoin and etretinate: 30 cases (1990–1994). *Journal of the American Veterinary Medical Association* 207:197–200.

Yager JA, Willcock BP (eds). 1994. *Surgical Pathology of the Dog and Cat.* London: Mosby Year Book.

Index